I0320186

HISTORY OF THE SECOND WORLD WAR

UNITED KINGDOM MEDICAL SERIES

This volume of the Official Medical History of the Second World War has been prepared under the direction of an Editorial Board appointed by Her Majesty's Government, but the authors alone are responsible for the method of presentation of the facts and the opinions expressed.

CASUALTIES AND MEDICAL STATISTICS

EDITED BY

W. FRANKLIN MELLOR

The Naval & Military Press Ltd

Published by

The Naval & Military Press Ltd
Unit 10 Ridgewood Industrial Park,
Uckfield, East Sussex,
TN22 5QE England

Tel: +44 (0) 1825 749494
Fax: +44 (0) 1825 765701

www.naval-military-press.com
www.military-genealogy.com

EDITORIAL COMMITTEE

FOREWORD

By SIR AUSTIN BRADFORD HILL, C.B.E., F.R.S.,
Ph.D.(Econ.), D.Sc.(London), Hon. M.D.(Edin.)

IT IS A TRUISM that throughout history victory or defeat in war has been swayed not only by military skill and valour but by disease and, in particular, epidemic disease. The Second World War was no exception though on the whole its characteristic was the prevention rather than the promotion of illness. We experienced, both in civil and military life, nothing akin to the violence of the 1918–19 influenza pandemic of the First World War—one of the great pandemics of all history. On the other hand but for the virtual conquest of malaria many a campaign in the Far East would have foundered. Nearer home we saw the almost startling development of infective hepatitis as an epidemic phenomenon in the troops. From all the Services we saw invaliding rates no longer swollen by tuberculosis but by peptic ulcers and psychoneuroses and so on.

Many an earlier volume in this Official Medical History of the Second World War has sought these factual data in developing its story. Now in this present and final volume the statistics are all brought together and set out in detail, not only, one hopes, to record the past but to serve as a guide to future planning and research. For instance, in spite of all the changing conditions of warfare, they should continue to illuminate the problems of Service wastage—the invaliding that takes place at particular stages of life, in particular occupations and from specific causes. They should certainly indicate how essential is a good system of recording sickness and injury in peace-time, not only for administrative reasons but for the contribution that a knowledge of these events should be able to make to epidemiology and therapeutics. For, while statistics may not often solve problems they are one of the most fruitful starting points by merely portraying a problem and thus leading to research.

The statistics here presented are, of course, incomplete. Under the conditions of war they could hardly be else. Yet on the whole one is impressed by all that was done to compile returns, in situations often of great difficulty and hardship and by the skill with which, at the centre, sampling procedures were called to aid in analysing data that reached an almost astronomical scale.

Some of the results here set out certainly make surprising reading. Thus in an account of the work of the Royal Naval Hospital, Haslar (Portsmouth) it is reported that in the early years of the war it was under continuous threat of bombardment from the air and all but the most seriously ill patients were evacuated every night to cots in the cellars. Meanwhile the hospital staff went to their action stations during the fairly numerous air-raid alerts. Yet both patients and staff appeared to thrive under this routine!

In similar vein the Royal Air Force records that with a rapid increase in strength in the first months of the war peace-time standards of accommodation went by the board—the floor space per man in barrack room or hut was halved and many a hut was draughty, ill-ventilated and inadequately heated. The problem of providing a balanced and satisfying diet was considerable; the ordinary hygiene of sewage disposal on new sites was yet another. Increased hours of work were inevitable. The winter of 1940 was very severe. Yet the sickness rate in 1940 hardly rose above the previous year's peace-time level.

It is good to have the figures to illustrate such, and many other, remarkable events. In this volume, too, they relate not only to the Fighting Services as of yore but also to a civil population that had itself to face many of the dangers of total warfare. The statistics for the Emergency Medical Services round off this numerical account of the medical stresses and demands of the Second World War.

CONTENTS

PREFACE

THE PREPARATION of this volume, as with its counterpart after the First World War, was beset by many difficulties, some of which are referred to in the Introductions to the three Fighting Services' contributions. Among these difficulties were the loss of documents in transit owing to enemy action, fast-moving warfare leaving little time for medical recording and the inexperience of some Service Medical Officers. Moreover, in retreat or defeat, e.g. Norway, Greece, Crete and the early years in the Middle East campaign, adequate documentation could hardly be expected.

The Army statistics, based mainly on hospital admissions and not on the Field Medical Cards, many of which were lost, cannot in consequence present a complete picture. For it was to the Field Medical Units that most of the casualties and sick came in the first place. It is from their records that a more complete account of the numbers of casualties that occurred, the types of injury or ailment, the treatment given, disposal, etc., might have emerged. Treatment in Field Medical Units was such that a sizeable proportion of casualties did not need to be sent to hospital. Thus, treatment of casualties in the field—an important feature of the Army Medical Services' successful achievements during the Second World War—is not fully recorded here. Sample statistics of the work of some of the medical units will be found in *Army Medical Services, Campaigns*, Vols. I–V in this series; the evolution and changing functions of these units during the war years are described in *Medical Services in War* (pp. 104–142), the penultimate volume of this series.

In the United Kingdom, for the first time, it was found necessary to set up an organisation to deal with casualties and sickness among civilians and Service personnel in a population exposed to air attack and the threat of invasion. This organisation—the Emergency Medical Services—was unique and the review of its work here holds special interest.

A great deal is owed to the contributors to this volume for all the time and painstaking effort they devoted to the preparation of their respective sections. The result is an impressive overall picture of the diseases and injuries sustained by the members of the United Kingdom Armed Services and the civilian population during the war years. Other data concerning particular diseases and types of injuries in specific Commands and Campaigns will be found in the relevant Service volumes of this History.

The production of a work of this kind was not without its frustrations and complications. I am indebted to Miss F. E. E. Harney, of the

Department of Health and Social Security, for sharing the editorial work and for her help in piloting the volume through the press. As in the case of previous volumes of this History, her loyalty, ability and dedication to the work in hand have been of rare quality.

W.F.M.

The Royal Naval Medical Services

MEDICAL STATISTICS

by Surgeon Captain F. P. Ellis,
O.B.E., Q.H.P., M.D., F.R.C.P., R.N.

CONTENTS

INTRODUCTION

BEFORE the year 1830 the numbers of men voted and returns of naval personnel killed and wounded were the only official statistical documents published by the Admiralty. Regular annual returns of deaths in ships of the Fleet were not required until 1810. The best statistical account of mortality, during the War of 1793–1815, was that prepared by W. V. Hodge[1] who based his figures upon extracts of the log books of ships compiled by William James.[2] In 1840 the Admiralty published annual statistical reports on the rates of mortality, invaliding and sickness for the years 1830–36 and after 1856 these statistical reports were collated and published by Her Majesty's Stationery Office, with certain exceptions, in the form of an annual Report of the Health of the Navy. These Reports made possible comparisons over the years between death rates, invaliding rates, incidence rates of diseases and the loss of time from sickness of various kinds. The figures set out refer not merely to the Fleet as a whole, but also to the various Stations where the Fleet was employed.

Although this annual statement was prepared with increasing care with the passage of years there was no separate section which applied to naval officers; and it was not until the year 1938 that routine medical examinations were instituted and medical history documents maintained for naval officers and then only for aircrew. The naval officer had nothing similar to the Medical History Sheet of the rating. Thus, until a relatively short time ago it was possible for an officer to serve throughout the whole of his career with no medical examination apart from that carried out at the time when he was originally found fit to enter the Service. If he were to go sick in the course of his Service career there was no system for recording such an illness except in the medical returns of his ship or establishment, or in the books of any naval hospital in which he might be treated, and there was no system for the collation of officers' medical records in one single file which would be available for scrutiny.

The principal sources of data available to the Medical Director-General in compiling the annual Report of the Health of the Navy were the quarterly journals of medical officers. Regulations required the senior medical officer of every ship and establishment to forward a quarterly journal to the Medical Department of the Admiralty through his commanding officer. This journal was divided into various tables, which included the movements of the ship, alphabetical sick list, clinical details of cases sent to hospital, injuries and general remarks on the state of health of the ship's company as a whole. Details of sickness from the various diseases were recorded in nosological tables covering the total number of cases, the number invalided, the number dead, the number sent to hospital and the total days' sickness according to an approved system of nomenclature.

It was inevitable, especially during war-time, that for various reasons (the medical officer himself might have been a casualty) some quarterly journals were incomplete or the journals themselves might be lost or destroyed by enemy action. In the case of some casualties the only notification received in the Medical Department would be a signal sent from the surviving naval authorities in the area. Such signals, required for notification of next-of-kin, pension awards, etc., would contain little or nothing in the way of clinical details; they would in general also contain the numbers of only the more seriously injured or dead. The figures given in Table 6 of Command Paper 6832 (Casualties of the Armed Forces, 1939 to 1945)* which shows the number of seriously wounded and killed in the Royal Navy in the Second World War were in fact culled from these signals. These totals vary from the totals shown in Tables 4–10, derived from the more detailed medical officers' quarterly journals. When ships were lost in action no records of the actual causes of death would be available for many of the casualties. In view of this the numbers who died in action were excluded from the above mentioned tables except for the years 1939 and 1940 and even these should be regarded as only approximations.

At the beginning of this survey it was stated that annual medical statistical reports were made since the year 1856 'with certain exceptions'. The first documentary reference in the present century to such an 'exception' occurs in September 1915. At that time, the question of security was raised and the Board of Admiralty concluded that such annual statistics might disclose to an enemy valuable information about the organisation and movements of the Fleet. It was agreed that although medical statistics would still be compiled they would not be published until after the end of hostilities and no naval medical statistics were published during the First World War. Unfortunately owing to administrative difficulties, not the least of which was shortage of clerical man-power, problems also arose concerning the collation of naval medical statistics during the later years of the war and led to the indefinite postponement of publication of the figures for the years 1916–18. These figures were never abstracted from the journals which were ordered to be stored as permanent records. The system having broken down, it took some time to resuscitate it once the First World War was ended.

During the period between the wars the Statistical Report of the Health of the Navy was published annually in the normal way from 1921 onwards. In June 1938, the suspension of publication during the

---

* *See* Annexure, p. 827.

course of the First World War was noted and the question of the future was raised. After consultations with the Army and the Royal Air Force Medical Departments, it was agreed by September 1938 that in the event of war the official Statistical Report on the Health of the Navy would be withdrawn from publication and sale, but a report in modified form would be prepared in conformity with the approved procedures of the War Office and Air Ministry.

THE SECOND WORLD WAR

With the outbreak of the Second World War it was decided that:

(1) publication of the Report of the Health of the Navy for the years 1937 and 1938 would be held over until the end of hostilities;

(2) reports for the war years might be compiled inside the Medical Department of the Admiralty but their publication would also be held over until the end of hostilities.

During the next six months the Medical Director-General was able to gain some idea of the difficulties which lay ahead in compiling medical statistics under war-time conditions, particularly if the war should last any length of time. By the end of the year 1939, 1,020 Journals had been received from medical officers and a revised organisation was obviously needed if the figures for disease and injury were to be extracted expeditiously. At the same time, scrutiny of the numerous journals from medical officers serving afloat revealed the difficulty of allocating any particular ship to a specified fleet or station in any given part of the year.

In peace-time, the journal of every medical officer included a table showing the movements of the ship. This permitted outbreaks of sickness in a ship to be associated with a particular station or port. As a security measure in the Second World War, the movements table was eliminated and it thus became impossible to study endemic or epidemic illnesses on a geographical basis.

In May, 1943, a Naval Medical Statistics Committee was appointed to review the situation. This Committee, which consisted of five members and included Surgeon Rear-Admiral R. A. Rowlands, as Chairman, Professor Major Greenwood and Surgeon Commander J. A. Fraser Roberts, was given wide terms of reference. It concluded that the existing system in the Navy was inadequate to meet modern administrative and scientific demands and that only a small portion of the information available was in fact utilised in compiling naval medical statistics. While appreciating that every effort had been made to compile medical statistics under the system then in existence the Committee considered that the time had come to make drastic changes and to recommend the introduction of a new system and new statistical procedures at the end of the war. At the same time it was suggested that steps be taken immediately without radical changes in the existing system to permit a better use of the records available and to initiate the task of their analysis.

Matters which, in the opinion of the Committee, called for attention were lack of expert statistical guidance, lack of administrative coordination and lack of sufficient clerical staff. The Committee was aware of the difficulties and was reluctant to make any recommendation which would involve the employment of additional man-power for statistical work. This was, perhaps, the most significant observation for the problem of man-power was one which had become vital to the maintenance of naval medical statistics at this particular time. Without adequate clerical assistance the work could not proceed.

The Committee presented its report towards the end of 1943. Its recommendations were approved in principle, but it proved impossible to take immediate steps towards implementing them all, as it was the general policy of all Government Departments that no task should be undertaken which was not essential to the successful prosecution of the war. This work was not considered to be essential.

At the end of the war in November 1945, a further Committee was appointed with the following terms of reference:

(1) To prepare a scheme for the future organisation of the medical statistical services for the Royal Navy and to make recommendations regarding its implementation.

(2) To make proposals on the number and qualifications required for the statistical staff in the Department of the Medical Director-General for the satisfactory operation of the new scheme.

(3) To consider the administration and non-statistical consequences likely to be involved in the adoption of the new scheme and to recommend accordingly.

This Committee completed its investigations and presented its final report in July 1946 and came to be known as the Royal Naval Medical Statistics Committee, 1946. Its detailed recommendations were:

(1) That a statistical and research file should be set up comprising an individual record for each officer and rating in the Navy.

(2) That such a file should be a current one so that should an officer or rating leave the Navy his medical records would be transferred to a 'dead' file.

(3) That such a statistical and research file could not form part of the more ample records required for administrative purposes.

(4) That the statistical and research file should not contain any information not included in the administrative records.

(5) That the statistical and research file should include:

 (a) General personal particulars of each individual on entry into the Navy which would periodically be kept up to date.

 (b) Medical particulars of each individual at the time of entry.

(c) Records of sickness.

(d) Additional medical information, such as records of routine medical examinations, the results of routine chest X-rays, records of inoculations and vaccinations, etc.

(e) A record of the movements of an individual from ship to ship during the course of his Service career.

(6) That a card recording as much of the information as practicable should form part of the statistical and research file.

(7) That the statistical and research file should be linked to one or more punched card indexes.

(8) The complete revision of medical history documents to ensure that copies of records of sickness of the individual accompany him throughout his Service career and are made available to the Medical Officer.

(9) Central control, in the Department of the Medical Director-General, of the complete medical statistical data of the whole of naval personnel, through which it would become possible to acquaint the Board of Admiralty and the public with facts relating to the health of the Navy far more fully and quickly than had been possible in the past (once the system was running satisfactorily).

(10) That new measures would call for adequate trained staff to work the new statistical machine.

Most of these recommendations of the '1946 Committee', in addition to a number of others, were fully implemented and co-ordinated with the post-war reorganisation of the medical records and statistical departments of the Army and the Royal Air Force. But, although great progress was thus made in reorganising the basic system for compiling naval medical statistics for the future, the Committee had not yet closed the gap which existed in the naval medical records of the past, and particularly for that period covered by the Second World War. The existence of this gap meant that even as late as 1948 those who were responsible for the production of the Official Naval History of the War were unable to produce any official figures. In November 1948, this subject was discussed by the Medical Director-General of the Navy, Surgeon Vice-Admiral Sir Henry St. Clair Colson, and the Senior Civil Consulting Physician to the Navy, Sir Alun Rowlands (previously Surgeon Rear-Admiral R. A. Rowlands) who had been closely associated with the activities of the 1943 and 1946 Committees. The chief points established by this discussion were as follows:

(1) It was essential for the production of the Official Naval Medical History of the War that certain naval medical statistics should be compiled and made available as soon as possible.

(2) It was agreed that work upon naval medical statistics as a whole should be recommenced immediately to cover the war period.

(3) It was felt that the production of a complete 'Report on the Health of the Navy' as previously published would not be necessary for the purposes of the Official History. Instead, it was considered that a tabular statement should be compiled to show:

(a) The total number of cases according to sickness and injury.

(b) The total number of final invalidings.

(c) The total number of deaths.

(d) The total number of days sickness on board ship and in hospital.

(e) The average number of persons sick daily.

(f) The ratio per 1,000 of total force sick daily.

(g) The ratio per 1,000 of total force of (a), (b) and (c) above. The whole of the above tabular statement was to be classified in accordance with the nomenclature of diseases as set out in the nosological tables in the journals of medical officers.

(4) It was also agreed that a serving medical officer on the staff of the Medical Director-General should act in a consulting capacity while the work was being carried out.

As a result a tabular statement was compiled for the war years in the Medical Department, Admiralty, under the supervision of Mr. W. G. Grant, which was based on figures from 20,537 medical officers' journals. The work of abstracting the information for the years 1939–45 was thus deferred until 1948. The figures which were made available eventually are contained in Tables 4–10. Condensed versions of these tables were published and discussed in the *Journal of the Royal Naval Medical Service* in 1966.[3] They provide the most accurate record available of the causes of man-power wastage due to sickness and injury in the Total Force during the years of the Second World War. It was only after the war that statistical reports were prepared which allowed a comparison to be made between the overall case incidence of the men in the Navy and that of the Women's Royal Naval Service.

The only action to compile vital statistics for the Total Force during the course of hostilities was the completion by Dr. (then Surgeon Commander) J. A. Fraser Roberts of an 'Analysis of Invalidings due to Disease and Deaths due to Disease for the years 1934–43' which was afforded only a limited circulation as an Admiralty Book of Reference.* This is reproduced in Section II. The figures for officers are excluded from most of the tables and the invaliding and death rates for certain diseases therefore vary from the rates for the Total Force

* Admiralty Book of Reference 1235 (1944).

which are shown in Tables 4–10 which are the rates for ratings and officers combined. Within the limitations imposed by war-time security and the lack of adequate statistical machinery this report, which has remained buried in the archives until recently, provided for the first time reliable figures for major diseases of officers and ratings separately and for the women as well as the men who served in the Navy. Fraser Roberts also showed the importance of adjusting the crude rates for diseases to allow for the different distributions of the age groups in the peace-time and war-time navies. In the words of Professor Major Greenwood, F.R.S., a member of the 1943 and 1946 Committees on Medical Statistics who wrote the Foreword, it attained 'a scientific standard which would justify its publication in the transactions of any learned society'. It is complete and provides the only uninterrupted account of disease trends in the Navy for the years preceding the Second World War and during the first four years of the war. The figures for invalidings in 1944 which are shown in Tables 11–23 and 29 were added after the book was published.

A comprehensive register of all cases admitted to the Royal Naval Hospital, Haslar, the largest British naval hospital, during the years 1939 to 1945, with the final diagnoses in each case, was maintained throughout the war by the Senior Consultant in Medicine, Surgeon Rear-Admiral R. A. (later Sir Alun) Rowlands. Sir Alun also arranged for the abstraction of similar information from the Hospital Muster Books for the years 1914–18 inclusive which provides the only valid comparison which can be made of the patterns of disease at a home-based naval hospital during the two wars.[3] The case numbers and the cases per 1,000 admissions are tabulated in Tables 33–38 according to a nosological index based on Table 3 of the Medical Officers' Journal.

I. THE TOTAL FORCE

In Table 1 the broad picture during the Second World War is compared with that for 1936,[4] the last year for which the Report on the Health of the Navy compiled by the old system was published, and 1953,[5] the first post-war year for which the Report was compiled by a new system of centralised medical recording with machine analysis of the coded data.

TABLE 1

Morbidity, Invaliding and Mortality Rates for Diseases and Injuries for the years 1936, 1939–45 and 1953 (excluding casualties in action)

	Fresh Cases per 1,000 Strength	Sick Daily per 1,000 Strength (non-effective rate)	Final Invalidings per 1,000 Strength	Deaths per 1,000 Strength
1936	437	19·5	11·7	2·0
1939	504	19·9	13·7	4·6
1940	473	19·3	17·9	3·2
1941	434	18·1	20·9	3·2
1942	409	17·2	16·1	2·9
1943	412	15·2	14·0	3·4
1944	361	15·1	14·5	2·8
1945	377	16·1	25·9	2·6
1953	378	15·6	18·7	1·7

During the war years the Navy expanded greatly. The age, constitution and the general physical status of its personnel were influenced and these changes affected the rates of sickness and death. With this proviso (excluding all casualties in action) the Navy would not appear to have been much less healthy in war-time than in these two years of peace. In fact it would appear that, except for deaths, in war the health of the Navy compared favourably with that during the years 1936 and 1953.

In Table 2 a comparison is made for certain of the more prominent disease groups. The sickness rates for 1953 are not included as the diseases included under these headings in the World Health Organisation's nomenclature which was adopted in 1953 and the succeeding years differ from those included under similar headings in the previous Reports. The incidence for different diseases is shown separately for officers and ratings and the total case incidence is not usually given in the reports prepared after the war.

Venereal disease rates were considerably reduced compared with the rate in 1936 partly as a result of advances in chemotherapy, partly because of extended spells of service at sea with less leave in foreign ports and partly because urethritis non-venereal, the incidence of which increased during the war, was shown not under venereal diseases but

TABLE 2
Common Disease Groups for Officers and Ratings
Rates per 1,000. 1936, 1939–45

Disease	1936	1939	1940	1941	1942	1943	1944	1945
Venereal Disease	57·0	56·6	33·6	33·0	28·9	20·8	22·6	31·7
Malaria	2·2	2·4	4·6	6·3	9·0	10·8	7·6	3·1
Diseases of the Eye	4·9	4·4	4·5	4·0	3·6	2·9	2·9	3·3
Diseases of the Ear	8·5	9·4	6·7	6·8	6·3	5·5	5·9	8·8
Diseases of the Veins	1·3	2·1	2·6	2·4	2·8	2·7	2·7	3·5
Diseases of the Stomach and Duodenum	9·1	16·8	20·9	20·8	16·7	15·0	15·8	17·8
Diseases of the Generative System and of Urinary Organs	11·7	12·1	12·0	11·4	10·9	11·4	12·0	14·6
Appendicitis	5·9	6·4	5·7	5·2	4·9	4·9	4·4	4·2
Hernia	4·5	3·5	4·6	4·4	4·3	4·4	3·4	3·6
Injuries	70·9	85·9	83·9	66·5	50·2	45·1	41·4	40·1
Diseases of the Liver	2·1	2·6	1·6	2·2	2·8	4·6	3·6	3·8

under diseases of the urinary and generative systems although most of these infections were acquired as the result of sexual intercourse.

By 1943 there had been nearly a five-fold increase in the rate of malaria. The war-time rates for diseases of the stomach and duodenum increased above the peace-time rate, but the surprising fact is that the overall picture in war-time did not change very greatly so far as one can discern from these gross statistics.

The increase in diseases of the liver was almost entirely due to the increased incidence of hepatitis. With the swollen war-time population and the long periods of convalescence frequently necessary, the actual demands on hospitals for beds for cases of hepatitis were greater than is suggested by the increase in rates in 1943 and 1944 shown above. Reference to Table 8 shows that the ratio per 1,000 'sick daily' with diseases of the liver of 0·29 per 1,000 in 1943 was only exceeded for injuries and the respiratory tract infections, pulmonary tuberculosis, the common cold, bronchitis and tonsillitis.

In Table 3 the invaliding rates for 1936 and 1953 are shown to illustrate the wastage sustained in this way before and after the war together with the losses during the war by reference to four of the most prominent causes of ill-health—pulmonary tuberculosis, psycho-neurotic illness, peptic ulcer and diseases of the eye.

There was a considerable increase in the invaliding rate for psycho-neurotic disease during the war. The invaliding rate for pulmonary tuberculosis showed a slight increase but this was primarily the result of the introduction of mass fluorography and more careful discrimination in eliminating those with early active infections from the Service. The incidence of disease detected clinically was declining during these years, a steady decline which, as Brooks[6] has reported, eventually

TABLE 3

Invalidings—Respiratory Tuberculosis, Psychoneuroses and Psychoses, Peptic Ulcer, Diseases of the Eye. Rates per 1,000

	Respiratory Tuberculosis	Psychoneuroses, Psychoses, etc.	Peptic Ulcer	Diseases of Eye
1936	1·9	1·5	0·5	1·1
1939	1·6	2·3	1·2	0·9
1940	1·7	4·2	1·6	1·0
1941	2·1	5·7	2·7	1·0
1942	2·6	3·5	1·7	0·6
1943	2·5	3·3	1·4	0·4
1944	2·4	3·6	1·2	0·4
1945	2·4	5·4	2·9	1·0
1953	2·5	2·8	2·3	1·1

resulted in a marked reduction of 'clinical' pulmonary tuberculosis between the years 1939 and 1953.

The invaliding rate for peptic ulcer was considerably in excess of the pre-war rate. A high rate was still maintained in 1953, eight years after the end of the war. It is not possible to say whether the increased invaliding rates for psychiatric disease and peptic ulcer were due to a real increase in disease or to revised medical standards. Perhaps the average pre-war man accepted more in the way of dyspepsia as a matter of course than the post-war individual without allowing it to disrupt his life and his work; perhaps the naval authorities were less inclined to retain the chronic dyspeptic than before the war. Undoubtedly many factors played their part.

TABLE 4

Number of Cases of Disease and Injury under the various Classes, the Number of Invalidings and Deaths; and the Average Number of Men Sick Daily in the Total Force, with Ratios per 1,000 of Average Strength for the Year 1939
(Average Strength 131,858)

DISEASE OR INJURY	Cases	In-valided	Dead	Days' Sickness			Average Number of Men Sick Daily	Ratio per 1,000 of Strength			
				On board	In Hospital	Total		Cases	In-valided	Dead	Sick Daily
DISEASES CAUSED BY INFECTION:											
Chicken-pox	96	—	—	2,953	575	3,528	9·7	·7	—	—	·07
Common Cold	11,194	—	—	43,979	31,814	75,793	207·7	84·9	—	—	1·57
Cow-pox	1,463	—	—	10,216	1,541	11,757	32·2	11·1	—	—	·24
Dengue	189	—	—	1,089	212	1,301	3·6	1·4	—	—	·02
Diphtheria	164	—	2	2,461	8,633	11,094	30·4	1·2	—	·0	·23
Dysentery	113	—	1	318	1,146	1,464	4·0	·9	—	·0	·03
Enteric Fever, Typhoid	1	—	—	1	202	203	·6	·0	—	—	·00
Enteric Fever, Paratyphoid	6	—	1	42	152	194	·5	·0	—	·0	·00
Erysipelas	55	—	—	756	202	958	2·6	·4	—	—	·01
Influenza	1,243	—	—	11,620	1,334	12,954	35·5	9·4	—	—	·26
Malaria	316	—	—	2,764	1,709	4,473	12·2	2·4	—	—	·09
Measles	86	—	1	520	965	1,485	4·1	·7	—	·0	·03
Meningococcal Infection	37	—	4	168	1,378	1,546	4.2	·3	—	·0	·03
Mumps	163	—	—	1,098	2,243	3,341	9·2	1·2	—	—	·06
Pneumococcal Infection (Lungs)	330	—	10	2,698	10,825	13,523	37·0	2·5	—	·1	·28
Pneumococcal Infection (Other Organs)	9	—	—	121	—	121	·3	·1	—	—	·00
Pyogenic Infection	18	—	3	370	303	673	1·8	·1	—	·0	·01
Pyrexia of Uncertain Origin	103	—	—	485	1,347	1,832	5·0	·8	—	—	·03
Rheumatic Fever	227	48	1	2,543	35,191	37,734	103·4	1·7	·4	·0	·78
Rheumatism, sub-acute	317	—	—	3,113	4,780	7,893	21·6	2·4	—	—	·16
Rubella	1,294	—	—	3,140	9,015	12,155	33·3	9·8	—	—	·25
Sandfly Fever	69	—	—	415	167	582	1·6	·6	—	—	·01
Scarlet Fever	249	—	1	1,635	6,003	7,638	20·9	1·9	—	·0	·15
Smallpox	10	—	—	4	204	208	·6	·1	—	—	·00

TABLE 4 (*contd.*)

Number of Cases of Disease and Injury under the various Classes, the Number of Invalidings and Deaths; and the Average Number of Men Sick Daily in the Total Force, with Ratios per 1,000 of Average Strength for the year 1939
(Average Strength 131,858)

DISEASE OR INJURY	Cases	In-valided	Dead	Days' Sickness			Average Number of Men Sick Daily	Ratio per 1,000 of Strength			
				On board	In Hospital	Total		Cases	In-valided	Dead	Sick Daily
Tonsillitis	5,599	—	—	27,705	29,167	56,872	155·8	42·5	—	—	1·18
Tuberculosis, Pulmonary*	228	216	16	1,797	10,292	12,089	33·1	1·7	1·6	·1	·25
Tuberculosis, Non-pulmonary	29	21	8	207	2,500	2,707	7·4	·2	·2	·1	·05
Undulant Fever	6	—	—	95	233	328	·9	·0	—	—	·00
Chancroid	1,027	—	—	2,049	4,461	6,510	17·8	7·8	—	—	·13
Chancroid, Sequelae	173	—	—	1,995	299	2,294	6·3	1·3	—	—	·04
Syphilis, First record	563	—	1	2,369	6,475	8,844	24·2	4·3	—	·0	·18
Syphilis, Later record	148	2	1	346	2,269	2,615	7·2	1·1	·0	·0	·05
Gonococcal Infection, Acute	4,250	1	—	7,358	26,168	33,526	91·9	32·2	·0	—	·69
Gonococcal Infection, Sequelae	707	28	—	3,618	7,978	11,596	31·8	5·4	·2	—	·24
Lympho-granuloma Inguinale	69	—	—	944	705	1,649	4·5	4·5	—	—	·03
Other Diseases caused by Infection	311	5	—	1,765	1,186	2,951	8·1	2·4	·0	—	·06
Diseases Caused by Metazoan Parasites	2,035	—	—	7,595	2,700	10,295	28·2	15·4	—	—	·21
DISEASES OF THE NERVOUS SYSTEM:											
Diseases of Spinal Cord	26	11	—	192	950	1,142	3·1	·2	·1	—	·02
Diseases of Brain	43	17	11	273	670	943	2·6	·3	·1	·1	·01
Apoplexy	5	—	5	—	—	—	—	·0	—	·0	—
Paralysis	46	9	1	465	1,553	2,018	5·5	·3	·1	·0	·04
Epilepsy	92	72	—	440	3,029	3,469	9·5	·7	·5	—	·07
Neurasthenia	122	19	—	777	1,544	2,321	6·4	·9	·1	—	·04

Other Nervous Diseases (including Mental)	1,046	288	3	4,638	23,750	28,388	77·8	7·9	2·2	·0	·58
DISEASES OF THE EYE	574	119	—	3,051	8,034	11,085	30·4	4·4	·9	—	·23
DISEASES OF THE EAR	1,241	81	—	6,766	16,682	23,448	64·2	9·4	·6	—	·48
DISEASES OF THE NOSE	333	5	—	1,245	5,338	6,583	18·0	2·5	·0	—	·13
DISEASES OF THE CIRCULATORY SYSTEM:											
Diseases of the Heart (Organic)	148	82	10	952	5,416	6,368	17·4	1·1	·6	·1	·13
Diseases of the Heart (Functional)	139	21	12	649	3,094	3,743	10·3	1·1	·2	·1	·07
Diseases of the Arteries	106	42	10	598	2,596	3,194	8·8	·8	·3	·1	·06
Diseases of the Veins	275	8	—	1,608	4,676	6,284	17·2	2·1	·1	—	·13
Diseases of the Blood and Blood-forming Organs	316	8	5	2,372	4,460	6,832	18·7	2·4	·1	·0	·14
Diseases of Glands of Internal Secretion	26	17	—	304	1,796	2,100	5·8	·2	·1	—	·04
Diseases of the Breast	14	—	—	37	38	75	·2	·1	—	—	·00
DISEASES OF THE RESPIRATORY SYSTEM:											
Diseases of the Larynx	344	—	—	1,831	1,125	2,956	8·1	2·6	—	—	·06
Bronchial Catarrh	653	—	—	3,536	4,127	7,663	21·0	5·0	—	—	·15
Bronchitis	1,195	49	2	9,256	9,731	18,987	52·0	9·1	·4	·0	·39
Asthma	124	19	—	601	1,625	2,226	6·1	·9	·1	—	·04
Fibrosis of Lung	50	15	—	264	1,264	1,528	4·2	·4	·1	—	·03
Pleurisy	274	14	2	1,792	7,720	9,512	26·1	2·1	·1	·0	·19
Other Diseases	238	35	10	1,835	8,438	10,273	28·1	1·8	·3	·1	·21
DISEASES OF TEETH AND GUMS	484	—	—	1,468	2,901	4,369	12·0	3·7	—	—	·09
HERNIA	468	33	1	1,264	13,805	15,069	41·3	3·5	·3	·0	·31
HERNIA (Recurrent)	78	—	—	379	1,565	1,944	5·3	·6	—	—	·04
DISEASES OF THE DIGESTIVE SYSTEM:											
Mouth, Palate, Fauces, Pharynx	766	—	1	4,044	3,393	7,437	20·4	5·8	—	·0	·15
Peptic Ulcer, Gastric	293	61	4	1,072	8,139	9,211	25·2	2·2	·5	·0	·19

* As a general rule all cases of Pulmonary Tuberculosis were either invalided from the Navy or died. Many cases, however, were treated in the Service for many months at a time so that the number of cases shown in the tables for each Calendar Year may not correspond to the sum of the number of cases invalided and the number of deaths.

TABLE 4 (*contd.*)

Number of Cases of Disease and Injury under the various Classes, the Number of Invalidings and Deaths; and the Average Number of Men Sick Daily in the Total Force, with Ratios per 1,000 of Average Strength for the year 1939
(Average Strength 131,858)

DISEASE OR INJURY	Cases	In-valided	Dead	Days' Sickness			Average Number of Men Sick Daily	Ratio per 1,000 of Strength			
				On board	In Hospital	Total		Cases	In-valided	Dead	Sick Daily
Peptic Ulcer, Duodenal	270	90	2	1,161	11,862	13,023	35·7	2·0	·7	·0	·27
Appendicitis	848	4	6	3,628	17,608	21,236	58·2	6·4	·0	·0	·44
Other Diseases of the Stomach	1,668	35	3	7,827	13,071	20,898	57·3	12·6	·3	·0	·43
Other Diseases of the Intestines	1,432	12	5	6,168	6,305	12,473	34·2	10·9	·1	·0	·25
Diseases of Rectum and Anus	459	1	—	2,492	9,751	12,243	33·5	3·5	·0	—	·25
Diseases of the Liver	344	2	2	2,868	5,382	8,250	22·6	2·6	·0	·0	·17
Other Diseases	104	4	5	630	2,443	3,073	8·4	·8	·0	·0	·06
DISEASES OF NUTRITION OR METABOLISM:											
Scurvy	4	—	—	20	—	20	·1	·0	—	—	·00
Beri-Beri	—	—	—	—	—	—	—	—	—	—	—
Gout	40	2	—	307	369	676	1·9	·3	·0	—	·01
Diabetes	33	24	—	138	1,396	1,534	4·2	·3	·2	—	·03
Other Diseases	27	—	—	208	273	481	1·3	·2	—	—	·00
DISEASES OF GENERATIVE SYSTEM:											
Stricture	6	—	—	16	150	166	·5	·0	—	—	·00
Varicocele	36	—	—	105	399	504	1·4	·3	—	—	·01
Orchitis	45	—	—	191	117	308	·8	·3	—	—	·00
Other Diseases	980	3	—	3,083	12,253	15,336	42·0	7·4	·0	—	·31
DISEASES OF BONES, JOINTS, MUSCLES, FASCIAE AND BURSAE:											
Periosteum and Bone	71	9	—	612	3,274	3,886	10·6	·5	·1	—	·08
Cartilage and Joints	382	37	1	2,869	7,455	10,324	28·3	2·9	·3	·0	·21

Spine	17	10	—	45	429	474	1·3	·1	·1	—	·00
Muscles, Fasciae, Tendons, Bursae	935	12	—	7,023	6,319	13,342	36·6	7·1	·1	—	·27
Deformities and Congenital Malformations	124	53	1	614	3,119	3,733	10·2	·9	·4	·0	·07
DISEASES OF AREOLAR TISSUE AND SKIN:											
Abscess	817	—	—	5,372	5,134	10,506	28·8	6·2	—	—	·21
Boil	1,666	—	—	9,609	2,494	12,103	33·2	12·6	—	—	·25
Eczema	167	2	—	1,910	2,270	4,180	11·5	1·3	·0	—	·08
Impetigo	562	—	—	5,617	4,289	9,906	27·1	4·3	—	—	·20
Other Diseases	2,866	17	2	19,556	28,230	47,786	130·9	21·7	·1	·0	·99
DISEASES OF URINARY ORGANS:											
Kidneys	304	28	8	2,115	7,580	9,695	26·6	2·3	·2	·1	·20
Ureter and Bladder	122	2	—	619	3,004	3,623	9·9	·9	·0	—	·07
Urinary Disorders	118	—	—	499	2,182	2,681	7·3	·9	—	—	·05
NEW GROWTHS, MALIGNANT	45	11	6	169	1,186	1,355	3·7	·3	·1	·0	·02
NEW GROWTHS, NON-MALIGNANT	206	3	—	667	3,048	3,715	10·2	1·6	·0	—	·07
ALCOHOLISM	45	—	—	74	276	350	1·0	·3	—	—	·00
POISONING, VARIOUS	223	—	—	1,390	300	1,690	4·6	1·7	—	—	·03
GENERAL INJURIES:											
Multiple Injuries	171	1	37	769	3,119	3,888	10·7	1·3	·0	·3	·08
Multiple Burns and Scalds	34	—	6	223	276	499	1·4	·3	—	·0	·01
Heat Stroke	121	—	2	457	144	601	1·6	·9	—	·0	·01
Suffocation—Drowning	236	—	236	—	—	—	—	1·8	—	1·8	—
Suffocation—Effects of	117	—	114	38	40	78	·2	·9	—	·9	·00
Compressed Air Disease	1	—	1	—	—	—	—	·0	—	·0	—
LOCAL INJURIES:											
Burns and Scalds	571	—	—	4,645	3,232	7,877	21·6	4·3	—	—	·16
Injuries and Wounds	7,766	104	24	56,163	76,744	132,907	364·1	58·9	·8	·2	2·76
WOUNDS AND INJURIES IN ACTION	2,310	—	1,885	1,595	5,549	7,144	19·6	17·5	—	14·3	·14
SUICIDES	15	—	15	—	—	—	—	·1	—	·1	—
TOTALS	68,724	1,812	2,488	353,553	612,905	966,458	2647·8	521·2	13·7	18·9	20·08

TABLE 5

Number of Cases of Disease and Injury under the various Classes, the Number of Invalidings and Deaths; and the Average Number of Men Sick Daily in the Total Force, with Ratios per 1,000 of Average Strength for the year 1940

(Average Strength 270,000)

DISEASE OR INJURY	Cases	In-valided	Dead	Days' Sickness			Average Number of Men Sick Daily	Ratio per 1,000 of Strength			
				On Board	In Hospital	Total		Cases	In-valided	Dead	Sick Daily
DISEASES CAUSED BY INFECTION:											
Chicken-pox	165	—	—	836	1,677	2,513	6·9	·6	—	—	·02
Common Cold	17,065	—	—	74,521	36,581	111,102	303·6	63·2	—	—	1·12
Cow-pox	2,498	—	—	11,032	2,282	13,314	36·4	9·3	—	—	·13
Dengue	67	—	—	179	499	678	1·9	·2	—	—	·00
Diphtheria	213	—	2	875	8,679	9,554	26·1	·8	—	·0	·09
Dysentery	137	—	1	568	1,671	2,239	6·1	·5	—	·0	·02
Enteric Fever, Typhoid	10	—	1	23	468	491	1·3	·0	—	·0	·00
Enteric Fever, Paratyphoid	16	—	2	115	354	469	1·3	·1	—	·0	·00
Erysipelas	69	—	—	624	670	1,294	3·5	·3	—	—	·01
Influenza	6,253	—	1	59,534	13,356	72,890	199·2	23·2	—	·0	·73
Malaria	1,240	—	7	6,409	5,308	11,717	32·0	4·6	—	·0	·11
Measles	204	—	—	1,612	4,380	5,992	16·4	·8	—	—	·06
Meningococcal Infection	162	—	—	1,562	3,150	4,712	12·9	·6	—	—	·04
Mumps	202	—	—	1,633	3,092	4,725	12·9	·7	—	—	·04
Pneumococcal Infection (Lungs)	669	6	21	7,622	19,219	26,841	73·3	2·5	·0	·1	·27
Pneumococcal Infection (Other Organs)	12	—	—	148	1,157	1,305	3·6	·0	—	—	·01
Pyogenic Infection	22	—	5	237	541	778	2·1	·1	—	·0	·00
Pyrexia of Uncertain Origin	218	1	1	1,561	1,526	3,087	8·4	·8	·0	·0	·03
Rheumatic Fever	306	58	—	4,796	7,992	12,788	34·9	1·1	·2	—	·12
Rheumatism, sub-acute	697	32	1	9,019	8,306	17,325	47·3	2·6	·1	·0	·17
Rubella	3,780	—	—	16,370	25,319	41,689	113·9	14·0	—	—	·42
Sandfly Fever	128	—	—	715	257	972	2·7	·5	—	—	·00
Scarlet Fever	316	—	—	1,999	17,440	19,439	53·1	1·2	—	—	·19
Small-pox	—	—	—	—	—	—	—	—	—	—	—
Tonsillitis	9,761	—	1	58,970	34,624	93,594	255·7	36·2	—	·0	·94

Tuberculosis, Pulmonary*	563	448	29	2,229	21,146	23,375	63·9	2·1	1·7	·1	·23
Tuberculosis, Non-pulmonary	53	43	13	458	2,000	2,458	6·7	·2	·2	·0	·02
Undulant Fever	4	—	—	26	101	127	·3	·0	—	—	·00
Chancroid	1,008	—	—	2,882	2,257	5,139	14·0	3·7	—	—	·05
Chancroid, Sequelae	127	—	—	—	—	—	—	·5	—	—	—
Syphilis, First record	881	1	—	3,341	8,959	12,300	33·6	3·3	·0	—	·12
Syphilis, Later record	178	—	—	556	2,639	3,195	8·7	·7	—	—	·03
Gonococcal Infection, Acute	6,097	1	—	13,530	28,815	42,345	115·7	22·6	·0	—	·42
Gonococcal Infection, Sequelae	667	39	—	3,807	19,284	23,091	63·1	2·5	·1	—	·23
Lympho-granuloma Inguinale	77	—	—	543	639	1,182	3·2	·3	—	—	·01
Other Diseases caused by Infection	820	12	1	4,567	6,641	11,208	30·6	3·0	·0	·0	·11
Diseases caused by Metazoan Parasites	5,874	—	—	9,942	9,886	19,828	54·2	21·8	—	—	·20
DISEASES OF THE NERVOUS SYSTEM:											
Diseases of the Spinal Cord	56	28	3	355	2,011	2,366	6·5	·2	·1	·0	·02
Diseases of Brain	82	37	45	418	9,862	10,280	28·1	·3	·1	·2	·10
Apoplexy	11	—	—	82	—	82	·2	·0	—	—	·00
Paralysis	98	35	1	729	3,522	4,251	11·6	·4	·1	·0	·04
Epilepsy	296	212	—	1,655	9,146	10,801	29·5	1·1	·8	—	·10
Neurasthenia	326	27	—	3,011	2,054	5,065	13·8	1·2	·1	—	·05
Other Nervous Diseases (including Mental)	3,753	1,114	—	22,009	104,918	126,927	346·8	13·9	4·1	—	1·28
DISEASES OF THE EYE	1,208	267	—	7,407	18,729	26,136	71·4	4·5	1·0	—	·26
DISEASES OF THE EAR	1,805	206	1	9,750	21,065	30,815	84·2	6·7	·8	·0	·31
DISEASES OF THE NOSE	833	7	—	3,481	9,804	13,285	36·3	3·1	·0	—	·13
DISEASES OF THE CIRCULATORY SYSTEM:											
Diseases of the Heart (Organic)	353	149	54	2,462	9,588	12,050	32·9	1·3	·6	·2	·12

* As a general rule all cases of Pulmonary Tuberculosis were either invalided from the Navy or died. Many cases, however, were treated in the Service for many months at a time so that the number of cases shown in the tables for each Calendar Year may not correspond to the sum of the number of cases invalided and the number of deaths.

TABLE 5 (*contd.*)

Number of Cases of Disease and Injury under the various Classes, the Number of Invalidings and Deaths; and the average Number of Men Sick Daily in the Total Force, with Ratios per 1,000 of Average Strength for the year 1940
(Average Strength 270,000)

DISEASE OR INJURY	Cases	In-valided	Dead	Days' Sickness			Average Number of Men Sick Daily	Ratio per 1,000 of Strength			
				On Board	In Hospital	Total		Cases	In-valided	Dead	Sick Daily
Diseases of the Heart (Functional)	294	47	30	2,535	3,556	6,091	16·6	1·1	·2	·1	·06
Diseases of the Arteries	310	182	28	1,944	7,626	9,570	26·1	1·1	·7	·1	·09
Diseases of the Veins	702	37	3	4,055	11,883	15,938	43·5	2·6	·1	·0	·16
Diseases of the Blood and Blood-forming Organs	587	13	9	4,445	6,759	11,204	30·6	2·2	·0	·0	·11
Diseases of Glands of Internal Secretion	81	35	2	450	3,380	3,830	10·5	·3	·1	·0	·03
Diseases of the Breast	27	1	—	106	167	273	·7	·1	·0	—	·00
DISEASES OF THE RESPIRATORY SYSTEM:											
Diseases of the Larynx	767	2	—	6,303	2,921	9,224	25·2	2·8	·0	—	·09
Bronchial Catarrh	1,380	2	—	11,717	4,906	16,623	45·4	5·1	·0	—	·16
Bronchitis	4,100	210	4	34,763	39,930	74,693	204·1	15·2	·8	·0	·75
Asthma	336	55	—	2,331	4,100	6,431	17·6	1·2	·2	—	·06
Fibrosis of Lung	151	63	—	1,017	4,620	5,637	15·4	·6	·2	—	·05
Pleurisy	729	22	—	6,330	3,909	10,239	28·0	2·7	·1	—	·10
Other Diseases	656	100	39	5,752	20,697	26,449	72·3	2·4	·4	·1	·26
DISEASES OF THE TEETH AND GUMS	1,235	4	—	5,110	7,685	12,795	35·0	4·6	·0	—	·12
HERNIA	1,255	28	1	2,938	32,490	35,428	96·8	4·6	·1	·0	·35
HERNIA (Recurrent)	103	—	—	407	1,636	2,043	5·6	·4	—	—	·02
DISEASES OF THE DIGESTIVE SYSTEM:											
Mouth, Palate, Fauces, Pharynx	2,095	—	—	11,686	6,744	18,430	50·4	7·8	—	—	·18
Peptic Ulcer, Gastric	652	127	2	4,445	17,195	21,640	59·1	2·4	·5	·0	·21

Peptic Ulcer, Duodenal	770	293	4	4,957	27,017	31,974	87·4	2·9	1·1	·0	·32
Appendicitis	1,549	3	15	6,931	31,790	38,721	105·8	5·7	·0	·1	·39
Other Diseases of the Stomach	4,218	80	3	28,680	33,399	62,079	169·6	15·6	·3	·0	·62
Other Diseases of the Intestines	2,500	34	21	13,153	11,655	24,808	67·8	9·3	·1	·1	·25
Diseases of the Rectum and Anus	1,005	8	1	4,602	17,599	22,201	60·7	3·7	·0	·0	·22
Diseases of the Liver	419	9	7	3,858	7,057	10,915	29·8	1·6	·0	·0	·11
Other Diseases	196	17	5	1,239	4,864	6,103	16·7	·7	·1	·0	·06
DISEASES OF NUTRITION OR METABOLISM:											
Scurvy	19	—	—	129	89	218	·6	·1	—	—	·00
Beri-Beri	—	—	—	—	—	—	—	—	—	—	—
Gout	126	6	—	1,204	1,055	2,259	6·2	·5	·0	—	·02
Diabetes	43	32	—	1,189	1,982	3,171	8·7	·2	·1	—	·03
Other Diseases	59	2	—	197	898	1,095	3·0	·2	·0	—	·01
DISEASES OF THE GENERATIVE SYSTEM:											
Stricture	15	—	2	36	105	141	·4	·1	—	·0	·00
Varicocele	105	1	—	254	1,361	1,615	4·4	·4	·0	—	·01
Orchitis	90	—	—	701	469	1,170	3·2	·3	—	—	·01
Other Diseases	1,825	5	—	5,380	13,042	18,422	50·3	6·8	·0	—	·18
DISEASES OF BONES, JOINTS, MUSCLES, FASCIAE, BURSAE:											
Periosteum and Bone	129	27	1	1,185	6,988	8,173	22·3	·5	·1	·0	·08
Cartilage and Joints	726	179	—	5,353	26,115	31,468	86·0	2·7	·7	—	·31
Spine	60	19	—	345	2,229	2,574	7·0	·2	·1	—	·02
Muscles, Fasciae, Tendons, Bursae	2,037	28	—	16,391	15,786	32,177	87·9	7·5	·1	—	·32
Deformities and Congenital Malformations	317	80	—	1,438	6,703	8,141	22·2	1·2	·3	—	·08
DISEASES OF AREOLAR TISSUE AND SKIN:											
Abscess	1,141	1	—	7,972	6,690	14,662	40·1	4·2	·0	—	·14
Boil	2,174	—	—	13,294	2,267	15,561	42·5	8·1	—	—	·15
Eczema	340	—	—	3,336	2,716	6,052	16·5	1·3	—	—	·06
Impetigo	794	—	—	6,931	4,846	11,777	32·2	2·9	—	—	·11
Other Diseases	5,103	37	2	35,371	42,135	77,506	211·8	18·9	·1	·0	·78

TABLE 5 (*contd.*)

Number of Cases of Disease and Injury under the various Classes, the Number of Invalidings and Deaths; and the Average Number of Men Sick Daily in the Total Force, with Ratios per 1,000 of Average Strength for the year 1940
(Average Strength 270,000)

DISEASE OR INJURY	Cases	In-valided	Dead	Days' Sickness			Average Number of Men Sick Daily	Ratio per 1,000 of Strength			
				On board	In Hospital	Total		Cases	In-valided	Dead	Sick Daily
DISEASES OF URINARY ORGANS:											
Kidneys	642	56	23	2,204	12,247	14,451	39·5	2·4	·2	·1	·14
Ureter and Bladder	338	16	1	1,718	4,114	5,832	15·9	1·3	·1	·0	·05
Urinary Disorders	199	6	—	1,013	2,880	3,893	10·6	·7	·0	—	·03
NEW GROWTHS, MALIGNANT	102	36	28	592	3,293	3,885	10·6	·4	·1	·1	·03
NEW GROWTHS, NON-MALIGNANT	329	2	—	1,219	3,036	4,255	11·6	1·2	·0	—	·04
ALCOHOLISM	62	5	1	121	461	582	1·6	·2	·0	·0	·00
POISONING, VARIOUS	248	1	7	1,184	215	1,399	3·8	·9	·0	·0	·01
GENERAL INJURIES:											
Multiple Injuries	324	7	245	1,333	9,109	10,442	28·5	1·2	·0	·9	·10
Multiple Burns and Scalds	65	—	9	527	3,313	3,840	10·5	·2	—	·0	·03
Heat Stroke	218	—	1	912	183	1,095	3·0	·8	—	·0	·01
Suffocation—Drowning	122	—	122	—	290	290	·8	·5	—	·5	·00
Suffocation—Effects of	32	—	9	45	52	97	·3	·1	—	·0	·00
Compressed Air Disease	—	—	—	—	—	—	—	—	—	—	—
LOCAL INJURIES:											
Burns and Scalds	929	18	—	8,648	15,804	24,452	66·8	3·4	·1	—	·24
Injuries and Wounds	13,600	172	27	97,184	168,659	265,843	726·3	50·4	·6	·1	2·69
WOUNDS AND INJURIES IN ACTION	7,383	19	3,854	11,321	25,769	37,090	101·3	27·3	·1	14·3	·37
SUICIDES	24	—	24	—	—	—	—	·1	—	·1	—
TOTALS	135,220	4,850	4,720	752,681	1,190,100	1,942,781	5,308·1	500·8	18·0	17·5	19·65

TABLE 6

Number of Cases of Disease and Injury under the various Classes, the Number of Invalidings and Deaths; and the Average Number of Men Sick Daily in the Total Force, with the Ratios per 1,000 of Average Strength for the year 1941
(Average Strength 396,000)

DISEASE OR INJURY	Cases	In-valided	Dead	Days' Sickness			Average Number of Men Sick Daily	Ratio per 1,000 of Strength			
				On Board	In Hospital	Total		Cases	In-valided	Dead	Sick Daily
DISEASES CAUSED BY INFECTION:											
Chicken-pox	148	—	—	1,084	1,322	2,406	6·6	·4	—	—	·01
Common Cold	17,373	—	—	87,732	26,051	113,783	311·7	43·9	—	—	·78
Cow-pox	2,559	—	—	9,574	2,457	12,031	33·0	6·5	—	—	·08
Dengue	322	—	—	1,571	647	2,218	6·1	·8	—	—	·01
Diphtheria	399	—	6	1,681	14,206	15,887	43·5	1·0	—	·0	·10
Dysentery	465	1	—	1,007	4,213	5,220	14·3	1·2	·0	—	·03
Enteric Fever, Typhoid	11	1	2	72	804	876	2·4	·0	·0	·0	·00
Enteric Fever, Paratyphoid	15	—	—	253	1,110	1,363	3·7	·0	—	—	·00
Erysipelas	75	—	—	423	624	1,047	2·9	·2	—	—	·00
Influenza	5,310	—	5	53,793	4,217	58,010	158·9	13·4	—	·0	·40
Malaria	2,502	1	16	13,973	10,880	24,853	68·1	6·3	·0	·0	·17
Measles	493	—	—	3,543	5,817	9,360	25·6	1·2	—	—	·06
Meningococcal Infection	150	—	7	1,241	2,211	3,452	9·5	·4	—	·0	·02
Mumps	365	—	—	2,542	3,783	6,325	17·3	·9	—	—	·04
Pneumococcal Infection (Lungs)	915	3	26	9,846	22,405	32,251	88·4	2·3	·0	·1	·22
Pneumococcal Infection (Other Organs)	36	—	14	120	—	120	·3	·1	—	·0	·00
Pyrogenic Infection	46	1	10	530	603	1,133	3·1	·1	·0	·0	·00
Pyrexia of Uncertain Origin	310	—	—	1,840	2,900	4,740	13·0	·8	—	—	·03
Rheumatic Fever	245	16	—	2,987	4,900	7,887	21·7	·6	·0	—	·05
Rheumatism, sub-acute	864	22	—	10,975	9,580	20,555	56·3	2·2	·1	—	·14
Rubella	953	—	—	3,655	4,758	8,413	23·0	2·4	—	—	·05
Sandfly Fever	825	—	—	1,348	2,525	3,873	10·7	2·1	—	—	·02
Scarlet Fever	252	—	—	2,180	8,192	10,372	28·4	·6	—	—	·07
Small-pox	3	—	2	—	82	82	·2	·0	—	·0	·00
Tonsillitis	12,065	—	—	65,031	50,802	115,833	317·4	30·5	—	—	·80

TABLE 6 (*contd.*)

Number of Cases of Disease and Injury under Various Classes, the Number of Invalidings and Deaths; and the Average Number of Men Sick Daily in the Total Force, with the Ratios per 1,000 of Average Strength for the Year 1941
(Average Strength 396,000)

DISEASE OR INJURY	Cases	In-valided	Dead	Days' Sickness			Average Number of Men Sick Daily	Ratio per 1,000 of Strength			
				On Board	In Hospital	Total		Cases	In-valided	Dead	Sick Daily
Tuberculosis, Pulmonary*	825	822	44	5,600	39,582	45,182	123·8	2·1	2·1	·1	·31
Tuberculosis, Non-pulmonary	125	121	20	854	4,225	5,079	13·9	·3	·3	·1	·03
Undulant Fever	5	—	—	17	77	94	·3	·0	—	—	·00
Chancroid	1,258	1	—	4,437	5,714	10,151	27·8	3·2	·0	—	·07
Chancroid, Sequelae	107	—	—	—	—	—	—	·3	—	—	
Syphilis, First record	1,790	8	—	9,803	18,211	28,014	76·8	4·6	·0	—	·19
Syphilis, Later record	276	5	—	1,102	3,774	4,876	13·4	·7	·0	—	·03
Gonococcal Infection, Acute	8,661	14	—	29,087	38,055	67,142	184·0	21·9	·0	—	·46
Gonococcal Infection, Sequelae	842	17	—	4,014	24,229	28,243	77·4	2·1	·0	—	·19
Lympho-granuloma Inguinale	92	—	—	833	865	1,698	4·7	·2	—	—	·01
Other Diseases caused by Infection	1,122	6	4	6,660	12,981	19,641	53·8	2·8	·0	·0	·13
Diseases caused by Metazoan Parasites	15,291	1	—	32,462	22,989	55,451	151·9	38·6	·0	—	·38
DISEASES OF THE NERVOUS SYSTEM:											
Diseases of Spinal Cord	106	33	4	423	2,651	3,074	8·4	·3	·1	·0	·02
Diseases of Brain	114	63	33	640	5,875	6,515	17·8	·3	·2	·1	·04
Apoplexy	6	—	6	28	—	28	·1	·0	—	·0	·00
Paralysis	136	17	1	204	4,715	4,919	13·5	·3	·0	·0	·03
Epilepsy	390	230	—	1,671	10,006	11,677	32·0	1·0	·6	—	·08
Neurasthenia	309	6	—	4,112	1,174	5,286	14·5	·8	·0	—	·03
Other Nervous Diseases (including Mental)	5,176	2,248	4	31,688	151,923	183,611	503·0	13·1	5·7	·0	1·27

DISEASES OF THE EYE	1,576	409	—	10,120	29,290	39,410	108·0	4·0	1·0	—	·27
DISEASES OF THE EAR	2,702	373	—	13,641	39,190	52,831	144·7	6·8	·9	—	·36
DISEASES OF THE NOSE	1,386	21	—	5,761	19,268	25,029	68·6	3·5	·1	—	·17
DISEASES OF THE CIRCULATORY SYSTEM:											
Diseases of the Heart (Organic)	419	160	28	3,204	8,895	12,099	33·1	1·0	·4	·1	·08
Diseases of the Heart (Functional)	409	35	16	3,099	4,339	7,438	20·4	1·0	·1	·0	·05
Diseases of the Arteries	405	210	60	2,539	9,450	11,989	32·8	1·0	·5	·2	·08
Diseases of the Veins	945	34	1	6,150	16,235	22,385	61·3	2·4	·1	·0	·15
Diseases of the Blood and Blood-forming Organs	840	33	6	5,862	10,415	16,307	44·7	2·1	·1	·0	·11
Diseases of Glands of Internal Secretion	132	28	6	753	3,883	4,636	12·7	·3	·1	·0	·03
Diseases of the Breast	27	—	—	176	300	476	1·3	·1	—	—	·00
DISEASES OF THE RESPIRATORY SYSTEM:											
Diseases of the Larynx	601	1	1	4,785	1,711	6,496	17·8	1·5	·0	·0	·04
Bronchial Catarrh	1,099	—	1	5,988	2,492	8,480	23·2	2·8	—	·0	·05
Bronchitis	5,461	334	5	53,938	38,742	92,680	253·9	13·8	·8	·0	·64
Asthma	470	97	1	3,855	6,519	10,374	28·4	1·2	·2	·0	·07
Fibrosis of Lung	436	5	—	961	2,891	3,852	10·6	1·1	·0	—	·02
Pleurisy	951	9	—	9,415	10,932	20,347	55·7	2·4	·0	—	·14
Other Diseases	842	184	23	7,683	29,927	37,610	103·0	2·1	·5	·1	·26
DISEASES OF TEETH AND GUMS	2,041	—	—	9,637	10,088	19,725	54·0	5·1	—	—	·13
HERNIA	1,735	28	—	4,654	44,311	48,965	134·2	4·4	·1	—	·33
HERNIA (Recurrent)	134	6	—	489	1,169	1,658	4·5	·3	·0	—	·01
DISEASES OF THE DIGESTIVE SYSTEM:											
Mouth, Palate, Fauces, Pharynx	2,554	1	—	14,304	8,682	22,986	63·0	6·4	·0	—	·15
Peptic Ulcer, Gastric	1,108	290	11	6,350	25,168	31,518	86·4	2·8	·7	·0	·21
Peptic Ulcer, Duodenal	1,178	788	6	6,663	40,137	46,800	128·2	3·0	2·0	·0	·32
Appendicitis	2,055	2	16	11,327	31,335	42,662	116·9	5·2	·0	·0	·29
Other Diseases of the Stomach	5,932	151	1	43,997	48,225	92,222	252·7	15·0	·4	·0	·63

* As a general rule all cases of Pulmonary Tuberculosis were either invalided from the Navy or died. Many cases, however, were treated in the Service for many months at a time so that the number of cases shown in the tables for each Calendar Year may not correspond to the sum of the number of cases invalided and the number of deaths.

TABLE 6 (*contd.*)

Number of Cases of Disease and Injury under the Various Classes, the Number of Invalidings and Deaths; and the Average Number of Men Sick Daily in the Total Force, with the Ratios per 1,000 of Average Strength for the Year 1941
(Average Strength 396,000)

DISEASE OR INJURY	Cases	In-valided	Dead	Days' Sickness			Average Number of Men Sick Daily	Ratio per 1,000 of Strength			
				On Board	In Hospital	Total		Cases	In-valided	Dead	Sick Daily
Other Diseases of the Intestines	4,580	40	20	20,232	24,040	44,272	121·3	11·6	·1	·1	·30
Diseases of Rectum and Anus	1,425	16	—	7,199	21,302	28,501	78·1	3·6	·0	—	·19
Diseases of the Liver	858	8	8	9,400	18,306	27,706	75·9	2·2	·0	·0	·19
Other Diseases	290	9	8	1,859	4,107	5,966	16·3	·7	·0	·0	·04
DISEASES OF NUTRITION OR METABOLISM:											
Scurvy	6	—	—	49	53	102	·3	·0	—	—	·00
Beri-Beri	3	—	—	10	—	10	·0	·0	—	—	·00
Gout	101	8	—	894	1,404	2,298	6·3	·2	·0	—	·01
Diabetes	80	9	1	685	3,249	3,934	10·8	·2	·0	·0	·02
Other Diseases	84	26	—	237	925	1,162	3·2	·2	·1	—	·00
DISEASES OF GENERATIVE SYSTEM:											
Stricture	26	—	—	73	142	215	·6	·1	—	—	·00
Varicocele	160	—	—	555	2,876	3,431	9·4	·4	—	—	·02
Orchitis	128	—	—	974	668	1,642	4·5	·3	—	—	·01
Other Diseases	2,484	7	—	10,220	22,799	33,019	90·5	6·3	·0	—	·22
DISEASES OF BONES, JOINTS, MUSCLES, FASCIAE AND BURSAE:											
Periosteum and Bone	199	59	—	1,837	9,343	11,180	30·6	·5	·1	—	·07
Cartilage and Joints	1,148	255	—	8,570	43,506	52,076	142·7	2·9	·6	—	·36
Spine	89	46	—	627	3,600	4,227	11·6	·2	·1	—	·02
Muscles, Fasciae, Tendons, Bursae	2,725	72	—	21,049	20,444	41,493	113·7	6·9	·2	—	·28
Deformities and Congenital Malformations	546	185	—	3,440	12,276	15,716	43·1	1·4	·5	—	·10

DISEASES OF AREOLAR TISSUE AND SKIN:											
Abscess	1,528	2	—	11,301	10,136	21,437	58·7	3·8	·0	—	·14
Boil	2,947	—	—	19,032	2,954	21,986	60·2	7·4	—	—	·15
Eczema	516	7	—	5,226	4,840	10,066	27·6	1·3	·0	—	·06
Impetigo	1,714	—	—	15,149	11,051	26,200	71·8	4·3	—	—	·18
Other Diseases	7,820	82	—	69,722	75,307	145,029	397·3	19·7	·2	—	1·00
DISEASES OF URINARY ORGANS:											
Kidneys	921	60	20	4,673	15,579	20,252	55·5	2·3	·2	·1	·14
Ureter and Bladder	453	6	—	2,481	11,027	13,508	37·0	1·1	·0	—	·09
Urinary Disorders	340	15	—	1,715	4,723	6,438	17·6	·9	·0	—	·04
NEW GROWTHS, MALIGNANT	131	26	52	516	5,127	5,643	15·5	·3	·1	·1	·03
NEW GROWTHS, NON-MALIGNANT	523	21	—	1,714	5,634	7,348	20·1	1·3	·1	—	·05
ALCOHOLISM	83	2	6	155	561	716	2·0	·2	·0	·0	·00
POISONING, VARIOUS	444	1	14	1,862	605	2,467	6·8	1·1	·0	·0	·01
GENERAL INJURIES:											
Multiple Injuries	520	23	299	1,814	11,627	13,441	36·8	1·3	·1	·8	·09
Multiple Burns and Scalds	116	1	24	903	6,307	7,210	19·8	·3	·0	·1	·04
Heat Stroke	529	—	2	1,509	351	1,860	5·1	1·3	—	·0	·01
Suffocation—Drowning	234	—	234	100	—	100	·3	·6	—	·6	·00
Suffocation—Effects of	15	—	4	—	65	65	·2	·0	—	·0	·00
Compressed Air Disease	8	—	—	31	—	31	·1	·0	—	—	·00
LOCAL INJURIES:											
Burns and Scalds	1,380	6	6	12,325	10,377	22,702	62·2	3·5	·0	·0	·15
Injuries and Wounds	17,801	454	126	148,817	238,073	386,890	1,060·0	45·0	1·1	·3	2·67
WOUNDS AND INJURIES IN ACTION	5,739	67	—	11,898	28,351	40,249	110·3	14·5	·2	—	·27
SUICIDES	55	—	55	—	—	—	—	·1	—	·1	·00
TOTALS	177,519	8,341	1,265	1,044,840	1,607,494	2,652,334	7,266·7	448·3	21·1	3·2	18·35

TABLE 7

Number of Cases of Disease and Injury under the Various Classes, the Number of Invalidings and Deaths; and the Average Number of Men Sick Daily in the Total Force, with the Ratios per 1,000 of Average Strength for the Year 1942
(Average Strength 516,000)

DISEASE OR INJURY	Cases	In-valided	Dead	Days' Sickness			Average Number of Men Sick Daily	Ratio per 1,000 of Strength			
				On Board	In Hospital	Total		Cases	In-valided	Dead	Sick Daily
DISEASES CAUSED BY INFECTION:											
Chicken-pox	279	—	—	1,554	3,095	4,649	12·7	·5	—	—	·02
Common Cold	16,828	—	—	69,858	18,614	88,472	242·4	32·6	—	—	·46
Cow-pox	3,195	—	—	13,443	2,527	15,970	43·8	6·2	—	—	·08
Dengue	827	—	—	3,683	2,596	6,279	17·2	1·6	—	—	·03
Diphtheria	421	3	6	2,047	17,465	19,512	53·5	·8	·0	·0	·10
Dysentery	918	2	4	2,371	13,094	15,465	42·4	1·8	·0	·0	·08
Enteric Fever, Typhoid	45	—	3	263	1,623	1,886	5·2	·1	—	·0	·01
Enteric Fever, Paratyphoid	17	—	1	173	1,187	1,360	3·7	·0	—	·0	·00
Erysipelas	90	—	—	401	695	1,096	3·0	·2	—	—	·00
Influenza	2,950	1	—	26,797	4,138	30,935	84·8	5·7	·0	—	·16
Malaria	4,619	5	22	35,010	16,124	51,134	140·1	9·0	·0	·0	·27
Measles	190	—	—	924	2,764	3,688	10·1	·4	—	—	·01
Meningococcal Infection	156	—	—	511	3,635	4,146	11·4	·3	—	—	·02
Mumps	785	—	—	3,763	11,859	15,622	42·8	1·5	—	—	·08
Pneumococcal Infection (Lungs)	1,093	6	29	10,836	26,178	37,014	101·4	2·1	·0	·1	·19
Pneumococcal Infection (Other Organs)	19	—	—	104	302	406	1·1	·0	—	—	·00
Pyogenic Infection	137	1	23	538	1,062	1,600	4·4	·3	·0	·0	·00
Pyrexia of Uncertain Origin	627	1	—	4,402	4,531	8,933	24·5	1·2	·0	—	·04
Rheumatic Fever	203	47	—	2,644	4,525	7,169	19·6	·4	·1	—	·03
Rheumatism, sub-acute	816	52	1	9,259	19,028	28,287	77·5	1·6	·1	·0	·15
Rubella	562	—	—	3,241	1,999	5,240	14·4	1·1	—	—	·02
Sandfly Fever	1,504	—	—	6,170	1,873	8,043	22·0	2·9	—	—	·04
Scarlet Fever	217	—	—	626	7,472	8,098	22·2	·4	—	—	·04
Small-pox	16	—	2	127	90	217	·6	·0	—	·0	·00
Tonsillitis	14,421	—	1	75,093	61,396	136,489	373·9	27·9	—	·0	·72

Tuberculosis, Pulmonary*	1,202	1,348	64	9,166	69,500	78,666	215·5	2·3	2·6	·1	·41
Tuberculosis, Non-pulmonary	131	96	5	1,154	5,431	6,585	18·0	·3	·2	·0	·03
Undulant Fever	11	—	—	158	173	331	·9	·0	—	—	·00
Chancroid	1,425	—	—	8,336	4,456	12,792	35·0	2·8	—	—	·06
Chancroid, Sequelae	94	—	—	—	—	—	—	·2	—	—	—
Syphilis, First record	2,432	1	—	18,623	19,463	38,086	104·3	4·7	·0	—	·20
Syphilis, Later record	351	18	—	2,267	5,425	7,692	21·1	·7	·0	—	·04
Gonococcal Infection, Acute	9,322	1	—	41,917	35,080	76,997	211·0	18·1	·0	—	·40
Gonococcal Infection, Sequelae	1,151	11	—	7,623	10,463	18,086	49·6	2·2	·0	—	·09
Lympho-granuloma Inguinale	104	—	1	1,314	956	2,270	6·2	·2	—	·0	·01
Other Diseases caused by Infection	1,468	5	11	7,734	8,723	16,457	45·1	2·8	·0	·0	·08
Diseases caused by Metazoan Parasites	31,102	—	—	43,389	30,091	73,480	201·3	60·3	—	—	·39
DISEASES OF THE NERVOUS SYSTEM:											
Diseases of Spinal Cord	115	52	9	390	2,866	3,256	8·9	·2	·1	·0	·01
Diseases of Brain	104	45	70	716	5,922	6,638	18·2	·2	·1	·1	·03
Apoplexy	13	—	—	7	—	7	·0	·0	—	—	·00
Paralysis	144	20	3	777	2,798	3,575	9·8	·3	·0	·0	·01
Epilepsy	427	261	1	2,173	9,901	12,074	33·1	·8	·5	·0	·06
Neurasthenia	233	2	—	2,031	434	2,465	6·8	·5	·0	—	·01
Other Nervous Diseases (including Mental)	6,130	1,818	2	31,327	231,039	262,366	718·8	11·9	3·5	·0	1·39
DISEASES OF THE EYE	1,832	289	—	9,951	24,120	34,071	93·3	3·6	·6	—	·18
DISEASES OF THE EAR	3,237	371	1	15,333	45,084	60,417	165·5	6·3	·7	·0	·32
DISEASES OF THE NOSE	1,751	20	1	6,972	32,743	39,715	108·8	3·4	·0	·0	·21
DISEASES OF THE CIRCULATORY SYSTEM:											
Diseases of the Heart (Organic)	396	151	41	3,826	4,599	8,425	23·1	·8	·3	·1	·04
Diseases of the Heart (Functional)	450	15	33	2,731	14,002	16,733	45·8	·9	·0	·1	·08

* As a general rule all cases of Pulmonary Tuberculosis were either invalided from the Navy or died. Many cases, however, were treated in the Service for many months at a time so that the number of cases shown in the tables for each Calendar Year may not correspond to the sum of the number of cases invalided and the number of deaths.

TABLE 7 (*contd.*)

Number of Cases of Disease and Injury under the Various Classes, the Number of Invalidings and Deaths; and the Number of Men Sick Daily in the Total Force, with the Ratios per 1,000 of Average Strength for the Year 1942
(Average Strength 516,000)

DISEASE OR INJURY	Cases	In-valided	Dead	Days' Sickness			Average Numbero Men Sick Daily	Ratio per 1,000 of Strength			
				On Board	In Hospital	Total		Cases	In-valided	Dead	Sick Daily
Diseases of the Arteries	542	257	59	3,073	14,172	17,245	47·2	1·1	·5	·1	·09
Diseases of the Veins	1,436	16	2	7,944	21,753	29,697	81·4	2·8	·0	·0	·15
Diseases of the Blood and Blood-forming Organs	1,007	14	11	6,571	12,999	19,570	53·6	2·0	·0	·0	·10
Diseases of Glands of Internal Secretion	155	25	4	998	10,049	11,047	30·3	·3	·0	·0	·05
Diseases of the Breast	49	—	—	219	550	769	2·1	·1	—	—	·00
DISEASES OF THE RESPIRATORY SYSTEM:											
Diseases of the Larynx	641	3	—	4,427	2,360	6,787	18·6	1·2	·0	—	·03
Bronchial Catarrh	915	1	—	7,397	1,886	9,283	25·4	1·8	·0	—	·04
Bronchitis	5,850	325	2	46,638	52,230	98,868	270·9	11·3	·6	·0	·52
Asthma	541	137	1	4,242	7,937	12,179	33·4	1·0	·3	·0	·06
Fibrosis of Lung	1,068	38	—	2,043	18,184	20,227	55·4	2·1	·1	—	·10
Pleurisy	1,143	82	2	9,929	18,436	28,365	77·7	2·2	·2	·0	·15
Other Diseases	1,306	112	31	6,973	45,269	52,242	143·1	2·5	·2	·1	·27
DISEASES OF TEETH AND GUMS	2,597	—	—	12,726	7,375	20,101	55·1	5·0	—	—	·10
HERNIA	2,209	25	—	10,365	63,447	73,812	202·2	4·3	·0	—	·39
HERNIA (Recurrent)	195	9	—	855	2,074	2,929	8·0	·4	·0	—	·01
DISEASES OF THE DIGESTIVE SYSTEM:											
Mouth, Palate, Fauces, Pharynx	2,777	2	—	16,387	12,260	28,647	78·5	5·4	·0	—	·15
Peptic Ulcer, Gastric	880	263	12	3,530	25,935	29,465	80·7	1·7	·5	·0	·15
Peptic Ulcer, Duodenal	1,141	635	7	6,212	52,438	58,650	160·7	2·2	1·2	·0	·31
Appendicitis	2,508	8	11	13,146	49,525	62,671	171·7	4·9	·0	·0	·33
Other Diseases of the Stomach	6,606	156	3	39,729	66,748	106,477	291·7	12·8	·3	·0	·56

Other Diseases of the Intestines	5,116	59	24	24,327	30,487	54,814	150·2	9·9	·1	·0	·29
Diseases of Rectum and Anus	1,785	12	—	8,421	37,249	45,670	125·1	3·5	·0	—	·24
Diseases of the Liver	1,427	10	16	12,384	34,023	46,407	127·1	2·8	·0	·0	·24
Other Diseases	315	22	11	1,780	6,707	8,487	23·3	·6	·0	·0	·04
DISEASES OF NUTRITION OR METABOLISM:											
Scurvy	—	—	—	—	46	46	·1	—	—	—	·00
Beri-Beri	3	—	—	—	38	38	·1	·0	—	—	·00
Gout	110	4	—	1,218	720	1,938	5·3	·2	·0	—	·01
Diabetes	58	42	1	216	3,169	3,385	9·3	·1	·1	·0	·01
Other Diseases	88	5	1	335	586	921	2·5	·2	·0	·0	·00
DISEASES OF GENERATIVE SYSTEM:											
Stricture	34	—	—	59	1,091	1,150	3·2	·1	—	—	·00
Varicocele	169	—	—	350	2,795	3,145	8·6	·3	—	—	·01
Orchitis	164	4	—	1,132	2,010	3,142	8·6	·3	·0	—	·01
Other Diseases	3,211	7	—	16,385	36,681	53,066	145·4	6·2	·0	—	·28
DISEASES OF BONES, JOINTS, MUSCLES, FASCIAE AND BURSAE:											
Periosteum and Bone	285	41	3	2,240	8,835	11,075	30·3	·6	·1	·0	·05
Cartilage and Joints	1,268	214	—	7,780	38,561	46,341	127·0	2·5	·4	—	·24
Spine	147	85	2	638	8,836	9,474	26·0	·3	·2	·0	·05
Muscles, Fasciae, Tendons, Bursae	2,751	44	—	21,464	28,162	49,626	136·0	5·3	·1	—	·26
Deformities and Congenital Malformations	751	168	—	3,047	19,136	22,183	60·8	1·5	·3	—	·11
DISEASES OF AREOLAR TISSUE AND SKIN:											
Abscess	1,902	2	—	13,581	3,013	16,594	45·5	3·7	·0	—	·08
Boil	3,233	—	—	20,044	5,098	25,142	68·9	6·3	—	—	·13
Eczema	602	20	—	6,102	9,988	16,090	44·1	1·2	·0	—	·08
Impetigo	2,637	1	—	25,068	25,992	51,060	139·9	5·1	·0	—	·27
Other Diseases	10,026	138	—	76,813	111,216	188,029	515·1	19·4	·3	—	·99
DISEASES OF URINARY ORGANS:											
Kidneys	1,088	63	27	7,565	27,151	34,716	95·1	2·1	·1	·1	·18
Ureter and Bladder	524	16	—	3,328	11,889	15,217	41·7	1·0	·0	—	·08
Urinary Disorders	490	7	3	1,933	5,516	7,449	20·4	·9	·0	·0	·03

TABLE 7 (*contd.*)

Number of Cases of Disease and Injury Under the Various Classes, the Number of Invalidings and Deaths; and the Average Number of Men Sick Daily in the Total Force, with the Ratios per 1,000 of Average Strength for the Year 1942

(Average Strength 516,000)

DISEASE OR INJURY	Cases	In-valided	Dead	Days' Sickness			Average Number of Men Sick Daily	Ratio per 1,000 of Strength			
				On Board	In Hospital	Total		Cases	In-valided	Dead	Sick Daily
NEW GROWTHS, MALIGNANT	163	59	68	714	8,603	9,317	25·5	·3	·1	·1	·04
NEW GROWTHS, NON-MALIGNANT	658	7	—	2,550	11,069	13,619	37·3	1·3	·0	—	·07
ALCOHOLISM	71	2	8	403	777	1,180	3·2	·1	·0	·0	·00
POISONING, VARIOUS	891	—	10	3,870	5,194	9,064	24·8	1·7	—	·0	·04
GENERAL INJURIES:											
Multiple Injuries	641	42	148	2,246	32,681	34,927	95·7	1·2	·1	·3	·18
Multiple Burns and Scalds	130	14	27	1,075	9,015	10,090	27·6	·3	·0	·1	·05
Heat Stroke	344	—	8	2,389	492	2,881	7·9	·7	—	·0	·01
Suffocation—Drowning	347	—	347	171	—	171	·5	·7	—	·7	·00
Suffocation—Effects of	35	—	—	—	65	65	·2	·1	—	—	·00
Compressed Air Disease	3	—	1	39	29	68	·2	·0	—	·0	·00
LOCAL INJURIES:											
Burns and Scalds	1,572	9	—	13,684	14,985	28,669	78·5	3·0	·0	—	·15
Injuries and Wounds	19,968	456	266	151,730	299,833	451,563	1,237·2	38·7	·9	·5	2·39
WOUNDS AND INJURIES IN ACTION	2,818	128	—	11,916	46,528	58,444	160·1	5·5	·2	—	·31
SUICIDES	52	—	52	—	—	—	—	·1	—	·1	—
TOTALS	214,003	8,431	1,502	1,142,154	2,165,034	3,307,188	9,060·8	414·8	16·3	2·9	17·55

TABLE 8

Number of Cases of Disease and Injury under the various Classes, the Number of Invalidings and Deaths; and the Average Number of Men Sick Daily in the Total Force, with the Ratios per 1,000 of Average Strength for the Year 1943
(Average Strength 670,000)

DISEASE OR INJURY	Cases	In-valided	Dead	Days' Sickness			Average Number of Men Sick Daily	Ratio per 1,000 of Strength			
				On Board	In Hospital	Total		Cases	In-valided	Dead	Sick Daily
DISEASES CAUSED BY INFECTION:											
Chicken-pox	618	—	—	3,317	4,733	8,050	22·1	·9	—	—	·03
Common Cold	33,451	—	—	150,803	28,505	179,308	491·3	49·9	—	—	·73
Cow-pox	2,728	—	—	12,304	458	12,762	35·0	4·1	—	—	·05
Dengue	1,478	—	—	5,865	7,574	13,439	36·8	2·2	—	—	·05
Diphtheria	378	1	4	1,357	20,898	22,255	61·0	·6	·0	·0	·09
Dysentery	1,812	5	4	7,612	18,006	25,618	70·2	2·7	·0	·0	·10
Enteric Fever, Typhoid	55	2	4	497	2,775	3,272	9·0	·1	·0	·0	·01
Enteric Fever, Paratyphoid	35	—	—	227	308	535	1·5	·1	—	—	·00
Erysipelas	108	—	—	502	601	1,103	3·0	·2	—	—	·00
Influenza	6,814	—	—	50,493	7,871	58,364	160·0	10·2	—	—	·23
Malaria	7,216	1	20	44,845	25,527	70,372	192·8	10·8	·0	·0	·28
Measles	546	—	—	2,375	8,763	11,138	30·5	·8	—	—	·04
Meningococcal Infection	142	—	—	792	3,273	4,065	11·1	·2	—	—	·01
Mumps	541	—	—	2,992	8,021	11,013	30·2	·8	—	—	·04
Pneumococcal Infection (Lungs)	1,393	18	33	12,377	34,014	46,391	127·1	2·1	·0	·0	·18
Pneumococcal Infection (Other Organs)	16	—	1	64	217	281	·8	·0	—	·0	·00
Pyogenic Infection	116	11	32	678	1,653	2,331	6·4	·2	·0	·0	·00
Pyrexia of Uncertain Origin	1,068	—	—	5,111	4,689	9,800	26·8	1·6	—	—	·04
Rheumatic Fever	270	79	2	3,320	8,220	11,540	31·6	·4	·1	·0	·04
Rheumatism, sub-acute	782	45	—	7,612	20,616	28,228	77·3	1·2	·1	—	·11
Rubella	1,671	—	—	6,508	6,458	12,966	35·5	2·5	—	—	·05
Sandfly Fever	2,752	—	—	10,152	3,521	13,673	37·5	4·1	—	—	·05
Scarlet Fever	324	—	—	1,485	9,844	11,329	31·0	·5	—	—	·04
Small-pox	41	—	7	195	880	1,075	2·9	·1	—	·0	·00
Tonsillitis	19,729	—	—	101,208	56,373	157,581	431·7	29·4	—	—	·64

TABLE 8 (*contd.*)

Number of Cases of Disease and Injury under the various Classes, the Number of Invalidings and Deaths; and the Average Number of Men Sick Daily in the Total Force, with the ratios per 1,000 of Average Strength for the year 1943
(Average Strength 670,000)

DISEASE OR INJURY	Cases	In-valided	Dead	Days' Sickness			Average Number of Men Sick Daily	Ratio per 1,000 of Strength			
				On Board	In Hospital	Total		Cases	In-valided	Dead	Sick Daily
Tuberculosis, Pulmonary*	1,564	1,672	59	7,919	83,908	91,827	251·6	2·3	2·5	·1	·37
Tuberculosis, Non-pulmonary	141	112	14	784	9,922	10,706	29·3	·2	·2	·0	·04
Undulant Fever	19	—	—	412	346	758	2·1	·0	—	—	·00
Chancroid	1,296	—	—	5,321	3,808	9,129	25·0	1·9	—	—	·03
Chancroid, Sequelae	65	—	—	—	—	—	—	·1	—	—	—
Syphilis, First record	2,008	2	—	12,770	15,991	28,761	78·8	3·0	·0	—	·11
Syphilis, Later record	424	6	—	2,169	4,555	6,724	18·4	·6	·0	—	·02
Gonococcal Infection, Acute	9,667	—	—	39,387	30,176	69,563	190·6	14·4	—	—	·28
Gonococcal Infection, Sequelae	420	22	—	6,924	26,064	32,988	90·4	·6	·0	—	·13
Lympho-granuloma Inguinale	123	—	—	1,137	390	1,527	4·2	·2	—	—	·00
Other Diseases Caused by Infection	1,963	15	15	8,914	12,122	21,036	57·6	2·9	·0	·0	·08
Diseases caused by Metazoan Parasites	37,063	—	—	33,129	20,804	53,933	147·8	55·3	—	—	·22
DISEASES OF THE NERVOUS SYSTEM:											
Diseases of Spinal Cord	128	66	18	594	4,700	5,294	14·5	·2	·1	·0	·02
Diseases of Brain	158	53	71	554	9,490	10,044	27·5	·2	·1	·1	·04
Apoplexy	11	—	2	16	46	62	·2	·0	—	·0	·00
Paralysis	191	28	2	836	3,680	4,516	12·4	·3	·0	·0	·01
Epilepsy	499	204	2	2,100	10,604	12,704	34·8	·7	·3	·0	·05
Neurasthenia	216	—	—	1,474	251	1,725	4·7	·3	—	—	·00
Other Nervous Diseases (including Mental)	6,890	2,206	2	31,322	245,759	277,081	759·1	10·3	3·3	·0	1·13

DISEASES OF THE EYE . . .	1,921	265	—	9,424	24,382	33,806	92·6	2·9	·4	—	·13
DISEASES OF THE EAR . . .	3,686	361	—	16,291	45,728	62,019	169·9	5·5	·5	—	·25
DISEASES OF THE NOSE . . .	2,133	33	—	7,008	31,180	38,188	104·6	3·2	·0	—	·15
DISEASES OF THE CIRCULATORY SYSTEM:											
Diseases of the Heart (Organic) .	416	127	34	3,180	4,652	7,832	21·5	·6	·2	·1	·03
Diseases of the Heart (Functional)	447	35	27	2,390	13,420	15,810	43·3	·7	·1	·0	·06
Diseases of the Arteries . .	646	273	78	3,042	14,529	17,571	48·1	1·0	·4	·1	·07
Diseases of the Veins . . .	1,835	42	—	9,789	23,188	32,977	90·3	2·7	·1	—	·13
Diseases of the Blood and Blood-forming Organs . . .	1,278	35	18	7,620	11,927	19,547	53·6	1·9	·1	·0	·07
Diseases of Glands of Internal Secretion.	161	30	7	815	8,255	9,070	24·8	·2	·0	·0	·03
Diseases of the Breast . . .	62	—	—	374	796	1,170	3·2	·1	—	—	·00
DISEASES OF THE RESPIRATORY SYSTEM:											
Diseases of the Larynx . .	645	—	—	4,085	4,484	8,569	23·5	1·0	—	—	·03
Bronchial Catarrh . . .	1,029	—	—	7,232	2,144	9,376	25·7	1·5	—	—	·03
Bronchitis	6,608	320	2	49,258	53,608	102,866	281·8	9·9	·5	·0	·42
Asthma	682	108	1	4,697	9,313	14,010	38·4	1·0	·2	·0	·05
Fibrosis of Lung	1,484	42	1	1,378	24,308	25,686	70·4	2·2	·1	·0	·10
Pleurisy	1,351	28	—	10,060	18,744	28,804	78·9	2·0	·0	—	·11
Other Diseases	1,819	222	33	10,742	52,814	63,556	174·1	2·7	·3	·0	·25
DISEASES OF TEETH AND GUMS . .	2,496	1	—	10,745	8,011	18,756	51·4	3·7	·0	—	·07
HERNIA	2,959	18	1	15,116	77,562	92,678	253·9	4·4	·0	·0	·37
HERNIA (Recurrent)	270	4	—	664	3,611	4,275	11·7	·4	·0	—	·01
DISEASES OF THE DIGESTIVE SYSTEM:											
Mouth, Palate, Fauces, Pharynx .	3,850	—	—	20,715	21,102	41,817	114·6	5·7	—	—	·17
Peptic Ulcer, Gastric . . .	894	250	14	4,513	23,580	28,093	77·0	1·3	·4	·0	·11
Peptic Ulcer, Duodenal . .	1,309	653	17	7,608	48,443	56,051	153·6	2·0	1·0	·0	·22

* As a general rule all cases of Pulmonary Tuberculosis were either invalided from the Navy or died. Many cases, however, were treated in the Service for many months at a time so that the number of cases shown in the tables for each Calendar Year may not correspond to the sum of the number of cases invalided and the number of deaths.

TABLE 8 (*contd.*)

Number of Cases of Disease and Injury under the various Classes, the Number of Invalidings and Deaths; and the Average Number of Men Sick Daily in the Total Force, with the ratios per 1,000 of Average Strength for the year 1943
(Average Strength 670,000)

DISEASE OR INJURY	Cases	In-valided	Dead	Days' Sickness			Average Number of Men Sick Daily	Ratio per 1,000 of Strength			
				On Board	In Hospital	Total		Cases	In-valided	Dead	Sick Daily
Appendicitis	3,271	3	22	15,620	48,321	63,941	175·2	4·9	·0	·0	·26
Other Diseases of the Stomach	7,821	62	6	39,858	63,182	103,040	282·3	11·7	·1	·0	·42
Other Diseases of the Intestines	6,823	64	19	33,521	34,272	67,793	185·7	10·2	·1	·0	·27
Diseases of Rectum and Anus	2,310	11	—	9,407	33,993	43,400	118·9	3·4	·0	—	·17
Diseases of the Liver	3,095	21	21	25,305	47,411	72,716	199·2	4·6	·0	·0	·29
Other Diseases	480	7	18	3,158	10,919	14,077	38·6	·7	·0	·0	·05
DISEASES OF NUTRITION OR METABOLISM:											
Scurvy	1	—	—	8	—	8	·0	·0	—	—	·00
Beri-Beri	3	—	3	33	32	65	·2	·0	—	·0	·00
Gout	125	4	—	1,428	888	2,316	6·3	·2	·0	—	·00
Diabetes	84	57	1	427	2,558	2,985	8·2	·1	·1	·0	·01
Other Diseases	165	—	—	588	1,266	1,854	5·1	·2	—	—	·00
DISEASES OF GENERATIVE SYSTEM:											
Stricture	39	—	—	225	640	865	2·4	·1	—	—	·00
Varicocele	186	—	—	573	3,330	3,903	10·7	·3	—	—	·01
Orchitis	232	—	—	1,532	2,060	3,592	9·8	·3	—	—	·01
Other Diseases	4,665	6	—	18,002	47,113	65,115	178·4	7·0	·0	—	·26
DISEASES OF BONES, JOINTS, MUSCLES, FASCIAE AND BURSAE:											
Periosteum and Bone	331	64	4	1,766	13,975	15,741	43·1	·5	·1	·0	·06
Cartilage and Joints	1,563	256	—	9,645	40,382	50,027	137·1	2·3	·4	—	·20
Spine	192	97	—	778	14,767	15,545	42·6	·3	·1	—	·06
Muscles, Fasciae, Tendons, Bursae	3,196	57	—	20,745	27,509	48,254	132·2	4·8	·1	—	·19

Deformities and Congenital Malformations	920	181	—	4,515	23,397	27,912	76·5	1·4	·3	—	·11
DISEASES OF AREOLAR TISSUE AND SKIN:											
Abscess	2,639	1	—	16,946	13,526	30,472	83·5	3·9	·0	—	·12
Boil	3,864	—	—	23,630	4,813	28,443	77·9	5·8	—	—	·11
Eczema	766	34	—	7,945	14,111	22,056	60·4	1·1	·1	—	·09
Impetigo	3,229	—	—	29,617	18,475	48,092	131·8	4·8	—	—	·19
Other Diseases	12,602	171	—	90,602	127,179	217,781	596·7	18·8	·3	—	·89
DISEASES OF URINARY ORGANS:											
Kidneys	1,264	94	37	7,984	30,255	38,239	104·8	1·9	·1	·1	·15
Ureter and Bladder	689	20	—	3,619	30,887	34,506	94·5	1·0	·0	—	·14
Urinary Disorders	526	3	—	1,957	6,464	8,421	23·1	·8	·0	—	·03
NEW GROWTHS, MALIGNANT	181	88	67	877	9,230	10,107	27·7	·3	·1	·1	·04
NEW GROWTHS, NON-MALIGNANT	890	4	—	2,132	12,106	14,238	39·0	1·3	·0	—	·05
ALCOHOLISM	107	8	5	373	708	1,081	3·0	·2	·0	·0	·00
POISONING, VARIOUS	1,123	1	10	4,676	10,598	15,274	41·8	1·7	·0	·0	·06
GENERAL INJURIES:											
Multiple Injuries	658	22	153	3,321	9,268	12,589	34·5	1·0	·0	·2	·05
Multiple Burns and Scalds	216	6	23	1,435	4,349	5,784	15·8	·3	·0	·0	·02
Heat Stroke	314	—	1	1,431	342	1,773	4·9	·5	—	·0	·00
Suffocation—Drowning	632	—	632	—	—	—	—	·9	—	·9	—
Suffocation—Effects of	44	—	—	117	185	302	·8	·1	—	—	·00
Compressed Air Disease	2	1	—	16	—	16	·0	·0	·0	—	·00
LOCAL INJURIES:											
Burns and Scalds	1,737	9	43	13,277	18,075	31,352	85·9	2·6	·0	·1	·12
Injuries and Wounds	24,090	649	614	160,316	355,696	516,012	1,413·7	36·0	1·0	·9	2·11
WOUNDS AND INJURIES IN ACTION	2,475	140	38	4,103	41,522	45,625	125·0	3·7	·2	·1	·18
SUICIDES	62	—	62	1	2	3	·0	·1	—	·1	·00
TOTALS	278,420	9,535	2,304	1,356,708	2,416,001	3,772,709	10,336·2	415·6	14·2	3·4	15·42

TABLE 9

Number of Cases of Disease and Injury under the various Classes, the Number of Invalidings and Deaths; and the Average Number of Men Sick Daily in the Total Force, with Ratios per 1,000 of Average Strength for the year 1944
(Average Strength 792,000)

DISEASE OR INJURY	Cases	In-valided	Dead	Days' Sickness			Average Number of Men Sick Daily	Ratio per 1,000 of Strength			
				On Board	In Hospital	Total		Cases	In-valide d	Dead	Sick Daily
DISEASES CAUSED BY INFECTION:											
Chicken-pox	484	—	—	1,202	5,376	6,578	18·0	·6	—	—	·02
Common Cold	21,505	—	—	253,644	11,692	265,336	725·0	27·2	—	—	·91
Cow-pox	1,240	—	—	6,660	586	7,246	19·8	1·6	—	—	·02
Dengue	3,886	—	1	18,077	11,125	29,202	79·8	4·9	—	·0	·10
Diphtheria	346	—	6	1,645	17,460	19,105	52·2	·4	—	·0	·06
Dysentery	2,715	11	8	10,863	24,801	35,664	97·4	3·4	·0	·0	·12
Enteric Fever, Typhoid	56	—	10	914	2,844	3,758	10·3	·1	—	·0	·01
Enteric Fever, Paratyphoid	42	—	1	487	1,196	1,683	4·6	·1	—	·0	·00
Erysipelas	128	—	—	667	845	1,512	4·1	·2	—	—	·00
Influenza	3,406	—	2	33,023	3,806	36,829	100·6	4·3	—	·0	·12
Malaria	6,028	2	24	39,363	28,390	67,753	185·1	7·6	·0	·0	·23
Measles	255	—	—	1,326	4,315	5,641	15·4	·3	—	—	·01
Meningococcal Infection	122	—	5	600	1,399	1,999	5·5	·2	—	·0	·00
Mumps	559	—	—	2,692	6,880	9,572	26·2	·7	—	—	·03
Pneumococcal Infection (Lungs)	1,529	18	29	15,623	42,752	58,375	159·5	1·9	·0	·0	·20
Pneumococcal Infection (Other Organs)	14	—	6	102	766	868	2·4	·0	—	·0	·00
Pyrogenic Infection	100	—	11	668	2,996	3,664	10·0	·1	—	·0	·01
Pyrexia of Uncertain Origin	1,644	—	—	7,381	5,898	13,279	36·3	2·1	—	—	·04
Rheumatic Fever	346	70	2	5,081	11,272	16,353	44·7	·4	·1	·0	·05
Rheumatism, Sub-Acute	930	34	—	9,757	21,879	31,636	86·4	1·2	·0	—	·10
Rubella	2,354	—	—	11,472	9,597	21,069	57·6	3·0	—	—	·07
Sandfly Fever	4,423	—	—	15,824	8,004	23,828	65·1	5·6	—	—	·08
Scarlet Fever	636	—	—	1,973	13,553	15,526	42·4	·8	—	—	·05
Small-pox	100	—	14	276	1,580	1,856	5·1	·1	—	·0	·00
Tonsillitis	22,536	—	2	125,278	66,236	191,514	523·3	28·5	—	·0	·66

Tuberculosis, Pulmonary*	2,017	1,903	81	8,400	154,791	163,191	445·9	2·5	2·4	·1	·56
Tuberculosis, Non-pulmonary	140	122	28	1,090	12,120	13,210	36·1	·2	·2	·0	·04
Undulant Fever	5	—	—	16	239	255	·7	·0	—	—	·00
Chancroid	1,422	1	—	7,165	5,903	13,068	35·7	1·8	·0	—	·04
Chancroid, Sequelae	60	—	—	—	—	—	—	·1	—	—	—
Syphilis, First record	2,404	16	—	16,444	22,227	38,671	105·7	3·0	·0	—	·13
Syphilis, Later record	506	2	2	1,761	6,197	7,958	21·7	·6	·0	·0	·02
Gonococcal Infection, Acute	11,900	6	—	51,838	53,853	105,691	288·8	15·0	·0	—	·36
Gonococcal Infection, Sequelae	1,495	—	1	6,560	13,499	20,059	54·8	1·9	—	·0	·06
Lympho-granuloma Inguinale	160	—	—	1,304	517	1,821	5·0	·2	—	—	·00
Other Diseases caused by Infection	2,184	12	13	10,777	13,240	24,017	65·6	2·8	·0	·0	·08
Diseases caused by Metazoan Parasites	32,803	1	—	22,243	10,011	32,254	88·1	41·4	·0	—	·11
DISEASES OF THE NERVOUS SYSTEM:											
Diseases of Spinal Cord	144	89	17	498	7,146	7,644	20·9	·2	·1	·0	·02
Diseases of Brain	171	65	66	1,017	9,336	10,353	28·3	·2	·1	·1	·03
Apoplexy	6	—	—	17	—	17	·0	·0	—	—	·00
Paralysis	200	36	—	1,233	5,787	7,020	19·2	·3	·0	—	·02
Epilepsy	468	260	3	1,751	11,455	13,206	36·1	·6	·3	·0	·04
Neurasthenia	210	5	—	1,790	518	2,308	6·3	·3	·0	—	·00
Other Nervous Diseases (including Mental)	8,620	2,828	5	40,547	299,815	340,362	930·0	10·9	3·6	·0	1·17
DISEASES OF THE EYE	2,285	348	—	11,328	27,267	38,595	105·5	2·9	·4	—	·13
DISEASES OF THE EAR	4,674	462	3	25,908	47,438	73,346	200·4	5·9	·6	·0	·25
DISEASES OF THE NOSE	2,177	41	—	8,277	32,621	40,898	111·7	2·7	·1	—	·14
DISEASES OF THE CIRCULATORY SYSTEM:											
Diseases of the Heart (Organic)	405	236	34	2,861	8,570	11,431	31·2	5	·3	·0	·03
Diseases of the Heart (Functional)	428	113	15	2,556	10,988	13,544	37·0	·5	·1	·0	·04

* As a general rule all cases of Pulmonary Tuberculosis were either invalided from the Navy or died. Many cases, however, were treated in the Service for many months at a time so that the number of cases shown in the tables for each Calendar Year may not correspond to the sum of the number of cases invalided and the number of deaths.

TABLE 9 (*contd.*)

Number of Cases of Disease and Injury under the various Classes, the Number of Invalidings and Deaths; and the Average Number of Men Sick Daily in the Total Force, with ratios per 1,000 of Average Strength for the year 1944
(Average Strength 792,000)

DISEASE OR INJURY	Cases	In-valided	Dead	Days' Sickness			Average Number of Men Sick Daily	Ratio per 1,000 of Strength			
				On Board	In Hospital	Total		Cases	In-valided	Dead	Sick Daily
Diseases of the Arteries	691	238	82	3,723	16,521	20,244	55·3	·9	·3	·1	·06
Diseases of the Veins	2,136	65	2	11,307	28,122	39,429	107·7	2·7	·1	·0	·13
Diseases of the Blood and Blood-forming Organs	1,345	20	12	8,840	11,785	20,625	56·4	1·7	·0	·0	·07
Diseases of Glands of Internal Secretion	206	18	1	861	8,458	9,319	25·5	·3	·0	·0	·03
Diseases of the Breast	104	—	—	444	1,301	1,745	4·8	·1	—	—	·00
DISEASES OF THE RESPIRATORY SYSTEM:											
Diseases of the Larynx	608	1	—	3,872	2,387	6,259	17·1	·8	·0	—	·02
Bronchial Catarrh	806	7	—	6,283	1,219	7,502	20·5	1·0	·0	—	·02
Bronchitis	6,854	414	4	53,890	52,812	106,702	291·5	8·7	·5	·0	·36
Asthma	795	134	1	5,950	10,500	16,450	44·9	1·0	·2	·0	·05
Fibrosis of Lung	1,268	120	—	1,490	18,452	19,942	54·5	1·6	·2	—	·06
Pleurisy	1,506	106	7	12,390	34,846	47,236	129·1	1·9	·1	·0	·16
Other Diseases	2,080	297	39	12,025	47,878	59,903	163·7	2·6	·4	·0	·20
DISEASES OF TEETH AND GUMS	2,070	—	—	9,844	6,671	16,515	45·1	2·6	—	—	·05
HERNIA	2,677	33	1	11,029	78,251	89,280	243·9	3·4	·0	·0	·30
HERNIA (Recurrent)	332	5	—	998	8,508	9,506	26·0	·4	·0	—	·03
DISEASES OF THE DIGESTIVE SYSTEM:											
Mouth, Palate, Fauces, Pharynx	3,691	1	2	22,915	16,406	39,321	107·4	4·7	·0	·0	·13
Peptic Ulcer, Gastric	977	211	14	6,084	25,420	31,504	86·1	1·2	·3	·0	·10
Peptic Ulcer, Duodenal	1,723	706	13	10,290	80,645	90,935	248·5	2·2	·9	·0	·31
Appendicitis	3,521	3	13	15,073	59,717	74,790	204·3	4·4	·0	·0	·25
Other Diseases of the Stomach	9,786	135	6	56,735	56,090	112,825	308·3	12·4	·2	·0	·38

Other Diseases of the Intestines	8,785	28	17	44,770	36,861	81,631	223·0	11·1	·0	·0	·28
Diseases of Rectum and Anus	2,315	6	1	10,240	34,579	44,819	122·5	2·9	·0	·0	·15
Diseases of the Liver	2,812	19	11	22,846	43,411	66,257	181·0	3·6	·0	·0	·22
Other Diseases	490	13	22	2,836	12,564	15,400	42·1	·6	·0	·0	·05
DISEASES OF NUTRITION OR METABOLISM:											
Scurvy	—	—	—	—	—	—	—	—	—	—	—
Beri-Beri	3	—	3	23	—	23	·1	·0	—	·0	·00
Gout	132	8	—	1,412	10,931	12,343	33·7	·2	·0	—	·04
Diabetes	66	64	1	470	4,520	4,990	13·6	·1	·1	·0	·01
Other Diseases	202	5	—	780	2,055	2,835	7·7	·3	·0	—	·00
DISEASES OF GENERATIVE SYSTEM:											
Stricture	41	2	—	102	378	480	1·3	·1	·0	—	·00
Varicocele	188	—	—	931	2,438	3,369	9·2	·2	—	—	·01
Orchitis	303	—	—	1,856	3,977	5,833	15·9	·4	—	—	·02
Other Diseases	6,128	14	—	26,563	56,306	82,869	226·4	7·7	·0	—	·28
DISEASES OF BONES, JOINTS, MUSCLES, FASCIAE AND BURSAE:											
Periosteum and Bone	413	51	3	3,094	12,559	15,653	42·8	·5	·1	·0	·05
Cartilage and Joints	1,893	366	—	11,204	49,963	61,167	167·1	2·4	·5	—	·21
Spine	208	94	—	1,097	9,403	10,500	28·7	·3	·1	—	·03
Muscles, Fasciae, Tendons, Bursae	3,796	53	—	25,393	31,400	56,793	155·2	4·8	·1	—	·19
Deformities and Congenital Malformations	1,032	256	—	6,599	25,157	31,756	86·8	1·3	·3	—	·10
DISEASES OF AREOLAR TISSUE AND SKIN:											
Abscess	2,924	14	—	19,622	16,210	35,832	97·9	3·7	·0	—	·12
Boil	4,828	4	—	32,065	6,845	38,910	106·3	6·1	·0	—	·13
Eczema	872	63	—	9,318	14,825	24,143	66·0	1·1	·1	—	·08
Impetigo	3,042	4	—	28,007	18,091	46,098	126·0	3·8	·0	—	·15
Other Diseases	15,563	310	2	132,065	151,948	284,013	776·0	19·7	·4	·0	·97
DISEASES OF URINARY ORGANS:											
Kidneys	1,425	109	20	8,975	29,900	38,875	106·2	1·8	·1	·0	·13
Ureter and Bladder	711	6	—	3,547	15,571	19,118	52·2	·9	·0	—	·06
Urinary Disorders	711	6	—	2,972	9,872	12,844	35·1	·9	·0	—	·04

TABLE 9 (*contd.*)

Number of Cases of Disease and Injury under the Various Classes, the Number of Invalidings and Deaths; and the Average Number of Men Sick Daily in the Total Force, with ratios per 1,000 of Average Strength for the year 1944
(Average Strength 792,000)

DISEASE OR INJURY	Cases	In-valided	Dead	Days' Sickness			Average Number of Men Sick Daily	Ratio per 1,000 of Strength			
				On Board	In Hospital	Total		Cases	In-valided	Dead	Sick Daily
NEW GROWTHS, MALIGNANT	178	85	93	998	10,566	11,564	31·6	·2	·1	·1	·03
NEW GROWTHS, NON-MALIGNANT	1,100	5	—	4,111	15,555	19,666	53·7	1·4	·0	—	·06
ALCOHOLISM	123	2	6	506	876	1,382	3·8	·2	·0	·0	·00
POISONING VARIOUS	970	2	28	4,499	7,432	11,931	32·6	1·2	·0	·0	·04
GENERAL INJURIES:											
Multiple Injuries	948	41	595	4,012	7,513	11,525	31·5	1·2	·1	·8	·03
Multiple Burns and Scalds	209	5	29	1,859	3,161	5,020	13·7	·3	·0	·0	·01
Heat Stroke	575	—	6	2,658	609	3,267	8·9	·7	—	·0	·01
Suffocation—Drowning	443	—	443	—	—	—	—	·6	—	·6	—
Suffocation—Effects of	53	—	16	203	108	311	·8	·1	—	·0	·00
Compressed Air Disease	3	—	—	26	53	79	·2	·0	—	—	·00
LOCAL INJURIES:											
Burns and Scalds	1,815	17	6	17,044	17,636	34,680	94·8	2·3	·0	·0	·11
Injuries and Wounds	26,774	603	267	149,302	454,448	603,750	1,649·6	33·8	·8	·3	2·08
WOUNDS AND INJURIES IN ACTION	1,880	126	—	782	17,262	18,044	49·3	2·4	·2	—	·06
SUICIDES	53	—	53	8	—	8	·0	·1	—	·1	·00
TOTALS	287,451	11,576	2,208	1,626,817	2,759,758	4,386,575	11,985·2	362·9	14·6	2·8	15·13

TABLE 10

Number of Cases of Disease and Injury under the Various Classes, the Number of Invalidings and Deaths; and the Average Number of Men Sick Daily in the Total Force, with Ratios per 1,000 of Average Strength for the Year 1945
(Average Strength 772,000)

DISEASE OR INJURY	Cases	In-valided	Dead	Days' Sickness			Average Number of Men Sick Daily	Ratio per 1,000 Strength of			
				On Board	In Hospital	Total		Cases	In-valided	Dead	Sick Daily
DISEASES CAUSED BY INFECTION:											
Chicken-pox	496	—	—	2,164	3,820	5,984	16·4	·6	—	—	·02
Common Cold	19,395	—	—	95,484	12,298	107,782	295·3	25·1	—	—	·38
Cow-pox	2,203	—	—	9,842	—	9,842	27·0	2·9	—	—	·03
Dengue	2,328	—	—	11,656	6,203	17,859	48·9	3·0	—	—	·06
Diphtheria	227	5	5	1,297	8,523	9,820	26·9	·3	·0	·0	·03
Dysentery	3,142	25	1	18,572	40,450	59,022	161·7	4·1	·0	·0	·20
Enteric Fever, Typhoid	71	2	18	166	6,296	7,062	19·3	·1	·0	·0	·02
Enteric Fever, Paratyphoid	65	2	—	560	2,730	3,290	9·0	·1	·0	—	·01
Erysipelas	123	—	—	416	600	1,016	2·8	·2	—	—	·00
Influenza	2,832	—	—	26,828	1,879	28,707	78·6	3·7	—	—	·10
Malaria	2,412	11	7	17,538	19,271	36,809	100·8	3·1	·0	·0	·13
Measles	326	—	—	2,566	4,756	7,322	20·1	·4	—	—	·02
Meningococcal Infection	91	9	4	373	1,276	1,649	4·5	·1	·0	·0	·00
Mumps	723	—	—	4,195	8,711	12,906	35·4	·9	—	—	·04
Pneumococcal Infection (Lungs)	1,449	45	23	15,192	41,873	57,065	156·3	1·9	·1	·0	·20
Pneumococcal Infection (Other Organs)	32	1	1	199	—	199	·5	·0	·0	·0	·00
Pyogenic Infection	169	7	7	1,055	6,473	7,528	20·6	·2	·0	·0	·02
Pyrexia of Uncertain Origin	1,655	—	—	8,157	7,261	15,418	42·2	2·1	—	—	·05
Rheumatic Fever	316	91	2	4,208	17,219	21,427	58·7	·4	·1	·0	·07
Rheumatism, sub-acute	805	83	—	6,440	16,335	22,775	62·4	1·0	·1	—	·08
Rubella	814	—	—	4,343	1,808	6,151	16·9	1·1	—	—	·02
Sandfly Fever	2,493	—	—	7,925	6,315	14,240	39·0	3·2	—	—	·05
Scarlet Fever	401	1	1	2,700	8,003	10,703	29·3	·5	·0	·0	·03
Small-pox	41	—	2	71	198	269	·7	·1	—	·0	·00
Tonsillitis	23,672	1	3	129,882	79,258	209,140	573·0	30·7	·0	·0	·74

TABLE 10 (*Contd.*)

Number of Cases of Disease and Injury under the Various Classes, the Number of Invalidings and Deaths; and the Average Number of Men Sick Daily in the Total Force, with Ratios per 1,000 of Average Strength for the year 1945
(Average Strength 772,000)

DISEASE OR INJURY	Cases	In-valided	Dead	Days' Sickness			Average Number of Men Sick Daily	Ratio per 1,000 Strength			
				On Board	In Hospital	Total		Cases	In-valided	Dead	Sick Daily
Tuberculosis, Pulmonary*	2,790	1,859	78	15,557	255,466	271,023	742·5	3·6	2·4	·1	·96
Tuberculosis, Non-pulmonary	160	105	17	980	11,053	12,033	33·0	·2	·1	·0	·04
Undulant Fever	16	—	—	99	709	808	2·2	·0	—	—	·00
Chancroid	1,650	3	—	7,101	3,527	10,628	29·1	2·1	·0	—	·03
Chancroid, Sequelae	54	—	—	—	—	—	—	·1	—	—	—
Syphilis, First record	3,020	17	—	14,086	27,844	41,930	114·9	3·9	·0	—	·14
Syphilis, Later record	1,270	35	—	2,018	8,964	10,982	30·1	1·6	·0	—	·03
Gonococcal Infection, Acute	16,411	5	—	44,807	32,058	76,865	210·6	21·3	·0	—	·27
Gonococcal Infection, Sequelae	1,777	10	—	8,066	15,700	23,766	65·1	2·3	·0	—	·08
Lympho-granuloma Inguinale	283	3	—	2,181	2,073	4,254	11·7	·4	·0	—	·01
Other Diseases caused by Infection	2,526	11	9	11,969	18,127	30,096	82·5	3·3	·0	·0	·10
Diseases caused by Metazoan Parasites	31,092	5	—	16,751	8,064	24,815	68·0	40·3	·0	—	·08
DISEASES OF THE NERVOUS SYSTEM:											
Diseases of Spinal Cord	152	81	16	642	10,472	11,114	30·4	·2	·1	·0	·03
Diseases of Brain	186	60	84	732	8,119	8,851	24·2	·2	·1	·1	·03
Apoplexy	4	—	—	135	—	135	·4	·0	—	—	·00
Paralysis	210	58	4	1,032	9,840	10,872	29·8	·3	·1	·0	·03

* As a general rule all cases of Pulmonary Tuberculosis were either invalided from the Navy or died. Many cases, however, were treated in the Service for many months at a time so that the number of cases shown in the tables for each Calendar Year may not correspond to the sum of the number of cases invalided and the number of deaths.

Epilepsy	433	286	2	1,957	12,788	14,745	40·4	·6	·4	·0	·05
Neurasthenia	171	7	—	1,333	771	2,104	5·8	·2	·0	—	·00
Other Nervous Diseases (including Mental)	8,282	4,181	4	40,226	327,702	367,928	1,008·0	10·7	5·4	·0	1·30
DISEASES OF THE EYE	2,538	757	—	10,980	33,419	44,399	121·6	3·3	1·0	—	·15
DISEASES OF THE EAR	6,803	1,713	1	36,158	67,782	103,940	284·8	8·8	2·2	·0	·36
DISEASES OF THE NOSE	2,552	115	1	9,319	40,433	49,752	136·3	3·3	·1	·0	·17
DISEASES OF THE CIRCULATORY SYSTEM:											
Diseases of the Heart (Organic)	401	162	42	2,600	9,152	11,752	32·2	·5	·2	·1	·04
Diseases of the Heart (Functional)	413	89	25	2,279	7,141	9,420	25·8	·5	·1	·0	·03
Diseases of the Arteries	678	553	66	2,932	19,578	22,510	61·7	·9	·7	·1	·07
Diseases of the Veins	2,670	106	—	11,256	36,744	48,000	131·5	3·5	·1	—	·17
Diseases of the Blood and Blood-forming Organs	1,432	42	34	9,280	10,834	20,114	55·1	1·9	·1	·0	·07
Diseases of Glands of Internal Secretion.	248	63	3	1,174	10,819	11,993	32·9	·3	·1	·0	·04
Diseases of the Breast	129	—	—	387	1,635	2,022	5·5	·2	—	—	·00
DISEASES OF THE RESPIRATORY SYSTEM:											
Diseases of the Larynx	636	1	1	4,423	1,857	6,280	17·2	·8	·0	·0	·02
Bronchial Catarrh	754	3	—	7,114	1,836	8,950	24·5	1·0	·0	—	·03
Bronchitis	6,656	805	—	55,658	47,083	102,741	281·5	8·6	1·0	—	·36
Asthma	771	260	3	5,000	11,971	16,971	46·5	1·0	·3	·0	·06
Fibrosis of Lung	689	97	—	1,197	7,487	8,684	23·8	·9	·1	—	·03
Pleurisy	1,410	219	2	11,359	25,462	36,821	100·9	1·8	·3	·0	·13
Other Diseases	2,303	256	37	14,960	60,565	75,525	206·9	3·0	·3	·0	·26
DISEASES OF TEETH AND GUMS	1,759	2	—	8,609	7,218	15,827	43·4	2·3	·0	—	·05
HERNIA	2,780	104	1	10,746	95,748	106,494	291·8	3·6	·1	·0	·37
HERNIA (Recurrent)	349	44	—	532	6,014	6,546	17·9	·5	·1	—	·02
DISEASES OF THE DIGESTIVE SYSTEM:											
Mouth, Palate, Fauces, Pharynx	4,267	3	—	23,815	11,490	35,305	96·7	5·5	·0	—	·12
Peptic Ulcer, Gastric	1,079	533	11	4,827	22,177	27,004	74·0	1·4	·7	·0	·09
Peptic Ulcer, Duodenal	1,867	1,666	8	8,261	81,355	89,616	245·5	2·4	2·2	·0	·31
Appendicitis	3,244	20	10	11,896	61,788	73,684	201·9	4·2	·0	·0	·26
Other Diseases of the Stomach	10,837	382	8	67,680	70,824	138,504	379·5	14·0	·5	·0	·49

TABLE 10 (*Contd.*)

Number of Cases of Disease and Injury under the Various Classes, the Number of Invalidings and Deaths; and the Average Number of Men Sick Daily in the Total Force, with Ratios per 1,000 of Average Strength for the year 1945
(Average Strength 772,000)

DISEASE OR INJURY	Cases	In-valided	Dead	Days' Sickness			Average Number of Men Sick Daily	Ratio per 1,000 Strength			
				On Board	In Hospital	Total		Cases	In-valided	Dead	Sick Daily
Other Diseases of the Intestines	9,034	218	13	44,084	38,119	82,203	225·2	11·7	·3	·0	·29
Diseases of Rectum and Anus	2,499	14	1	10,249	37,891	48,140	131·9	3·2	·0	·0	·17
Diseases of the Liver	2,944	27	19	23,758	52,309	76,067	208·4	3·8	·0	·0	·26
Other Diseases	557	61	40	2,321	9,907	12,228	33·5	·7	·1	·1	·04
DISEASES OF NUTRITION OR METABOLISM:											
Scurvy	—	—	—	—	—	—	—	—	—	—	—
Beri-Beri	6	2	4	154	1,726	1,880	5·2	·0	·0	·0	·00
Gout	84	14	—	807	812	1,619	4·4	·1	·0	—	·00
Diabetes	89	126	1	317	6,114	6,431	17·6	·1	·2	·0	·02
Other Diseases	381	15	3	1,249	6,788	8,037	22·0	·5	·0	·0	02
DISEASES OF GENERATIVE SYSTEM:											
Stricture	35	4	—	104	1,244	1,348	3·7	·0	·0	—	·00
Varicocele	158	1	—	768	2,361	3,129	8·6	·2	·0	—	·01
Orchitis	338	1	—	2,447	4,088	6,535	17·9	·4	·0	—	·02
Other Diseases	7,924	18	2	30,703	69,243	99,946	273·8	10·2	·0	·0	·35
DISEASES OF BONES, JOINTS, MUSCLES, FASCIAE AND BURSAE:											
Periosteum and Bone	465	128	—	2,356	16,175	18,531	50·8	·6	·2	—	·06
Cartilage and Joints	2,260	706	—	12,326	93,788	106,114	290·7	2·9	·9	—	·37
Spine	257	174	—	971	18,838	19,809	54·3	·3	·2	—	·07
Muscles, Fasciae, Tendons, Bursae	3,652	127	—	26,294	26,715	53,009	145·2	4·7	·2	—	·18
Deformities and Congenital Malformations	1,063	401	1	4,250	26,423	30,673	84·0	1·4	·5	·0	·10

DISEASES OF AREOLAR TISSUE AND SKIN:											
Abscess	3,177	—	1	18,824	26,927	45,751	125·3	4·1	—	·0	·16
Boil	5,196	—	—	32,573	11,779	44,352	121·5	6·7	—	—	·15
Eczema	975	87	—	9,389	17,864	27,253	74·7	1·3	·1	—	·09
Impetigo	2,921	5	—	26,148	16,286	42,434	116·3	3·8	·0	—	·15
Other Diseases	17,761	552	1	126,018	183,549	309,567	848·1	23·0	·7	·0	1·09
DISEASES OF URINARY ORGANS:											
Kidneys	1,459	223	30	7,184	29,245	36,429	99·8	1·9	·3	·0	·12
Ureter and Bladder	790	37	—	3,686	20,179	23,865	65·4	1·0	·0	—	·08
Urinary Disorders	724	11	1	2,336	9,194	11,530	31·6	·9	·0	·0	·04
NEW GROWTHS, MALIGNANT	170	117	131	829	16,242	17,071	46·8	·2	·2	·2	·06
NEW GROWTHS, NON-MALIGNANT	1,242	31	1	3,920	20,340	24,260	66·5	1·6	·0	·0	·08
ALCOHOLISM	98	1	9	272	990	1,262	3·5	·1	·0	·0	·00
POISONING, VARIOUS	701	2	24	3,284	2,140	5,424	14·9	·9	·0	·0	·01
GENERAL INJURIES:											
Multiple Injuries	1,220	134	419	4,169	12,208	16,377	44·9	1·6	·2	·5	·05
Multiple Burns and Scalds	282	32	19	2,101	6,298	8,399	23·0	·4	·0	·0	·02
Heat Stroke	854	—	14	3,620	1,108	4,728	13·0	1·1	—	·0	·01
Suffocation—Drowning	327	—	327	—	—	—	—	·4	—	·4	—
Suffocation—Effects of	20	—	20	155	10	165	·5	·0	—	·0	·00
Compressed Air Disease	1	—	—	6	1	7	·0	·0	—	—	·00
LOCAL INJURIES:											
Burns and Scalds	1,509	32	8	11,855	16,714	28,569	78·3	2·0	·0	·0	·10
Injuries and Wounds	25,697	1,660	323	162,268	472,264	634,532	1,738·4	33·3	2·2	·4	2·25
WOUNDS AND INJURIES IN ACTION	1,032	250	—	1,692	6,756	8,448	23·1	1·3	·3	—	·02
SUICIDES	47	—	47	—	—	—	—	·1	—	·1	—
TOTALS	291,982	20,215	2,000	1,448,030	3,087,880	4,535,910	12,427·2	378·2	26·2	2·6	16·09

II. INVALIDINGS DUE TO DISEASE AND DEATHS DUE TO DISEASE

Some time after the first draft of Section I—Total Force—was prepared the following masterly analysis of invalidings due to disease and deaths due to disease in the Royal Navy for the years 1934–1943 (1944 added later), which had been completed by Surgeon Commander J. A. Fraser Roberts, R.N.V.R., when he was on the Staff of the Medical Director-General during the war, and which had formerly been a Restricted Document, was declassified. This made it possible to include this notable milestone in Naval medical statistics *in toto* in this contribution, preceded by a Foreword by the late Professor Major Greenwood, F.R.S., Consultant in Medical Statistics to the Royal Navy during the war years.

FOREWORD

by

Major Greenwood, F.R.S., D.Sc., F.R.C.P.

It has been suggested that, as civilian consultant to the Board of Admiralty and a member of the Committee which advised an immediate analysis of available statistical data of mortality and invaliding rates from disease, I might appropriately submit to you some general observations on the following report.

In the first place, I wish to say emphatically that this report reflects the greatest credit on those members of your Headquarters staff who, under conditions of great difficulty, have produced a document which attains a scientific standard which would justify its publication in the transactions of any learned society. Further, I would say that the inferences drawn by the compiler are of practical importance to the Board, for they not only set out the causes and numerical importance of wastage down to the end of 1943, but permit reasonable forecasts to be made under service conditions of the future.

The inferences in the report are so clearly stated that it may seem superfluous to say more, but I may perhaps underline those conclusions which are of particular interest to executive officers. From the point of view of Service wastage, rates of invaliding out and of dying have the same effect, they can be added together. Taking the gross figures, *viz.*, rates not adjusted to age composition, there is no change in death rates when pre-war and war-time figures are compared; roughly, the death rates were about 1·1 per 1,000 immediately before and during the war. The invaliding rate increased from a little more than 12·0 per 1,000 to between 17 and 18 per 1,000. The total wastage rate, therefore, increased by about 45 per cent. As a matter of merely archaeological interest, I infer that the *death* rate in Nelson's fleet in the two years August 1803, to August 1805, which Gillespie (rightly) contrasted with earlier fleet experience as a triumph of sanitary organisation, was about five times that of naval ratings in 1940–43.

If we used the crude wastage rate as a measure of the intake needed to compensate for wastage from disease, the result would be of little value because of changes in the age composition of the fleet and of the wholly different wastage rates in age groups. The figures shown in Table 11 for age groups are those needed and it will be seen that in all groups of age above 20 those of 1943 show improvement, although the rates at ages over 30 continue greatly in excess of pre-war rates. It is, however, evident that even in the highest age group, ratings over 39 years of age, wastage is not calamitous; for, adding invaliding to mortality rates, we have a round figure of 34·0 per 1,000; a group suffering this annual wastage would not be reduced to 90 per cent. of its original strength in less than three years. These data provide a wholly adequate picture of the *general* position, but what in civilian statistics would be called an occupational analysis would be needed to inform the executive officer of the amount of important variation. It is obvious that the strain imposed on the crew of a submarine or upon fleet air arm pilots may be much greater than upon ratings employed in office work ashore. But, even if Service conditions permitted such an analysis, its *immediate* value for practical purposes might be small. Even the war-time Navy is not, statistically speaking, a very large aggregate. If occupationally subdivided not merely into arms of the Service, but further into occupational groups within each arm, the resultant special wastage rates would often be based on such small numbers that their reliability would be small.

In the past this fundamental principle has often been violated in Service publications which have included hundreds of rates based upon figures so small that no thoughtful person would trust them as measures of Service conditions. This, of course, does not mean that a naval statistician is to refuse to advise an executive officer on the inferences to be drawn from a statistical statement unless the data are reckoned in thousands; he would indeed be an unprofitable public servant if he took that course. One can easily imagine Service problems (such, for instance, as those which are on the borderline between medicine and training) of great importance for the study of which large numbers could not be available. Modern statistical methods enable us to draw conclusions from samples which a generation ago would have been regarded as hopelessly inadequate. But these methods do not lend themselves to brief statement or expression in simple averages intelligible to a hasty reader. To reach these one must have large numbers.

The reasons just given explain the restrictions of analysis by causes of wastage to a small number of groups. For rapid comparison the age adjusted rates of Table 12 should be used. An executive officer will naturally look at the items of greatest numerical importance, which are Pulmonary Tuberculosis, Psychoses, etc., and Peptic Ulcer. In 1934–38 these three causes accounted for about 35 per cent. of the whole invaliding rate (age adjusted); in 1942 they accounted for more than half the total. The compiler's comments should be noted. I merely remark that here we have a striking example of the influence on bodily health of psychological factors. Pulmonary Tuberculosis is affected, as the compiler points out, by special factors, *viz.*, new methods of ascertainment; even here, however, mental strain is not irrelevant. The connexion between the other two groups—a connexion, not, of course, an identity—is manifest. Once again the importance of personnel selection is indicated.

For, I think, the first time some comparison has been instituted between the experience of officers and ratings. For reasons stated in the report, this can only be rough, but is suggestive. The proportion borne by the three above-named groups of the total invaliding rate has changed less between 1934–38 and 1942 than among ratings; but age standardisation might greatly modify this impression. These are, I think, some of the most interesting points made. This is not the place to discuss a general reform of record taking, which was the subject-matter of Surgeon Rear Admiral Rowlands's committee's recent report. I hope, however, that enough has been said to satisfy the Board that further analysis of existing data would be of value in war-time and that co-operation between other branches (especially those concerned with wastage during or immediately after training) and your medical-statistical staff is desirable.

R.N.

An Analysis of Invalidings due to Disease and Deaths due to Disease, 1934–1944

by Surgeon Commander J. A. Fraser Roberts, R.N.V.R.

GENERAL SUMMARY

1. The tables show invalidings due to disease and deaths due to disease as annual rates per 1,000 strength borne, of officers or of ratings respectively, for each of the war years 1939 to 1943. They also show, for comparison, the corresponding average annual rates for the five-year period, 1934–38, immediately preceding the war.

2. *The tables are themselves the summary of this enquiry.*—It is impossible to do more in this general summary than direct attention to some of the more important values and trends.

3. *The danger of comparing the invaliding rates of peace and war.*—Table 11 shows that the average annual invaliding rate among ratings for the period 1934–38 was 10·4 per 1,000. This is not greatly different from the figure of 12·8 in 1943; yet when examined age group by age group they are seen to be very differently made up. In peace-time there is a wide margin for selection and the emphasis is upon the early elimination of those unlikely to stay the course. Therefore the invaliding rate for those under 20 is no less than 16·3 per 1,000; with the further consequence of a fall to 5·9 by the time the age of 30–34 is attained.

In war-time, once a man has commenced his service, all the emphasis is upon keeping him at duty as long as possible. The true biological relationship then emerges: the older the man the smaller his chances of remaining fit. In 1943 the invaliding rate rose steadily from 9·4 per 1,000 in the under-twenties to 30·3 in the over-forties.

Thus, although the total rates for all ages are so similar in the two periods, the pre-war rate is nearly 75 per cent. greater for those under 20, while the war-time rate is nearly 300 per cent. greater among the over-forties.

With this caution, the comparison with pre-war rates is useful for some purposes, e.g., in connexion with pulmonary tuberculosis.

4. *The magnitude of differences in invaliding rates at different ages.*—Some diseases show little change with age, e.g., pulmonary tuberculosis (Table 13); in others it is very great. In circulatory diseases, for example, the rate at advanced ages may be anything up to 20 times what it is among the young.

The effect on total figures has been indicated in paragraph 3 above. The problem of wastage caused by invalidings due to disease cannot be properly investigated without taking age into account.

5. *The importance of studying rates adjusted so as to allow for changes in the age structure of the Service.*—It follows from what has been said that changes in the age composition of the Service could easily lead to wide variations in invaliding rates without any marked change when corresponding age groups are compared. Consequently the tables showing invaliding rates give both crude and age-adjusted rates. The latter are simply the rates that would have been observed had the age composition of the Navy remained constant at the average figure for the period 1934–38.

Two important and opposed trends have affected the age composition of the Royal Navy during the war. First, the intake of reservists in 1939–40 brought in a group which, though not very large numerically compared with the whole force, nevertheless had such a high invaliding rate that age-adjusted rates for these years are substantially lower than the crude rates (*see* Table 11). Thereafter this effect diminished, while the great intake of the very young has produced the opposite effect. By 1942 the age-adjusted rate is appreciably higher than the crude rate.

Table 18 (circulatory diseases) illustrates the most extreme effects of age adjustment.

6. *The general trend of invaliding rates throughout the war.*—The total figures (Table 11) show that the rate rose to a peak in 1941 and thereafter declined.

Taking the age groups separately, however, it is noteworthy that the peak was attained in 1941 among those under 35, there was little difference between 1940 and 1941 at 35–39, while among those over 39 the peak occurred in 1940, not in 1941. These tendencies appear in some of the tables showing individual disease groups, very notably in the case of mental diseases (Table 15). It is probably reasonable to deduce that among younger men the highest invaliding rates correspond to the period of maximum operational stress, whereas the older men, the reservists of 1939–40, rapidly showed that a substantial proportion were unable to stand the strain of any form of naval service.

The invaliding rate among officers (Tables 22 and 23) varied very little throughout the war except for a very high figure in 1940. Unfortunately, age adjustment cannot be carried out on the figures for officers. It is likely, however, that the peak (again specially notable in mental diseases) is to be attributed to the cause mentioned in the previous paragraph.

7. *The closely parallel trend of mental diseases and peptic ulcer* (Tables 15 and 20).—The trends are very similar throughout the period, except

that peptic ulcer does not show the marked peak in 1940 among older men.

8. *Death rates due to disease.*—In contrast to the invaliding rate, the death rate due to disease has remained remarkably constant throughout the whole period. In fact, when changes in the age composition of the Service are allowed for, there is no significant variation. It can be concluded that apart from fluctuations due simply to this cause and a fall in deaths from pulmonary tuberculosis in 1943 the rate has not varied throughout the war and is no higher in war than peace.

Officers have almost double the death rate of ratings. This is to be attributed almost entirely, in all probability, to their greater age. Greater reluctance to invalid officers is probably a contributory factor. As mentioned above, however, age adjustments cannot be made; nor can it be shown (as is probably the case) that fluctuations in the death rate among officers, shown in Table 27, are to be attributed to variations in age composition of the officer population.

9. *Pulmonary Tuberculosis.*—This requires a special word as the trends are entirely different from those of any other disease group shown. To take one comparison, in 1940 mental diseases were twice as important as pulmonary tuberculosis as a cause of invaliding. In 1942–43 there is little difference.

The invaliding rate among ratings (Table 13) remained constant till 1940. A sharp rise occurred in 1941 and a further sharp rise in 1942. Among officers the rate of invaliding remained constant for a year longer, the rise taking place in 1942.

A fall among ratings took place in 1943. On the relatively large numbers involved this attains high significance when compared with the rate for 1942. It will be interesting to see whether this favourable tendency continued in 1944.* Over so short a period and on the basis of these figures alone no definite statement can be made as to the possible effect of miniature mass fluorography in bringing about the fall. This much, however, can be said: a change in the hoped for direction has taken place at the time at which it would have been expected.

Officers have not shared the fall of 1943.

It is known in civilian practice and confirmed in these tables that age adjustment has little effect on figures for pulmonary tuberculosis. Hence it is reasonable to compare the absolute rates of officers and ratings. The rate among officers is only half what it is among ratings, the same proportionate rise having taken place in both during the war.

---

* Reference to Table 13, however, shows that this was not the case. (Ed.)

The death rate from tuberculosis (Table 25) among ratings remained constant till 1943, when it fell almost to half. It is difficult not to conclude that this is the direct result of mass fluorography, which has led to the earlier detection and invaliding of those who otherwise would have died while still in the Service.

The figures for officers are too small to support any conclusion.

GENERAL NOTES ON TABLES 11–32

1. *Population concerned.*—Those classes of Royal Navy and Royal Marine personnel have been included which were similarly included in 'The Health of the Navy', last published in 1936.

2. *Choice of disease groups.*—It is impossible to discern trends and detect changes unless numbers are sufficient. This severely limits the number of disease groups which it is profitable to show separately. The choice of disease groups has been largely determined by this, but a number of other factors were also borne in mind: first, that the disease groups should be reasonably homogeneous; secondly, that they should be separable from one another with fair efficiency; thirdly, that any separation should be likely to have some practical importance; lastly, that as it might be desired to condense the list further, additional groups, not themselves important, would be needed to ensure completeness.

Invalidings due to disease have been classified under 17 headings; deaths, owing to the smaller numbers involved, under 6.

3. *Basis of classification into disease group.*—The classification used to determine the group into which invalidings and deaths fell was the Medical Research Council Morbidity Code (1944). One departure, not numerically important, was, however, made. In the Code deformities resulting from injury are classified as disease not injury. It is easy to see why this should be done in civilian practice. In a fighting Service, however, the great majority of injuries producing subsequent deformity have been incurred in the Service; hence it seemed preferable to classify the resulting disability as due to injury and these cases do not appear in the analysis.

4. *The significance of a difference between two rates.*—When the rates for two periods differ it is important to know whether the difference could have arisen simply by chance, i.e., owing to the accidents of sampling, or whether this is unlikely. If the former there is nothing to discuss; if the latter it is permissible to speculate on possible causes for the change.

The logic of the procedure adopted in the tables showing invaliding rates is as follows. In comparing the rates for two periods one inquires how often from a population showing the joint pooled rate of the two periods one could expect to draw samples of the sizes concerned which differ by at least the amount observed. Arbitrary levels must then be selected. If the difference could arise by chance in this way more often than once in 20 times it is judged non-significant, for it could so easily have arisen by the accidents of sampling that any further discussion is profitless. If, however, the observed difference would occur by chance less often than once in 20 times it is becoming unlikely that it has arisen in this way; there is something to explain. Such a difference is termed significant in these tables. If the observed difference would occur by the accidents of sampling less often than once in 100 times it is judged highly unlikely to have arisen in this way and the difference is termed highly significant.

The larger the numbers observed the smaller the change in rate that we can detect. For example, the invaliding rate due to pulmonary tuberculosis at all ages in 1942 was 2·93 per annum per 1,000 strength. The corresponding rate in 1943 was 2·54. Because of the relatively large numbers concerned, this fall, though moderate, is nevertheless highly significant.

As a contrast in the age group 25–29 in 1939 the invaliding rate for peptic ulcer was 0·53; in 1940 it was 1·05. Although the rate has doubled, the difference, owing to the relatively small numbers involved, is not significant. In the absence of additional evidence based on other years and other age groups discussion would be a waste of time.

In the tables showing invaliding rates each figure is compared with the corresponding figure for 1940, the first complete war year. A significant difference is indicated by the sign +; a highly significant difference by + +. (The comparison is based on the ratio of the difference to its standard error, the latter being calculated on the pooled rate. This is equivalent to a 2 × 2 test for homogeneity. Yates's correction for continuity has been used. Where the expected number in either group was less than 5, odds were calculated exactly.)

The death rates, owing to their greater constancy, lend themselves to the direct question—has there been any significant variation at all? The answer will be found in the notes appended to the tables.

TABLE 11

Total Invalidings due to Disease. Annual Rates per 1,000 Strength by Age Groups. (Officers Excluded)

	1934–38	1939	1940	1941	1942	1943	1944
Age Group— Under 20	16·32 ++	12·12	10·92	13·49 ++	9·16 ++	9·39 ++	11·46
20–24	12·18 ++	9·09	10·02	13·44 ++	11·36 ++	9·39	10·38
25–29	9·05 ++	6·60 ++	13·01	19·70 ++	16·37 ++	11·86	13·69
30–34	5·85 ++	7·42 ++	15·68	23·71 ++	20·78 ++	14·67	15·31
35–39	6·99 ++	10·74 ++	23·63	26·45 +	26·08	20·49 ++	21·33
Over 39	11·85 ++	31·25 ++	44·25	35·34 ++	36·70 ++	30·28 ++	35·08 ++
40–44	9·83 ++	16·69 ++	35·63	29·55 ++	—	—	—
Over 44	18·18 ++	43·83 ++	52·41	40·78 ++	—	—	—
TOTAL—Crude Rate	10·44 ++	11·46 ++	17·12	19·70 ++	16·42 +	12·81 ++	14·33 ++
TOTAL—Age Adjusted Rate	10·44 ++	9·80 ++	15·10	19·30 ++	16·86 ++	13·38 ++	14·84

NOTES ON TABLE 11

1. + indicates a significant difference from the corresponding rate for 1940. ++ indicates a highly significant difference from the corresponding rate for 1940.
2. Age-adjusted rates are the rates which would have been observed had the age composition of the Navy remained constant at the average for the period 1934–38.
3. The large differences between the invaliding rates of peace and war at corresponding ages illustrate the peace-time emphasis on early elimination and the war-time emphasis on keeping as many men as possible at duty. Comparisons between peace and war should be made with much caution (*see* General Summary, page 55).
4. Under the age of 35 the peak invaliding rates were attained in 1941, presumably the year of maximum stress. Over 39 the peak occurred in 1940; this is doubtless due to the intake of reservists, a proportion of whom proved unfit for any kind of naval service.
5. The crude rates for 1939–40 are substantially higher than the age-adjusted rates. This is due to the intake of relatively elderly reservists. By 1942–43 this effect had diminished and an opposite tendency, due to the influx of large numbers of the very young, make the crude rates lower than they would have been had the age composition of the Navy remained constant at the pre-war figure.

TABLE 12

Invalidings due to Disease. Annual Rates per 1,000 Strength. (Officers Excluded)

	1934–38	1939	1940	1941	1942	1943	1944
Tuberculosis, Pulmonary—							
Crude Rate	1·74	1·54	1·79	2·26 ++	2·93 ++	2·54 ++	2·55 ++
Age Adjusted Rate	1·74	1·58 +	1·87	2·27 ++	3·01 ++	2·52 ++	2·57 ++
Tuberculosis, Non-Pulmonary—							
Crude Rate	0·13	0·13	0·14	0·20	0·19	0·18	0·17
Age Adjusted Rate	0·13	0·12	0·14	0·20	0·19	0·18	0·16
Epilepsy—							
Crude Rate	0·31 ++	0·52 ++	0·80	0·72	0·56 ++	0·49 ++	0·35 ++
Age Adjusted Rate	0·31 ++	0·47 ++	0·84	0·84	0·56 ++	0·46 ++	0·33 ++
Other Diseases of the Nervous System—							
Crude Rate	0·15 ++	0·27 +	0·43	0·41	0·30 ++	0·23 ++	0·30 ++
Age Adjusted Rate	0·15 ++	0·22 +	0·37	0·38	0·33	0·24 ++	0·35
Psychoses, Psychoneuroses and Mental Deficiency—							
Crude Rate	1·47 ++	1·65 ++	3·68	5·00 ++	3·46	2·76 ++	3·48
Age Adjusted Rate	1·47 ++	1·45 ++	3·37	5·10 ++	3·68 +	3·00 ++	3·70 +
Diseases of the Eye—							
Crude Rate	1·24 ++	0·83	1·00	0·85	0·62 ++	0·35 ++	0·53 ++
Age Adjusted Rate	1·24 ++	0·74 +	0·94	0·94	0·62 ++	0·35 ++	0·53 ++
Diseases of the Ear—							
Crude Rate	0·99 +	0·59 +	0·81	0·99 +	0·78	0·54 ++	0·66 +
Age Adjusted Rate	0·99 ++	0·54 +	0·75	0·96 ++	0·84	0·60 +	0·73
Disease of the Circulatory System—							
Crude Rate	0·64 ++	0·97 ++	1·42	0·94 ++	0·81 ++	0·68 ++	0·72 ++
Age Adjusted Rate	0·64 +	0·69	0·80	0·62 +	0·54 ++	0·52 ++	0·58 ++
Bronchitis—							
Crude Rate	0·09 ++	0·38 ++	0·84	0·87	0·70 +	0·46 ++	0·60 ++
Age Adjusted Rate	0·09 ++	0·19 ++	0·52	0·70 ++	0·71 ++	0·47	0·61
Asthma—							
Crude Rate	0·07 ++	0·13	0·21	0·32 +	0·29	0·18	0·18
Age Adjusted Rate	0·07 ++	0·11 +	0·21	0·28	0·29	0·20	0·20
Other Diseases of the Respiratory System—							
Crude Rate	0·35 ++	0·40 ++	0·73	0·63	0·54 ++	0·48 ++	0·66
Age Adjusted Rate	0·35 ++	0·33 ++	0·62	0·57	0·53	0·48 +	0·62

	1934–38	1939	1940	1941	1942	1943	1944
Peptic Ulcer—							
Crude Rate	0·46 ++	1·06 ++	1·77	2·93 ++	2·15 ++	1·38 ++	1·24 ++
Age Adjusted Rate	0·46 ++	0·90 ++	1·71	3·00 ++	2·32 ++	1·64	1·43 ++
Other Diseases of the Digestive System—							
Crude Rate	0·42 +	0·53	0·54	0·61	0·58	0·33 ++	0·31 ++
Age Adjusted Rate	0·42	0·46	0·42	0·54 +	0·65 ++	0·39	0·35
Arthritis—							
Crude Rate	0·12 ++	0·17 ++	0·57	0·48	0·45 +	0·35 ++	0·43 ++
Age Adjusted Rate	0·12 ++	0·11 ++	0·34	0·35	0·46 +	0·37	0·44 +
Deformities and Malformations of the Locomotory System—							
Crude Rate	0·52 +	0·37	0·38	0·55 ++	0·36	0·26 ++	0·37
Age Adjusted Rate	0·52 ++	0·33	0·35	0·59 ++	0·40	0·29	0·42
Other Diseases of the Locomotory System—							
Crude Rate	0·18 +	0·22	0·27	0·40 ++	0·36 +	0·37 +	0·32
Age Adjusted Rate	0·18 +	0·19	0·26	0·39 ++	0·41 ++	0·40 ++	0·35
Other Diseases—							
Crude Rate	1·56	1·70	1·74	1·54	1·34 ++	1·23 ++	1·46 ++
Age Adjusted Rate	1·56	1·37	1·59	1·57	1·32 ++	1·27 ++	1·47
TOTAL—ALL DISEASES—							
Crude Rate	10·44 ++	11·46 ++	17·12	19·70 ++	16·42 +	12·81 ++	14·33 ++
Age Adjusted Rate	10·44 ++	9·80 ++	15·10	19·30 ++	16·86 ++	13·38 ++	14·84

NOTES ON TABLE 12

1. + indicates a significant difference from the corresponding rate for 1940. ++ indicates a highly significant difference from the corresponding rate for 1940.

2. Age adjusted rates are the rates which would have been observed had the age composition of the Navy remained constant at the average for the period 1934–38.

3. The trends in pulmonary tuberculosis are quite different from those of any other disease group. As in civilian experience age adjustment makes practically no difference. (*See* General Notes, page 59, and Table 13.)

4. In a number of disease groups the rates rise to a maximum about 1941, declining thereafter. In epilepsy, other nervous diseases and diseases of the ear, age adjustment makes little difference. In the important groups of mental diseases and peptic ulcer (whose parallelism is striking) age adjustment somewhat reduces the magnitude of the changes.

5. Some disease groups show relatively little change during wartime and are little affected by age adjustment. Included in this category are non-pulmonary tuberculosis, deformities of the locomotory system and other diseases of the locomotory system. Rather surprisingly perhaps, asthma too, tends to behave this way.

6. Other diseases of the respiratory and digestive systems, and also arthritis, show a moderate rise and fall, which, as the age-adjusted figures reveal, is almost entirely due to variation in the age composition of the Navy.

7. Circulatory diseases provide a striking example of the effect of changes in age composition. The very large changes in the crude figures are greatly reduced, though not eliminated, in the age-adjusted figures. Bronchitis behaves in the same way.

8. The heterogeneous group, other diseases, shows a moderate fall in 1942–43.

9. Diseases of the eye, which consist largely of errors of refraction, show the effect of administrative action. The acceptance of lower standards has produced a notable fall by 1943.

TABLE 13

Pulmonary Tuberculosis. Annual Invaliding Rates per 1,000 Strength by Age Groups. (Officers Excluded)

	1934–38	1939	1940	1941	1942	1943	1944
Age Group— Under 20	1·03	0·82 +	1·43	2·26 +	2·49 ++	2·47 ++	2·54 ++
20–24	1·81 ++	1·27	1·28	2·06 ++	2·64 ++	2·39 ++	2·25 ++
25–29	2·05	1·48	1·79	2·10	2·84 ++	2·13	2·76 ++
30–34	1·72	2·27	2·28	2·55	3·00	2·35	2·34
35–39	1·94 +	2·27	2·85	2·40	4·18 +	3·14	2·72
Over 39	2·36	2·36	2·47	2·76	3·96 ++	3·87 ++	3·75 ++
40–44	2·05	1·82	2·32	2·87	—	—	—
Over 44	3·33	2·96	2·61	2·66	—	—	—
TOTAL—Crude Rate	1·74	1·54	1·79	2·26 ++	2·93 ++	2·54 ++	2·55 ++
TOTAL—Age Adjusted Rate	1·74	1·58 +	1·87	2·27 ++	3·01 ++	2·52 ++	2·57 ++

NOTES ON TABLE 13

1. + indicates a significant difference from the corresponding rate for 1940. ++ indicates a highly significant difference from the corresponding rate for 1940.
2. Age-adjusted rates are the rates which would have been observed had the age composition of the Navy remained constant at the average for the period 1934–38.
3. As in civilian experience the rates do not differ greatly over the age range concerned. Consequently age adjustment makes very little difference to the crude rates.
4. There has been a striking increase in invalidings due to pulmonary tuberculosis in 1941 and again in 1942. In 1943 a fall occurred. The difference between the rates for 1942 and 1943 is highly significant.
5. *See* General Summary, page 55, for a brief discussion. A possible indication that miniature mass fluorography had begun to affect the figures is the high rate in 1942–43 amongst those over 39. It is older men of high resistance, with symptomless but nevertheless active disease, whom, it might be anticipated mass fluorography would particularly detect. It is also they who provide sources of infection in their ships and whose removal may perhaps lead to improvement in the figures for the Navy as a whole. At present, however, this should not be regarded as more than speculation.

TABLE 14

Epilepsy. Annual Invaliding Rates per 1,000 Strength by Age Groups. (Officers Excluded)

	1934–38	1939	1940	1941	1942	1943	1944
Age Group— Under 20	0·74	0·97	0·95	1·32	0·77	0·78	0·63
20–24	0·38 ++	0·42 +	0·83	0·67	0·60 +	0·42 ++	0·30 ++
25–29	0·16 ++	0·10 ++	0·77	0·86	0·52	0·29 ++	0·30 ++
30–34	0·05 ++	0·36 +	1·03	0·61	0·58 +	0·35 ++	0·27 ++
35–39	0·18 ++	0·52	0·65	0·86	0·40	0·50	0·11 ++
Over 39	0·21	0·55	0·53	0·26	0·14 ++	0·30	0·14 ++
40–44	0·21	0·45	0·61	0·23	—	—	—
Over 44	0·22	0·66	0·46	0·30	—	—	—
TOTAL—Crude Rate	0·31 ++	0·52 ++	0·80	0·72	0·56 ++	0·49 ++	0·35 ++
TOTAL—Age Adjusted Rate	0·31 ++	0·47 ++	0·84	0·84	0·56 ++	0·46 ++	0·33 ++

NOTES ON TABLE 14

1. + indicates a significant difference from the corresponding rate for 1940. ++ indicates a highly significant difference from the corresponding rate for 1940.
2. Age-adjusted rates are the rates which would have been observed had the age composition of the Navy remained constant at the average for the period 1934–38.
3. The rates, which are little affected by age adjustment, rise to a maximum in 1940–41 and fall sharply thereafter.
4. The somewhat erratic changes at different ages may well be an indication of the difficulty of diagnosing and classifying these cases. Electro-encephalography has not yet provided the assistance that was hoped for at one time.

TABLE 15

Psychoses, Psychoneuroses, and Mental Deficiency. Annual Invaliding Rates per 1,000 Strength by Age Groups. (Officers Excluded)

	1934–38	1939	1940	1941	1942	1943	1944
Age Group— Under 20	2·44	1·90	1·89	3·86 ++	2·15	2·30	2·94 ++
20–24	2·09 +	1·88 +	2·64	4·12 ++	2·87	2·24 +	3·03
25–29	1·03 ++	1·15 ++	3·57	5·73 ++	4·00	3·18	3·59
30–34	0·84 ++	0·84 ++	3·70	6·21 ++	4·34	3·34	4·12
35–39	0·77 ++	0·99 ++	4·49	5·83 +	5·38	4·22	5·08
Over 39	1·07 ++	3·15 ++	7·96	5·69 ++	4·78 ++	3·59 ++	4·74 ++
40–44	0·92 ++	2·57 ++	7·87	5·76 +	—	—	—
Over 44	1·55 ++	3·78 ++	8·04	5·63 ++	—	—	—
TOTAL—Crude Rate	1·47 ++	1·65 ++	3·68	5·00 ++	3·46	2·76 ++	3·48
TOTAL—Age Adjusted Rate	1·47 ++	1·45 ++	3·37	5·10 ++	3·68 +	3·00 ++	3·70 +

NOTES ON TABLE 15

1. + indicates a significant difference from the corresponding rate for 1940. ++ indicates a highly significant difference from the corresponding rate for 1940.
2. Age-adjusted rates are the rates which would have been observed had the age composition of the Navy remained constant at the average for the period 1934–38.
3. Mental diseases reveal in more marked form the tendencies shown by the invaliding rates as a whole (*see* General Summary, page 55, and notes on Table 11). Amongst the younger men there is a very marked peak in 1941. In older men 1940 is equally clearly the peak year. Officers also show a pronounced peak in that year (*see* Table 23)
4. Age Adjustment reduces somewhat the fall in 1942–43.

TABLE 16

Diseases of the Eye. Annual Invaliding Rates per 1,000 Strength by Age Groups. (Officers Excluded)

	1934–38	1939	1940	1941	1942	1943	1944
Age Group— Under 20	1·77 +	0·97	1·13	1·13	0·41 ++	0·38 ++	0·58 ++
20–24	1·45 ++	0·87	0·71	0·62	0·50 +	0·24 ++	0·41 ++
25–29	1·81 ++	0·86	0·69	0·82	0·67	0·44	0·54
30–34	0·51	0·36	0·64	1·13	0·65	0·37	0·58
35–39	0·39 ++	0·35 ++	1·50	1·09	0·83 +	0·26 ++	0·46 ++
Over 39	0·59 ++	1·58	1·89	1·01 ++	1·18 +	0·62 ++	0·97 ++
40–44	0·28 ++	0·76	1·54	1·14	—	—	—
Over 44	1·55	2·47	2·22	0·90 ++	—	—	—
TOTAL—Crude Rate	1·24 ++	0·83	1·00	0·85	0·62 ++	0·35 ++	0·53 ++
TOTAL—Age Adjusted Rate	1·24 ++	0·74 +	0·94	0·94	0·62 ++	0·35 ++	0·53 ++

NOTES ON TABLE 16

1. + indicates a significant difference from the corresponding rate for 1940. ++ indicates a highly significant difference from the corresponding rate for 1940.
2. Age-adjusted rates are the rates which would have been observed had the age composition of the Navy remained constant at the average for the period 1934–38.
3. Most of the cases falling into this group are defective vision, i.e., errors of refraction. The acceptance of lower standards has led to a notable reduction of rates by 1943.

TABLE 17

Diseases of the Ear. Annual Invaliding Rates per 1,000 Strength by Age Groups. (Officers Excluded)

	1934–38	1939	1940	1941	1942	1943	1944
Age Group— Under 20	2·09 ++	0·73	0·51	0·32	0·41	0·44	0·54
20–24	1·34 ++	0·55	0·55	0·74	0·59	0·39	0·45
25–29	0·64	0·48	0·75	1·12	0·82	0·59	0·78
30–34	0·39 ++	0·66	0·88	1·50 +	1·38	0·60	0·94
35–39	0·39 ++	0·17 ++	1·01	1·12	1·15	1·03	1·01
Over 39	0·43 ++	1·02	1·70	1·43	1·16	0·88 ++	1·11 +
40–44	0·28 ++	0·61	1·23	1·59	—	—	—
Over 44	0·89	1·48	2·16	1·28 +	—	—	—
TOTAL—Crude Rate	0·99 +	0·59 +	0·81	0·99 +	0·78	0·54 ++	0·66 +
TOTAL —Age Adjusted Rate	0·99 ++	0·54 +	0·75	0·96 ++	0·84	0·60 +	0·73

NOTES ON TABLE 17

1. + indicates a significant difference from the corresponding rate for 1940. ++ indicates a highly significant difference from the corresponding rate for 1940.
2. Age-adjusted rates are the rates which would have been observed had the age composition of the Navy remained constant at the average for the period 1934–38.
3. As in several other disease groups the total crude rates show a rise to a maximum in 1941, followed by a fall. The magnitude of these changes is considerably reduced, though not abolished, by age adjustment.
4. As in the figures for all diseases (Table 11) and for mental diseases (Table 15), the peak for those over 44 occurred in 1940.

TABLE 18

Diseases of the Circulatory System. Annual Invaliding Rates per 1,000 Strength by Age Groups. (Officers Excluded)

	1934–38	1939	1940	1941	1942	1943	1944
Age Group— Under 20	1·64 ++	0·79	0·57	0·35	0·17 ++	0·20 ++	0·33 +
20–24	0·66	0·53	0·48	0·22 ++	0·25 ++	0·20 ++	0·27 ++
25–29	0·25 ++	0·39	0·61	0·38	0·22 ++	0·24 ++	0·23 ++
30–34	0·08 ++	0·54	0·85	0·72	0·39 +	0·45 +	0·43 +
35–39	0·36 +	0·76	0·80	1·08	0·70	0·62	0·74
Over 39	1·23 ++	4·53 +	6·58	4·53 ++	5·70	5·26 +	5·27 +
40–44	0·78 ++	1·38	2·59	2·22	—	—	—
Over 44	2·66 ++	7·96	10·36	6·70 ++	—	—	—
TOTAL—Crude Rate	0·64 ++	0·97 ++	1·42	0·94 ++	0·81 ++	0·68 ++	0·72 ++
TOTAL—Age Adjusted Rate	0·64 +	0·69	0·80	0·62 +	0·54 ++	0·52 ++	0·58 ++

NOTES ON TABLE 18

1. + indicates a significant difference from the corresponding rate for 1940. ++ indicates a highly significant difference from the corresponding rate for 1940.

2. Age-adjusted rates are the rates which would have been observed had the age composition of the Navy remained contant at the average for the period 1934–38.

3. In no disease group is the increase with advancing age so pronounced. Consequently age adjustment gives very different rates from the crude figures. The latter show, even at all ages taken together, a marked peak in 1940. Age adjustment greatly reduces the fluctuations.

4. So great is the increase with age that in this disease group the great influx of the very young does not compensate, even by 1943, for the intake of far smaller numbers of older men.

5. Age adjustment does not eliminate all variation. As in several other disease groups there is a rise and a fall. The very high rate for those over 44 in 1940 shows that as regards circulatory diseases also, a considerable proportion of reservists were unable to stand the stress of naval life.

TABLE 19

Bronchitis. Annual Invaliding Rates per 1,000 Strength by Age Groups. (Officers Excluded)

	1934–38	1939	1940	1941	1942	1943	1944
Age Group— Under 20	0·17	0·12	0·11	0·13	0·11	0·09	0·13
20–24	0·09	0·13	0·14	0·20	0·14	0·13	0·12
25–29	0·02 ++	0·05	0·27	0·43	0·59 +	0·19	0·34
30–34	0·04 ++	0·00 ++	0·52	0·96	0·92	0·54	0·64
35–39	0·13 ++	0·17 ++	1·13	1·64	1·64	1·20	1·43
Over 39	0·27 ++	3·07	4·20	3·58	3·07 ++	2·72 ++	3·93
40–44	0·21 ++	1·66	2·98	2·40	—	—	—
45–49	0·44 ++	4·61	5·36	4·68	—	—	—
TOTAL—Crude Rate	0·09 ++	0·38 ++	0·84	0·87	0·70 +	0·46 ++	0·60 ++
TOTAL—Age Adjusted Rate	0·09 ++	0·19 ++	0·52	0·70 ++	0·71++	0·47	0·61

NOTES ON TABLE 19

1. + indicates a significant difference from the corresponding rate for 1940. ++ indicates a highly significant difference from the corresponding rate for 1940.
2. Age-adjusted rates are the rates which would have been observed had the age composition of the Navy remained constant at the average for the period 1934–38.
3. Somewhat like circulatory diseases (Table 18) though in not quite so pronounced a way, invalidings due to bronchitis rise sharply with increasing age. Similarly age adjustment eliminates much of the variation shown by the crude rates.
4. Under 25 the rates are very small and also fairly constant. From 25 to 39 there is the usual rise and fall, with the peak in 1941 ,though spreading over to 1942. Over 39 the peak occurs in 1940.

TABLE 20

Peptic Ulcer. Annual Invaliding Rates per 1,000 Strength by Age Groups. (Officers Excluded)

	1934–38	1939	1940	1941	1942	1943	1944
Age Group— Under 20	0·06	0·27	0·06	0·29 +	0·26 +	0·29 +	0·34 ++
20–24	0·43	0·24	0·43	1·30 ++	0·82 ++	0·77 ++	0·72 ++
25–29	0·55 ++	0·53	1·05	3·23 ++	2·36 ++	1·56 +	1·51 +
30–34	0·43 ++	1·02 ++	2·48	4·45 ++	3·69 ++	2·37	1·14 ++
35–39	0·74 ++	1·98 ++	4·69	6·26 +	4·42	3·32 ++	3·27 ++
Over 39	1·18 ++	5·28	5·51	5·79	6·82 +	4·06 ++	4·20 ++
40–44	1·27 ++	4·54	5·94	5·92	—	—	—
Over 44	0·89 ++	6·09	5·11	5·65	—	—	—
TOTAL—Crude Rate	0.46 ++	1·06 ++	1·77	2·93 ++	2·15 ++	1·38 ++	1·24 ++
TOTAL—Age Adjusted Rate	0·46 ++	0·90 ++	1·71	3·00 ++	2·32 ++	1·64	1·43 ++

NOTES ON TABLE 20

1. + indicates a significant difference from the corresponding rate for 1940. ++ indicates a highly significant difference from the corresponding rate for 1940.
2. Age-adjusted rates are the rates which would have been observed had the age composition of the Navy remained constant at the average for the period 1934–38.
3. The rise and fall are very marked and the trends closely parallel to those for mental diseases (Table 15). One particular in which these two groups resemble each other and differ from other disease groups is a fairly considerable rise with age up to a certain point only. In both groups the rates for those over 44 do not exceed those for the age group 40–44.
4. The rise to 1941 and fall thereafter are notable. The rate for 1943 is only half that for 1941. Age adjustment minimises somewhat the fall in 1942–43.
5. The rates for Officers are very different. Not only are they lower, but Officers show little variation throughout the period of the war (*see* Table 23).

Table 21

Arthritis. Annual Invaliding Rates per 1,000 Strength by Age Groups. (Officers Excluded)

	1934–38	1939	1940	1941	1942	1943	1944
Age Group— Under 20	0·12	0·03	0·06	0·03	0·07	0·06	0·06
20–24	0·08	0·05	0·09	0·09	0·09	0·11	0·12
25–29	0·08	0·00	0·17	0·28	0·36	0·28	0·25
30–34	0·11	0·06	0·24	0·55	0·56	0·47	0·54
35–39	0·14 ++	0·35 +	0·88	0·72	1·14	0·80	0·99
Over 39	0·59 ++	1·10 ++	2·88	2·04 +	2·05 +	1·76 ++	2·57
40–44	0·64 ++	0·30 ++	2·04	1·11 +	—	—	—
Over 44	0·44 ++	1·97 +	3·68	2·91	—	—	—
TOTAL—Crude Rate	0·12 ++	0·17 ++	0·57	0·48	0·45 +	0·35 ++	0·43 ++
TOTAL—Age Adjusted Rate	0·12 ++	0·11 ++	0·34	0·35	0·46 +	0·37	0·44 +

NOTES ON TABLE 21

1. + indicates a significant difference from the corresponding rate for 1940. ++ indicates a highly significant difference from the corresponding rate for 1940.
2. Age-adjusted rates are the rates which would have been observed had the age composition of the Navy remained constant at the average for the period 1934–38.
3. Arthritis, like some of the more heterogeneous disease groups, not analysed separately, does not show much variation during the war-time period. What little variation there s from 1940 to 1943 is eliminated by age adjustment. The only change of any note is a fall among those over 39.

Table 22

Officers. Invalidings due to Disease. Total Annual Rates per 1,000 Strength

1934–38	1939	1940	1941	1942	1943	1944
3·50 ++	7·42 ++	13·01	9·94 ++	9·50 ++	9·49 ++	12·97

NOTES ON TABLE 22

1. ++ indicates a highly significant difference from the corresponding rate for 1940.
2. Owing to the fact that the ages of officers are often omitted from documents reaching the Medical Department it is unfortunately impossible to analyse the figures by age groups or to calculate age-adjusted rates. For this reason little can be deduced from a comparison of the rates for officers and ratings.
3. The invaliding rate has remained remarkably constant throughout the war, apart from the pronounced rise in 1940. Doubtless this is to be ascribed to the proportion of reservists, many of advanced years, who proved unable to stand the stress of naval life.

TABLE 23

Officers. Invalidings due to Disease. Annual Rates per 1,000 Strength.

	1934–38	1939	1940	1941	1942	1943	1944
Tuberculosis, Pulmonary	0·84	0·84	1·09	0·87	1·46	1·52	2·08 ++
Tuberculosis, Non-Pulmonary	0·19	0·15	0·04	0·00	0·07	0·05	0·07
Epilepsy	0·12	0·23	0·11	0·11	0·07	0·07	0·19
Other Diseases of the Nervous System	0·02 ++	0·53	0·51	0·40	0·20 +	0·26	0·41
Psychoses and Psychoneuroses	0·65 ++	2·52 ++	5·11	3·34 ++	2·55 ++	3·01 ++	4·56
Diseases of the Eye	0·36	0·08	0·25	0·42	0·35	0·42	0·66 ++
Diseases of the Ear	0·14	0·23	0·22	0·16	0·17	0·23	0·21
Diseases of the Circulatory System	0·36 ++	1·14 ++	2·65	1·72 +	1·50 ++	1·10 ++	1·42 ++
Bronchitis	0·00 +	0·08	0·14	0·37	0·28	0·35	0·37
Asthma	0·07	0·08	0·07	0·11	0·17	0·09	0·19
Other Diseases of the Respiratory System	0·05 +	0·15	0·25	0·13	0·26	0·16	0·25
Peptic Ulcer	0·07 ++	0·46	0·47	0·50	0·61	0·72	0·63
Other Diseases of the Digestive System	0·10 +	0·08	0·33	0·37	0·37	0·21	0·38
Arthritis	0·05 ++	0·08	0·36	0·16	0·22	0·14	0·29
Deformities and Malformations of the Locomotory System	0·00 +	0·00	0·18	0·11	0·09	0·05	0·00 +
Other Diseases of the Locomotory System	0·00	0·08	0·00	0·24 ++	0·15 +	0·10	0·12
Other Diseases	0·48 ++	0·69	1·23	0·93	0·98	1·01	1·14
TOTAL—All Diseases	3·50 ++	7·42 ++	13·01	9·94 ++	9·50 ++	9·49 ++	12·97

NOTES ON TABLE 23

1. + indicates a significant difference from the corresponding rate for 1940. ++ indicates a highly significant difference from the corresponding rate for 1940.

2. For the sake of completeness the same disease groups are shown as in the corresponding table for ratings (Table 12). The relatively small numbers involved, however, do not permit trends to be examined in much detail; few differences from the 1940 rates are significant. The usefulness of the table is further limited by the impossibility of calculating age-adjusted rates (*see* notes on Table 22).

3. As amongst ratings, invalidings are very different in peace and war.

4. Mental diseases show a striking rise and fall, with a peak in 1940. Circulatory diseases show a rise and fall which is more marked than among ratings. In both instances the explanation is probably the same as in ratings, i.e., in mental diseases the intake of reservists; in circulatory diseases chiefly the changes in the age composition of the officer population.

5. Invalidings due to pulmonary tuberculosis rose in 1942–43 (cf. Table 13). The difference between the periods 1934–41 and 1942–43 is significant.

6. If these three groups are deducted, i.e., pulmonary tuberculosis, mental diseases, and circulatory diseases, the remainder show considerably lower rates than they do among ratings. Furthermore, there is no indication of change throughout the years 1940–43, the rates being respectively 4·2, 4·0, 4·0 and 3·9.

TABLE 24

Deaths due to Disease. Total Annual Rates per 1,000 Strength. (Officers Excluded)

	1934–38	1939	1940	1941	1942	1943
Crude Rates	1·17	1·10	1·31	1·28	1·21	1·00
Age Adjusted Rates	1·17	0·99	1·08	1·13	1·10	0·96

NOTES ON TABLE 24

1. Age-adjusted rates are the rates which would have been observed had the age composition of the Navy remained constant at the average for the period 1934–38.

2. The crude rates show a slight rise to a maximum in 1940–41, followed by a fall. The figures for the six periods shown are highly significantly heterogeneous. When, however, age-adjusted rates are compared the variation almost vanishes. If, in addition, allowance is made for the fall in 1943 in deaths due to pulmonary tuberculosis (*see* Table 25) there is no significant departure from homogeneity.

3. It can be concluded that apart from a slight rise in 1940–41, due entirely to changes in the age composition of the Navy, there has been no significant variation in the death rate due to disease throughout the war and that the death rate of war-time is no higher than that of peace.

TABLE 25

Deaths due to Disease. Annual Rates per 1,000 Strength by Disease Groups. (Officers Excluded)

	1934–38	1939	1940	1941	1942	1943
Tuberculosis, Pulmonary	0·12	0·12	0·10	0·15	0·14	0·08
Diseases of the Nervous System	0·08	0·09	0·10	0·08	0·11	0·08
Diseases of the Circulatory System—						
Crude Rate	0·11	0·13	0·23	0·19	0·15	0·15
Age Adjusted Rate	0·11	0·13	0·14	0·12	0·11	0·12
Diseases of the Respiratory System	0·21	0·19	0·22	0·21	0·17	0·10
Diseases of the Digestive System	0·21	0·20	0·23	0·21	0·18	0·18
Other Diseases	0·44	0·37	0·43	0·44	0·46	0·41
TOTAL—ALL DISEASES—						
Crude Rate	1·17	1·10	1·31	1·28	1·21	1·00
Age Adjusted Rate	1·17	0·99	1·08	1·13	1·10	0·96

NOTES ON TABLE 25

1. Age-adjusted rates are the rates which would have been observed had the age composition of the Navy remained constant at the average for the period 1934–38.

2. This table shows death rates separately for six broad groups of diseases.

3. Deaths from pulmonary tuberculosis, which hardly varied at all from 1934 to 1942, fell sharply in 1943. The difference between the rates for 1942 and 1943 is highly significant. It is very probable that the fall is due to minature mass fluorography, by means of which a number of men who would otherwise have died in the Service were detected and invalided before this could occur.

4. Apart from a fall in 1943 in deaths due to respiratory diseases (for which it is difficult to offer any explanation) the rates for the other individual disease groups are remarkably constant, if circulatory diseases are omitted.

5. The crude rates for circulatory diseases are highly significantly heterogeneous, but this effect entirely disappears in the age-corrected figures. It is this diseases group which is largely responsible for the age effect in the total figures, mentioned in the notes on Table 24.

TABLE 26

Deaths due to Disease for Whole Period 1934–43. Annual Rates per 1,000 Strength by Age and Disease Groups. (Officers Excluded)

	Tuberculosis, Pulmonary	Diseases of the Nervous System	Diseases of the Circulatory System	Diseases of the Respiratory System	Diseases of the Digestive System	Other Diseases	Total all Diseases
Age Group— Under 20	0·09	0·06	0·04	0·10	0·15	0·36	0·80
20–24	0·10	0·05	0·03	0·10	0·14	0·30	0·72
25–29	0·12	0·07	0·06	0·08	0·15	0·36	0·84
30–34	0·10	0·07	0·07	0·21	0·18	0·40	1·03
35–39	0·16	0·11	0·29	0·28	0·25	0·56	1·65
Over 39	0·20	0·34	0·99	0·58	0·57	1·09	3·77
40–44 (1934–41 only)	0·11	0·21	0·51	0·37	0·35	0·74	2·29
Over 44 (1934–41 only)	0·19	0·46	1·34	0·74	0·80	1·37	4·90
TOTAL—All Ages	0·12	0·09	0·15	0·17	0·20	0·43	1·16

NOTES ON TABLE 26

1. The numbers involved are too small for any useful separation by age groups to be made year by year as was done for invaliding rates. The remarkable constancy of the death rates throughout the period, however, as revealed in Tables 24 and 25, make it reasonable to analyse by age groups for the complete ten-year period.
2. The rising death-rate with advancing age is well illustrated ,this change being smallest for pulmonary tuberculosis and greatest for circulatory diseases.

TABLE 27

Officers. Deaths due to Disease. Total Annual Rates per 1,000 Strength

1934–38	1939	1940	1941	1942	1943
1·51	1·83	2·72	2·25	2·33	1·85

NOTES ON TABLE 27

1. Owing to the fact that ages of officers are often omitted in documents reaching the Medical Department, age relationships cannot be investigated.

2. The rate among officers is only 30 per cent. higher than among ratings (Table 24) during the peace-time period 1934–38.

3. During war-time the rate among officers is about double that of ratings. This is chiefly due, in all probability, to the much larger proportion of older officers. This is confirmed by the fact that over the whole period deaths due to circulatory disease, a sensitive indicator of age, are nearly four times more frequent among officers. A contributory cause may be the greater reluctance to invalid officers.

4. The annual death rates for officers are markedly variable, with a peak in 1940. This, too, may well be due to changes in the age composition of the officer population

TABLE 28

Officers. Deaths due to Disease for the Whole Period 1939–43. Annual Rates per 1,000 Strength by Disease Groups

Pulmonary Tuberculosis	0·09
Diseases of the Nervous System	0·18
Diseases of the Circulatory System	0·57
Diseases of the Respiratory System	0·24
Diseases of the Digestive System	0·30
Other Diseases	0·69
Total—All Diseases	2·07

NOTES ON TABLE 28

1. The numbers involved are too small to show figures for the years separately.

2. The death rate from pulmonary tuberculosis is distinctly lower than among ratings (*see* Table 26).

3. In the other disease groups it is higher, being no less than four times as high in circulatory diseases.

W.R.N.S.

An Analysis of Invalidings due to Disease and Deaths due to Disease, 1941-44

NOTES ON THE TABLES

1. The general notes (pp. 59–60) refer to these tables also.

2. Age censuses are not available for officers and ratings separately. Consequently the joint figures have had to be used for ratings. Officers are, of course, older, but as they constitute only 5 per cent. of the W.R.N.S., the calculation of age-adjusted rates would not be seriously affected.

For the year 1941 only one age census, that of December 31, is available. This has been applied to the whole year.

3. Table 29 shows that the total invaliding rate fell sharply from 1941 to 1942 and that there is practically no difference between 1942 and 1943. The numbers borne, particularly in 1941, were small, so that hardly any of the differences in the rates for individual disease groups are significant.

4. In Table 31 the rates are adjusted for both sexes to the same standard population In addition the rates for women are further adjusted to what they would have been had the numbers borne in the three years respectively been in the same proportion as among the men.

The total invaliding rates do not differ substantially, though the rate for women is highly significantly lower than for men.

Men show rates which are highly significantly greater than among women in pulmonary tuberculosis, epilepsy, diseases of the eye, diseases of the ear, peptic ulcer and other diseases of the digestive system. They are significantly higher in bronchitis, other respiratory diseases and deformities.

Women are highly significantly higher in mental diseases and circulatory diseases and significantly higher in non-pulmonary tuberculosis.

The most striking difference is peptic ulcer, with a rate 12 times greater in men than women.

TABLE 29

W.R.N.S. Invalidings due to Disease. Annual Rates per 1,000 Strength. (Officers Excluded)

	1941	1942	1943	1944
Tuberculosis, Pulmonary				
Crude Rate	1·94	1·65	1·82	1·77
Age Adjusted Rate . . .	2·21	1·41	1·76	1·51
Tuberculosis, Non-Pulmonary				
Crude Rate	0·20	0·49	0·33	0·27
Age Adjusted Rate . . .	0·22	0·45	0·26	0·27
Epilepsy				
Crude Rate	0·74	0·39	0·17	0·34
Age Adjusted Rate . . .	0·71	0·31	0·15	0·27
Psychoses, Psychoneuroses and Mental Deficiency				
Crude Rate	5·43	4·28	4·26	4·96
Age Adjusted Rate . . .	5·48	4·27	4·72	6·46 ++
Diseases of the Circulatory System				
Crude Rate	0·94	1·05	0·74	0·43 ++
Age Adjusted Rate . . .	0·92	1·05	0·92	0·56 +
Diseases of the Respiratory System				
Crude Rate	1·34	0·81	0·79	1·01
Age Adjusted Rate . . .	1·42 +	0·73	1·03	0·94
Diseases of the Digestive System				
Crude Rate	0·54	0·32	0·21	0·53
Age Adjusted Rate . . .	0·54	0·37	0·42	0·61
Diseases of the Locomotory System				
Crude Rate	1·41	0·74	0·58	0·83
Age Adjusted Rate . . .	1·37	0·77	0·70	0·98
Menopause				
Crude Rate	0·47	0·42	0·46	0·43
Age Adjusted Rate . . .	0·37	0·29	0·42	0·56
Other Gynaecological Diseases				
Crude Rate	1·14	0·63	0·37	0·55
Age Adjusted Rate . . .	1·23	0·64	0·48	0·91
Other Diseases				
Crude Rate	4·02	2·98	2·60	2·24 +
Age Adjusted Rate . . .	4·26 +	2·91	2·84	2·45
TOTAL—All Diseases				
Crude Rate	18·17 ++	13·76	12·33	13·36
Age Adjusted Rate . . .	18·73 ++	13·20	13·70	15·52 ++

\+ indicates a significant difference from the rate for 1942.
++ indicates a highly significant difference from the rate for 1942.

TABLE 30

W.R.N.S. Invalidings due to Disease, 1941–43, by Age Groups, Rates per 1,000 Strength (Officers Excluded)

Under 20	8·66
20–24	10·83
25–29	13·42
30–34	15·22
35–39	17·05
Over 39	47·50

TABLE 31

R.N. Comparisons of Men and Women in regard to Invalidings due to Disease, 1941–43. Annual Rates per 1,000 Strength. Figures adjusted for Age and Relative Proportions in the Three Years. (Officers Excluded).

	Women	Men	Significance of Difference
Tuberculosis, Pulmonary	1·76	2·62	++
Tuberculosis, Non-Pulmonary	0·31	0·19	+
Epilepsy	0·34	0·59	++
Other Diseases of the Nervous System	0·33	0·31	—
Psychoses, Psychoneuroses and Mental Deficiency	4·76	3·75	++
Diseases of the Eye	0·23	0·58	++
Diseases of the Ear	0·13	0·77	++
Diseases of the Circulatory System	0·96	0·55	++
Bronchitis	0·40	0·61	+
Asthma	0·30	0·25	—
Other Diseases of the Respiratory System	0·33	0·52	+
Peptic Ulcer	0·17	2·20	++
Other Diseases of the Digestive System	0·26	0·51	++
Arthritis	0·32	0·40	—
Deformities and Malformations of the Locomotory System	0·25	0·40	+
Other Diseases of the Locomotory System	0·32	0·40	—
Menopause	0·36	—	—
Other Gynaecological Diseases	0·72	—	—
Other Diseases	2·53	1·36	++
TOTAL—All Diseases	14·78	16·01	++

TABLE 32

W.R.N.S. Deaths due to Disease, 1941–43. Annual Rates per 1,000 Strength (Officers Excluded)

Crude Rate	0·55
Age Adjusted Rate	0·63
Corresponding Age Adjusted Rate for Men	1·05

(Difference between sexes is highly significant)

III THE ROYAL NAVAL HOSPITAL, HASLAR

The numbers of patients admitted with different diseases or injuries to the Royal Naval Hospital, Haslar, from 1914 to 1918 were obtained from the Hospital Muster Books for those years and the numbers admitted from 1939 to 1945 were recorded according to a nosological index based on Table 3 of the Medical Officers' Journal. They are shown in Table 38. The proportions of each type of case per 1,000 total admissions provide a contrast in this hospital's experience in the two wars and add to knowledge of the distribution of diseases (particularly as from 1916 to 1918 there are otherwise no naval statistical data available, as far as we are aware). The Statistical Reports of the Health of the Navy for the years 1914 and 1915[7,8] published retrospectively after the First World War provide a further basis for comparison for some diseases.

This was the largest Naval hospital in both wars and the main clearing station for cases invalided from abroad. The total numbers admitted are shown in Table 33.

TABLE 33

Total Admissions to the Royal Naval Hospital, Haslar, in the First and Second World Wars

1914–18 (bed complement = 1,300)		*1939–45* (bed complement = 1,100 at times reduced to 400)	
1914 (5 months)	1,362	1939 (4 months)	2,715
1915	11,306	1940	12,491
1916	13,169	1941	13,688
1917	14,956	1942	15,823
1918	14,149	1943	16,163
		1944	14,382
		1945	16,399
Total	54,942	Total	91,661

The numbers were consistently greater during the Second World War than the First, which is somewhat surprising in view of the lower—and during the air-raid years very much lower—bed complement; but the turnover of cases was brisker in the Second World War because of an effective arrangement for evacuating cases to Emergency Medical Services Hospitals. The cases per thousand admissions for the more prominent groups of diseases and injuries are given in Table 34.

These figures, being proportions of the total admissions, indicate differences in the disease patterns at this hospital. They should not be confused with incidence rates in the population at risk.

TABLE 34

Admissions to the Royal Naval Hospital, Haslar, during the First and Second World Wars
Proportion of cases per 1,000 admissions in certain disease groups.

	1914–18	1939–45
Chicken Pox	0·9	2·6
Common Cold	16·3	45·7
Dysentery	22·6	2·4
Typhoid	14·0	0·2
Paratyphoid	2·5	0·2
Influenza	35·3	1·2
Malaria	9·9	3·3
Measles	16·0	2·9
Meningococcal Infection	4·2	1·8
Pneumococcal Infection (lungs)	17·4	11·7
Rheumatic Fever	4·9	4·4
Rheumatism, sub-acute	1·4	3·0
Rubella	19·4	15·6
Tonsillitis	14·1	42·5
Tuberculosis—Pulmonary	19·2	25·2
Tuberculosis—Non-pulmonary	2·3	2·6
Chancroid*	11·4	0·5
Syphilis*	107·0	7·3
Gonococcal Infection, Acute*	33·6	7·6
Gonococcal Infection, Sequelae*	11·6	2·3
Neurasthenia*	22·3	0·4
Other Nervous Diseases (including Mental)*	40·9	47·5
Diseases of the Heart (Organic)	19·0	4·5
Diseases of the Heart (Functional)	7·2	4·9
Bronchitis	15·5	24·8
Pleurisy	10·8	6·1
Appendicitis	15·4	22·4
Peptic Ulcer (Gastric)	2·5	9·7
Peptic Ulcer (Duodenal)	2·1	21·3
Hernia	28·7	34·0
Diseases of Muscles, Fasciae, etc.	21·5	11·1
Other Diseases of the Skin*	13·5	41·3
General Injuries	89·7	135·4
Injuries in Action	30·2	43·4

* *See* p. 82.

Whereas the proportion of illnesses designated as common cold and tonsillitis in the Second World War was thrice that in the First, the figure for influenza in the Second was only one thirtieth of that in the First World War. 'Catarrh' was *not* a frequent diagnosis in this hospital in the First World War in contrast with the Total Force figures for 1915 (the only year for which Total Force figures for 'catarrh' *are* available). A prominent cause for the high influenza figure was undoubtedly the epidemic in 1918 during which 1,942 cases were admitted. Naval personnel in the Port suffered lightly from influenza during the Second World War—only in 1944 were there more than 20 admissions—but the admission rate for the 'common cold' was always high, with a particularly heavy epidemic—1,533 admissions—in 1940.

A notable improvement was to be seen in the relative frequency of dysentery in the Second World War which was one tenth of that in the First.

The marked reduction in venereal disease at this hospital during the Second World War was primarily due to the fact that most of these cases were treated at another hospital in the Portsmouth area.

Similarly, the proportions of admissions for neurasthenia and mental illness together were smaller in the Second World War when the more serious cases in these categories were treated at the Royal Naval Auxiliary Hospital, Knowle, not at Haslar.

Proportionately, ten times as many men were admitted with duodenal ulcer during the Second as in the First World War partly because opaque-meal examinations, which permitted a radiological diagnosis to be made as a matter of routine in the Second World War, were not carried out so frequently in the earlier war. It is possible that revised medical standards and stress during the 'blitzes' were contributory factors. Some indication of the latter is given in Table 35 by the peptic ulcer admissions during 1941 when Portsmouth was heavily bombed and in 1945 after the flying-bomb attacks and the invasion of Europe in the previous year and this impression is reinforced by the invaliding figures for digestive diseases for the Total Force.

TABLE 35

Peptic Ulcer admissions to the Royal Naval Hospital, Haslar

Year	Total Admissions, All Causes	Gastric Ulcer	Perforated Gastric Ulcer	Duodenal Ulcer	Perforated Duodenal Ulcer
1939	2,715	54	None	55	None
1940	12,491	114	5	248	3
1941	13,688	184	30	316	19
1942	15,823	97	7	296	2
1943	16,163	112	15	259	13
1944	14,382	103	19	299	26
1945	16,399	223	48	479	24
Total	91,661	887	124	1,952	87

Proportionately, more patients with 'diseases of the areolar tissue and skin' were treated at Haslar during the Second World War than in the First. The cases under this heading per 1,000 total admissions are summarised in Table 36. This may be partly because skin cases were admitted more freely to hospital rather than because of a true increase in skin disease, particularly as the rates for the Total Force were greater for the years 1914 and 1915 than for the years 1939–45.

TABLE 36

Skin diseases. Cases per 1,000 admissions

	1914–18	1939–45
Abscess	7·8	6·4
Boil	2·3	4·0
Eczema	3·9	0·8
Impetigo	1·3	6·5
Other Diseases	13·5	41·3

The larger proportion of 'general injuries' admitted during the Second World War was due in part to the greater use of motor cycles and other forms of motor vehicle, while the increased proportion of 'injuries in action' were, perhaps, a natural result of the hospital being in the 'front line' more than it was in the First World War.

Table 37 below shows, for certain other diseases of topical interest, the numbers of admissions to Haslar from 1939 to 1945 with the proportions per 1,000 admissions and the rates per 1,000 strength of the Portsmouth Command (excluding visiting ships).

TABLE 37

Diseases of topical interest at the Royal Naval Hospital, Haslar, 1939–45

	1939	1940	1941	1942	1943	1944	1945	Total
Total Admissions	2,715	12,491	13,688	15,823	16,163	14,382	16,399	91,661
Av. Complement Ports. Command	21,177	29,625	36,223	48,634	66,451	91,641	70,641	364,392
Hypertension	26	45	58	71	78	74	91	443
	*(9·6)	(3·6)	(4·2)	(4·5)	(4·8)	(5·2)	(5·6)	(4·8)
	**(1·2)	(1·5)	(1·6)	(1·5)	(1·2)	(0·8)	(1·3)	(1·2)
Catarrhal or Toxic Hepatitis	9	37	70	76	185	89	186	652
	(3·3)	(3·0)	(5·1)	(4·8)	(11·5)	(6·2)	(11·3)	(7·1)
	(0·4)	(1·2)	(1·9)	(1·6)	(2·8)	(1·0)	(2·6)	(1·8)
Arsenical Hepatitis	1	5	57	106	100	50	17	336
	(0·4)	(0·4)	(4·2)	(6·7)	(6·2)	(3·5)	(1·0)	(3·7)
	(0·5)	(0·2)	(1·6)	(2·2)	(1·5)	(0·5)	(0·2)	(0·9)
Glandular Fever	—	4	7	21	33	23	27	115
	—	(0·3)	(0·5)	(1·3)	(2·0)	(1·6)	(1·7)	(1·3)
	—	(0·1)	(0·2)	(0·4)	(0·5)	(0·3)	(0·4)	(0·3)
Carcinoma of Bronchus	1	1	3	5	1	2	—	13
Leukaemia	—	—	3	1	2	2	5	13
Lymphadenoma	1	—	2	7	1	7	4	22

* Proportions per 1,000 admissions. **Rates per 1,000 strength.

The rates per 1,000 understate the true incidence since all cases in the Command were not admitted to Haslar. They should be regarded rather as indicators of the trend over the years. The average strengths are those given in the Annual Reports of Naval Medical Officers of Health, Portsmouth.

The increasing numbers of cases of hypertension during the first four years of the war was due primarily to the increasing size of the population at risk.

The increase in 'catarrhal' (or infective) hepatitis and 'arsenical' hepatitis during the early years of the war was real, although the latter trend was reversed after 1942 when those responsible for the treatment of syphilis became more aware of the dangers of transmitting the hepatitis agent by contaminated syringes or needles. Evidence has been provided to show that some cases of infective hepatitis in the Navy may also have been due to 'syringe-transmission' as a result of routine immunisation procedures.[9,10] The admission rates for glandular fever show a similar trend to those for hepatitis.

There were only 13 patients with carcinoma of the bronchus and 13 patients with leukaemia among 91,661 cases admitted to this hospital but nearly twice as many were admitted with lymphadenoma.

In summary, the types of cases treated in the two wars differed in several important respects, some of which are mentioned above. The conditions under which the work was done were probably more rigorous in the Second World War, particularly during the early years, when the Port was under continuous threat of bombardment from the air and all but the most seriously ill patients were evacuated to cots in the cellars every night, while the hospital staff went to their action stations during the fairly numerous air-raid alerts. It was, perhaps, surprising that most of them, patients and staff, appeared to thrive under this routine.

TABLE 38

Nosological Table showing the Number of Patients treated in the Royal Naval Hospital, Haslar, Gosport during the First World War 1914–1918 and the Second World War 1939–1945

DISEASE OR INJURY	Aug. to Dec. 1914	1915	1916	1917	1918	Total	Cases per 1,000 of Total Admitted	Sept. to Dec. 1939	1940	1941	1942	1943	1944	1945	Total	Cases per 1,000 of Total Admitted
DISEASES CAUSED BY INFECTION:																
Chicken Pox	1	4	18	13	13	49	0·9	3	8	22	55	44	62	43	237	2·6
Common Cold	26	79	171	201	418	895	16·3	227	1,533	794	775	552	166	146	4,193	45·7
Cow-pox	4	10	23	29	11	77	1·4	5	32	44	90	43	6	13	233	2·5
Dengue	—	—	—	—	—	—	—	—	—	—	—	—	—	—	—	—
Diphtheria	6	14	17	19	12	68	1·2	3	31	23	16	54	61	14	202	2·2
Dysentery	—	821	220	101	97	1,239	22·6	3	6	5	26	18	39	127	224	2·4
Enteric Fever, Typhoid	4	478	219	46	24	771	14·0	—	—	1	2	—	2	13	18	0·2
Enteric Fever, Paratyphoid	1	44	76	15	3	139	2·5	—	4	1	2	—	2	13	22	0·2
Erysipelas	1	13	17	10	11	52	0·9	—	17	8	8	5	3	6	47	0·5
Influenza	10	67	115	89	1,661	1,942	35·3	—	19	9	11	11	40	20	110	1·2
Malaria	5	38	115	256	134	548	9·9	—	10	13	56	79	80	62	300	3·3
Measles	1	194	409	118	158	880	16·0	7	31	90	32	53	10	42	265	2·9
Meningococcal Infection	1	12	87	115	14	229	4·2	6	46	38	18	36	17	7	168	1·8
Mumps	4	99	102	158	55	418	7·6	—	24	35	146	118	79	39	441	4·8
Pneumococcal Infection (Lungs)	28	126	171	161	470	956	17·4	30	75	144	171	230	193	227	1,070	11·7
Pneumococcal Infection (Other Organs)	—	—	1	—	—	1	0·0	—	1	—	—	—	—	1	2	0·0
Pyogenic Infection	14	56	40	50	53	213	3·9	102	3	1	31	52	47	84	320	3·5
Pyrexia of Uncertain Origin	3	33	42	47	37	162	2·9	1	11	10	8	5	27	22	84	0·9
Rheumatic Fever	14	73	80	58	46	271	4·9	5	76	62	48	59	59	90	399	4·4
Rheumatism, sub-acute	1	6	26	10	35	78	1·4	8	44	24	45	31	52	68	272	3·0
Rubella	—	256	333	307	171	1,067	19·4	60	924	242	53	60	76	10	1,425	15·6
Sandfly Fever	—	1	1	—	—	2	0·0	—	—	—	—	—	—	2	2	0·0
Scarlet Fever	12	63	81	112	36	304	5·5	6	73	62	27	74	45	11	298	3·3
Small-pox	—	—	—	—	—	—	—	—	—	—	—	—	—	—	—	—
Tonsillitis	26	146	183	234	187	776	14·1	212	549	593	676	687	533	643	3,893	42·5
Tuberculosis, Pulmonary	23	193	293	248	296	1,053	19·2	39	121	186	311	475	392	790	2,314	25·2
Tuberculosis, Pulmonary (Observation)	17	81	125	138	108	469	8·5	—	—	—	—	—	—	—	—	—
Tuberculosis, Non-pulmonary	4	16	36	31	40	127	2·3	1	16	35	49	42	40	52	235	2·6
Undulant Fever	—	7	—	5	12	24	0·4	—	—	—	3	—	—	2	5	0·1
Chancroid	32	97	134	199	167	629	11·4	5	9	32	2	—	—	—	48	0·5
Syphilis	116	602	1,153	2,405	1,603	5,879	107·0	23	202	265	56	49	49	29	673	7·3
Gonococcal Infection, Acute	68	269	331	613	563	1,844	33·6	91	241	300	12	9	22	18	693	7·6
Gonococcal Infection, Sequelae	9	89	202	219	119	638	11·6	23	60	56	19	25	16	10	209	2·3
Lympho-granuloma Inguinale	22	41	70	72	61	266	4·8	—	—	1	2	—	—	—	3	0·0
Other Diseases caused by Infection	32	2	13	18	3	68	1·2	9	101	25	45	64	49	44	337	3·7

TABLE 38 (*contd.*)

Nosological Table showing the Number of Patients treated in the Royal Naval Hospital, Haslar, Gosport during the First World War 1914–1918 and the Second World War 1939–1945

DISEASE OR INJURY	Aug. to Dec. 1914	1915	1916	1917	1918	Total	Cases per 1,000 of Total Admitted	Sept. to Dec. 1939	1940	1941	1942	1943	1944	1945	Total	Cases per 1,000 of Total Admitted
Diseases Caused by Metazoan Parasites	4	20	30	61	67	182	3·3	3	350	839	463	197	92	49	1,993	21·7
DISEASES OF THE NERVOUS SYSTEM:																
Diseases of Spinal Cord	1	3	3	9	10	26	0·5	—	10	19	27	24	20	40	140	1·5
Diseases of Brain	3	7	5	12	8	35	0·6	10	5	6	23	17	17	29	107	1·2
Apoplexy	—	—	1	2	2	5	0·1	—	—	—	—	—	—	—	—	—
Paralysis	4	35	31	44	39	153	2·8	—	13	15	11	20	14	26	99	1·1
Epilepsy	21	79	100	103	104	407	7·4	17	55	59	60	81	51	78	401	4·4
Neurasthenia	10	156	245	336	476	1,223	22·3	7	8	5	3	6	3	2	34	0·4
Other Nervous Diseases (including Mental)	53	411	533	624	625	2,246	40·9	174	796	842	606	600	480	852	4,350	47·5
DISEASES OF THE EYE	26	329	430	418	340	1,543	28·1	45	154	190	222	172	157	212	1,152	12·6
DISEASES OF THE EAR	16	211	263	343	312	1,145	20·8	41	199	309	373	391	305	456	2,074	22·6
DISEASES OF THE NOSE	8	51	74	106	93	332	6·0	24	114	190	239	293	192	260	1,312	14·3
DISEASES OF THE CIRCULATORY SYSTEM:																
Diseases of the Heart (Organic)	19	210	278	274	262	1,043	19·0	27	67	66	60	66	57	69	412	4·5
Diseases of the Heart (Functional)	8	57	103	145	84	397	7·2	21	52	68	101	95	60	49	446	4·9
Diseases of the Arteries	6	12	29	34	22	103	1·9	27	87	96	105	112	123	157	707	7·7
Diseases of the Veins	17	145	156	190	130	638	11·6	31	100	99	193	165	198	467	1,253	13·7
Diseases of the Blood and Blood-forming Organs	2	27	31	40	20	120	2·2	9	41	73	68	25	33	66	315	3·4
Diseases of Glands of Internal Secretion	4	14	33	11	16	78	1·4	6	26	25	28	23	17	37	162	1·8
Diseases of the Breast	—	—	2	—	—	2	0·0	—	7	6	5	5	6	16	45	0·5
DISEASES OF THE RESPIRATORY SYSTEM:																
Diseases of the Larynx	1	11	20	16	9	57	1·0	11	38	15	36	18	16	9	143	1·6
Bronchial Catarrh	—	3	8	7	15	33	0·6	26	36	14	6	17	12	19	130	1·4
Bronchitis	27	130	238	238	221	854	15·5	98	346	337	485	393	275	335	2,269	24·8
Asthma	4	30	30	46	44	154	2·8	11	53	68	72	61	81	113	459	5·0
Fibrosis of Lung	—	—	—	3	2	5	0·1	1	19	193	540	1,324	1,200	297	3,574	39·0
Pleurisy	18	103	171	149	153	594	10·8	17	57	68	125	131	97	65	560	6·1
Other Diseases	4	40	68	56	92	260	4·7	6	151	180	347	478	417	454	2,033	22·2
DISEASES OF TEETH AND GUMS	11	152	219	211	124	717	13·1	1	83	64	113	144	143	161	709	7·7
HERNIA	47	299	389	468	372	1,575	28·7	64	278	423	655	669	424	599	3,112	34·0
HERNIA (Recurrent)	—	2	13	8	9	32	0·6	4	26	21	48	64	41	85	289	3·2

DISEASES OF THE DIGESTIVE SYSTEM:																
Mouth, Palate, Fauces, Pharynx	—	40	21	19	31	111	2·0	59	106	172	165	117	89	67	775	8·5
Peptic Ulcer, Gastric	5	25	50	23	35	138	2·5	54	114	184	97	112	103	223	887	9·7
Peptic Ulcer, Duodenal	5	11	34	25	40	115	2·1	55	248	316	296	259	299	479	1,952	21·3
Appendicitis	21	180	248	214	182	845	15·4	52	180	219	311	448	425	416	2,051	22·4
Other Diseases of the Stomach	20	157	196	240	163	776	14·1	46	267	409	667	508	396	528	2,821	30·8
Other Diseases of the Intestines	21	263	169	114	74	641	11·7	38	182	118	202	198	186	270	1,194	13·0
Diseases of Rectum and Anus	44	182	236	270	238	970	17·7	37	124	170	282	280	191	202	1,286	14·0
Diseases of the Liver	4	122	66	46	28	266	4·8	18	47	145	222	330	168	227	1,157	12·6
Other Diseases	—	23	12	14	22	71	1·3	11	33	20	35	26	43	99	267	2·9
DISEASES OF NUTRITION OR METABOLISM:																
Scurvy	—	3	—	—	—	3	0·1	—	—	1	—	—	—	—	1	0·0
Beri-Beri	—	6	8	11	8	33	0·6	—	—	—	—	—	—	6	6	0·1
Gout	3	20	17	27	10	77	1·4	6	5	10	7	10	7	10	55	0·6
Diabetes	4	12	11	8	8	43	0·8	7	10	23	17	24	28	43	152	1·7
Other Diseases	—	1	13	4	3	21	0·4	1	2	6	3	19	12	48	91	1·0
DISEASES OF GENERATIVE SYSTEM:																
Stricture	14	36	55	58	35	198	3·6	—	—	2	11	10	12	14	49	0·5
Varicocele	1	28	44	93	63	229	4·2	—	12	22	27	26	11	12	110	1·2
Orchitis	—	14	17	16	14	61	1·1	8	7	23	38	14	4	16	110	1·2
Other Diseases	11	50	106	159	128	454	8·3	11	168	205	168	278	239	400	1,469	16·0
DISEASES OF BONES, JOINTS, MUSCLES, FASCIAE AND BURSAE:																
Periosteum and Bone	3	38	44	37	23	145	2·6	11	17	31	26	31	27	60	203	2·2
Cartilage and Joints	22	101	110	128	109	470	8·6	61	129	115	191	133	144	204	977	10·7
Spine	1	7	13	20	10	51	0·9	—	15	20	54	58	23	58	228	2·5
Muscles, Fasciae, Tendons, Bursae	41	355	291	327	170	1,184	21·5	32	104	151	207	172	151	204	1,021	11·1
Deformities and Congenital Malformations	2	53	50	53	48	206	3·7	5	80	159	214	184	94	186	922	10·1
DISEASES OF AREOLAR TISSUE AND SKIN																
Abscess	19	100	102	114	93	428	7·8	—	40	88	152	119	78	112	589	6·4
Boil	5	19	27	42	34	127	2·3	8	29	59	88	65	65	57	371	4·0
Eczema	13	44	56	48	52	213	3·9	10	7	5	9	7	4	34	76	0·8
Impetigo	3	15	17	22	13	70	1·3	4	60	131	132	138	67	62	594	6·5
Other Diseases	14	122	175	246	186	743	13·5	206	314	476	674	696	582	837	3,785	41·3
DISEASES OF URINARY ORGANS:																
Kidneys	13	112	95	135	132	487	8·9	27	95	143	140	169	183	277	1,034	11·3
Ureter and Bladder	6	20	43	43	30	142	2·6	27	72	54	87	79	80	114	513	5·6
Urinary Disorders	2	26	42	49	34	153	2·8	12	16	18	47	44	37	63	237	2·6
NEW GROWTHS, MALIGNANT	—	21	35	31	21	108	2·0	—	35	28	57	69	61	90	340	3·7
NEW GROWTHS, NON-MALIGNANT	—	20	34	40	31	125	2·3	3	77	102	141	184	162	222	891	9·7
ALCOHOLISM	3	18	9	11	6	47	0·9	—	8	3	2	3	7	3	26	0·3
POISONING, VARIOUS	3	6	12	12	42	75	1·4	7	10	16	10	9	3	22	77	0·8

TABLE 38 (cont.)

Nosological Table showing the Number of Patients treated in the Royal Naval Hospital, Haslar, Gosport during the First World War 1914–1918 and the Second World War 1939–1945

DISEASE OR INJURY	Aug. to Dec. 1914	1915	1916	1917	1918	Total	Cases per 1,000 of Total Admitted	Sept. to Dec. 1939	1940	1941	1942	1943	1944	1945	Total	Cases per 1,000 of Total Admitted
GENERAL INJURIES:																
Injuries	213	1,094	1,247	1,219	1,155	4,928	89·7	339	1,466	1,788	2,164	2,223	2,075	2,352	12,407	135·4
Burns and Scalds	18	36	77	59	56	246	4·5	8	31	55	65	86	109	100	454	5·0
Heat Stroke	—	2	24	18	3	47	0·9	—	2	3	2	2	2	2	13	0·1
Sun Stroke	—	14	—	—	—	14	0·3	—	—	—	—	—	—	—	—	—
Effects of Suffocation	—	—	—	—	—	—	—	—	—	—	—	—	—	—	—	—
Compressed Air Disease	—	—	—	—	—	—	—	—	—	—	—	2	1	—	3	0·0
Trench Feet	—	—	—	3	3	6	0·1	—	—	—	—	—	1	—	1	0·0
Trench Fever	—	—	5	4	4	13	0·2	—	—	—	—	—	—	—	—	—
Exposure	—	2	13	4	4	23	0·4	—	—	—	—	—	—	—	—	—
WOUNDS AND INJURIES IN ACTION:	15	824	365	242	212	1,658	30·2	2	802	607	758	344	1,210	257	3,980	43·4
SUICIDES	—	5	1	5	1	12	0·2	—	1	—	1	9	4	1	16	0·2
NO APPRECIABLE DISEASE	—	273	330	375	50	1,028	18·7	—	138	180	245	212	173	372	1,320	14·4
NOT YET DIAGNOSED	14	239	242	277	276	1,048	19·1	—	—	—	—	—	—	—	—	—
PRISONERS OF WAR (REPATRIATED)	—	—	—	—	—	—	—	—	—	—	—	—	128	—	128	1·4
TOTALS	1,362	11,306	13,169	14,956	14,149	54,942	—	2,715	12,491	13,688	15,823	16,163	14,382	16,399	91,661	—

CONCLUSION

Apart from any other factor the disruption of the machinery for producing the Annual Reports on the Health of the Navy during the two World Wars of the 20th Century makes a retrospective comparison of the causes of morbidity, invaliding and deaths in these two wars a somewhat precarious undertaking. The figures for admissions to the Royal Naval Hospital, Haslar, provide the only data which permit one to contrast the pattern of diseases in the Navy throughout the two wars. Those who wish to take the matter further might consult the numerous Medical Officers' Journals or the Death and Invaliding Registers for the war years which are preserved in storage, but this would be a formidable task. There are no intermediate records.

The deliberations of the war-time Committees on Naval Medical Statistics were penetrating and exhaustive and their reports should be consulted in the original by those who have to consider the Navy's needs in the future. For example, the 1946 Committee was well aware that any report on the health of the Navy based on the nosological tables of the Medical Officers' Journals would be at least two years behind the times by the time it was published and furthermore the nosological tables and, therefore, the health of the Navy reports did not include returns for those cases which were not placed on the sick list. Thus, their Report stated:

> 'Summary returns are essential to the work of the Statistics Branch for they alone can provide prompt information on which immediate action can be taken. They enable the Medical Director-General to survey at any moment the health of the fleet and the availability of accommodation for the sick. They have, however, another and most important function, for they are capable of research uses which cannot be met by detailed individual records. . . . A ship is a self-contained community with a relatively stationary population. Hence sickness rates can be readily worked out and related to such factors as ship-design, climatic conditions and the like. . . . While the individual records relate only to sickness sufficiently severe to warrant the excuse of duty, summary returns can incorporate minor sickness which, as it is ten times more frequent, is a far more sensitive indicator of living conditions. . . . We would stress the fact that the standard monthly sickness return can be, and most emphatically should be, a simple document. Very few disease headings are needed and when appropriate books for record-keeping and appropriate forms are available, the rendering of accurate and valuable returns should be a matter of the utmost simplicity. In this connection we would recommend a census system of returns, i.e., the numbers in

any category are counted at a fixed time each week... We recommend that the returns should be made monthly in writing.'

It is significant that 1946 was the year when the first ENIAC computer became available—a development which was eventually to make the central management of such returns not only a more practical proposition but also infinitely less liable to clerical inaccuracies—although this, of course, does not diminish the clerical labour necessary on the periphery to produce summary returns and the need for simplicity in the form of the latter.

REFERENCES

1. Hodge, W. V. (1855), *J.R.Statist.Soc.*, 201 *et seq.*
2. James, W., *Naval History, 1822–1824.*
3. Ellis, F. P. and Rowlands, R. A. (1966), *J. Roy.Nav.Med.Serv.* 52, 5.
4. *Statistical Report of the Health of the Navy for the year 1936* (H.M.S.O., London).
5. *Statistical Report of the Health of the Navy for the years 1953–1956, Admiralty Book of Reference* (B.R.26(I), 1960).
6. Brooks, W. D. W. (1957), *Lancet*, i, 541.
7. *Statistical Report of the Health of the Navy for the year 1914* (H.M.S.O., London).
8. *Statistical Report of the Health of the Navy for the year 1915* (H.M.S.O., London).
9. Ellis, F. P. (1953), *J.Hyg., Camb.* 51, 145.
10. Ellis, F. P. (1955), *J.Hyg., Camb.* 53, 124.

The Army Medical Services

MEDICAL STATISTICS

by Major H. G. Mayne

CONTENTS

Note: In some of the tables, the total of the detail does not agree with that shown. This is due to rates being calculated to the nearest decimal point. The differences are small.

ABBREVIATIONS, TERMS, ETC. USED IN THIS VOLUME

A.D.M.S.	Assistant Director of Medical Services
A.F.	Army Form
A.T.S.	Auxiliary Territorial Service
B.A.	British Army
B.E.F.	British Expeditionary Force
B.N.A. and C.M.F.	British North African and Central Mediterranean Force
B.O.R.	British Other Rank
D.D.M.S.	Deputy Director of Medical Services
D.M.S.	Director of Medical Services
E.A.	Enemy Action (Applied herein to Injuries)
E.A.R.	Equivalent Annual Rate. An annual rate calculated from quarterly rates or from less than twelve months of the year.
E.A.O.R.	East African Other Rank
E.M.S.	Emergency Medical Services
E.N.T.	Ear, Nose and Throat
G.H.Q.	General Headquarters
Hallux V. etc.	Includes *Hallux Valgus, Varus, Flexus and Rigidus*
I.A.	Indian Army
I.A.T.	Inflammation of the Areolar Tissue
I.D.K.	Internal Derangement of the knee. Includes: Internal Derangement of the knee and other joints. Subluxation of the intra-articular cartilage. Rupture of the intra-articular cartilage. Ruptured crucial ligament of the knee, and loose body.
I.M.N.S.	Indian Military Nursing Service
I.O.R.	Indian Other Rank
Malaria, B.T.	Malaria—Benign Tertian
Malaria, M.T.	Malaria—Malignant Tertian
Malaria, Q.	Malaria,—Quartan
M.E.F.	Middle East Force
M.M.R.	Mean Monthly Rate. A rate adjusted to correspond with that for a month of fixed length 30·5 days, almost one-twelfth of a calendar year.
Morbidity	Sickness from disease as opposed to injury.
N.A.	Not applicable
N.Cs.(E.)	Non Combatants (enrolled). Menials employed in the Indian Army and formerly known as Followers.
N.E.A.	Non-Enemy Action. Applied herein to Injuries
N.V.	Non-Venereal

N.W.E.	North West Europe
N.Y.D.	Not yet diagnosed
O.2.E.	Officer in charge of Second Echelon
O.R.	Other Rank
P.A.I.C.	Persia and Iraq Command
P.U.O.	Pyrexia of Unknown Origin
Q.A.I.M.N.S.	Queen Alexandra's Imperial Military Nursing Service
S.E.A.C.	South East Asia Command
V.A.D.	Voluntary Aid Detachment
V.C.O.	Viceroy's Commissioned Officer. Roughly analogous to a Warrant Officer in the British Army.
V.D.	Venereal Disease
W.A.C.(I.)	Women's Auxiliary Corps (India)
W.A.O.R.	West African Other Ranks

INTRODUCTION

Health statistics of the civilian population as a whole are limited to the diagnoses of deaths and certain notifiable infectious diseases. This is primarily due to the fact that no machinery has as yet been devised for the collection of the relevant statistical raw material. In the army, however, medical statistics are limited only by the efficiency of the administrative machine in ensuring that medical documents are correctly completed and sent to their destination promptly and safely.

For the following reasons, the Army can offer far more avenues for fruitful medical statistical research than does the civilian population:

(a) Every medical unit which treats a soldier completes a *standard* form which is available for statistical purposes. (Statistics in respect of those treated in civil hospitals have hitherto been virtually unobtainable for the whole civilian population due in great part to their basic material being so diverse in character and content that collection, collation, interpretation and publication were not possible.)

(b) Soldiers are admitted to military medical units for minor diseases which, in a civilian population, would be treated at home.

The work of the Army Medical Services is at the same time more limited and more specialised, being restricted with regard to age, physique and, to a certain degree, sex. It is more extensively concerned with those tropical and sub-tropical diseases which are encountered so seldom, if at all, by doctors in civil life.

For convenience, the functions of Army Medical Statistics may be grouped under three heads:

(a) *Current Administration*, e.g. incidence of disease; bedstate information, allocation of hospital accommodation; the assessment of non-effectiveness of personnel on medical grounds.

(b) *Long term planning*, e.g. determination of major sources of medical wastage among different types of personnel in different countries; the relation of age and sex to wastage, special risks associated with different trades, arms of service, and ethnic groups.

(c) *Research*, e.g. the assessment of the efficacy of therapeutic measures; research in aetiology and epidemiology of diseases.

Before the reorganisation of the Army medical statistical machinery in 1943, its activities were confined almost exclusively to current administration. Compared with the major developments which were then instituted, the evolution of these statistics was slow. The Army was a pioneer in this field and it will not be uninteresting to trace its development.

Two early works which deserve attention are Sir John Pringle's *On the Diseases of the Army*, published in 1752, which drew attention to the connexion between dirt and disease, and Munro's *Account of the Diseases which were most frequent in British Military Hospitals in Germany from 1761 to 1763*, published in 1764. It was through the initiative of Munro that admission and discharge books were introduced into Army hospitals.

Some years later, Alexander Tulloch became interested in Army mortality in connexion with the problem of Army pensions. He extended his interests and, in collaboration with Thomas Balfour, published a series of reports dealing with the health of troops serving in different countries. These published reports were among the earliest British vital statistics; they were certainly the earliest among the Armed Forces. The Navy followed the Army's lead, as did, in due course, the American, French, Italian and Prussian forces.

The public clamour over the conditions in Army hospitals in the Crimea led to the establishment of an investigating committee, among the members of which were Sidney Herbert and Alexander Tulloch. Their conclusions, which were published in 1861 as the *Report of the Committee on the preparaticn of A1my Medical Statistics and on the duties to be performed by the Statistical Branch of the Army Medical Department* outlined the statistical policy to be followed. The first Annual Report on the Health of the Army for that year was produced. Such reports have been published for each succeeding year, except during the First World War and during the years 1938 to 1945.

Although the reforms introduced were a considerable achievement, the Army medical statistical machine was not devised to cope with the conditions which arose early in the Second World War. Many serious problems obtruded themselves and it is of interest to investigate the difficulties of the organisation, examine the methods by which they were overcome and trace the development of the system throughout the war.

Before the outbreak of war, the very few soldiers who were admitted to civilian hospitals were transferred to military hospitals as soon as circumstances permitted. With the creation of the Emergency Medical Services, civilian hospitals, from late in 1939, played an increasingly greater part in the medical care of Service men and women, until a high proportion of military patients in the United Kingdom were in civil hospitals.

At the outset, these hospitals were entirely outside the control of the army medical authorities. They were thus not obliged to comply with the army methods of medical documentation and system of returns and it became necessary to obtain information regarding admissions, discharges and transfers of military patients. This was done by means of E.M.S. Form 105 (Form 404 in Scotland), an administrative form completed by E.M.S. hospitals. Except for a diagnosis, the forms contained no medical data. As they were rendered for discharges as well as admissions, and as regimental particulars were often incorrect, the task of collating the many thousands of forms received was formidable. The information from this source was entirely unsuitable and insufficient from a medical point of view.

In addition to the receipt of these forms, Medical Record Cards (A.F. I.1220) were submitted for all Army patients in military hospitals at home and abroad. These cards were initiated when a patient was received as a direct admission or transferred to a military hospital and sent to the War Office when discharged or transferred. There would thus be in existence more than one card for a patient transferred from the military hospital which originally admitted him. The cards contained, in addition to regimental particulars, medical case notes.

The sorting of the Army and E.M.S. forms provided another problem. Manual sorting, hitherto employed and suitable for small numbers, was hopelessly inadequate for the greatly increased numbers arriving daily at the War Office. The introduction of the Hollerith punched card system, with the formulation of the necessary codes to cover all the items of administrative and medical interest, assisted in some measure the task of sorting and collating information. Because the forms did not always represent complete hospital cases, all methods of collation which were tried failed to produce satisfactory results.

It was clear that adequate medical statistics could not be obtained unless E.M.S. hospitals were persuaded to adopt the army method of documentation for their military patients and unless arrangements could be made for one set of Medical Record Cards for one patient to be submitted on final discharge from hospital irrespective of the number of transfers between hospitals. In so far as military hospitals were concerned, the latter was purely a medical administrative problem and easily resolved. Negotiations with the E.M.S. authorities for their hospitals to adopt military documentation for military patients were successful, arrangements being made for the new system to commence in September 1942.

From then, it became possible to produce more reliable statistics, but due to a variety of reasons, a deficiency of Hollerith cards existed, *vis à vis* patients admitted to hospitals. Among these may be instanced,

(a) Losses in transit from overseas of A.Fs. I.1220, due to enemy action.

(b) The highly mobile conditions of warfare.

(c) Failure through enemy action or other causes to send record cards to the War Office.

(d) The lack of experience, from an administrative point of view, of many medical officers and their omission to initiate the cards.

(e) The impossibility, at least initially, of complete and effective control over the administration of military patients in civil hospitals.

There was also the possibility of a slight leakage in the War Office.

A further difficulty arose in that labour problems caused a serious backlog in coding of documents and the punching of Hollerith cards. From September 1944, and throughout the remainder of the war, coding was restricted, in the case of the United Kingdom to ten per cent. of cases, and for other major commands twenty or fifty per cent.

Because of these deficiencies and restrictions, in the following chapters where statistics emanating from the punched card system are used, some assessment is made of the deficiency involved.

The above refers to personal medical records, complete statistics from which cannot be prepared until patients have been discharged from hospital, in some cases many months after admission. To provide a rapid flow of medical statistics regarding the incidence of disease, deaths, and bedstates, military hospitals before the war were required to submit, monthly, a return (A.F. A31) giving, *inter alia*, the numbers admitted, by disease, deaths, etc. This return, at least in the United Kingdom, was cancelled early in the war in an over-enthusiastic attempt to save paper work. No adequate substitutes were introduced until after the war, although many returns were initiated, modified and subsequently cancelled.

In some commands overseas, where A.F. A31, or modified versions thereof, obtained before the war, notably in India and Egypt, the form continued to be used and was the basic medical statistical return throughout the war. Indeed, it was adapted for use in a new command, South-East Asia, on the Indo-Burma Front and in Ceylon. In other overseas commands, e.g. North Africa and Central Mediterranean Force and North-West Europe, medical statistical returns were of local pattern and bore little or no resemblance to A.F. A31 either in format or content. The difficulties in checking and consolidating forms of such differing patterns were many and it does not seem unreasonable to suggest that the same form of medical statistics could have been used throughout the world wherever British soldiers were stationed. This practice obtains to-day. One disadvantage of the lack of a standard return is illustrated in the following pages where the make-up of tabulations presented for the Middle East (based on A.F. A31) differs from those for South-East Asia Command (modified A.F. A31) and again from those for the North Africa and Central Mediterranean Force (based on local returns).

Basic military medical statistics required from hospitals and other medical units fall into four main categories:

(a) Bedstate information (not available for inclusion in this volume).

(b) Admissions (but not transfers) by diagnoses.

(c) Deaths, by causes.

(d) (in overseas commands only) Transfers to the United Kingdom on medical grounds, by diagnoses.

Returns from Commands and Forces lacked much of this information. Those from one force contained numbers (without diagnoses) recommended for transfer to the United Kingdom on medical grounds and however valuable the information was at force headquarters its usefulness at the War Office was questionable. Statistics now received in the War Office contain all the above information on forms standard in all Commands.

Statistics relating to discharges from the Army on medical grounds presented little difficulty in their collection. All such discharges took place in the United Kingdom following military medical boards. They were carried out by military medical authorities either at military or E.M.S. hospitals, the latter under the administration of Military Registrars. In 1942 a special report (A.F. B3978) was introduced to record information regarding each discharge. This form was completed by the presidents of medical boards and sent to the War Office. It formed the basic data for the punched card index of medical discharges. This index was the only exception to the restriction on coding, and from its inception there was a full coding of the reports until the end of the war, and subsequently.

The Director-General, Army Medical Services, in 1943, called for a special report on the existing statistical machine and for the purpose the services of Professor Lancelot Hogben, F.R.S., was placed at the disposal of the War Office by the University of Birmingham. Consequent upon the report submitted, the statistical branch was merged into the Directorate of Biological Research (later renamed the Directorate of Medical (Statistical) Research) with Brigadier F. A. E. Crew, F.R.S., as Director and Professor Hogben as Deputy Director. The directorate was given wider terms of reference with a greatly increased technical staff. It was then increasingly possible to deal with statistical matters other than current medical administration and a programme of research was initiated. Results of these activities in the extended field were published in monthly Bulletins of Army Health Statistics inaugurated in January 1945. Included therein were also statistics relating to current administration. The main papers in these Bulletins were later incorporated in the *Statistical Report on the Health of the Army, 1943–45*, published by H.M.S.O. in 1948.

As previously noted, annual reports on the Health of the Army were not published during the war years. The 1943–45 Report did not bridge the gap from a statistical point of view in that it covered only three years and was not a comprehensive work with a detailed morbidity survey covering, at least, all the large commands. For the same reason it could not be accepted, important as it was, as the Army contribution to the statistical volume in the Official Medical History of the War series.

The present contribution includes as much material as possible that was not published in the 1943–45 Report. In compiling morbidity statistics, it was the intention to use, whenever the basic data so lent itself, the conventional yardstick of medical statistics, the rate for 1,000 of the population at risk (the Report dealt mainly with relative rates). This was found possible for all Commands dealt with herein, except for West Africa. Here, the basic materials were the Annual Hygiene Reports which contained no crude figures for admissions to hospitals, etc., but only relative rates. In passing, it may be mentioned that only in the chapter relating to West Africa are there some tables identical with those in the 1943–45 Report. This is due to the somewhat limited annual reports for that Command being used as basic data for both purposes.

Because of the limitations inherent in the medical index of punched cards at the War Office, it was felt that, wherever possible, reliance should be placed upon returns and reports and only where no adequate or reliable statistics could be obtained from these sources should calculations based on Hollerith tabulations be used. Sufficient data was found to provide material for the chapters relating to the Middle East Force, North Africa and Central Mediterranean Force, East and West Africa Commands, India, the Indo-Burma Front and Ceylon. The search for records relating to other spheres of activities proved disappointing and a combination of Hollerith tabulations and other data is used for chapters relating to the B.E.F. France and North-West Europe. Only for the United Kingdom and the chapter relating to discharges from the Army on medical grounds are statistics based on Hollerith tabulations. It was disappointing, too, that no reliable, accurate, and complete statistical data existed for such campaigns as Greece and Crete (1941), Greece (1944), Norway, Arakan, etc. Statistics in respect of these were merged into those of the Force or Command which supplied the forces operating there.*

---

* Some statistical data for these campaigns may be found in the Army Medical Services, Campaigns volumes in this series.

The geographical disposition of the Army and the channels of communication, suggest that the logical manner of treatment of Army Medical Statistics would be on similar lines. This has been followed in the present volume. In dealing with the Middle East Force, it was found to be possible to divide the statistics into smaller geographical (command) groups. Further, in some commands, where Colonial and Dominion troops were serving with British, it has been possible to discuss the special medical risks which attach to each different ethnic group.

It may not be out of place to mention here some of the outstanding features recorded in the following pages. In so far as admissions for diseases are concerned, the highest recorded rate among British Troops occurred in 1943 on the Indo-Burma Front when the exceptionally high figure of 1,746 per 1,000 other ranks was registered. In the following year the rate fell to 1,334 and, in 1945, to 780, less than half the peak rate. Admissions for disease in Ceylon also registered a high rate, that of 1,094 per 1,000 in 1942, but by 1945 it had fallen to just over one-half at 584. Perhaps the healthiest of the larger overseas commands was the Middle East where the rate of admission for disease ranged from a peak of 677 in 1941 to 380 per 1,000 in 1945.

The remarkable decline in admissions on the Indo-Burma Front and in Ceylon were mainly due to the dramatic reduction in the incidence of malaria, which was not confined to these two Commands. Admission rates per 1,000 strength for malaria among British Troops were as follows:

	1942	1943	1944	1945
Indo-Burma Front	335	628	406	128
Ceylon	278	254	82	36
India	164	198	248	131
North Africa and Central Mediterranean . .	—	—	76	19
Middle East . . .	27	24	42	22

On the Indo-Burma Front, the peak rate of 628 per 1,000 in 1943 was reduced by four-fifths in two years. In Ceylon the peak figure of 278 in 1942 was reduced to approximately one-eighth by 1945. The decline in India in 1945 was nearly fifty per cent. of the rate obtaining in the previous year. A record low rate of 34 per 1,000 was reached in 1946 which compares very favourably with the pre-war figure of 50 per 1,000 in 1938. The figures from the Middle East and Central Mediterranean also show reductions in 1945, the former by one-half and the latter by three-quarters of the peak rates, both of which occurred in 1944. These striking results are not only a tribute to medical science but also to the Army Medical Services through anti-malaria training and discipline among all ranks, the suppressive treatment enforced and to the work of Anti-Malaria Units of which one hundred and fifteen were operating in India, Burma and Ceylon when the war ended.

Another factor in the decline of admissions on the Indo-Burma Front was the reduction in the number of dysentery cases by fifty per cent. in two years. The peak rate of 132 per 1,000 was followed by 97 in 1944 and 65 in 1945. A reduction in admissions for dysentery also occurred in the Central Mediterranean where a rate of 4 in 1945 was preceded by 12 per 1,000. In the other tropical and sub-tropical commands no reduction was witnessed.

In all major commands except one, the incidence of admissions for mental diseases increased annually with the peak rate in 1945. The exception was in the Middle East where yearly declines followed the peak rate in 1942. Rates per 1,000 were as follows:

	1940	1942	1945
Indo-Burma Front . .	—	3	23
India	3	5	13
Ceylon	—	5	10
Middle East . . .	6	20	5
United Kingdom . .	4	7	8

The reasons for these increases were probably the cumulative effect of the stress and strain of war coupled with more accurate diagnoses following the increase in the number of psychiatrists available.

In Chapter XI is discussed the recovery rate of those other ranks wounded in North-West Europe from the landings in Normandy to the cessation of fighting. It is noted there that deaths from wounds was seven per cent., so that the chances of survival after being wounded were ninety-three per cent. Invalidings from the Army of these soldiers accounted for fourteen per cent., so that from the Army point of view of wastage, the recovery rate was seventy-nine per cent. Many of those wounded were, however, fit for some degree of civil employment and if a disability of forty per cent. or less is taken as the criterion for a reasonably wide range of employment, one third of the injured made a good recovery. Thus, with deaths from wounds at seven per cent. and invalids fit for no employment or in a restricted capacity at nine per cent., the recovery rate was eighty four per cent.

The first chapter deals with diseases and injuries of British troops in the United Kingdom. This is followed by one relating to the British Expeditionary Force to France in 1939 and those to other commands and forces overseas according to their proximity to England. Finally, a chapter on discharges from the Army on medical grounds is presented. Due to the non-availability of data, it is not possible to include an account of the morbidity of the entire British Army for the war years.

CHAPTER I

THE UNITED KINGDOM

THE STATISTICS which follow emanate from tabulations produced by the Hollerith Section of the War Office. In spite of the known limitations of these tabulations, this course was inevitable, and was entirely due to there being no other sources from which the information could be obtained. Up to 1940, statistical data regarding admissions to and deaths in hospital, etc., were received in the War Office monthly. In 1940 these returns were cancelled and no satisfactory substitute was provided.

From the outbreak of war, Service patients were admitted to hospitals under the aegis of the Emergency Medical Services as well as to Service hospitals. No returns or Hospital Record Cards (A.F.I.1220) in respect of Army patients were received from E.M.S. Hospitals until 1942, when such hospitals were persuaded to compile A.Fs. I.1220 for these patients. As these cards are the basic data from which information is transferred to Hollerith punched cards, it follows that the Hollerith tabulations for 1940 to 1942 contain data relating only to:

(*a*) those admitted to Military Hospitals and

(*b*) those transferred from other types of hospitals in the United Kingdom, including those of the E.M.S.

They do not include patients treated exclusively in E.M.S. Hospitals.* The tabulations for the years 1943 to 1945 include all known Army patients admitted to all types of hospitals in the United Kingdom.

The number of Army patients admitted to E.M.S. Hospitals in 1943 and 1944 are known and the following analysis shows these admissions as a percentage of those recorded on Hollerith cards.

Class of Troops	1943	1944
Males . .	57	55
Females . .	68	66
All . . .	58	57

The tabulations relating to admissions to hospitals do not include any patients transferred from hospitals outside the United Kingdom. Such casualties are rightly included in the statistics of the overseas command in which they originated. On the other hand, any such patients

* *See* Emergency Medical Services, Part I. Service Patients, pp. 647 *et seq.*

transferred who subsequently died while still serving are included in the mortality tabulations in this section.

Initially, a Hollerith card was punched for all A.Fs. I.1220 received in the War Office. As from September 1, 1944, however, in an effort to conserve labour and supplies, it was decided to code and punch only ten per cent. of these forms. Furthermore, the amount of information to be transferred to the Hollerith cards was restricted to ten items, instead of the twenty-one previously coded.

The decision to restrict the punching of cards to a ten per cent. sample was implemented by selecting A.Fs. I.1220 of those patients, the Army or personal number of whom ended with the digit 5.

Among the information not now coded under the new procedure was 'Result on Discharge'. This stated whether the patient was returned to his unit, died, or was discharged from the Army as an invalid. Consequent upon this, it is not possible to present annual mortality rates after 1943.

As there are no data in existence to act as controls, it cannot be ascertained what discrepancy exists, if any, in the number of A.Fs. I.1220 received, and that appearing in the Hollerith tabulations, neither is it possible to proffer any estimate, within reasonable limits. For what it is worth, however, it has been calculated that the deficiency in Hollerith cards *vis à vis* A.Fs. I.1220 relating to patients admitted to hospitals in North-West Europe, was in the region of twenty per cent. (*see* 'North-West Europe', Chapter III). It is known that the number of admissions during 1946 in the United Kingdom listed in the Hollerith tabulations was less than that enumerated in returns from hospitals by approximately thirty per cent. of the total recorded in the tabulations.

In calculating annual rates, annual strengths obtained from the mean of average quarterly strengths were used. These annual strengths fluctuated somewhat, being highest in 1941 and 1942 and lowest in 1945. If the 1940 strength is taken as 100, variations are as below:

Variations in Strength of British Troops in the United Kingdom

	Male			Female
Year	Officers	Other Ranks	All Ranks	All Ranks
1940	100	100	100	100
1941	157	137	138	173
1942	163	134	136	447
1943	147	118	119	652
1944	135	101	102	655
1945	99	79	80	537

To summarise, Hollerith tabulations for admissions to, and deaths in, hospitals in the United Kingdom suffer from the following defects, which apply to members of both the male and female Services:

(*a*) Admissions to, and deaths in, E.M.S. Hospitals from the outbreak of war to some time in 1942 are not included.

(*b*) An unknown number of transfers from E.M.S. to Military Hospitals from January 1940 to August 1942 and included in the Hollerith tabulations tends to reduce the overall discrepancy.

(*c*) From September 1944, only ten per cent. of admissions were coded.

(*d*) There is a strong possibility that the Hollerith tabulations are deficient by at least twenty per cent.

(*e*) Deaths were not coded from September 1944.

(*f*) There may be a small deficiency in Hollerith cards, *vis à vis* A.Fs. I.1220 received in the War Office.

Any discussion on the statistics which follow must necessarily be limited by these factors.

Tabulations, separately for the male and female Services, are presented in respect of:

(*a*) Rates of admissions to hospitals per 1,000 strength annually, 1940 to 1945, by causes.

(*b*) Relative rates of admissions annually, by causes.

(*c*) Comparative rates of admissions annually, by causes.

(*d*) Breakdown of admissions to hospitals for injuries.

(*e*) Average rates of admissions to hospitals, by causes, for the six years 1940 to 1945.

(*f*) Relative Mortality Rates, annually, 1940–43.

In the tabulations relating to comparative rates of admissions, 1943 has been taken as the base year, because this year was the first full year in which admissions to all types of hospitals are known.

It is emphasised that the statistics in this chapter deal with admissions to and deaths in hospitals only. Admissions to other medical units, except where they result in transfers to hospitals are not included. Care should therefore be exercised in comparing rates herein with those in post-war annual reports which sometimes include in their totals admissions to all medical units.

Advantage is being taken of including herein a tabulation of admissions to hospitals in 1939, hitherto unpublished.

BRITISH MALE TROOPS

Rates of admission to hospitals in the United Kingdom of British Army males, based on Hollerith tabulations, are presented in Tables 1 to 6. Table 2 records rates per 1,000 strength, Table 3 cites relative rates and Table 4 compares admissions in 1943 with those of the other years under review. Table 4 records the average rates of admission for the six years, while Tables 5 and 6 present a breakdown of admissions through injury. Mortality rates for the years 1940 to 1945 are exhibited in Tables 7 and 8. Admission rates for 1939 are included as Table 16.

Because of the limitations mentioned in the preamble to this chapter, it is not considered advisable to use the rates cited as morbidity rates without adjustment. For this purpose, and as a rough guide, it is suggested that the following correction factors will neutralise the deficiencies to a great extent.

1940 and 1941—between 2·0 and 2·5
1942 —between 1·5 and 2·0
1943 to 1945 —1·3

Exceptions to this are the rates for Mental and Venereal Diseases. Patients suffering from these diseases passed through military hospitals during the course of their treatment and are thus recorded in the tabulations. Because of this the correction factor of 1·3 should be applied to these disease rates in all years.

Admissions for diseases only ranged from 103 per 1,000 in 1941 to 153 in 1945, while those for injuries varied from 5 in 1940 to 19 in 1943. Admissions on account of injuries comprised from five to eleven per cent. of the total.

Relevant rates, to the nearest whole number, were as follows:

United Kingdom, 1940–45
Rates of Admissions to Hospitals, British Troops, Male

Source: Hollerith Tabulations

Year	Rates per 1,000 Strength			Relative Rates			Comparative Rates		
	Disease	Injury	Totals	Disease	Injury	Totals	Disease	Injury	Totals
1940	105	5	110	95	5	100	72	29	67
1941	103	6	109	94	6	100	71	34	66
1942	137	16	152	90	10	100	94	83	93
1943	146	19	164	89	11	100	100	100	100
1944	129	16	144	89	11	100	88	83	88
1945	153	18	170	90	10	100	105	94	104

The highest recorded annual rate was in 1945 at 170 per 1,000. In the same year was registered the highest rate of admissions for diseases only, 153 per 1,000, while the peak of admissions on account of injuries occurred in 1943 at 19 per 1,000. Injuries were responsible for five and six per cent. of admissions in 1940 and 1941 and ten and eleven per cent. for the remainder of the years. Over the period there was recorded an average rate of 129 for disease and 13 for injury, a total of 142 per 1,000.

Applying the correction factors noted above, adjusted admission rates per 1,000 strengths would be in the region of

1940—between 220 and 275
1941—between 220 and 275
1942—between 230 and 305
1943—213
1944—187
1945—221

DISEASES OF THE DIGESTIVE SYSTEM

Of individual diseases and disease groups, Diseases of the Digestive System were responsible for the highest rates of admissions, being fifty per cent. more than those for Diseases of the Skin, which followed in order of numerical importance. Recorded rates ranged from 14 per 1,000 in 1940 and 1941 to 23 in 1945. Expressed as a percentage of admissions for disease, these rates represent 13 in 1940, and 15 per cent. in 1943 and 1945. The average rate of admission over the six years was 19 per 1,000. An analysis of admissions for this group of diseases follows on page 112.

Numerically, HERNIAS were the most important contributory cause of admissions in this group of diseases. Rates varied from 3 per 1,000 in 1940 to 7 in 1945. The 1943 rate of 5·8 fell to 4·4 in the following year but increased to 6·9 in 1945. Expressed as percentages of the total of the group, the 1940 and 1944 admissions represent twenty-four, the 1941 and 1943 admissions twenty-six, those for 1942 twenty-seven, while admissions in 1945 were some thirty per cent. The average rate over the six years at just under 5 per 1,000 was slightly in excess of one quarter the total of the group. Admissions in 1944 were three quarters of and, in 1945, one-fifth more than the rates for 1943.

Next in order of numerical importance were admissions in respect of DYSPEPSIA and GASTRITIS. Rates which varied slightly throughout the six years, increased from 2·8 in 1940 to 3·8 in 1942 then declined each year to a final 2·7 per 1,000 in 1945. The relative rates are interesting in that they exhibit a decline each year from twenty one per cent. in 1941 to eleven in 1945. Admission rates for 1944 and 1945 were slightly less than three-quarters that for 1943.

Admissions for APPENDICITIS were, on the average, one half those for HERNIAS. Apart from slight declines in 1941 and 1944, rates increased annually from 1·8 in 1940 to 3·7 in 1945. The rate in 1943 was a little under 1 per 1,000 less than that in 1945. Admissions over the period were some thirteen per cent. of the group total. In 1944 the relative rate increased by one per cent. to fourteen and this was followed by sixteen

United Kingdom, 1940–45

Admissions to Hospitals for Diseases of the Digestive System. British Troops, Male Annual Rates per 1,000 Strength with Relative and Comparative Rates

Source: Hollerith Tabulations

1. *Annual Rates per 1,000 Strength*	1940	1941	1942	1943	1944	1945	Averages
Gastric Ulcers	0·44	0·30	0·22	0·31	0·27	0·35	0·32
Duodenal Ulcers	1·44	1·23	1·07	1·43	1·41	1·70	1·38
Peptic Ulcers, Unspecified	0·40	0·18	0·08	0·08	0·10	0·20	0·17
Perforation of Ulcers	0·07	0·11	0·11	0·17	0·17	0·25	0·15
Dyspepsia and Gastritis	2·80	2·87	3·79	3·69	2·67	2·67	3·08
Hernia	3·27	3·61	5·68	5·82	4·40	6·93	4·95
Appendicitis	1·80	1·58	2·66	2·77	2·55	3·66	2·50
Haemorrhoids	0·88	1·18	2·26	2·39	1·89	2·13	1·79
Other Causes	2·66	2·85	5·31	5·30	4·75	5·57	4·41
Totals	13·76	13·91	21·18	21·96	18·21	23·46	18·75
Percentages of total admissions for diseases	13	14	15	15	14	15	15
2. *Relative Rates*							
Gastric Ulcers	3	2	1	1	1	1	2
Duodenal Ulcers	11	9	5	7	8	7	7
Peptic Ulcers, Unspecified	3	1	0·4	0·4	1	1	1
Perforation of Ulcers	1	1	0·5	1	1	1	1
Dyspepsia and Gastritis	20	21	18	17	15	11	16
Hernia	24	26	27	26	24	30	26
Appendicitis	13	11	13	13	14	16	13
Haemorrhoids	6	8	11	11	10	9	10
Other Causes	19	21	25	24	26	24	24
Totals	100	100	100	100	100	100	100
3. *Comparative Rates* (1943 = 100)							
Gastric Ulcers	142	97	73	100	87	113	
Duodenal Ulcers	101	86	75	100	99	119	
Peptic Ulcers, Unspecified	500	225	100	100	125	150	
Perforation of Ulcers	41	65	65	100	100	147	
Dyspepsia and Gastritis	76	78	103	100	72	72	
Hernia	56	62	98	100	76	119	
Appendicitis	65	57	96	100	92	132	
Haemorrhoids	37	49	95	100	79	89	
Other Causes	50	54	100	100	90	105	
Totals	63	63	96	100	83	107	

per cent. In contrast to this the comparative rate in 1944 fell from 100 to 92 and increased to 132 in 1945.

Rates of admissions on account of HAEMORRHOIDS increased from an initial low figure of just under 1 per 1,000 to 2·4 in 1943, declined to 1·9 in 1944 and finally registered 2·1 per 1,000 in 1945. The average rate of 1·8 was ten per cent. of the group total. The admission rate in 1944 was slightly over three-quarters that in the previous year and the rate in 1945 was also lower, by approximately one-tenth.

Of admissions for Ulcers, those for DUODENAL ULCERS were the more numerous, being twice the total of the remainder. Admissions declined from 1·4 in 1940 to 1·1 in 1942, then increased to 1·7 in 1945. They contributed, on the average, some seven per cent. of the total admissions of the group. A similar trend in admissions was exhibited by both GASTRIC and UNSPECIFIED PEPTIC ULCERS in that a decline from 1940 to the mid-years of the period was followed by annual increases. The average rate of admissions for Gastric Ulcers was 0·3 per 1,000, while that for unspecified Peptic Ulcers was 0·2. Admissions for PERFORATED ULCERS increased steadily from 0·07 in 1940 to 0·25 in 1945 with an average rate of 0·17 per 1,000 which represented one per cent. of the group total.

DISEASES OF THE SKIN

Following diseases of the Digestive System in order of numerical importance came Diseases of the Skin, admission rates for which increased from 8 per 1,000 in 1940 to 16 in 1943, then fell to 14 in 1945. These admissions, which averaged approximately ten per cent. of all admissions for diseases are analysed in the tables on page 114.

One quarter of admissions of this group were attributable to IMPETIGO, rates for which increased from 2·5 per 1,000 in 1940 to a peak of 4·5 in 1942. Thereafter admissions declined from 4·2 in 1943 to 2·2 in 1945. They were approximately one-third of the total for the group in the first three years, one-quarter in 1943 and one-sixth in 1945. With admissions for Dermatitis, they accounted for nearly one-half of the total for the group.

DERMATITIS was responsible for one-fifth of admissions for the group. Apart from a slight fall in 1944, rates increased steadily over the years from 1·5 in 1940 to 3·3 in 1943 and 3·7 in 1945, with an average of 2·6 per 1,000. Relative rates ranged between 15 in 1942 and 26 in 1943. Compared with 1943, admissions were seven per cent. lower in 1944, but twelve per cent. higher in 1945.

Although admissions for BOILS fluctuated between 0·6 in 1940 to 1·35 in 1943, expressed as a proportion of group admissions, they were stable at eight per cent. in the first two and nine per cent. each in the following four years. The rate in 1944 (1·17) was six-sevenths that in 1943 and in 1945 it was slightly less, by two per cent., of 1943 admissions, at 1·32. The average rate for the six years was 1 per 1,000.

Diseases of the SEBACEOUS GLANDS were responsible for seven per cent. of the group admissions at rates which, commencing at 0·4 reached 1·3 in 1943 before declining to 1·1 in 1945, averaging 0·9 per 1,000 over the six years. ECZEMA, next in numerical importance, caused an average rate of 0·8 over the period. Annual rates commenced at 0·5 in 1940 and increased annually to just over 1 per 1,000 in 1945.

United Kingdom, 1940–45
Admissions to Hospitals for Diseases of the Skin. British Troops, Male
Annual Rates per 1,000 Strength with Relative and Comparative Rates

Source: Hollerith Tabulations

1. *Annual Rates per 1,000 Strength*	1940	1941	1942	1943	1944	1945	Averages
Impetigo	2·51	3·21	4·47	4·19	2·91	2·23	3·25
Dermatitis	1·53	1·90	2·09	3·34	3·09	3·73	2·61
Boils	0·64	0·79	1·16	1·35	1·17	1·32	1·07
Carbuncles	0·26	0·27	0·60	0·72	0·60	0·84	0·55
Eczema	0·47	0·56	0·77	1·00	0·98	1·06	0·81
Warts	0·14	0·29	0·45	0·61	0·57	0·69	0·46
Psoriasis	0·25	0·31	0·45	0·53	0·37	0·63	0·42
Tinea	0·53	0·67	0·79	0·71	0·38	0·39	0·58
Diseases of the:							
Sebaceous Glands	0·41	0·60	1·05	1·29	1·06	1·13	0·92
Sweat Glands and Ducts	0·03	0·03	0·05	0·13	0·08	0·14	0·08
Hair and Follicles	0·26	0·38	0·48	0·48	0·42	0·38	0·40
Nails	0·02	0·01	0·01	0·02	0·02	0·03	0·02
Other Causes	0·73	0·80	1·23	1·51	1·32	1·59	1·20
Totals	7·78	9·82	13·60	15·88	12·97	14·16	12·37
Percentages of total admissions for diseases	7	10	9	11	10	9	10
2. *Relative Rates*							
Impetigo	32	33	33	26	22	16	26
Dermatitis	20	19	15	21	24	26	21
Boils	8	8	9	9	9	9	9
Carbuncles	3	3	4	5	5	6	4
Eczema	6	6	6	6	8	7	7
Warts	2	3	3	4	4	5	4
Psoriasis	3	3	3	3	3	4	3
Tinea	7	7	6	4	3	3	5
Diseases of the:							
Sebaceous Glands	5	6	8	8	8	8	7
Sweat Glands and Ducts	0·4	0·3	0·4	0·8	0·6	1	1
Hair and Follicles	3	4	4	3	3	3	3
Nails	0·2	0·1	0·1	0·1	0·2	0·2	0·2
Other Causes	9	8	9	10	10	11	10
Totals	100	100	100	100	100	100	100
3. *Comparative Rates* (1943 = 100)							
Impetigo	60	77	107	100	69	53	
Dermatitis	46	57	63	100	93	112	
Boils	47	59	86	100	87	98	
Carbuncles	36	38	83	100	83	117	
Eczema	47	56	77	100	98	106	
Warts	23	48	74	100	93	113	
Psoriasis	47	58	85	100	70	119	
Tinea	75	94	111	100	54	55	
Diseases of the:							
Sebaceous Glands	32	47	81	100	82	88	
Sweat Glands and Ducts	23	23	38	100	62	108	
Hair and Follicles	54	79	100	100	88	79	
Nails	100	50	50	100	100	150	
Other Causes	48	53	81	100	87	105	
Totals	49	62	86	100	82	89	

Rates of admission increased over the years for the following:

	which increased from	*with an average of*
CARBUNCLES	0·26 to 0·84	0·55
WARTS	0·14 to 0·69	0·46
PSORIASIS	0·25 to 0·63	0·42
Diseases of the		
HAIR AND FOLLICLES	0·26 to 0·38	0·40
SWEAT GLANDS AND DUCTS	0·03 to 0·14	0·08

In contrast to these, admissions for TINEA increased from 0·5 to 0·8 in 1942 before declining to 0·4 in 1945, with an average rate of 0·6 per 1,000.

DISEASES OF THE EAR, NOSE AND THROAT

Recorded admissions to hospitals on account of this group of diseases averaged 12 per 1,000 over the years 1940–45. In two years the average was exceeded, by 2 and 1 per 1,000 in 1943 and 1945 respectively. In 1940, 1942 and 1944 annual rates were slightly (from 0·02 to 0·39) lower than the average, but in 1941 it was 2·5 per 1,000 less. Annual rates ranged from 9 to an increase of fifty per cent. at 14. Admissions are analysed in the tables presented hereunder.

United Kingdom, 1940–45
Admissions to Hospitals for Diseases of the Ear, Nose and Throat.
British Troops, Male
Annual Rates per 1,000 Strength with Relative and Comparative Rates

Source: Hollerith Tabulations

1. *Annual Rates per 1,000 Strength*	1940	1941	1942	1943	1944	1945	Averages
Otitis Media	0·89	0·86	1·26	1·60	1·41	1·38	1·23
Tonsillitis	5·23	4·65	5·99	6·97	5·65	6·42	5·82
Deformities of the Nasal Septum	0·43	0·77	0·82	0·78	0·59	0·93	0·72
Laryngitis	0·52	0·28	0·32	0·29	0·18	0·29	0·30
Pharyngitis	2·76	1·04	0·84	0·97	0·53	0·67	1·13
Other Causes	1·74	1·70	2·60	3·36	3·10	3·37	2·65
Totals	11·57	9·30	11·83	13·97	11·46	12·97	11·85
Percentages of total admissions for diseases	11	9	9	10	9	9	9
2. *Relative Rates*							
Otitis Media	7·70	9·24	10·64	11·48	12·29	10·67	10
Tonsillitis	45·19	49·99	50·63	49·88	49·31	49·47	49
Deformities of the Nasal Septum	3·72	8·33	7·02	5·54	5·19	7·16	6
Laryngitis	4·48	3·01	2·67	2·06	1·53	1·54	3
Pharyngitis	23·87	11·20	7·07	6·96	4·65	5·19	10
Other Causes	15·04	18·23	21·97	24·08	27·03	25·97	22
Totals	100	100	100	100	100	100	100
3. *Comparative Rates* (1943 = 100)							
Otitis Media	71	54	79	100	88	86	
Tonsillitis	75	67	86	100	81	92	
Deformities of the Nasal Septum	55	99	105	100	76	119	
Laryngitis	179	97	110	100	62	69	
Pharyngitis	285	107	87	100	55	69	
Other Causes	52	51	77	100	92	100	
Totals	83	67	85	100	82	93	

Admissions for this group of diseases were, on the average, some nine per cent. of the total admissions for diseases. TONSILLITIS was responsible for approximately one half the group total, and admissions on this account ranged from 5 per 1,000 in 1941 to a peak of 7 in 1943. Rates in 1944 and 1945, at 5·7 and 6·4 respectively, were eighty and ninety per cent. of those recorded in 1943.

OTITIS MEDIA accounted for admissions at rates varying from 0·9 in 1940 and 1941 to 1·6 in 1943, with an average of 1·2 per 1,000. These admissions were from eight to twelve per cent. of the total for the group and in 1944 and 1945, at approximately 1·4, they were somewhat less than ninety per cent. the rate in 1943.

Admissions for PHARYNGITIS were only slightly less than those for Otitis Media and one-fifth the rates for Tonsillitis. They were notable for the comparatively high rate of 2·8 per 1,000 in 1940, over three times the average for the following five years. In 1941 the rate had fallen to 1 per 1,000 and by 1945 had declined to 0·7, some seventy per cent. of that in 1943.

DEFORMITIES of the NASAL SEPTUM caused admissions which increased from 0·4 per 1,000 in 1940 to 0·9 in 1945, with an average of 0·7. They were some six per cent. of the group total. Admissions for LARYNGITIS were comparatively high in 1940 at 0·5 per 1,000. They declined to 0·29 by 1945, the average rate being 0·3 per 1,000.

DISEASES OF THE MUSCULO-SKELETAL SYSTEM

Rates of admission on account of this group of diseases ranged from slightly under 8 per 1,000 in 1941 to just over 14 in 1943, an increase of eighty per cent. These rates represented eight and ten per cent. of all admissions for disease, while the average rate of 11 per 1,000 was between eight and nine per cent. of such admissions.

A breakdown to component diseases is given below:

United Kingdom, 1940–45
Admissions to Hospital for Diseases of the Musculo-Skeletal System
British Troops, Male
Annual Rates per 1,000 Strength with Relative and Comparative Rates

Source: Hollerith Tabulations

1. *Annual Rates per 1,000 Strength* *Diseases of the Joints:*	1940	1941	1942	1943	1944	1945	Averages
Synovitis	0·91	0·84	1·36	1·51	1·13	1·07	1·14
Arthritis	0·30	0·25	0·43	0·56	0·49	0·50	0·42
I.D.K.*	1·32	1·22	2·45	2·66	2·11	2·47	2·04
Others	0·15	0·56	0·28	0·31	0·21	0·27	0·29
Diseases of the Bone	0·36	0·32	0·46	0·49	0·32	0·59	0·42
Diseases of the Spine	0·09	0·12	0·20	0·26	0·19	0·31	0·20
Diseases of the Muscle	0·03	0·04	0·11	0·08	0·05	0·03	0·06
Diseases of the Fasciae, Tendons, Tendon Sheath and Bursae:							
Bursitis	0·26	0·28	0·50	0·65	0·50	0·48	0·44
Others	0·22	0·24	0·42	0·53	0·41	0·49	0·39
Diseases and Deformities of the Limbs:							
Ingrowing Toenails	0·32	0·31	0·49	0·54	0·46	0·38	0·42
Infected fingers	0·45	0·58	1·31	2·01	1·97	1·38	1·28
Hallux V., etc.†	0·39	0·26	0·23	0·14	0·08	0·08	0·19
Hammer Toe	0·30	0·20	0·22	0·17	0·11	0·08	0·18
Others	0·57	0·25	0·94	0·62	0·47	0·49	0·56
Rheumatic Conditions:‡							
Non-Articular	2·13	1·99	2·94	3·11	2·57	2·19	2·49
Articular	0·29	0·32	0·48	0·60	0·49	0·67	0·48
Totals	8·09	7·78	12·82	14·24	11·56	11·48	11·00
Percentages of total admissions for diseases	8	8	9	10	9	8	9

Admission to Hospital for Diseases of the Musculo-Skeletal System—continued

2. *Relative Rates*

Diseases of the Joints:							
Synovitis	11·31	10·73	10·62	10·67	9·82	9·29	10·36
Arthritis	3·73	3·26	3·37	3·91	4·20	4·37	3·82
I.D.K.*	16·27	15·71	19·14	18·67	18·23	21·51	18·55
Others	1·80	7·26	2·21	2·16	1·84	2·38	2·64
Diseases of the Bone	4·39	4·00	3·59	3·47	2·73	5·16	3·82
Diseases of the Spine	1·16	1·60	1·54	1·81	1·65	2·70	1·82
Diseases of the Muscle	0·37	0·57	0·84	0·55	0·39	0·24	0·55
Diseases of the Fasciae, Tendons, Tendon Sheath and Bursae:							
Bursitis	3·25	3·56	3·85	4·58	4·37	4·13	4·00
Others	2·73	3·12	3·25	3·73	3·55	4·28	3·55
Diseases and Deformities of the Limbs:							
Ingrowing Toenails	3·90	3·87	3·78	3·79	3·96	3·33	3·82
Infected fingers	5·58	7·49	10·25	14·11	17·08	11·98	11·63
Hallux V., etc.†	4·81	3·32	1·77	0·97	0·70	0·71	1·73
Hammer Toe	3·66	2·62	1·71	1·16	0·92	0·71	1·63
Others	7·07	3·20	7·34	4·38	4·09	4·29	5·09
Rheumatic Conditions:‡							
Non-Articular	26·34	25·57	22·94	21·86	22·20	19·05	22·63
Articular	3·63	4·12	3·78	4·18	4·27	5·87	4·36
Totals	100	100	100	100	100	100	100

3. *Comparative Rates* (1943 = 100)

Diseases of the Joints:						
Synovitis	60	56	90	100	75	71
Arthritis	54	45	77	100	88	89
I.D.K.*	50	46	92	100	79	93
Others	48	181	90	100	68	87
Diseases of the Bone	73	65	94	100	65	120
Diseases of the Spine	44	46	77	100	73	119
Diseases of the Muscle	38	50	138	100	63	38
Diseases of the Fasciae, Tendons, Tendon Sheath and Bursae:						
Bursitis	40	43	77	100	77	74
Others	42	45	79	100	77	92
Diseases and Deformities of the Limbs:						
Ingrowing Toenails	59	57	91	100	85	70
Infected fingers	22	29	65	100	98	69
Hallux V., etc.†	279	186	164	100	57	57
Hammer Toe	176	118	129	100	65	47
Others	92	40	152	100	76	79
Rheumatic Conditions:‡						
Non-Articular	68	64	95	100	83	70
Articular	48	53	80	100	82	112
Totals	57	55	90	100	81	81

* I.D.K. includes: Internal derangement of knee and other joints, Subluxation of intra-articular cartilage, Rupture of intra-articular cartilage, Ruptured crucial ligament of knee, and loose body.
† Hallux V, etc. includes: *Hallux valgus, varus, flexus* or *rigidus.*
‡ Rheumatic Conditions *excludes* Rheumatic Fever.

One-third of the admissions in this group was due to Diseases of the JOINTS of which INTERNAL DERANGEMENT of the KNEE constituted over fifty per cent. Admissions for the latter ranged between 1·2 in 1941 and 2·7 in 1943 with an average of 2 per 1,000. They were approximately nineteen per cent. of the total of the group. SYNOVITIS was responsible for admissions at the average rate of slightly over 1, ARTHRITIS for 0·4 and OTHER DISEASES of the JOINTS for 0·3, per 1,000.

RHEUMATIC CONDITIONS (excluding Rheumatic Fever) caused admissions at 3 per 1,000, approximately one quarter of the group. The non-articular type accounted for five times the admissions for the articular type. The former commenced at 2·1 per 1,000 in 1940 and increased to 3·1 in 1943 before subsiding to 2·2 in 1945. The latter, on the other hand, increased steadily from 0·29 to 0·67 over the period.

Admissions due to DISEASES and DEFORMITIES of the LIMBS were slightly under one quarter of the total admissions of the group. INFECTED FINGERS caused rates which, commencing at 0·45 in 1940, rose to 2·01 in 1943 and declined to 1·38 in 1945, with an average of 1·28. These represented nearly twelve per cent. of group admissions. Admissions for INGROWING TOENAILS experienced a similar trend in rising from 0·32 in 1940 to 0·54 in 1943 and subsiding to 0·38 in 1945. The rates for HALLUX VALGUS *et al,* as well as those for HAMMER TOES exhibited a somewhat different tendency with declining annual rates from 0·39 and 0·30 respectively in 1940 to 0·08 in 1945.

VENEREAL DISEASES

Army personnel contracting Venereal Diseases were normally treated in Military Hospitals, and only a comparative few were cared for in E.M.S. Hospitals. Admissions on account of Venereal Disease in 1940 were at the rate of 7 per 1,000, representing some seven per cent. of the total admissions due to diseases. A rise of 3 per 1,000 in 1941 was followed by a further rise of 3 in the following year, bringing the rate to a peak of 14, equivalent to ten per cent. of the total disease rate. In 1943 and 1944 admissions declined to 11 and 9 per 1,000 respectively, but in the next year they increased to 13. The average rate of slightly under 11 represents some eight per cent. of the admissions for all diseases. Admissions are analysed in the tables on page 119.

As could be expected, admissions for GONORRHOEA were much more numerous than those for the other classes, being nearly three-quarters of the total of the group. This being so, the trend of admissions is that of all Venereal Disease admissions. Rates at 6 in 1940 increased to 9 in 1941 and 11 in 1942. A decline of 3 per 1,000 occurred in 1943 and this was followed by a similar fall to 5 in 1944 before increasing to 9 in 1945. The average rate of admissions was 8 per 1,000. In spite of the increases in admissions, relative rates decreased from 86 in 1940 to 58 in 1944 with an increase to a final rate of 67 in 1945.

Admissions for SYPHILIS increased annually from 0·9 in 1940 to between three and four times at over 3 per 1,000 in 1945 with an average of 2 per 1,000. Expressed as percentages of all admissions for the group, they increased from twelve per cent. in 1940 to twenty-eight in 1944 and were on the average twenty per cent. of all admissions for Venereal Disease.

The comparatively few admissions due to SOFT CHANCRE recorded rates of 0·06 in 1941 to 0·02 in 1945 with an average of 0·04 per 1,000.

United Kingdom, 1940–45

Admissions to Hospitals for Venereal Diseases
British Troops, Male
Annual Rates per 1,000 Strength with Relative and Comparative Rates

Source: Hollerith Tabulations

1. *Annual Rates per 1,000 Strength*	1940	1941	1942	1943	1944	1945	Averages
Gonorrhoea	6·35	8·84	11·27	8·04	5·08	8·85	8·07
Syphilis	0·89	1·41	2·45	2·88	2·42	3·15	2·20
Soft Chancre	0·04	0·06	0·04	0·03	0·03	0·02	0·04
Other Causes and Unspecified	0·12	0·19	0·18	0·32	1·17	1·12	0·52
Totals	7·40	10·50	13·94	11·27	8·70	13·14	10·83
Percentages of total admissions for diseases	7	10	10	8	7	9	8
2. *Relative Rates*							
Gonorrhoea	85·81	84·19	80·84	71·34	58·39	67·35	74·52
Syphilis	12·03	13·43	17·58	25·55	27·82	23·97	20·31
Soft Chancre	0·54	0·57	0·29	0·27	0·34	0·15	0·37
Other Causes and Unspecified	1·62	1·81	1·29	2·84	13·45	8·52	4·80
Totals	100	100	100	100	100	100	100
3. *Comparative Rates* (1943 = 100)							
Gonorrhoea	79	110	140	100	63	110	
Syphilis	31	49	85	100	84	109	
Soft Chancre	133	200	133	100	100	67	
Other Causes and Unspecified	38	59	56	100	366	350	
Totals	66	93	124	100	77	117	

DISEASES OF THE GENITO-URINARY SYSTEM

Admissions for this group of diseases showed a steady increase, interrupted by a very slight decline only in 1944, from an initial rate of 4 in 1940 to 10 in 1945 with an average of 6 per 1,000. In 1944 they were very slightly lower (by 0·05 per 1,000) than those in 1943, but 1945 admissions recorded an increase of nearly 3 per 1,000. They were between four and seven per cent. of all admissions for disease, averaging at five per cent. The tables on page 120 analyse the admissions.

Over seventy per cent. of the admissions in this group were caused by Diseases of the ORGANS OF GENERATION. Recorded admissions of this sub-group increased annually from under 3 in 1940 to 5 in 1943 and finally to between 7 and 8 per 1,000 in 1945, with an average of 4·7 which represented over three per cent. of all admissions for disease. Of the average of nearly 5 per 1,000 in the sub-group, N.V. URETHRITIS was responsible for sixty per cent. Admissions climbed from 0·76 in 1940 to 3·92 in 1945, a range of slightly over 3. The growing numerical importance of this disease is emphasised by its relative rates within the group, which increased from 19 to 39 per cent. over the six years.

Admissions for N.V. EPIDIDYMITIS also recorded increases over the period, the rate of 0·84 in 1945 being six times that in 1940. Increases in

United Kingdom, 1940–45

Admissions to Hospitals for Diseases of the Genito-Urinary System
British Troops, Male
Annual Rates per 1,000 Strength with Relative and Comparative Rates

Source: Hollerith Tabulations

1. *Annual Rates per 1,000 Strength*	1940	1941	1942	1943	1944	1945	Averages
Diseases of the Kidneys:							
Pyelitis	0·18	0·07	0·18	0·27	0·22	0·26	0·20
Renal Colic	0·14	0·15	0·16	0·16	0·17	0·26	0·17
Others	0·34	0·30	0·40	0·48	0·51	0·75	0·46
Diseases of the Ureter	0·04	0·05	0·05	0·05	0·07	0·09	0·06
Diseases of the Bladder:							
Cystitis	0·26	0·30	0·39	0·46	0·42	0·39	0·37
Others	0·03	0·04	0·06	0·07	0·07	0·08	0·06
Urinary Disorders	0·32	0·40	0·58	0·62	0·55	0·56	0·50
Diseases of the Organs of Generation:							
Balanitis, N.V.	0·56	0·01	0·63	0·51	0·35	0·59	0·44
Urethritis, N.V.	0·76	1·20	1·68	1·78	2·38	3·92	1·95
Prostatitis	0·02	0·05	0·06	0·06	0·06	0·15	0·07
Varicocele	0·25	0·21	0·26	0·22	0·10	0·15	0·20
Hydrocele	0·23	0·23	0·35	0·38	0·32	0·36	0·31
Orchitis, N.V.	0·06	0·05	0·09	0·11	0·09	0·14	0·09
Epididymitis, N.V.	0·14	0·14	0·42	0·54	0·59	0·84	0·45
Paraphimosis	0·07	0·12	0·21	0·18	0·18	0·27	0·17
Phimosis	0·20	0·30	0·52	0·54	0·42	0·55	0·42
Others	0·35	0·41	0·68	0·70	0·58	0·56	0·55
Totals	3·95	4·03	6·72	7·13	7·08	9·92	6·47
Percentages of total admissions for diseases	4	4	5	5	5	7	5
2. *Relative Rates*							
Diseases of the Kidneys:							
Pyelitis	4·67	1·83	2·63	3·76	3·05	2·66	3·09
Renal Colic	3·49	3·80	2·37	2·27	2·38	2·66	2·63
Others	8·57	7·48	5·98	6·69	7·22	7·53	7·11
Diseases of the Ureter	0·97	1·19	0·76	0·70	0·94	0·92	0·93
Diseases of the Bladder:							
Cystitis	6·60	7·36	5·72	6·39	5·94	3·95	5·72
Others	0·69	1·07	0·94	0·90	1·03	0·83	0·93
Urinary Disorders	8·15	10·01	8·56	8·71	7·79	5·60	7·73
Diseases of the Organs of Generation:							
Balanitis, N.V.	14·15	0·33	9·42	7·20	4·92	5·97	6·80
Urethritis, N.V.	19·29	29·87	25·07	24·94	33·63	39·49	30·14
Prostatitis	0·52	0·98	0·87	0·87	0·86	1·47	1·08
Varicocele	6·22	5·09	3·80	3·11	1·45	1·56	3·09
Hydrocele	5·94	5·78	5·21	5·35	4·57	3·67	4·79
Orchitis, N.V.	1·62	1·28	1·35	1·52	1·26	1·38	1·39
Epididymitis, N.V.	3·46	3·54	6·29	7·55	8·39	8·45	6·95
Paraphimosis	1·75	2·84	3·10	2·57	2·47	2·75	2·63
Phimosis	4·95	7·48	7·79	7·60	5·89	5·51	6·49
Others	8·96	10·07	10·14	9·87	8·21	5·60	8·50
Totals	100	100	100	100	100	100	100
3. *Comparative Rates* (1943 = 100)							
Diseases of the Kidneys:							
Pyelitis	67	26	67	100	81	96	
Renal Colic	88	94	100	100	106	163	
Others	71	63	83	100	106	156	
Diseases of the Ureter	80	100	100	100	140	180	
Diseases of the Bladder:							
Cystitis	57	65	85	100	91	85	
Others	43	57	86	100	100	114	
Urinary Disorders	52	65	94	100	89	90	
Diseases of the Organs of Generation:							
Balanitis, N.V.	110	2	124	100	69	116	
Urethritis, N.V.	43	67	94	100	134	220	
Prostatitis	33	83	100	100	100	250	
Varicocele	114	95	118	100	45	68	
Hydrocele	61	61	92	100	84	95	
Orchitis, N.V.	55	45	82	100	82	127	
Epididymitis, N.V.	26	26	78	100	109	156	
Paraphimosis	39	67	117	100	100	150	
Phimosis	37	56	96	100	78	102	
Others	50	59	97	100	83	80	
Totals	55	57	94	100	99	139	

admissions on account of N.V. BALANITIS from 1941 to 1945 were also recorded when rates rose from 0·01 to 0·59. This increase, however, was offset by admissions in 1940, which recorded 0·56 per 1,000, slightly under the peak rate in 1945. N.V. ORCHITIS was responsible for low rates of admissions which fluctuated from 0·05 in 1941 to 0·14 in 1945. Steady increases in admissions on account of diseases in this sub-group were also registered by:

PHIMOSIS from 0·20 in 1940 to 0·55 in 1945
HYDROCELE from 0·23 in 1940 to 0·36 in 1945
PARAPHIMOSIS from 0·07 in 1940 to 0·27 in 1945
PROSTATITIS from 0·02 in 1940 to 0·15 in 1945

In only one instance did admission rates decline. This was for VARICOCELE where admissions ranging from 0·10 to 0·26 fluctuated from 0·25 in 1940 to 0·15 in 1945.

Diseases of the KIDNEY accounted for admissions which averaged 0·8 per 1,000 over the six years. Of these, PYELITIS was responsible for one quarter and RENAL COLIC for slightly less. Both diseases followed the general trend of admissions for the group by recording increasing rates of admissions.

Diseases of the BLADDER caused admission rates at 0·43 per 1,000. Of this CYSTITIS was responsible for nearly ninety per cent. at rates which commenced at 0·26 in 1940, increased to 0·46 in 1943 and declined to 0·39 in 1945.

MENTAL DISEASES

Admissions on account of Mental Diseases, only a comparatively few of which were treated in E.M.S. hospitals, followed the trend exhibited by several individual and groups of diseases in recording rates which increased annually to 1943, declined in the following year and increased again in 1945. Rates for this group, which averaged five per cent. of all admissions for disease, commenced at under 4, increased to 8 by 1943, fell to slightly under 7 and finally, in 1945, reached 8 per 1,000. The average rate of admissions over the six years was 6 per 1,000. The tables on page 122 analyse these admissions.

Nearly three-quarters of the admissions in this group were caused by PSYCHONEUROSES, admissions for which naturally followed the pattern of the whole group with increasing annual rates, except in 1944 when there was a small diminution. Recorded rates were 2·4 in 1940 rising to 6 in 1943, 5 in 1944 and 6·6 in the final year of the period with an average of 4·6 per 1,000. They represented some sixty to eighty per cent. of all group admissions.

In this sub-group, admissions on account of ANXIETY STATE were by far the more numerous comprising over sixty per cent. of the total. Apart

United Kingdom, 1940–45
Admissions to Hospitals for Mental Diseases. British Troops, Male
Annual Rates per 1,000 Strength with Relative and Comparative Rates

Source: Hollerith Tabulations

1. *Annual Rates per 1,000 Strength*	1940	1941	1942	1943	1944	1945	Averages
Psychoses:							
Manic Depressive	0·26	0·32	0·56	0·49	0·28	0·24	0·36
Schizophrenia	0·23	0·28	0·34	0·39	0·49	0·38	0·35
Paranoid State	0·03	0·03	0·03	0·04	0·02	0·01	0·03
Others	0·02	0·02	0·02	0·02	0·02	0·03	0·02
Psychoneuroses:							
Anxiety State	1·29	1·33	2·39	3·76	3·45	4·89	2·85
Hysteria	0·66	0·83	1·64	1·96	1·47	1·44	1·33
Others	0·45	0·41	0·65	0·35	0·21	0·27	0·39
Psychopathic Personality	0·32	0·53	0·77	0·81	0·80	0·70	0·65
Mental Deficiency	0·30	0·18	0·18	0·15	0·13	0·08	0·17
Other Mental Diseases	0·03	0·02	0·02	0·06	0·01	0·01	0·03
Totals	3·59	3·95	6·60	8·03	6·89	8·05	6·18
Percentages of total admissions for diseases	3	4	5	5	5	5	5
2. *Relative Rates*							
Psychoses:							
Manic Depressive	7·24	8·18	8·51	6·15	4·10	2·94	5·82
Schizophrenia	6·37	7·22	5·13	4·85	7·09	4·76	5·66
Paranoid State	0·85	0·76	0·52	0·44	0·33	0·11	0·49
Others	0·68	0·43	0·36	0·15	0·25	0·34	0·32
Psychoneuroses:							
Anxiety State	35·83	33·72	36·14	46·86	50·04	60·70	46·12
Hysteria	18·25	20·92	24·87	24·40	21·39	17·89	21·52
Others	12·65	10·27	9·86	4·42	3·08	3·40	6·31
Psychopathic Personality	8·94	13·30	11·64	10·12	11·64	8·73	10·52
Mental Deficiency	8·25	4·67	2·73	1·88	1·93	1·02	2·75
Other Mental Diseases	0·91	0·53	0·24	0·73	0·15	0·11	0·49
Totals	100	100	100	100	100	100	100
3. *Comparative Rates* (1943 = 100)							
Psychoses:							
Manic Depressive	53	65	114	100	57	49	
Schizophrenia	60	72	87	100	126	97	
Paranoid State	75	75	75	100	50	25	
Others	100	100	100	100	100	150	
Psychoneuroses:							
Anxiety State	34	35	64	100	92	130	
Hysteria	34	42	84	100	75	73	
Others	129	117	186	100	60	77	
Psychopathic Personality	40	65	95	100	99	86	
Mental Deficiency	200	120	120	100	87	53	
Other Mental Diseases	50	33	33	100	17	17	
Totals	45	49	82	100	86	100	

from the slight decline in 1944, rates increased annually from 1·3 per 1,000 in 1940 to 4·9 in 1945, and were forty-six per cent. of the group total. Admissions due to HYSTERIA followed a slightly different trend, commencing at 0·7 in 1940, increasing annually to 2 in 1943, followed by a decline in each of the following years to 1·4 in 1945. The average rate over the six years was 1·3 per 1,000, representing twenty-two per cent. of all admissions for the group.

PSYCHOSES were the cause of approximately one-sixth of the admissions for Psychoneuroses and twelve per cent. of the whole group. Those for MANIC DEPRESSIVE state were only very slightly more numerous than were admissions for Schizophrenia, and reached a peak of 0·6 in 1942 (from 0·3 in 1940) before declining to 0·2 in 1945. Admissions for SCHIZOPHRENIA increased each year from 0·2 in 1940 to a peak of 0·5 in 1944. The rate in 1945 was slightly less than that in 1944 at 0·4 per 1,000.

PSYCHOPATHIC PERSONALITY produced admissions at rates which increased annually from 0·3 in 1940 to 0·8 in 1943 and 1944, declining to 0·7 in the final year. The average rate of 0·65 per 1,000 was some ten per cent. that of the whole group. Admissions due to MENTAL DEFICIENCY were at variance with the general trend of the group as a whole in that they declined year by year. Rates fell from 0·30 in 1940 to 0·08 in 1945, with an average of a little under 0·2 per 1,000.

DISEASES OF THE RESPIRATORY SYSTEM

This group of diseases was responsible for admission rates which varied from 4·95 in 1941 to a peak of 6·59 in 1943 with an average rate of 5·7 per 1,000. As percentages of admissions for all diseases, the rates

United Kingdom, 1940–45

Admissions to Hospitals for Diseases of the Respiratory System. British Troops, Male Annual Rates per 1,000 Strength with Relative and Comparative Rates

Source: Hollerith Tabulations

1. *Annual Rates per 1,000 Strength*	1940	1941	1942	1943	1944	1945	Averages
Bronchitis:							
Acute	1·21	0·84	1·02	1·31	0·73	0·87	1·00
Chronic	0·87	0·81	1·22	1·45	1·16	0·95	1·08
Unspecified	2·45	1·89	1·87	1·88	1·40	1·41	1·82
Asthma	0·41	0·43	0·69	0·53	0·46	0·62	0·52
Pleurisy	0·49	0·40	0·50	0·54	0·52	0·70	0·52
Other Causes	0·86	0·58	0·54	0·88	0·73	0·83	0·74
Totals	6·29	4·95	5·83	6·59	5·00	5·38	5·68
Percentages of total admissions for diseases	6	5	4	4	4	4	4
2. *Relative Rates*							
Bronchitis:							
Acute	19·20	16·89	17·48	19·95	14·56	16·24	17·61
Chronic	13·86	16·46	20·93	21·96	23·17	17·60	19·02
Unspecified	38·98	38·25	31·98	28·57	28·12	26·23	32·04
Asthma	6·50	8·65	11·75	7·97	9·26	11·50	9·15
Pleurisy	7·87	7·96	8·64	8·15	10·33	13·03	9·15
Other Causes	13·59	11·79	9·22	13·40	14·56	15·40	13·03
Totals	100	100	100	100	100	100	100
3. *Comparative Rates* (1943 = 100)							
Bronchitis:							
Acute	96	85	88	100	73	81	
Chronic	63	75	95	100	106	80	
Unspecified	136	134	112	100	98	92	
Asthma	77	81	130	100	87	117	
Pleurisy	91	74	93	100	96	130	
Other Causes	98	66	61	100	83	94	
Totals	95	75	88	100	76	82	

ranged from 3·5 to 6 per cent. The general tendency of these relative rates was to decline annually from the peak of 6 in 1940 to 3·5 in 1945. This was in distinct contrast to the rates per 1,000 which displayed undulating annual variations not in common with the majority of the diseases tabulated. An opening rate of 6·3 in 1940 was followed by a fall to 5 in 1941. Then two annual increments brought the rate to its peak of 6·6 in 1943. The rate in 1944 was less than in the previous year at 5, but another increase in 1945 raised the rate to 5·4 per 1,000. An analysis of admissions for the group is given on page 123.

Admissions due to BRONCHITIS were responsible for from sixty to over seventy per cent. of the total for Respiratory Diseases, being heaviest in 1940 and 1941 and declining annually during the following years. They varied from 3·3 to 4·6 per 1,000, the higher rates being experienced in 1940, 1942 and 1943. ACUTE Bronchitis recorded admissions which, averaging at 1 per 1,000, were one-quarter of the total for Bronchitis. Those for CHRONIC cases were only very slightly higher, while UNSPECIFIED Bronchitis registered the remainder at a little less than half the total.

ASTHMA and PLEURISY recorded identical average rates at 0·5 per 1,000, approximately ten per cent. of the total for the group. Rates for the former ranged from 0·4 in 1940 to a peak of 0·7 in 1942 with a final rate of 0·6. Those for Pleurisy exhibited an almost similar range varying from 0·4 in 1941 to 0·7 in 1945.

SCABIES

Next in numerical importance were admissions for Scabies, rates for which are listed below.

United Kingdom, 1940–45

Rates of Admissions to Hospitals for Scabies. British Troops, Male

Source: Hollerith Tabulations

	1940	1941	1942	1943	1944	1945	Averages
Rates per 1,000 Strength . .	9·33	11·37	7·82	1·10	0·71	1·00	5
Comparative Rates . .	848	1,034	711	100	65	91	—
Percentages of total admissions for diseases	9	11	6	1	1	1	4

Admissions were conspicuous for their dramatic decline from rates which were comparatively high in the first three years at 9, 11 and 8 per 1,000 respectively to 1 per 1,000 in each of the years 1943 to 1945. From being eleven per cent. of all admissions for disease in 1941, they registered slightly over one-half per cent. in 1945. In no other disease or group of diseases did admissions to hospitals in the United Kingdom exhibit such a remarkable decline.

DISEASES OF THE AREOLAR TISSUE

Admissions on account of Diseases of the Areolar Tissue varied from 2·8 in 1941 to 5·5 in 1943 with an average of 4 per 1,000. They constituted between three and four per cent. of all admissions for disease. In 1944 they were just over eighty per cent. of those recorded in 1943, while in 1945 they were ninety-four per cent. The tables below analyse the admissions.

United Kingdom, 1940–45

Admissions to Hospitals for Disease of the Areolar Tissue. British Troops, Male Annual Rates per 1,000 Strength with Relative and Comparative Rates

Source: Hollerith Tabulations

1. *Annual Rates per 1,000 Strength*	1940	1941	1942	1943	1944	1945	Averages
Cellulitis	2·46	2·14	2·64	4·08	3·13	3·52	2·99
Benign and Unspecified Tumours and Cysts	0·04	0·06	0·14	0·17	0·20	0·29	0·15
Unspecified Abscesses	0·50	0·60	1·01	1·25	1·17	1·33	0·98
Other Causes	0·00	0·00	0·01	0·01	0·01	0·03	0·01
Totals	3·00	2·80	3·80	5·51	4·51	5·17	4·13
Percentages of total admissions for diseases	3	3	3	4	4	3	3
2. *Relative Rates*							
Cellulitis	81·88	76·59	69·37	73·95	69·37	68·08	72·40
Benign and Unspecified Tumours and Cysts	1·24	2·13	3·70	3·08	4·44	5·64	3·63
Unspecified Abscesses	16·76	21·17	26·69	22·72	25·98	25·75	23·73
Other Causes	0·12	0·11	0·24	0·24	0·21	0·53	0·24
Totals	100	100	100	100	100	100	100
3. *Comparative Rates* (1943 = 100)							
Cellulitis	60	52	65	100	77	86	
Benign and Unspecified Tumours and Cysts	24	35	83	100	118	171	
Unspecified Abscesses	40	48	81	100	94	106	
Other Causes	23	27	77	100	59	260	
Totals	54	51	69	100	82	94	

Between seventy and eighty per cent. of the admissions of this group were on account of CELLULITIS, rates for which fluctuated between 2 and 4 per 1,000. The highest rate of admission occurred in 1943 followed by 3·1 and 3·5 respectively in 1944 and 1945. The average rate over the six years was 3 per 1,000.

Unspecified ABSCESSES accounted for nearly one quarter of all admissions for this group. Rates increased annually from 0·5 in 1940 to 1·3 in 1945 and averaged at very slightly under 1 per 1,000.

Rates for Benign and Unspecified TUMOURS and CYSTS increased each year from 0·04 in 1940 to 0·29 in 1945. They represented, on the average, under four per cent. of all admissions for the group. Admissions for Malignant Tumours and Cysts, which are included in 'Other causes' were very few, being some four per cent. only of the Benign and Unspecified types.

DISEASES OF THE CARDIO-VASCULAR SYSTEM

Admissions for this group of diseases were noticeable, in 1942, for the increase by over one hundred per cent., at 5·7, of those on the previous year (2·48 per 1,000). They then declined during the next two years to 3·7 in 1944, but increased to 4·7 in 1945. Admissions over the six years were equivalent to an average rate of 4 per 1,000 and are analysed in the tables presented below.

United Kingdom, 1940–45

Admissions to Hospitals for Diseases of the Cardio-Vascular System. British Troops, Male Annual Rates per 1,000 Strength with Relative and Comparative Rates

Source: Hollerith Tabulations

1. *Annual Rates per 1,000 Strength*	1940	1941	1942	1943	1944	1945	Averages
Valvular Disease of the Heart	0·17	0·10	0·95	0·13	0·06	0·06	0·24
Varicose Veins	1·33	1·75	3·84	3·97	2·69	3·59	2·86
Other Causes	0·86	0·63	0·95	1·09	0·91	1·02	0·91
Totals	2·36	2·48	5·74	5·19	3·66	4·67	4·01
Percentages of total admissions for diseases	2	2	4	4	3	3	3
2. *Relative Rates*							
Valvular Disease of the Heart	7·20	4·03	16·55	2·51	1·64	1·29	5·99
Varicose Veins	56·36	70·57	66·90	76·49	73·50	76·87	71·32
Other Causes	36·44	25·40	16·55	21·00	24·86	21·84	22·69
Totals	100	100	100	100	100	100	100
3. *Comparative Rates* (1943 = 100)							
Valvular Disease of the Heart	131	77	731	100	46	46	
Varicose Veins	34	44	97	100	68	90	
Other Causes	79	58	87	100	83	94	
Totals	45	48	111	100	71	90	

By far the majority (seventy per cent.) of admissions in the group was caused by VARICOSE VEINS, rates for which increased from 1·3 in 1940 to 4 in 1943 before subsiding to 3·6 in 1945. The largest increase in admissions occurred in 1942 when a rate of 3·8 was recorded, some 2 per 1,000 in excess of admissions in 1941. The average rate was 2·9 per 1,000.

A comparatively large increase in admissions occurred in 1942 on account of VALVULAR DISEASE of the HEART. A rate of 0·10 in 1941 rose to 0·95 in the following year. This was followed by 0·13 in 1943 and 0·06 per 1,000 in both 1944 and 1945.

MALARIA

Admissions for Malaria were remarkable for the dramatic increase in 1944. During 1940 and 1941 recorded cases produced rates of 0·08 and 0·07 respectively. In 1942 admissions increased to 0·21 and the following year witnessed a further rise to 0·54. In 1944 they were so numerous as to increase the rate to nearly 10 per 1,000. This was followed in 1945 by a twenty-five per cent. decrease to 7 per 1,000. Much of the increase can only be attributed to relapses occurring among troops returning to the United Kingdom from the Middle East and North Africa. Unfortunately, it is not possible to produce figures to support this hypothesis as the coding of Malaria for statistical purposes did not distinguish between fresh and relapse cases. Admissions are analysed in the tables below.

United Kingdom, 1940–45

Admissions to Hospitals for Malaria. British Troops, Males
Annual Rates per 1,000 Strength with Relative and Comparative Rates

Source: Hollerith Tabulations

1. *Annual Rates per 1,000 Strength*	1940	1941	1942	1943	1944	1945	Averages
Malaria:							
Benign Tertian	0·02	0·01	0·02	0·18	6·73	4·17	1·86
Sub-Tertian	0·00	0·01	0·06	0·09	0·13	0·07	0·06
Others and Unspecified	0·06	0·05	0·13	0·27	2·77	2·80	1·01
Totals	0·08	0·07	0·21	0·54	9·63	7·04	2·93
Percentages of total admissions for diseases	0·1	0·1	0·2	0·4	7	5	2
2. *Relative Rates*							
Malaria:							
Benign Tertian	21·62	12·60	11·89	34·20	69·92	59·25	63·48
Sub-Tertian	7·21	15·75	27·91	17·55	1·39	1·03	2·05
Others and Unspecified	71·17	71·65	60·20	48·25	28·69	39·72	34·47
Totals	100	100	100	100	100	100	100
3. *Comparative Rates* (1943 = 100)							
Malaria:							
Benign Tertian	11	6	11	100	3,739	2,317	
Sub-Tertian	5	11	67	100	144	78	
Others and Unspecified	22	19	48	100	1,026	1,037	
Totals	15	13	39	100	1,783	1,304	

Admissions for BENIGN TERTIAN Malaria were over sixty per cent. of all admissions in this group and, naturally, tended to conform to its overall pattern of admissions by increases from 0·02 in 1940 to 0·18 in 1943, followed by an exceptionally large rise to 6·7 with 4·2 as the rate in 1945.

Cases of SUB-TERTIAN Malaria produced rates which increased from 0·00 in 1940 to 0·13 in 1944 and declined to 0·07 in 1945. 'Others and

Unspecified Malaria' comprise on the average over one-third of all Malaria admissions and include the following:

QUARTAN Malaria —3 cases in 1942, 8 in 1943 and 32 in 1944

OVALE —1 case in 1941, 1942 and 1944, and 3 cases in 1943.

BLACKWATER FEVER—7 cases in 1941, 9 in 1942, and 5 in 1943.

Most of these numbers are so small that they would be shown as 0·00 per 1,000 if entered in the tabulations.

COMMON COLD

Following Malaria in numerical importance came admissions for Common Cold, rates for which are tabled hereunder.

United Kingdom, 1940–45

Admissions to Hospitals for Common Cold. British Troops, Male

Source: Hollerith Tabulations

	1940	1941	1942	1943	1944	1945	Averages
Rates per 1,000 Strength . .	2·61	2·77	2·02	4·12	1·36	1·82	2·45
Comparative Rates . .	63	67	49	100	33	44	—
Percentages of total admissions for diseases . . .	2	3	1	3	1	1	2

Admissions during the six years were erratic, increasing and decreasing in alternate years. The rate in 1940 was 2·6; in 1941 it had increased to 2·8, but during 1942 fell to 2·0. A hundred per cent. increase in 1943 brought the rate to slightly over 4 per 1,000. During the following year it fell to 1·4 but increased again in 1945 to 1·8. The average rate was slightly under 2·5 per 1,000. Admissions in 1941 and 1943 were three per cent. and in 1942, 1944 and 1945 one per cent. of all admissions for diseases.

DISEASES OF THE NERVOUS SYSTEM

Nearly two per cent. of all admissions for disease were attributable to Diseases of the Nervous System. Admissions fluctuated between 1·9 in 1941 and 2·8 in 1943, culminating in the slightly lower rate of 2·75 in 1945. The average over the period was 2·4 per 1,000. Tabulations showing analysis of admissions for this group are given on page 129.

Admissions on account of SCIATICA were more numerous than other causes within the group. Over the six years they averaged 0·76 per 1,000 and were approximately one-third of all the admissions for the group. Rates, which were higher during the last three years, commenced at 0·4 in 1940, rose to 1·0 by 1943 and remained comparatively stable during the next two years. Other cases of NEURITIS produced rates which were fairly steady, ranging from 0·11 to 0·16 per 1,000.

United Kingdom, 1940–45

Admissions to Hospitals for Diseases of the Nervous System. British Troops, Male Annual Rates per 1,000 Strength with Relative and Comparative Rates

Source: Hollerith Tabulations

1. *Annual Rates per 1,000 Strength*	1940	1941	1942	1943	1944	1945	Averages
Sciatica	0·43	0·43	0·73	1·00	0·98	1·01	0·76
Other Neuritis	0·14	0·11	0·15	0·16	0·15	0·14	0·14
Migraine	0·08	0·09	0·12	0·14	0·08	0·15	0·11
Epilepsy	0·49	0·31	0·30	0·26	0·22	0·26	0·31
Other Diseases of Uncertain Pathology	0·05	0·04	0·08	0·09	0·06	0·15	0·08
Effort Syndrome	0·27	0·27	0·34	0·30	0·16	0·16	0·25
Diseases of Cerebral Meninges	0·07	0·04	0·04	0·06	0·08	0·11	0·07
Diseases of Brain	0·07	0·06	0·07	0·06	0·09	0·14	0·08
Disorders of Cranial Nerves	0·22	0·35	0·40	0·46	0·30	0·37	0·35
Other Causes	0·20	0·20	0·24	0·27	0·23	0·26	0·23
Totals	2·02	1·90	2·47	2·80	2·35	2·75	2·38
Percentages of total admissions for diseases	2	2	2	2	2	2	2

2. *Relative Rates*	1940	1941	1942	1943	1944	1945	Averages
Sciatica	21·33	22·66	29·53	35·59	41·55	36·75	31·93
Other Neuritis	6·85	5·86	6·12	5·66	6·56	4·97	5·88
Migraine	6·80	4·59	4·97	5·12	3·48	5·63	4·62
Epilepsy	24·49	16·41	12·30	9·15	9·16	9·27	13·03
Other Diseases of Uncertain Pathology	2·47	2·16	3·08	3·32	2·57	5·65	3·36
Effort Syndrome	13·41	14·38	13·77	10·63	6·89	5·96	10·51
Diseases of Cerebral Meninges	3·30	2·13	1·78	2·32	3·54	3·97	2·94
Diseases of Brain	3·59	3·26	2·65	2·26	3·72	4·97	3·36
Disorders of Cranial Nerves	10·68	18·20	16·25	16·37	12·97	13·58	14·71
Other Causes	10·08	10·35	9·55	9·58	9·56	9·27	9·66
Totals	100	100	100	100	100	100	100

3. *Comparative Rates* (1943 = 100)	1940	1941	1942	1943	1944	1945
Sciatica	43	43	73	100	98	101
Other Neuritis	88	69	94	100	94	88
Migraine	57	64	86	100	57	107
Epilepsy	188	119	115	100	85	100
Other Diseases of Uncertain Pathology	56	44	89	100	67	167
Effort Syndrome	90	90	113	100	53	53
Diseases of Cerebral Meninges	117	67	67	100	133	183
Diseases of Brain	117	100	117	100	150	233
Disorders of Cranial Nerves	48	76	87	100	65	123
Other Causes	74	74	89	100	85	96
Totals	72	68	88	100	84	98

DISORDERS of CRANIAL NERVES accounted for an average rate of 0·35 per 1,000. Admissions increased from 0·2 in 1940 to nearly 0·5 in 1943, declined to 0·3 and increased to slightly under 0·4 in 1945. The trend of admissions for EPILEPSY was somewhat different in that rates decreased annually from 0·5 in 1940 to 0·2 in 1944. The rate in 1945 at 0·26 was identical to that recorded in 1943.

Admissions through EFFORT SYNDROME recorded identical rates in 1940 and 1941 at under 0·3 per 1,000. They rose slightly in 1942 and 1943 and, in 1944 and 1945, were again identical at under 0·2. The average rate was 0·25 per 1,000.

Other causes, admissions for which increased over the six years under review were:

MIGRAINE which rose from 0·08 in 1940 to 0·15 in 1945
DISEASE of the BRAIN which rose from 0·07 in 1940 to 0·14 in 1945
DISEASE of the CEREBRAL MENINGES
which rose from 0·07 in 1940 to 0·11 in 1945.

PNEUMONIA

Admissions for Pneumonia were responsible for rates which averaged over 2 per 1,000, equivalent to one and three-quarters per cent. of all admissions for disease. Apart from 1944, when there was a small decline, increases were experienced each year. Rates commenced at 0·85 in 1940 and ended at 3·89 per 1,000 in 1945. They are analysed in the tables below.

United Kingdom, 1940–45

Admissions to Hospitals for Pneumonia. British Troops, Male
Annual Rates per 1,000 Strength with Relative and Comparative Rates

Source: Hollerith Tabulations

1. *Annual Rates per 1,000 Strength*	1940	1941	1942	1943	1944	1945	Averages
Pneumonia:							
Lobar	0·26	0·36	0·81	1·01	0·87	1·45	0·79
Broncho-Pneumonia	0·27	0·37	0·42	0·43	0·35	0·53	0·40
Pneumonitis	0·02	0·10	0·32	0·57	0·52	0·77	0·38
Unspecified	0·30	0·29	0·60	0·79	0·90	1·14	0·67
Totals	0·85	1·12	2·15	2·80	2·64	3·89	2·24
Percentages of total admissions for diseases	1	1	2	2	2	3	2
2. *Relative Rates*							
Pneumonia:							
Lobar	30·80	31·78	37·43	36·01	33·11	37·23	35·27
Broncho-Pneumonia	31·57	33·10	19·74	15·38	13·26	13·82	17·86
Pneumonitis	2·65	8·86	14·98	20·46	19·85	19·67	16·96
Unspecified	34·98	26·26	27·85	28·15	33·78	29·28	29·91
Totals	100	100	100	100	100	100	100
3. *Comparative Rates* (1943 = 100)							
Pneumonia:							
Lobar	26	36	80	100	86	144	
Broncho-Pneumonia	63	86	98	100	81	123	
Pneumonitis	4	18	56	100	91	135	
Unspecified	38	37	76	100	114	144	
Totals	30	40	77	100	94	139	

One third of all the cases in this group were attributable to LOBAR PNEUMONIA. Admission rates increased from 0·26 in 1940 to 1·01 in 1943, declined to 0·87 during the following year, then increased to 1·45 in 1945. The average rate was 0·79 per 1,000.

BRONCHO-PNEUMONIA was responsible for a similar trend in admissions although increases were not so sharp. Rates began at 0·27, rose to 0·43 by 1943, fell slightly to 0·35 and increased to 0·53 in 1945. The average rate of 0·4 was one-half that for Lobar Pneumonia.

The average admission rate for PNEUMONITIS at 0·38 was only very slightly less than that for Broncho-Pneumonia but the rate of increase from 1940 to 1945 was much more pronounced in the former which began at 0·02 and ended at 0·77, a range of 0·75 as compared with 0·26 for Broncho-Pneumonia.

DISEASES OF THE MOUTH, TEETH AND GUMS

Admissions to hospitals for this group of diseases, on the average, were slightly less than those for Pneumonia. Recorded rates, which varied from 1·5 to 2·8 per 1,000, increased annually to the peak rate in 1942, declined in each of the two following years, then rose in the final year to the rate which obtained in 1941. The average rate of admissions was 2·2 per 1,000 representing two per cent. of all admissions for disease. In the tables which follow the rates for the group are recorded.

United Kingdom, 1940–45

Admissions to Hospitals for Diseases of the Mouth, Teeth and Gums
British Troops, Male
Annual Rates per 1,000 Strength with Relative and Comparative Rates

Source: Hollerith Tabulations

1. *Annual Rates per 1,000 Strength*	1940	1941	1942	1943	1944	1945	Averages
Diseases of the Mouth:							
Stomatitis	0·06	0·18	0·13	0·08	0·10	0·05	0·10
Vincent's Angina	0·71	0·87	1·14	1·23	0·65	0·82	0·90
Others	0·01	0·01	0·01	0·02	0·01	0·02	0·01
Diseases of the Teeth:							
Dental Caries	0·11	0·12	0·17	0·19	0·13	0·19	0·15
Periostitis	0·19	0·17	0·18	0·26	0·13	0·11	0·17
Others	0·32	0·42	0·56	0·52	0·54	0·81	0·53
Diseases of the Gums:							
Gingivitis	0·09	0·46	0·51	0·31	0·17	0·23	0·30
Others	0·04	0·03	0·05	0·05	0·03	0·03	0·04
Totals	1·53	2·26	2·75	2·66	1·76	2·26	2·20
Percentages of all admissions for diseases	1	2	2	2	1	1	2
2. *Relative Rates*							
Diseases of the Mouth:							
Stomatitis	4·03	7·78	4·66	3·08	5·48	2·42	4·54
Vincent's Angina	45·85	38·42	41·54	46·16	36·88	36·28	40·91
Others	0·47	0·44	0·51	0·87	0·64	0·80	0·45
Diseases of the Teeth:							
Dental Caries	6·55	5·48	6·35	7·18	7·61	8·47	6·82
Periostitis	12·25	7·50	6·60	9·76	7·61	4·84	7·73
Others	20·69	18·43	20·19	19·57	30·23	35·89	24·09
Diseases of the Gums:							
Gingivitis	5·60	20·46	18·45	11·40	9·74	10·08	13·64
Others	2·56	1·49	1·70	1·98	1·81	1·21	1·82
Totals	100	100	100	100	100	100	100

3. *Comparative Rates* (1943 = 100)

Diseases of the Mouth:						
Stomatitis . . .	75	225	163	100	125	63
Vincent's Angina .	58	71	93	100	53	67
Others . . .	50	50	50	100	50	100
Diseases of the Teeth:						
Dental Caries . .	58	63	89	100	68	100
Periostitis . . .	73	65	69	100	50	42
Others . . .	62	81	108	100	104	156
Diseases of the Gums:						
Gingivitis	29	148	165	100	55	74
Others	80	60	100	100	60	60
Totals	58	85	103	100	66	85

With an average rate of 1 per 1,000, Diseases of the Mouth were responsible for forty-five per cent. of all admissions for the group. Diseases of the Teeth, at 0·85 per 1,000, were responsible for nearly forty per cent. and Diseases of the Gums, with a rate of 0·3, some fifteen per cent.

Nine-tenths of the admissions for Diseases of the Mouth were attributable to VINCENT'S ANGINA. Rates rose in three years from 0·7 in 1940 to 1·2 in 1943. In 1944 they fell to just over one-half the peak rate to 0·65 and increased to 0·8 in 1945. The average rate of 0·9 per 1,000 was some forty per cent. of the total for the group. STOMATITIS accounted for one-tenth of the admissions for Diseases of the Mouth and just under five per cent. of all admissions for the group. Rates varied from 0·05 in 1945 to 0·18 in 1941 with an average of 0·1 per 1,000.

Of admissions for Diseases of the Teeth, PERIOSTITIS accounted for one-fifth and DENTAL CARIES for slightly less. The former produced rates averaging at 0·17 per 1,000 and which, apart from a rise to a peak rate of 0·26 in 1943, declined each year from 0·19 to 0·11 in 1945. The trend of admissions for Dental Caries was in distinct contrast in that, apart from a decline in 1944, rates rose from 0·11 in 1940 to 0·19 in 1945 with an average of 0·15 per 1,000.

Nearly ninety per cent. of admissions for Diseases of the Gums were caused by GINGIVITIS, rates for which increased from 0·1 in 1940 to 0·5 in 1942, declining to 0·2 per 1,000 in 1945 and averaging 0·3 over the six years.

INFLUENZA

Admission rates for INFLUENZA were distinguished by high rates of 3·4 per 1,000 in both 1940 and 1943 as against an average of 1·1 for the remaining four years. Rates are given on page 133.

Although the admission rates per 1,000 strength in 1940 and 1943 are practically identical, expressed as percentages of the total admissions for disease, the rate in 1940 is greater by one per cent. The average rate of 1·9 per 1,000 was slightly over one-half of one per cent. of that for all diseases. Following the high rates of admissions in 1940 and 1943, the

United Kingdom, 1940–45
Admissions to Hospitals for Influenza. British Troops, Male
Annual Rates per 1,000 Strength with Comparative Rates

Source: Hollerith Tabulations

	1940	1941	1942	1943	1944	1945	Averages
Annual Rates per 1,000 Strength	3·47	1·48	1·06	3·42	1·07	0·85	1·89
Percentage of total admissions for Diseases	3	1	1	2	1	1	1
Comparative Rates (1943 = 100)	101	43	31	100	31	25	—

decline in 1941 was some fifty-seven per cent. compared with sixty-nine per cent. in 1944. It is to be noted that 1943, one of the peak years for admissions for Influenza experienced also the highest rate for Common Cold, at 4, against a remaining average of 2 per 1,000.

DISEASES OF THE EYE

The trend of admissions for Diseases of the Eye was that of an annual increase from 1·2 in 1940 to a peak of 2·1 in 1943, followed by a decline in each of the two following years to 1·7 in 1945. The average rate of 1·7 per 1,000 was some 1·4 per cent. of the total admissions for disease. Rates analysed according to group components are given below.

United Kingdom, 1940–45
Admissions to Hospitals for Diseases of the Eye. British Troops, Male
Annual Rates per 1,000 Strength with Relative and Comparative Rates

Source: Hollerith Tabulations

1. *Annual Rates per 1,000 Strength*	1940	1941	1942	1943	1944	1945	Averages
Diseases of the Eye:							
Conjunctivitis	0·29	0·35	0·54	0·57	0·44	0·40	0·43
Keratitis	0·42	0·56	0·64	0·67	0·66	0·53	0·58
Iritis	0·06	0·07	0·10	0·09	0·11	0·06	0·08
Blepharitis	0·07	0·11	0·15	0·14	0·14	0·15	0·13
Other Causes	0·38	0·50	0·61	0·59	0·48	0·56	0·52
Totals	1·22	1·59	2·04	2·06	1·83	1·70	1·74
Percentages of total admissions for diseases	1	2	1	1	1	1	
2. *Relative Rates*							
Diseases of the Eye:							
Conjunctivitis	23·33	22·01	26·34	27·77	23·92	23·53	24·71
Keratitis	34·42	35·06	31·42	32·44	36·06	31·02	33·33
Iritis	5·02	4·50	4·88	4·49	6·09	3·74	4·60
Blepharitis	5·85	7·04	7·46	6·82	7·48	9·09	7·47
Other Causes	31·38	31·39	29·90	28·48	26·45	32·62	29·89
Totals	100	100	100	100	100	100	100
3. *Comparative Rates* (1943 = 100)							
Diseases of the Eye:							
Conjunctivitis	51	61	95	100	77	70	
Keratitis	63	84	96	100	99	79	
Iritis	67	78	111	100	122	67	
Blepharitis	50	79	107	100	100	107	
Other Causes	64	85	103	100	81	95	
Totals	59	77	99	100	89	83	

KERATITIS was responsible for one-third of the admissions for this group, which followed the group pattern by increasing annually to 1943, following which there was a decline. Rates were 0·4 in 1940, 0·7 in 1943 and 0·5 in 1945 with an average of 0·6 per 1,000, which represented one third the total for the group.

Admissions for CONJUNCTIVITIS also followed the trend of the group with admissions ranging from 0·3 in 1940 to 0·6 in 1943 and 0·4 in 1945. The average of 0·4 was one quarter of the group total. Other admission rates were 0·13 for BLEPHARITIS and 0·08 for IRITIS.

DIPHTHERIA

Admissions on account of DIPHTHERIA resulted in an average annual rate of 0·44 per 1,000 over the six years, with annual rates ranging from 0·37 in 1940 and 1944 to 0·54 in 1945. Analyses of these admissions are tabulated below.

United Kingdom, 1940–45

Admissions to Hospitals for Diphtheria. British Troops, Male
Annual Rates per 1,000 Strength and Relative Rates

Source: Hollerith Tabulations

1. *Annual Rates per 1,000 Strength*	1940	1941	1942	1943	1944	1945	Averages
Diphtheria:							
Faucial	0·02	0·03	0·02	0·03	0·02	0·07	0·03
Nasal	—	0·00	0·00	0·01	0·00	0·02	0·01
Paralysis	0·00	0·00	0·00	0·01	0·02	0·05	0·01
Unspecified and Others	0·35	0·44	0·41	0·39	0·32	0·40	0·39
Totals	0·37	0·48	0·44	0·44	0·37	0·54	0·44
Percentages of total admissions for diseases	0·4	0·5	0·3	0·3	0·3	0·4	0·3
2. *Relative Rates*							
Diphtheria:							
Faucial	4·68	5·58	4·01	7·67	6·18	13·56	6·82
Nasal	—	0·99	1·09	1·95	1·35	3·39	2·27
Paralysis	0·97	0·66	0·49	1·95	5·60	8·47	2·27
Unspecified and Others	94·35	92·77	94·41	88·43	86·87	74·58	88·64
Totals	100	100	100	100	100	100	100

The majority of the cases recorded above fall within the classification of 'Unspecified and Others'. Of 'Others', admissions were so few that inclusion in the tabulation of Annual Rates would have resulted in their being recorded as '0·00' per 1,000. Such admissions include the following:

LARYNGEAL 1 case in 1942, and 2 in 1943.

CUTANEOUS 1 case each in 1941 and 1942, 4 in 1943, and 3 in 1944.

GRAVIS 1 case each in 1940 and 1942.

OTHER DISEASES

Although admissions for DYSENTERY accounted for an average of slightly less than 0·5 per 1,000, they were conspicuous for their steady increase each year, from 0·03 in 1940 to 1·97 per 1,000 in 1945. In contrast to this, RUBELLA was responsible for the comparatively high rate of 4·34 in 1940, as against an average of 0·68 for the remainder of the period. Only in 1944 and 1945 did admissions reach 1 per 1,000 and in 1942 it was as low as 0·23.

Admissions for TUBERCULOSIS, in general, registered an increase over the six years, rates ranging from 1·15 in 1940 to 1·07 in 1942 and 1·67 in 1945. They accounted for one per cent. of all admissions for disease. Of the average rate of 1·29, PULMONARY Tuberculosis was responsible for 1·08 per 1,000. Disorders of NUTRITION and METABOLISM also recorded increasing rates of admission, for 0·17 in 1940 to 0·51 in 1945.

MEASLES recorded rates which declined from 0·6 in 1940 to 0·2 in 1942, increased to 0·6 in 1943 before subsiding to 0·4 in 1945. The rate of admissions for MENINGOCOCCAL INFECTION in 1945 at 0·25 was half that in 1940, although in 1943 it had declined to the lowest recorded rate of the period at 0·14.

INJURIES

Admissions for injuries increased from over 5 per 1,000 in 1940 to nearly 19 in 1943. They declined by 3 in the following year and rose to just under 18 per 1,000 in 1945. The largest increase in admissions occurred in 1942 when the rate rose from 6 to 15 per 1,000. This increase was largely due to the rise of 6·5 in the rate of admissions for injuries not due to enemy action.

For nearly thirty per cent. of the injuries recorded in the Hollerith tabulations it is not disclosed whether or not they were caused by enemy action, as are the remainder. Table 5 records the rates per 1,000 strength of injuries caused by enemy action (E.A.) and those not so caused (N.E.A.). It also gives the rates of admissions for injuries for which the cause was not specified. Assuming that all admissions for injuries were in the proportions of those indicated in the table each year by E.A. and N.E.A. injuries, and those unspecified so allocated, rates would be as indicated on pages 136 and 137.

Table 5 records the rates per 1,000 of admissions for Injuries classified according to Enemy Action, Non-Enemy Action and Cause Unspecified. They are further classified as to Head Injuries, Fractures (other than to the head), Burns, Old Injuries, and Other Injuries. In Table 6 the information recorded in the previous table has been converted

United Kingdom, 1940–45

Admissions to Hospitals for Injuries
British Troops, Male
Adjusted Annual Rates per 1,000 Strength with Comparative Rates

Source: Hollerith Tabulations

1. *Adjusted Annual Rates per 1,000 Strength*	Enemy Action	Non-Enemy Action	Totals
1940	0·15	5·29	5·44
1941	0·11	6·33	6·44
1942	0·17	15·35	15·52
1943	0·34	18·44	18·78
1944	1·50	14·12	15·62
1945	2·58	15·13	17·71
Averages	0·81	12·44	13·25
2. *Comparative Rates* (1943 = 100)			
1940	44	29	39
1941	32	34	34
1942	50	83	83
1943	100	100	100
1944	441	77	83
1945	759	82	94

to relative rates. A consolidation of these tables giving average rates per 1,000 with relative rates is presented below.

United Kingdom, 1940–45

Admissions to Hospitals for Injuries. British Troops, Male
Average Annual Rates per 1,000 Strength and Relative Rates

Source: Hollerith Tabulations

1. *Average Annual Rates per 1,000 Strength*	Enemy Action	Non-Enemy Action	Cause not specified	Totals
Head Injuries	0·02	0·64	0·16	0·82
Fractures (Other Sites)	0·08	3·57	1·12	4·76
Burns	0·01	0·29	0·15	0·45
Old Injuries	0·21	0·43	0·68	1·32
Other Injuries	0·27	3·96	1·67	5·90
Totals	0·59	8·89	3·78	13·25
Relative Rates				
Head Injuries	3·39	7·20	4·23	6·19
Fractures (Other Sites)	13·56	40·16	29·63	35·92
Burns	1·70	3·26	3·97	3·40
Old Injuries	35·59	4·84	17·99	9·96
Other Injuries	45·76	44·54	44·18	44·53
Totals	100	100	100	100

Assuming, as before, that all admissions for Injuries were distributed in the proportions indicated above for E.A. and N.E.A. Injuries and correspondingly allocating those for which no cause was specified, rates are as shown in the following table.

United Kingdom, 1940–45

Admissions to Hospitals for Injuries British Troops, Male
Adjusted Average Annual Rates per 1,000 Strength and Relative Rates

Source: Hollerith Tabulations

1. *Adjusted Average Annual Rates per 1,000 Strength*	Enemy Action	Non-Enemy Action	Totals
Head Injuries	0·03	0·79	0·82
Fractures (Other Sites)	0·10	4·66	4·76
Burns	0·02	0·43	0·45
Old Injuries	0·43	0·89	1·32
Other Injuries	0·37	5·53	5·90
Totals	0·95	12·30	13·25
2. *Relative Rates*			
Head Injuries	3·16	6·42	6·19
Fractures (Other Sites)	10·53	37·88	35·92
Burns	2·11	3·50	3·40
Old Injuries	45·26	7·24	9·96
Other Injuries	38·94	44·96	44·53
Totals	100	100	100

Admissions for Injuries caused through enemy action increased annually from 0·1 per 1,000 in 1941 to 2·6 in 1945. In comparison, non-enemy action admissions increased from 6 in 1941 to 15 in 1945, although the peak rate of 18 occurred in 1943. The largest annual increase in admissions for E.A. injuries occurred in 1944 when the rate rose from slightly over 0·3 to 1·5 per 1,000. This was accompanied by a reduction in admissions for N.E.A. injuries. In 1945, however, a further increase in E.A. injuries was attended by a similar increase in N.E.A. injuries.

Of the total adjusted average admission rate of over 13 per 1,000 for injuries, those caused through enemy action accounted for seven per cent. at slightly under 1 per 1,000. Forty-five per cent. of these admissions were due to Old Injuries, eleven per cent. to Fractures (other than to the head), three to Head Injuries and two per cent. to Burns. This trend is not followed by N.E.A. injuries among which thirty-eight per cent. were for Fractures, seven per cent. for Old Injuries, six for Head Injuries and nearly four per cent. for Burns. The relative rates for Old E.A. injuries are thus six times those for N.E.A., while N.E.A. Fractures are four times those caused through E.A. Head Injuries are double and

Burns fifty per cent. higher. It is possible that the rate quoted for Old Injuries caused through enemy action may be somewhat inflated by the inclusion of those who, having originally been injured in overseas theatres, particularly in North-West Europe, were re-admitted for further treatment to hospitals in the United Kingdom.

DEATHS

Statistics relating to deaths in hospitals in the United Kingdom are recorded in Table 7. Owing to the decision to restrict coding, in which 'Result on Discharge' was eliminated, it is possible to present only statistics relating to the years 1940 to 1943. In this table are shown deaths as percentages of admissions for diseases (or disease groups) and, separately, those for injuries. Relative rates within these classifications are also given. Rates per 1,000 strength for disease and injury are presented in the table which follows.

United Kingdom, 1940–43

Mortality Rates per 1,000 Strength. British Male Troops

Source: Hollerith Tabulations

CAUSES	1940	1941	1942	1943
Disease	0·20	0·17	0·20	0·26
Injury	0·04	0·03	0·06	0·06
Totals	0·24	0·20	0·26	0·32

Mortality rates were highest in 1943 at 0·32 per 1,000 and lowest in 1941 at 0·20. Deaths through disease ranged from 0·17 in 1941 to 0·26 in 1943, while those from injury varied between 0·03 in 1941 to 0·06 in 1942 and 1943. In 1942 deaths from disease accounted for seventy-eight per cent. of all deaths while in the remaining years they were between eighty and eighty-five per cent.

Although the admission rate was low (0·14 to 0·52 per 1,000), deaths from MENINGOCOCCAL INFECTION recorded the highest rate among diseases from just under four in 1941 to nearly seven per cent. of admissions in 1943. The years which witnessed the lower rates of admission also experienced the heavier percentages of deaths. *Per contra*, relative rates were lowest in 1942 and 1943.

Comparatively high mortality rates were also recorded for TUBERCULOSIS, between two and three per cent. of admissions, with relative rates at between thirteen and sixteen per cent. of all deaths from disease.

A diminution in rates occurred in PNEUMONIA. In 1940, nearly two and a half per cent. of admissions for this disease died. By 1943, this had been reduced to a little over one-half per cent. Diseases of the NERVOUS SYSTEM were responsible for rates which were remarkably constant at 0·93 per cent. of admissions except in 1941 when the percentage was 0·89.

The largest number of deaths which occurred among diseases was for Diseases of the DIGESTIVE SYSTEM which recorded from twenty to twenty-five per cent. of all deaths.

Rates for injuries ranged from 0·7 per cent. of admissions in 1940 to 0·3 in 1945. Those from E.A. injuries were noteworthy for their percentage diminution, from eleven per cent. of admissions for all injuries in 1940 to a little over one per cent. in 1943. Deaths from N.E.A. injuries expressed as percentages of admissions also declined from 0·53 in 1940 to 0·27 in 1943. As relative rates, however, they increased from 49 in 1940 to 81 in 1942 and declined to 57 in the following year. Relative mortality rates for unspecified injuries ranged from fifteen to thirty-eight.

BRITISH FEMALE TROOPS

Admission rates of the Women's Services of the British Army to Hospitals in the United Kingdom are cited in Tables 8 to 14. Rates per 1,000 strength, Relative Rates, and Comparative Rates are recorded in Tables 8, 9 and 10 respectively. The average rates of admission over the six years under review are presented in Table 11, while admission rates for females are compared with those for males in Table 12. Injury rates are exhibited in Tables 13 and 14, and mortality rates for the years 1940 to 1943 are recorded in Table 15. Admission rates cited in these tables are subject to the limitations discussed at the beginning of this section and it is suggested that the correction factors given on page 110 be used.

Admissions for diseases only varied from 84 per 1,000 strength in 1940 to a peak of 152 in 1943, while those for injuries ranged from 3 in 1940 to 9 in 1943. Admissions on account of injuries accounted for from three to six per cent. of all admissions. Relevant rates, to the nearest whole number, were as follows.

United Kingdom, 1940–45

Rates of Admissions to Hospitals. British Troops, Female

Source: Hollerith Tabulations

Years	Rates per 1,000 Strength			Relative Rates			Comparative Rates (1943 = 100)		
	Disease	Injury	Totals	Disease	Injury	Totals	Disease	Injury	Totals
1940	84	3	87	96	4	100	55	38	54
1941	102	3	105	97	3	100	67	37	65
1942	137	8	145	95	5	100	91	86	90
1943	152	9	161	94	6	100	100	100	100
1944	110	7	117	94	6	100	72	78	73
1945	106	6	112	95	5	100	70	65	70

The highest annual rates for disease and injury were recorded in 1943 at 152 and 9 per 1,000 respectively, with a peak total admission rate of 161. The lowest rates were registered in 1940 at 84 per 1,000 for disease and 3 for injury. Injuries accounted for slightly over three per cent. of all admissions in 1941 to a little more than six per cent. in 1944. Over the six years were recorded the average rates of 115 for disease and 6 for injury, a total of 121 per 1,000.

DISEASES OF THE EAR, NOSE AND THROAT

Of individual diseases and disease groups, diseases of the EAR, NOSE, and THROAT were responsible for the highest rate of admission at an average of slightly under 16 per 1,000, representing nearly fourteen per cent. of all admissions for disease. These admissions are analysed below.

United Kingdom, 1940–45

Admissions to Hospitals for Diseases of the Ear, Nose and Throat

British Troops, Female

Annual Rates per 1,000 Strength and Relative Raths

Source: Hollerith Tabulations

1. *Annual Rates per 1,000 Strength*	1940	1941	1942	1943	1944	1945	Averages
Otitis Media	0·92	0·68	1·18	1·58	1·14	1·17	1·11
Tonsillitis	5·93	8·54	11·10	13·23	9·46	8·78	9·51
Other Diseases	6·92	5·14	5·06	5·71	4·56	4·48	5·31
Totals	13·77	14·36	17·34	20·52	15·16	14·43	15·93
Percentages of total admissions for diseases	16	14	13	14	14	14	14
2. *Relative Rates*							
Otitis Media	6·68	4·74	6·81	7·70	7·52	8·10	6·97
Tonsillitis	43·06	59·47	64·01	64·47	62·40	60·85	59·70
Other Diseases	50·25	35·79	29·18	27·83	30·08	31·05	33·33
Totals	100	100	100	100	100	100	100

Admissions followed the general trend for all diseases, with annual increments to 1943, then decreases in the two following years. TONSILLITIS recorded a peak rate of over 13 per 1,000 in 1943. This represented nearly nine per cent. of all admissions for disease and sixty per cent. of group admissions. OTITIS MEDIA was responsible for an average rate of slightly over 1 per 1,000, some seven per cent. of group admissions. The relevant average rate for male troops for this group was 12 per 1,000.

DISEASES OF THE GENITO-URINARY SYSTEM

Next in order of numerical importance came admissions for diseases of the GENITO-URINARY System, with rates which rose from 5 per 1,000 in 1940 to over 20 in 1943, declining to slightly under 17 in 1945, with an average of 14 per 1,000—one eighth of all admissions for disease.

Admissions for this group in 1944 and 1945 were greater than those for diseases of the Ear, Nose and Throat. The increase in admissions from 1940 to 1943 is noteworthy, the rate in 1943 being four times that in 1940. Admissions were lower among male troops at an average of 6 per 1,000.

DISEASES OF THE DIGESTIVE SYSTEM

Following diseases of the Genito-Urinary System in admission rates came diseases of the DIGESTIVE System. An analysis of admissions for this group follows.

United Kingdom, 1940–45
Admissions to Hospitals for Diseases of the Digestive System
British Troops, Female
Annual Rates per 1,000 Strength and Relative Rates

Source: Hollerith Tabulations

1. *Annual Rates per 1,000 Strength*	1940	1941	1942	1943	1944	1945	Averages
Gastric Ulcers	0·10	0·04	0·04	0·06	0·02	0·31	0·10
Duodenal Ulcers	0·03	0·02	0·15	0·16	0·20	0·18	0·12
Peptic Ulcers, Unspecified	—	—	0·02	0·01	0·07	—	0·02
Perforation of Ulcers	—	0·02	0·02	0·01	0·01	—	0·01
Dyspepsia and Gastritis	1·48	1·69	1·89	2·00	1·29	1·17	1·59
Hernia	0·10	0·17	0·42	0·59	0·40	0·49	0·36
Appendicitis	3·29	3·65	7·30	8·99	7·02	7·06	6·22
Haemorrhoids	0·16	0·42	0·56	0·70	0·64	0·86	0·56
Other Causes	3·53	4·05	6·16	6·26	4·08	3·75	4·64
Totals	8·69	10·06	16·56	18·78	13·73	13·82	13·62
Percentages of total admissions for diseases	10	10	12	12	13	13	12
2. *Relative Rates*							
Gastric Ulcers	1·15	0·40	0·24	0·32	0·15	2·24	0·73
Duodenal Ulcers	0·35	0·20	0·91	0·85	1·45	1·30	0·88
Peptic Ulcers, Unspecified	—	—	0·12	0·05	0·51	—	0·15
Perforation of Ulcers	—	0·20	0·12	0·05	0·07	—	0·07
Dyspepsia and Gastritis	17·03	16·80	11·41	10·65	9·40	8·47	11·67
Hernia	1·15	1·69	2·54	3·14	2·91	3·55	2·64
Appendicitis	37·86	36·28	44·08	47·87	51·13	51·09	45·67
Haemorrhoids	1·84	4·18	3·38	3·73	4·66	6·22	4·11
Other Causes	40·62	40·26	37·20	33·33	29·72	27·13	34·07
Totals	100	100	100	100	100	100	100

Admission rates for this group, commencing at under 9 per 1,000 in 1940, more than doubled to 19 in 1943 before declining to slightly under 14 in 1945. Relative rates were 10 in 1940 and 1941, 12 in the two years which followed and, in spite of a fall of 5 per 1,000, rose to 13 in 1944 and 1945.

APPENDICITIS was responsible for nearly one half the admissions for the group at an average of 6 per 1,000. Annual rates rose from 3 in 1940 to 9 in 1943 and decreased to 7 in 1944 and 1945. They were nearly forty per cent. of group admissions in 1940, forty-eight in 1943 and 51 in 1945. As opposed to this, the relative rates of admissions on account of DYSPEPSIA and GASTRITIS declined annually from 17 in 1940 to 8 in 1945, while the rates per 1,000 strength increased from 1·5 to 2·0 in 1943, falling to slightly over 1 in 1945.

Apart from a small decline in 1944, admissions for HAEMORRHOIDS increased steadily over the years from 0·16 to 0·86 per 1,000. Rates for HERNIAS varied from 0·1 in 1940 to a peak of 0·6 in 1943 and ULCERS were responsible for an average rate of 0·25 per 1,000.

It is interesting to compare the female with the male rates of admissions for this group. These are tabulated below.

United Kingdom, 1940–45
Admissions to Hospitals for Diseases of the Digestive System
Comparison of Male and Female Rates

Source: Hollerith Tabulations

	Average Rates per 1,000 Strength		Comparative Rates (Male = 100)	
	Male	Female	Male	Female
Gastric Ulcer	0·32	0·10	100	31
Duodenal Ulcer	1·38	0·12	100	9
Peptic Ulcer	0·17	0·02	100	12
Perforation of Ulcer	0·15	0·01	100	7
Dyspepsia and Gastritis	3·08	1·59	100	52
Hernia	4·95	0·36	100	7
Appendicitis	2·50	6·22	100	249
Haemorrhoids	1·79	0·56	100	31
Other Causes	4·41	4·64	100	105
Totals	18·75	13·62	100	73

The total average rate of admissions of females was some three-quarters that of male troops. Apart from 'Other Causes', for which the female rate was only slightly more, admissions on account of APPENDICITIS only were in excess of the male rate. In this instance, it was two and a half times that for males. The range among females was nearly 6 per 1,000 and for males only two. The largest increase in female admissions occurred in 1941 when the rate of 7·3 was exactly double that in the previous year. Among male troops, the increase was much smaller, from 1·6 to 2·6 per 1,000. Admissions for DYSPEPSIA and GASTRITIS were one-half those for males, while for GASTRIC ULCERS and HAEMORRHOIDS they were approximately one-third.

DISEASES OF THE MUSCULO-SKELETAL SYSTEM

Rates of admission followed the general trend by increasing annually to 1943 with subsequent declines in the two ensuing years. They are:

	Annual Rate per 1,000 Strength	*Percentage of total admissions for disease*
1940	5·40	6
1941	6·14	6
1942	9·38	7
1943	12·64	8
1944	8·73	8
1945	7·92	7

The rate in 1943 was more than double that in 1940 and was half as much again as that in 1945. The average rate of slightly under 8·5 per 1,000 was some seven per cent. of all admissions for disease.

SCABIES

Admissions for SCABIES were notable for the remarkable increase in 1941 and for the equally dramatic decline in 1943. Rates, which are enumerated below, increased from 2 in 1940 to 14 in 1941 and fell from 13 to 4 in 1943:

	Annual Rate per 1,000 Strength	*Percentage of total admissions for disease*
1940	2·44	3
1941	14·08	14
1942	13·03	10
1943	3·97	3
1944	0·51	0·5
1945	0·25	0·2

The average rate over the six years was under 6 per 1,000, while that for the period other than 1941 and 1942 was one-quarter at 1·4. The rates experienced by male troops averaged less at 5 per 1,000; they were lower in 1941 and 1942 at 11 and 8 per 1,000, but in 1940 were four times the female rate, at 9 per 1,000.

DISEASES OF THE SKIN

Admissions which on the average were only very slightly lower than for Scabies, followed the general trend for all diseases, with the peak rate in 1943, and were as follows:

	Annual Rate per 1,000 Strength	*Percentage of total admissions for disease*
1940	3·36	4
1941	5·02	5
1942	7·94	6
1943	8·04	5
1944	5·74	5
1945	3·87	4

These admissions averaged at 5·66 per 1,000, equivalent to five per cent. of all admissions for disease and were sixth in order of numerical importance. Male rates, which averaged over 12 per 1,000 were second in order of precedence and represented ten per cent. of all disease admissions.

DISEASES OF THE RESPIRATORY SYSTEM

This group was responsible for admissions which ranged from 4·3 to 6·5 per 1,000. Rates are analysed in the table which follows.

United Kingdom, 1940–45
Admissions to Hospitals for Diseases of the Respiratory System. British Troops, Female. Annual Rates per 1,000 Strength and Relative Rates

Source: Hollerith Tabulations

1. *Annual Rates per 1,000 Strength*	1940	1941	1942	1943	1944	1945	Averages
Bronchitis	3·72	3·75	3·46	4·15	2·50	3·01	3·43
Pleurisy	0·23	0·15	0·48	0·45	0·32	0·12	0·29
Other Causes	1·25	0·84	1·39	1·87	1·48	1·23	1·34
Totals	5·20	4·74	5·33	6·47	4·30	4·36	5·07
Percentages of total admissions for diseases	6	5	4	4	4	4	—
2. *Relative Rates*							
Bronchitis	71·54	79·11	64·92	64·14	58·14	69·04	67·79
Pleurisy	4·42	3·16	9·00	6·96	7·44	2·75	5·73
Other Causes	24·04	17·72	26·08	28·90	34·42	28·21	26·48
Totals	100	100	100	100	100	100	100

BRONCHITIS at the average rate of 3·4 per 1,000 was some 0·5 less than the rate for males, although the relative rates were almost identical. Admissions for PLEURISY were at a little more than half the male rate.

MENTAL DISEASES

This group caused admissions at rates which averaged 4·4 per 1,000 over the six years. They increased from 1·8 in 1940 to 6·6 in 1943 and declined to 5·5 by 1945. Rates are shown in the following tables.

United Kingdom, 1940–45
Admissions to Hospitals for Mental Diseases. British Troops, Female. Annual Rates per 1,000 Strength and Relative Rates

Source: Hollerith Tabulations

1. *Annual Rates per 1,000 Strength*	1940	1941	1942	1943	1944	1945	Averages
Psychoses	0·49	0·40	1·19	1·34	0·84	0·92	0·86
Psychoneuroses	0·92	2·15	3·42	4·60	3·41	4·42	3·15
Other Causes	0·40	0·46	0·56	0·61	0·18	0·18	0·40
Totals	1·81	3·01	5·17	6·55	4·43	5·52	4·42
Percentages of total admissions for diseases	2	3	4	4	4	5	4
2. *Relative Rates*							
Psychoses	27·07	13·29	23·02	20·46	18·96	16·67	19·50
Psychoneuroses	50·83	71·43	66·15	70·23	76·98	80·07	71·43
Other Causes	22·10	15·28	10·83	9·31	4·06	3·26	9·07
Totals	100	100	100	100	100	100	100

Nearly three-quarters of the admissions for this group were on account of PSYCHONEUROSES, rates for which increased from 0·9 to 2·2 in 1941, to a peak of 4·6 in 1943. They declined to 4·4 in 1945. The average rate of 3 per 1,000 was two-thirds that for males. Admissions due to PSYCHOSES were slightly higher among women at 0·86 compared with 0·76. Group admissions were four per cent. of all admissions for diseases—in the case of males, it was five per cent.

RUBELLA

Admissions for this infectious disease were distinguished by the remarkably high rate, in 1940, of nearly 13 per 1,000, compared with the average of 1·5 for the following five years. It has already been observed that among male troops in the United Kingdom, there occurred a comparatively high rate of over 4 per 1,000 in 1940, as against the subsequent quinquennial average of 0·68. Rates for the sexes are presented in the table which follows.

United Kingdom, 1940–45
Admissions to Hospitals for Rubella
Comparison of Male and Female Rates per 1,000 Strength
Source: Hollerith Tabulations

Year	Males	Females
1940	4·34	12·78
1941	0·43	0·44
1942	0·23	0·69
1943	0·61	1·43
1944	1·14	3·92
1945	1·00	1·17
Average 1940–45	1·29	3·41
Average 1941–45	0·68	1·53

Normally, it would seem that admissions of females for Rubella are approximately twice those for males, but in 1940, when rates were much higher than the average, they were three times the male rate.

COMMON COLD AND INFLUENZA

Peak admissions for COMMON COLD occurred in 1941 and 1943, while those for INFLUENZA were in 1940 and 1943. It was previously noted among male troops that high admission rates for Common Cold and Influenza also occurred in 1943. The following table shows the relevant rates.

United Kingdom, 1940–45
Admissions to Hospitals for Common Cold and Influenza
British Troops, Male and Female
Annual Rates per 1,000 Strength

Source: Hollerith Tabulation

	Common Cold		Influenza	
	Males	Females	Males	Females
1940	2·61	2·50	3·47	4·12
1941	2·77	4·18	1·48	1·12
1942	2·02	2·71	1·06	1·13
1943	4·12	4·55	3·42	4·05
1944	1·36	1·48	1·07	0·85
1945	1·82	1·60	0·85	0·49
Average Rates	2·45	2·84	1·89	1·95

There was but little difference in the average rates of admission between the sexes for Influenza. In the case of Common Cold, the difference was 0·4 per 1,000, being higher among women and in only two of the six years were admission rates lower than for men, and then but little. Subject to standardisation, it would appear that the females were slightly more prone to Common Cold.

DISEASES OF THE CARDIO-VASCULAR SYSTEM

Admissions for this group of diseases averaged 2·2 per 1,000 as opposed to nearly twice that rate for males. They followed the trend exhibited by males by increasing annually to 1943, declining in 1944 and rising in the final year to a rate less than that recorded in the peak year of 1943. Rates are analysed hereunder.

United Kingdom, 1940–45
Admissions to Hospitals for Diseases of the Cardio-Vascular System
British Troops, Female
Annual Rates per 1,000 Strength

Source: Hollerith Tabulations

	1940	1941	1942	1943	1944	1945	Averages
Valvular Disease of the Heart	0·10	0·10	0·18	0·11	0·07	—	0·09
Varicose Veins	0·43	0·65	1·38	2·10	1·68	1·21	1·41
Other Causes	0·76	0·74	0·91	0·84	0·42	0·49	0·69
Totals	1·29	1·49	2·47	3·05	2·17	2·70	2·20
Percentages of total admissions for diseases	1·5	1·5	1·8	2·0	2·0	2·3	1·9

VARICOSE VEINS accounted for more than one-half of all group admissions (among males they were nearly three-quarters) at an average rate of 1·4 per 1,000 which was exactly one-half the male rate. Admissions for VALVULAR DISEASE of the HEART were comparatively low at 0·09 per 1,000 compared with the male rate of 0·24.

OTHER DISEASES

PNEUMONIA accounted for admission rates at 1·35 per 1,000 which were nearly 1 per 1,000 less than for males. Those for TUBERCULOSIS at 1·12 were also slightly lower. Of the latter, sixty per cent. of the cases were the Pulmonary type, compared with eighty per cent. in males. Cases of MENINGOCOCCAL INFECTION, which recorded average rates at two-thirds those of males, provided the only instance among diseases where admission rates decreased annually. There were no recorded admissions in 1945. For MUMPS and DIPHTHERIA rates of admission among females were greater than those of the opposite sex by over seventy per cent. in each case. The average rates for women were 1·01 and 0·78 respectively.

INJURIES

Admission rates to hospitals of females on account of injuries were approximately one-half those for males. They increased from 3 in 1940 to 9 per 1,000 in the peak year of 1943 and closed at 6 in 1945. On the average, they were some five per cent. of all admissions (males were ten per cent.).

As was the case with male troops, injuries were classified in the Hollerith tabulations according to whether the injuries were, or were not, the result of enemy action or the cause was not so specified. Rates per 1,000 strength are given in Table 13.

Those known to be caused by enemy action were only slightly less than for males in 1940 and 1941 but in the succeeding years the difference in rates was more marked for, while this type of injury among males rose from 0·1 per 1,000 in 1940 to 1·9 in 1945, the female rates declined from 0·07 in 1940 to 0·03 in 1943, rose to 0·12 in 1944, followed by no admissions in 1945.

Injuries not due to enemy action recorded rates which increased from 2 per 1,000 in 1940 to 6 in 1943, finally declining to 4 in 1945, with an average of 4 per 1,000 compared with 9 in the case of males.

In Table 14 are consolidated the rates of admission presented in the previous table and classified according to Head Injuries, Fractures (other than to head), Burns, Old Injuries, and Other Injuries.

Head injuries, with an average rate of 0·6 per 1,000, accounted for ten per cent. of all injuries and were more frequent in 1943 and 1944 when the rates exceeded 0·8 per 1,000. Fractures, other than those to the head, were responsible for more than a quarter of all injuries and recorded a comparatively high rate of 2·66 in 1943 against an average of 1·65. Rates for Burns were heaviest in 1944 and for Old Injuries in 1943. Burns accounted for ten per cent. and Old Injuries some six per cent. of all injuries.

DEATHS

As with mortality statistics for males, and for the same reason, it is possible to present rates for the years 1940 to 1943 only. These are recorded in Table 15 as percentages of admissions by diseases or disease groups. Relative rates are also included.

Because there were so few deaths, particularly in 1940 and 1941, and in view of the great disparity in the numerical strengths of the sexes in the Army, comparisons of mortality rates between males and females would serve no useful purpose.

The greater number of deaths occurred in 1943; indeed, more deaths are recorded for that year than during the triennium immediately preceding.

During each of the years 1941, 1942, and 1943, TUBERCULOSIS was responsible for one quarter of the deaths from disease, more than any other disease or group. In 1943, PNEUMONIA caused one-seventh of the deaths, and Diseases of the GENITO-URINARY System, one-ninth. It is perhaps worth recording that there were no deaths from Pneumonia prior to 1943.

TABLE 1

United Kingdom, 1940–45. Admissions to Hospitals. British Troops, Male
Annual Rates per 1,000 Strength

Source: Hollerith Tabulations

	CAUSES	1940	1941	1942	1943	1944	1945	
1	Common Cold	2·61	2·77	2·02	4·12	1·36	1·82	1
2	Diphtheria	0·37	0·48	0·44	0·44	0·37	0·54	2
3	Dysentery	0·03	0·08	0·21	0·53	0·89	1·97	3
4	Enteric Group of Fevers	0·04	0·02	0·02	0·02	0·01	0·03	4
5	Influenza	3·47	1·48	1·06	3·42	1·07	0·85	5
6	Jaundice, Catarrhal	0·27	0·42	1·23	2·27	1·62	2·19	6
7	Malaria	0·08	0·07	0·21	0·54	9·63	7·04	7
8	Measles	0·55	0·49	0·19	0·57	0·34	0·40	8
9	Meningococcal Infection	0·52	0·33	0·23	0·14	0·16	0·25	9
10	Mumps	0·28	0·42	0·01	0·58	0·45	0·75	10
11	Pneumonia	0·85	1·12	2·15	2·80	2·64	3·89	11
12	Rheumatic Fever	0·24	0·17	0·20	0·22	0·26	0·36	12
13	Rubella	4·34	0·43	0·23	0·61	1·14	1·00	13
14	Scarlet Fever	0·50	0·32	0·25	0·49	0·56	0·90	14
15	Tuberculosis	1·15	1·13	1·07	1·36	1·37	1·67	15
16	Venereal Diseases	7·40	10·50	13·94	11·27	8·70	13·14	16
17	P.U.O.	0·11	0·06	0·10	0·15	0·19	0·27	17
18	Other Diseases due to Infection	1·60	1·30	1·49	1·53	1·51	1·14	18
19	Scabies	9·33	11·37	7·82	1·10	0·71	1·00	19
20	Other Infestations	0·34	0·14	0·20	0·18	0·19	0·35	20
21	Diseases of the Nervous System	2·02	1·90	2·47	2·80	2·35	2·75	21
22	Mental Conditions	3·59	3·95	6·60	8·03	6·89	8·05	22
23	Diseases of the Eye	1·22	1·59	2·04	2·06	1·83	1·70	23
24	Diseases of the Ear, Nose and Throat	11·57	9·30	11·83	13·97	11·46	12·97	24
25	Diseases of the Cardio-Vascular System	2·36	2·48	5·74	5·19	3·66	4·67	25
26	Diseases of the Blood and Blood-forming Organs	0·57	0·56	0·78	0·89	0·79	1·08	26
27	Diseases of the Breast	0·14	0·13	0·20	0·19	0·19	0·22	27
28	Diseases of the Endocrine System	0·03	0·05	0·08	0·08	0·05	0·09	28
29	Diseases of the Respiratory System	6·29	4·95	5·83	6·59	5·00	5·38	29
30	Diseases of the Mouth, Teeth and Gums	1·53	2·26	2·75	2·66	1·76	2·26	30
31	Diseases of the Digestive System	13·76	13·91	21·18	21·96	18·21	23·46	31
32	Disorders of Nutrition and Metabolism	0·17	0·19	0·25	0·33	0·29	0·51	32
33	Diseases of the Genito-Urinary System	3·95	4·03	6·72	7·13	7·08	9·92	33
34	Diseases of the Musculo-Skeletal System	8·09	7·78	12·82	14·24	11·56	11·48	34
35	Diseases of the Areolar Tissue	3·00	2·80	3·80	5·51	4·51	5·17	35

36	Diseases of the Skin	7·78	9·82	13·60	15·88	12·97	14·16	36
37	Poisons	0·02	0·04	0·07	0·08	0·05	0·05	37
38	All Other Diseases	4·59	3·86	6·00	5·76	7·04	9·05	38
39	*Total Admissions for Diseases*	104·75	102·70	136·81	145·67	128·87	152·51	39
40	Injuries—E.A.	0·10	0·08	0·12	0·24	1·09	1·90	40
41	Injuries—N.E.A.	3·42	4·42	10·97	13·12	10·24	11·16	41
42	Injuries—Not Specified	1·92	1·94	4·43	5·42	4·29	4·66	42
43	*Total Admissions for Injuries*	5·44	6·44	15·52	18·78	15·62	17·71	43
44	*Total Admissions*	110·19	109·14	152·33	164·45	144·49	170·22	44

Note: For suggested correction factors *see* page 110.

TABLE 2

United Kingdom, 1940–45. Admissions to Hospitals. British Troops, Male
Relative Rates

Source: Hollerith Tabulations

	CAUSES	1940	1941	1942	1943	1944	1945	
1	Common Cold	2·49	2·70	1·48	2·83	1·06	1·19	1
2	Diphtheria	0·35	0·47	0·32	0·30	0·29	0·35	2
3	Dysentery	0·03	0·08	0·15	0·36	0·69	1·29	3
4	Enteric Group of Fevers	0·04	0·02	0·01	0·01	0·01	0·02	4
5	Influenza	3·31	1·44	0·77	2·35	0·83	0·56	5
6	Jaundice, Catarrhal	0·26	0·41	0·90	1·56	1·26	1·44	6
7	Malaria	0·08	0·07	0·15	0·37	7·47	4·62	7
8	Measles	0·53	0·48	0·14	0·39	0·26	0·26	8
9	Meningococcal Infection	0·50	0·32	0·17	0·10	0·12	0·16	9
10	Mumps	0·27	0·41	0·74	0·40	0·35	0·49	10
11	Pneumonia	0·81	1·09	1·57	1·92	2·05	2·55	11
12	Rheumatic Fever	0·23	0·17	0·15	0·15	0·20	0·24	12
13	Rubella	4·14	0·42	0·17	0·42	0·88	0·66	13
14	Scarlet Fever	0·48	0·31	0·18	0·34	0·43	0·59	14
15	Tuberculosis	1·10	1·10	0·78	0·93	1·07	1·09	15
16	Venereal Diseases	7·06	10·22	10·19	7·74	6·75	8·62	16
17	P.U.O.	0·10	0·06	0·07	0·10	0·15	0·18	17
18	Other Diseases due to Infection	1·53	1·26	1·09	1·06	1·17	0·75	18
19	Scabies	8·91	11·07	5·72	0·76	0·55	0·66	19
20	Other Infestations	0·32	0·14	0·15	0·12	0·15	0·23	20
21	Diseases of the Nervous System	1·93	1·85	1·81	1·92	1·82	1·80	21
22	Mental Conditions	3·43	3·85	4·82	5·51	5·35	5·28	22
23	Diseases of the Eye	1·16	1·55	1·49	1·41	1·42	1·11	23
24	Diseases of the Ear, Nose and Throat	11·04	9·05	8·64	9·59	8·89	8·50	24
25	Diseases of the Cardio-Vascular System	2·25	2·41	4·19	3·56	2·84	3·06	25
26	Diseases of the Blood and Blood-forming Organs	0·54	0·54	0·57	0·61	0·61	0·71	26
27	Diseases of the Breast	0·03	0·05	0·06	0·05	0·04	0·06	27
28	Diseases of the Endocrine System	0·13	0·13	0·15	0·13	0·15	0·14	28
29	Diseases of the Respiratory System	6·00	4·82	4·26	4·52	3·88	3·53	29
30	Diseases of the Mouth, Teeth and Gums	1·46	2·20	2·01	1·83	1·37	1·48	30
31	Diseases of the Digestive System	13·14	13·54	15·48	15·07	14·13	15·38	31
32	Disorders of Nutrition and Metabolism	0·16	0·19	0·18	0·23	0·23	0·33	32
33	Diseases of the Genito-Urinary System	3·77	3·92	4·91	4·89	5·49	6·51	33
34	Diseases of the Musculo-Skeletal System	7·72	7·57	9·37	9·78	8·97	7·53	34
35	Diseases of the Areolar Tissue	2·86	2·73	2·78	3·78	3·50	3·39	35

36	Diseases of the Skin	7·43	9·56	9·49	10·90	10·07	9·28	36
37	Poisons	0·02	0·04	0·05	0·05	0·04	0·03	37
38	All Other Diseases	4·38	3·76	4·39	3·95	5·46	5·93	38
39	*Total Admissions for Diseases*	100	100	100	100	100	100	39
40	Injuries—N.E.A.	62·87	68·63	70·68	69·86	65·56	63·02	40
41	Injuries—E.A.	1·84	1·24	0·78	1·28	6·98	10·67	41
42	Injuries—Not Specified	32·29	30·13	28·54	28·86	27·46	26·31	42
43	*Total Admissions for Injuries*	100	100	100	100	100	100	43

TABLE 3

United Kingdom 1940–45. Admissions to Hospitals. British Troops, Male
Comparative Rates (1943 = 100)

Source: Hollerith Tabulations

	CAUSES	1940	1941	1942	1943	1944	1945	
1	Common Cold	63	67	49	100	33	44	1
2	Diphtheria	84	109	100	100	84	123	2
3	Dysentery	6	15	40	100	168	37	3
4	Enteric Group of Fevers	200	100	100	100	50	150	4
5	Influenza	101	43	31	100	31	25	5
6	Jaundice, Catarrhal	12	19	54	100	71	96	7
7	Malaria	1	1	39	100	1,783	1,304	8
8	Measles	96	86	33	100	60	70	9
9	Meningococcal Infection	371	24	164	100	114	179	6
10	Mumps	48	72	174	100	78	129	10
11	Pneumonia	30	40	77	100	94	139	11
12	Rheumatic Fever	109	77	91	100	118	164	12
13	Rubella	711	70	38	100	187	164	13
14	Scarlet Fever	102	65	51	100	114	184	14
15	Tuberculosis	85	83	79	100	101	123	15
16	Venereal Diseases	66	93	124	100	77	117	16
17	P.U.O.	73	40	67	100	127	180	17
18	Other Diseases due to Infection	105	85	97	100	99	75	18
19	Scabies	848	1,034	711	100	65	91	19
20	Other Infestations	189	78	111	100	106	194	20
21	Diseases of the Nervous System	72	68	88	100	84	98	21
22	Mental Conditions	45	49	82	100	86	100	22
23	Diseases of the Eye	59	77	99	100	89	83	23
24	Diseases of the Ear, Nose, and Throat	83	67	85	100	82	93	24
25	Diseases of the Cardio-Vascular System	45	48	111	100	71	90	25
26	Diseases of the Blood and Blood-forming Organs	64	63	88	100	89	121	26
27	Diseases of the Breast	74	68	105	100	100	116	27
28	Diseases of the Endocrine System	38	63	100	100	63	113	28
29	Diseases of the Respiratory System	95	75	88	100	76	82	29
30	Diseases of the Mouth, Teeth and Gums	58	85	103	100	66	85	30
31	Diseases of the Digestive System	63	63	96	100	83	107	31
32	Disorders of Nutrition and Metabolism	52	58	76	100	88	155	32
33	Diseases of the Genito-Urinary Tract	55	57	94	100	99	139	33
34	Diseases of the Musculo-Skeletal System	57	55	90	100	81	81	34
35	Diseases of the Areolar Tissue	54	51	69	100	82	94	35

36	Diseases of the Skin	49	62	86	100	82	89	36
37	Poisons	25	50	88	100	63	63	37
38	All Other Diseases	80	67	104	100	122	157	38
39	*Total Admissions for Diseases*	72	71	94	100	88	105	39
40	Injuries—E.A.	42	33	50	100	454	792	40
41	Injuries—N.E.A.	26	30	84	100	78	85	41
42	Injuries—Not Specified	35	36	82	100	79	86	42
43	*Total Admissions for Injuries*	29	34	83	100	83	94	43
44	*Total Admissions*	67	66	93	100	88	104	44

Note: For suggested correction factors, *see* page 110.

TABLE 4

United Kingdom, 1940–45
Admissions to Hospitals for Diseases. British Troops, Male
Average Rates per 1,000 Strength in Order of Precedence, with Relative Rates

Source: Hollerith Tabulations

CAUSES	Average Rates	Order of Precedence	Relative Rates
Diseases of the Digestive System	18·75	1	14·59
Diseases of the Skin	12·37	2	9·62
Diseases of the Ear, Nose and Throat	11·85	3	9·22
Diseases of the Musculo-Skeletal System	11·00	4	8·56
Venereal Diseases	10·83	5	8·42
Diseases of the Genito-Urinary Tract	6·47	6	5·03
Mental Conditions	6·18	7	4·81
Diseases of the Respiratory System	5·68	8	4·42
Scabies	5·22	9	4·06
Diseases of the Areolar Tissue	4·13	10	3·21
Diseases of the Cardio-Vascular System	4·01	11	3·12
Malaria	2·93	12	2·28
Common Cold	2·45	13	1·91
Diseases of the Nervous System	2·38	14	1·85
Pneumonia	2·24	15	1·74
Diseases of the Mouth, Teeth and Gums	2·20	16	1·71
Influenza	1·89	17	1·47
Diseases of the Eye	1·74	18	1·35
Jaundice, Catarrhal	1·33	19	1·03
Rubella	1·29	20	1·00
Tuberculosis	1·29	21	1·00
Diseases of the Blood and Blood-forming Organs	0·78	22	0·61
Dysentery	0·62	23	0·48
Mumps	0·58	24	0·45
Scarlet Fever	0·50	25	0·39
Diphtheria	0·44	26	0·34
Measles	0·42	27	0·33
Disorders of Nutrition and Metabolism	0·29	28	0·23
Meningococcal Infection	0·27	29	0·21
Rheumatic Fever	0·24	30	0·19
Diseases of the Breast	0·18	31	0·14
P.U.O.	0·15	32	0·12
Diseases of the Endocrine System	0·06	33	0·05
Poisoning	0·05	34	0·04
Enteric Group of Fevers	0·02	35	0·02
All Other Diseases	7·71		6·00
Totals	128·55		100

Note: For suggested correction factors *see* page 110.

TABLE 5

United Kingdom, 1940–45
Admissions to Hospitals for Injuries. British Troops, Male
Rates per 1,000 Strength

Source: Hollerith Tabulations

1. *Enemy Action*	1940	1941	1942	1943	1944	1945
Head Injuries	0·02	0·01	0·01	0·02	0·05	0·03
Fractures (Other Sites)	0·01	0·01	0·01	0·05	0·18	0·21
Burns	0·00	0·00	0·00	0·00	0·01	0·01
Old Injuries	0·02	0·02	0·02	0·03	0·23	0·98
Other Injuries	0·06	0·04	0·08	0·14	0·62	0·66
Totals	0·10	0·08	0·12	0·24	1·09	1·90
2. *Non-Enemy Action*						
Head Injuries	0·25	0·26	0·67	0·85	0·78	1·04
Fractures (Other Sites)	1·19	1·78	4·34	5·13	4·92	4·04
Burns	0·10	0·13	0·30	0·42	0·41	0·43
Old Injuries	0·33	0·35	0·56	0·54	0·37	0·42
Other Injuries	1·56	1·91	5·11	6·18	3·77	5·24
Totals	3·42	4·42	10·97	13·12	10·24	11·16
3. *Cause Not Known*						
Head Injuries	0·10	0·08	0·19	0·24	0·17	0·16
Fractures (Other Sites)	0·44	0·44	1·46	1·65	1·31	1·41
Burns	0·06	0·07	0·15	0·23	0·24	0·17
Old Injuries	0·57	0·65	0·62	0·60	0·61	1·06
Other Injuries	0·76	0·71	2·01	2·71	1·95	1·86
Totals	1·92	1·94	4·43	5·42	4·29	4·66
Total admissions through injury	5·44	6·44	15·52	18·78	15·62	17·71
Percentage of admissions for all causes	5	6	10	11	11	10

Note: For suggested correction factors *see* page 110.

TABLE 6

United Kingdom, 1940–45
Admissions to Hospitals for Injuries. British Troops, Male
Relative Rates

Source: Hollerith Tabulations

1. *Enemy Action*	1940	1941	1942	1943	1944	1945
Head Injuries	14	10	9	6	5	4
Fractures (Other Sites)	7	9	9	20	17	13
Burns	1	5	2	1	1	1
Old Injuries	21	27	18	12	21	35
Other Injuries	57	49	62	61	56	47
Totals	100	100	100	100	100	100
2. *Non-Enemy Action*						
Head Injuries	7	6	6	7	8	7
Fractures (Other Sites)	35	40	40	39	48	40
Burns	3	3	3	3	4	3
Old Injuries	10	8	5	4	3	5
Other Injuries	45	43	46	47	37	45
Totals	100	100	100	100	100	100
3. *Cause Not Known*						
Head Injuries	5	4	4	5	4	3
Fractures (Other Sites)	23	23	33	30	31	30
Burns	3	3	3	4	6	4
Old Injuries	30	33	14	11	14	23
Other Injuries	39	37	46	50	45	40
Totals	100	100	100	100	100	100

TABLE 7

United Kingdom, 1940–43. Deaths in Hospitals. British Troops, Male Expressed as percentages of admissions with Relative Rates

Source: Hollerith Tabulations

	CAUSES	Deaths as percentages of admissions				Relative Rates				
		1940	1941	1942	1943	1940	1941	1942	1943	
1	Common Cold	—	—	—	—	—	—	—	—	1
2	Diphtheria	0·19	0·44	0·36	0·84	0·35	1·24	0·80	1·41	2
3	Dysentery	—	0·76	—	0·25	—	0·31	—	0·47	3
4	Enteric Group of Fevers	3·45	—	—	—	0·71	—	—	—	4
5	Influenza	—	—	0·05	0·02	—	—	0·26	0·24	5
6	Jaundice, Catarrhal	0·54	0·13	—	0·13	0·71	0·31	—	1·18	6
7	Malaria	1·80	—	1·29	0·45	0·71	—	1·34	0·94	7
8	Measles	—	—	—	—	—	—	—	—	8
9	Meningococcal Infection	5·33	3·85	6·13	6·61	13·47	7·45	6·95	3·54	9
10	Mumps	—	—	—	—	—	—	—	—	10
11	Pneumonia	2·30	0·85	0·30	0·63	9·56	5·59	3·21	6·84	11
12	Rheumatic Fever	—	—	0·27	0·55	—	—	0·26	0·47	12
13	Rubella	—	—	—	—	—	—	—	—	13
14	Scarlet Fever	—	0·17	—	—	—	0·31	—	—	14
15	Tuberculosis	2·33	2·13	2·95	2·60	13·12	14·29	15·78	13·68	15
16	Venereal Diseases	0·01	0·15	0·14	0·05	0·35	0·93	2·67	2·36	16
17	P.U.O.	—	—	—	—	—	—	—	—	17
18	Other Diseases due to Infection	0·32	0·69	0·71	0·62	2·48	5·28	5·35	3·77	18
19	Scabies	—	—	—	—	—	—	—	—	19
20	Other Infestations	—	—	—	—	—	—	—	—	20
21	Diseases of the Nervous System	0·93	0·89	0·93	0·93	9·22	9·94	11·50	10·14	21
22	Mental Conditions	0·10	0·53	0·02	0·03	1·77	1·24	0·53	0·94	22
23	Diseases of the Eye	—	0·03	—	0·03	—	0·31	—	0·24	23
24	Diseases of the Ear, Nose and Throat	0·03	0·03	0·03	0·03	1·77	1·86	1·60	1·89	24
25	Diseases of the Cardio-Vascular System	0·62	0·59	0·26	0·39	7·09	8·70	7·49	7·78	25
26	Diseases of the Blood and Blood-forming Organs	1·02	1·42	1·10	1·36	2·84	4·66	4·28	4·71	26
27	Diseases of the Breast	—	—	—	—	—	—	—	—	27
28	Diseases of the Endocrine System	—	1·77	0·54	0·94	—	0·93	0·53	0·71	28
29	Diseases of the Respiratory System	0·17	0·15	0·06	0·35	5·32	4·04	1·60	8·96	29
30	Diseases of the Mouth, Teeth and Gums	—	—	0·02	—	—	—	0·26	—	30

TABLE 7—*Continued*

United Kingdom, 1940–43. Deaths in Hospitals. British Troops, Male
Expressed as percentages of admissions with Relative Rates

Source: Hollerith Tabulations

	CAUSES	Deaths as percentages of admissions				Relative Rates				
		1940	1941	1942	1943	1940	1941	1942	1943	
31	Diseases of the Digestive System	0·30	0·27	0·24	0·26	20·21	22·05	25·67	22·17	31
32	Disorders of Nutrition and Metabolism	0·86	—	—	0·37	0·71	—	—	0·47	32
33	Diseases of the Genito-Urinary System	0·18	0·27	0·24	0·11	3·55	6·52	6·68	3·07	33
34	Diseases of the Musculo-Skeletal System	0·04	—	0·03	0·00	1·42	—	2·14	0·24	34
35	Diseases of the Areolar Tissue	0·02	0·04	0·04	0·03	0·35	0·62	0·80	0·71	35
36	Diseases of the Skin	0·01	—	0·00	0·02	0·35	—	0·26	1·18	36
37	Poisons	12·90	—	—	0·81	1·42	—	—	0·24	37
38	All Other Diseases	0·11	0·16	—	0·07	2·48	3·42	—	1·65	38
39	*Total Deaths from Diseases*	0·20	0·17	0·15	0·18	100	100	100	100	39
40	Injuries—E.A.	10·64	6·21	2·23	1·29	29·41	13·85	4·63	4·86	40
41	Injuries—N.E.A.	0·53	0·44	0·42	0·27	49·02	56·92	80·56	57·28	41
42	Injuries—Not Specified	0·42	0·52	0·19	0·44	21·57	29·23	14·81	37·86	42
43	*Total Deaths from Injuries*	0·68	0·53	0·37	0·33	100	100	100	100	43
44	*Total Deaths*	0·22	0·19	0·17	0·19	—	—	—	—	44

Note: For suggested correction factors *see* page 110.

TABLE 8

United Kingdom, 1940–45. Admissions to Hospitals. British Troops, Female
Annual Rates per 1,000 Strength

Source: Hollerith Tabulations

	CAUSES	1940	1941	1942	1943	1944	1945	
1	Common Cold	2·50	4·18	2·71	4·55	1·48	1·60	1
2	Diphtheria	0·65	1·10	1·05	1·03	0·24	0·61	2
3	Dysentery	0·03	0·55	0·39	0·78	1·53	1·35	3
4	Enteric Group of Fevers	0·23	0·04	0·01	0·02	—	—	4
5	Influenza	4·12	1·12	1·13	4·05	0·80	0·49	5
6	Jaundice, Catarrhal	0·10	0·17	1·00	1·65	0·12	1·41	6
7	Malaria	—	0·02	0·01	0·02	0·02	0·25	7
8	Measles	1·42	1·18	0·88	1·73	0·15	1·41	8
9	Meningococcal Infection	0·33	0·30	0·28	0·10	0·05	—	9
10	Mumps	0·49	0·82	2·06	1·16	0·30	1·23	10
11	Pneumonia	0·79	1·24	1·76	1·85	0·98	1·47	11
12	Rheumatic Fever	0·26	0·06	0·30	0·26	0·40	—	12
13	Rubella	12·78	0·44	0·69	1·43	3·92	1·17	13
14	Scarlet Fever	1·05	0·82	0·94	1·47	0·99	1·53	14
15	Tuberculosis	0·36	0·78	1·58	1·75	1·44	0·79	15
16	Venereal Diseases	0·16	1·52	2·43	2·51	1·41	1·47	16
17	P.U.O.	0·20	0·19	0·18	0·39	0·22	0·25	17
18	Other Diseases due to Infection	1·09	3·33	2·32	2·54	2·26	2·27	18
19	Scabies	2·44	14·08	13·03	3·97	0·51	0·25	19
20	Other Infestations	0·03	0·40	0·27	0·19	0·12	0·25	20
21	Diseases of the Nervous System	1·02	1·37	2·07	2·28	1·94	2·03	21
22	Mental Conditions	1·82	3·01	5·17	6·55	4·43	5·52	22
23	Diseases of the Eye	0·40	0·95	1·05	1·13	0·77	1·11	23
24	Diseases of the Ear, Nose and Throat	13·77	14·36	17·34	20·52	15·16	14·43	24
25	Diseases of the Cardio-Vascular System	1·29	1·49	2·47	3·05	2·17	2·70	25
26	Diseases of the Blood and Blood-forming Organs	1·15	1·27	1·43	1·94	1·38	1·04	26
27	Diseases of the Breast	0·26	0·34	0·68	0·88	0·76	0·74	27
28	Diseases of the Endocrine System	0·16	0·65	0·52	0·98	0·78	0·92	28
29	Diseases of the Respiratory System	5·20	4·74	5·33	6·47	4·30	4·36	29
30	Diseases of the Mouth, Teeth and Gums	1·93	2·74	3·14	3·03	2·10	2·89	30

TABLE 8—*Continued*

United Kingdom, 1940–45. Admissions to Hospitals. British Troops, Female
Annual Rates per 1,000 Strength

Source: Hollerith Tabulations

	CAUSES	1940	1941	1942	1943	1944	1945	
31	Diseases of the Digestive System	8·69	10·06	16·56	18·78	13·73	13·82	31
32	Disorders of Nutrition and Metabolism	0·07	0·23	0·29	0·39	0·24	0·12	32
33	Diseases of the Genito-Urinary System	4·83	8·67	16·67	20·48	18·86	16·88	33
34	Diseases of the Musculo-Skeletal System	5·40	6·14	9·38	12·64	8·73	7·92	34
35	Diseases of the Areolar Tissue	1·88	2·74	2·99	4·10	3·67	2·95	35
36	Diseases of the Skin	3·36	5·02	7·94	8·04	5·74	3·87	36
37	Poisons	—	0·04	0·12	0·18	0·10	0·12	37
38	All Other Diseases	3·85	5·52	11·02	8·73	7·97	7·24	38
39	*Total Admissions for Diseases*	84·11	101·66	137·19	151·59	109·77	106·46	39
40	Injuries—N.E.A.	2·17	2·34	5·21	5·92	4·99	4·23	40
41	Injuries—E.A.	0·07	0·06	0·04	0·03	0·12	—	41
42	Injuries—Not Specified	1·19	1·01	2·56	3·14	1·98	1·66	42
43	*Total Admissions for Injuries*	3·43	3·40	7·81	9·08	7·09	5·89	43
44	*Total Admissions*	87·54	105·07	145·01	160·67	116·86	112·35	44

Note: For suggested correction factors *see* page 110.

TABLE 9

United Kingdom 1940–45. Admissions to Hospitals. British Troops, Female
Relative Rates

Source: Hollerith Tabulations

	CAUSES	1940	1941	1942	1943	1944	1945	
1	Common Cold	2·97	4·11	1·98	3·00	1·35	1·50	1
2	Diphtheria	0·77	1·08	0·77	0·68	0·22	0·57	2
3	Dysentery	0·04	0·54	0·28	0·51	1·39	1·27	3
4	Enteric Group of Fevers	0·27	0·04	0·00	0·01	—	—	4
5	Influenza	4·90	1·10	0·82	2·67	0·73	0·46	5
6	Jaundice, Catarrhal	0·12	0·17	0·73	1·09	0·11	1·32	6
7	Malaria	—	0·02	0·00	0·01	0·02	0·23	7
8	Measles	1·69	1·16	0·64	1·14	0·14	1·32	8
9	Meningococcal Infection	0·39	0·30	0·20	0·07	0·05	—	9
10	Mumps	0·58	0·81	1·50	0·77	0·27	1·16	10
11	Pneumonia	0·94	1·22	1·28	1·22	0·89	1·38	11
12	Rheumatic Fever	0·31	0·06	0·22	0·17	0·36	—	12
13	Rubella	15·19	0·43	0·50	0·94	3·57	1·10	13
14	Scarlet Fever	1·25	0·81	0·69	0·97	0·90	1·44	14
15	Tuberculosis	0·43	0·77	1·15	1·15	1·31	0·74	15
16	Venereal Diseases	0·19	1·50	1·77	1·66	1·28	1·38	16
17	P.U.O.	0·24	0·18	0·13	0·26	0·20	0·23	17
18	Other Diseases due to Infection	1·30	3·27	1·69	1·68	2·06	2·13	18
19	Scabies	2·90	13·85	9·50	2·62	0·46	0·23	19
20	Other Infestations	0·04	0·39	0·20	0·13	0·11	0·23	20
21	Diseases of the Nervous System	1·21	1·35	1·51	1·50	1·77	1·91	21
22	Mental Conditions	2·16	2·96	3·77	4·32	4·04	5·19	22
23	Diseases of the Eye	0·48	0·93	0·77	0·75	0·70	1·04	23
24	Diseases of the Ear, Nose and Throat	16·37	14·12	12·64	13·54	13·81	13·56	24
25	Diseases of the Cardio-Vascular System	1·53	1·46	1·80	2·01	1·98	2·54	25
26	Diseases of the Blood and Blood-forming Organs	1·37	1·25	1·04	1·28	1·26	0·98	26
27	Diseases of the Breast	0·31	0·33	0·50	0·58	0·69	0·70	27
28	Diseases of the Endocrine System	0·19	0·64	0·38	0·65	0·71	0·86	28
29	Diseases of the Respiratory System	6·18	4·66	3·89	4·27	3·92	4·10	29
30	Diseases of the Mouth, Teeth and Gums	2·30	2·70	2·29	2·00	1·91	2·71	30

TABLE 9—*Continued*

United Kingdom 1940–45. Admissions to Hospitals. British Troops, Female
Relative Rates

Source: Hollerith Tabulations

	CAUSES	1940	1941	1942	1943	1944	1945	
31	Diseases of the Digestive System	10·33	9·90	12·07	12·39	12·51	12·98	31
32	Disorders of Nutrition and Metabolism	0·08	0·23	0·21	0·26	0·22	0·11	32
33	Diseases of the Genito-Urinary System	5·74	8·53	12·15	13·51	17·18	15·86	33
34	Disease of the Musculo-Skeletal System	6·42	6·04	6·84	8·34	7·95	7·44	34
35	Diseases of the Areolar Tissue	2·24	2·69	2·18	2·70	3·34	2·77	35
36	Diseases of the Skin	3·99	4·94	5·79	5·30	5·23	3·64	36
37	Poisons	—	0·04	0·09	0·12	0·09	0·11	37
38	All Other Diseases	4·58	5·43	8·03	5·76	7·26	6·80	38
39	*Total Admissions for Diseases*	100	100	100	100	100	100	39
40	Injuries—N.E.A.	63·27	68·62	66·71	65·13	70·38	71·82	40
41	Injuries—E.A.	2·04	1·76	0·51	0·33	1·69	—	41
42	Injuries—Not Specified	34·69	29·62	32·78	34·54	27·93	28·18	42
43	*Total Admissions for Injuries*	100	100	100	100	100	100	43

TABLE 10

United Kingdom, 1940–45. Admissions to Hospitals. British Troops, Female
Comparative Rates (1943 = 100)

Source: Hollerith Tabulations

	CAUSES	1940	1941	1942	1943	1944	1945	
1	Common Cold	55	92	60	100	32	35	1
2	Diphtheria	63	107	102	100	23	59	2
3	Dysentery	3	71	50	100	196	173	3
4	Enteric Group of Fevers	1,150	200	50	100	—	—	4
5	Influenza	102	28	28	100	20	12	5
6	Jaundice, Catarrhal	6	10	61	100	7	85	6
7	Malaria	—	100	50	100	100	1,250	7
8	Measles	82	68	51	100	9	82	8
9	Meningococcal Infection	330	300	280	100	50	—	9
10	Mumps	42	71	178	100	26	106	10
11	Pneumonia	43	67	95	100	53	79	11
12	Rheumatic Fever	100	23	115	100	154	—	12
13	Rubella	804	31	48	100	274	82	13
14	Scarlet Fever	71	56	64	100	67	104	14
15	Tuberculosis	21	45	90	100	82	45	15
16	Venereal Diseases	6	61	97	100	56	59	16
17	P.U.O.	51	49	46	100	56	64	17
18	Other Diseases due to Infection	43	131	91	100	89	89	18
19	Scabies	61	353	328	100	13	6	19
20	Other Infestations	16	211	142	100	63	132	20
21	Diseases of the Nervous System	49	60	91	100	85	89	21
22	Mental Conditions	28	46	79	100	68	84	22
23	Diseases of the Eye	35	84	93	100	68	98	23
24	Diseases of the Ear, Nose and Throat	67	70	85	100	74	70	24
25	Diseases of the Cardio-Vascular System	42	49	81	100	71	89	25
26	Diseases of the Blood, and Blood-forming Organs	59	65	74	100	71	54	26
27	Diseases of the Breast	30	39	77	100	86	84	27
28	Diseases of the Endocrine System	16	66	53	100	80	94	28
29	Diseases of the Respiratory System	80	73	82	100	66	67	29
30	Diseases of the Mouth, Teeth and Gums	64	90	103	100	69	95	30

TABLE 10—*Continued*

United Kingdom, 1940–45. Admissions to Hospitals. British Troops, Female
Comparative Rates (1943 = 100)

Source: Hollerith Tabulations

	CAUSES	1940	1941	1942	1943	1944	1945	
31	Diseases of the Digestive System	46	54	88	100	83	74	31
32	Disorders of Nutrition and Metabolism	18	59	74	100	62	31	32
33	Diseases of the Genito-Urinary System	24	42	81	100	92	82	33
34	Diseases of the Musculo-Skeletal System	43	49	74	100	69	63	34
35	Diseases of the Areolar Tissue	46	67	73	100	90	72	35
36	Diseases of the Skin	42	62	99	100	71	48	36
37	Poisons	—	22	66	100	56	66	37
38	All Other Diseases	44	63	126	100	91	83	38
39	*Total Admissions for Diseases*	55	67	91	100	72	70	39
40	Injuries—N.E.A.	37	40	88	100	84	71	40
41	Injuries—E.A.	233	200	133	100	400	—	41
42	Injuries—Not Specified	38	32	82	100	63	53	42
43	*Total Admissions for Injuries*	38	37	86	100	78	65	43
44	*Total Admission*	54	65	90	100	73	70	44

Note: For suggested correction factors *see* page 110.

TABLE 11

United Kingdom, 1940–45
Admissions to Hospitals for Diseases. British Troops, Female
Average Rates per 1,000 Strength, in Order of Precedence, with Relative Rates

Source: Hollerith Tabulations

CAUSES	Average Rates	Order of Precedence	Relative Rates
Diseases of the Ear, Nose and Throat	15·93	1	13·84
Diseases of the Genito-Urinary System	14·40	2	12·51
Diseases of the Digestive System	13·60	3	11·81
Diseases of the Musculo-Skeletal System	8·36	4	7·26
Scabies	5·71	5	4·96
Diseases of the Skin	5·66	6	4·92
Diseases of the Respiratory System	5·07	7	4·40
Mental Conditions	4·42	8	3·84
Rubella	3·41	9	2·96
Diseases of the Areolar Tissue	3·06	10	2·66
Common Cold	2·84	11	2·47
Diseases of the Mouth, Teeth and Gums	2·64	12	2·29
Diseases of the Cardio-Vascular System	2·20	13	1·91
Influenza	1·95	14	1·69
Diseases of the Nervous System	1·79	15	1·55
Venereal Diseases	1·58	16	1·37
Diseases of the Blood and Blood-forming Organs	1·37	17	1·19
Pneumonia	1·35	18	1·17
Measles Scarlet Fever }	1·13	19	0·98
Tuberculosis	1·12	21	0·97
Mumps	1·01	22	0·88
Diseases of the Eye	0·90	23	0·78
Diphtheria	0·78	24	0·68
Dysentery	0·77	25	0·67
Jaundice, Catarrhal	0·74	26	0·64
Diseases of the Endocrine System	0·67	27	0·58
Diseases of the Breast	0·61	28	0·53
P.U.O.	0·24	29	0·21
Disorders of Nutrition and Metabolism	0·22	30	0·19
Rheumatic Fever	0·21	31	0·18
Meningococcal Infection	0·18	32	0·16
Poisoning	0·08	33	0·07
Malaria Enteric Group of Fevers }	0·05	34	0·04
All Other Diseases	9·90		8·60
Total Admissions for Diseases	115·13		100·00

Note: For suggested correction factors *see* page 110.

TABLE 12

United Kingdom, 1940–45
Admissions to Hospitals for Diseases (over 1 per 1,000)
British Troops, Female. Comparative Rates (Male = 100).
Based on average admission rates

Source: Hollerith Tabulations

	DISEASES	Males	Females	
1	Measles	100	269	1
2	Rubella	100	264	2
3	Scarlet Fever	100	226	3
4	Diseases of the Genito-Urinary System	100	223	4
5	Diseases of the Blood and Blood-forming Organs	100	175	5
6	Mumps	100	174	6
7	Diseases of the Ear, Nose and Throat	100	134	
8	Diseases of the Mouth, Teeth and Gums	100	120	8
9	Common Cold	100	116	9
10	Scabies	100	109	10
11	Influenza	100	103	11
12	Diseases of the Respiratory System	100	89	12
13	Tuberculosis	100	87	13
14	Diseases of the Musculo-Skeletal System	100	76	14
15	Diseases of the Nervous System	100	75	15
16	Diseases of the Areolar Tissue	100	74	16
17	Diseases of the Digestive System	100	75	17
18	Mental Conditions	100	71	18
19	Pneumonia	100	60	19
20	Diseases of the Cardio-Vascular System	100	55	20
21	Diseases of the Skin	100	46	21
22	Venereal Diseases	100	15	22
23	*Total Admissions for Diseases*	100	90	23

TABLE 13

United Kingdom, 1940–45
Admissions to Hospitals for Injuries. British Troops, Female
Rates per 1,000 Strength

Source: Hollerith Tabulations

1. *Enemy Action*	1940	1941	1942	1943	1944	1945
Head Injuries	—	0·04	0·01	—	0·01	—
Fractures (Other Sites)	—	—	0·01	0·01	0·01	—
Burns	—	—	—	—	—	—
Old Injuries	—	0·02	0·01	—	0·01	—
Other Injuries	0·07	—	0·01	0·03	0·09	—
Totals	0·07	0·06	0·04	0·03	0·12	—

2. *Non-Enemy Action*

Head Injuries	0·26	0·40	0·55	0·61	0·69	0·49
Fractures (Other Sites)	0·59	0·49	1·49	1·90	1·43	1·35
Burns	0·23	0·30	0·46	0·49	0·61	0·55
Old Injuries	0·16	0·06	0·17	0·25	0·20	0·18
Other Injuries	0·92	1·08	2·53	2·67	2·06	1·66
Totals	2·17	2·34	5·21	5·92	4·99	4·23

3. *Cause Not Known*

Head Injuries	0·03	—	0·15	0·19	0·15	0·12
Fractures (Other Sites)	0·26	0·17	0·64	0·76	0·39	0·37
Burns	0·23	0·11	0·21	0·28	0·27	0·18
Old Injuries	0·13	0·08	0·24	0·29	0·22	0·12
Other Injuries	0·53	0·65	1·31	1·63	0·95	0·86
Totals	1·19	1·01	2·56	3·14	1·98	1·66
Total Admissions through Injuries	3·43	3·40	7·81	9·08	7·09	5·89
Percentages of Admissions for All Causes	4	3	5	6	6	5

Note: For suggested correction factors *see* page 110.

TABLE 14

United Kingdom, 1940–45
Admissions to Hospitals for Injuries. British Troops, Female
Annual Rates per 1,000 Strength and Relative Rates

Source: Hollerith Tabulations

1. *Annual Rates per 1,000 Strength*	1940	1941	1942	1943	1944	1945
Head Injuries	0·29	0·44	0·71	0·80	0·85	0·61
Fractures (Other Sites)	0·85	0·66	2·15	2·66	1·83	1·72
Burns	0·46	0·41	0·67	0·76	0·88	0·73
Old Injuries	0·29	0·16	0·43	0·54	0·43	0·30
Other Injuries	1·53	1·73	3·85	4·32	3·10	2·52
Totals	3·43	3·40	7·81	9·08	7·09	5·89

2. *Relative Rates*

Head Injuries	8·48	12·94	9·09	8·81	11·99	10·37
Fractures (Other Sites)	24·85	19·41	27·53	29·40	25·81	29·25
Burns	13·45	12·06	8·58	8·37	12·41	12·41
Old Injuries	8·48	4·71	5·51	5·95	6·06	5·10
Other Injuries	44·74	50·88	49·30	47·57	43·72	42·86
Totals	100	100	100	100	100	100

Note: For suggested correction factors *see* page 110.

TABLE 15

United Kingdom, 1940–43
Deaths in Hospitals, British Troops, Female
Expressed as percentages of admissions with Relative Rates

	CAUSES	Deaths as percentages of admissions of Individual Diseases/Injury Groups				Relative Rates				
		1940	1941	1942	1943	1940	1941	1942	1943	
	Diseases									
1	Diphtheria	—	1·72	1·40	0·49	—	25·00	14·29	2·94	1
2	Influenza	—	—	—	0·12	—	—	—	2·94	2
3	Meningococcal Infection	—	—	5·26	10·53	—	—	14·29	5·88	3
4	Pneumonia	—	—	—	1·36	—	—	—	14·72	4
5	Tuberculosis	—	3·22	1·88	2·60	—	25·00	28·57	26·47	5
6	Venereal Diseases	—	—	—	0·20	—	—	—	2·94	6
7	Other Diseases due to Infection	—	—	—	0·40	—	—	—	5·88	7
8	Diseases of the Nervous System	—	—	0·36	0·44	—	—	7·14	5·88	8
9	Mental Disorders	—	—	—	0·15	—	—	—	5·88	9
10	Diseases of the Ear, Nose and Throat	—	—	0·04	—	—	—	7·14	—	10
11	Diseases of the Cardio-Vascular System	2·56	—	0·30	—	33·33	—	7·14	—	11
12	Diseases of the Blood and Blood-forming Organs	5·71	—	—	0·26	66·67	—	—	2·94	12
13	Diseases of the Breast	—	—	1·09	—	—	—	7·14	—	13
14	Diseases of the Respiratory System	—	—	—	0·08	—	—	—	2·94	14
15	Diseases of the Digestive System	—	—	0·04	0·05	—	—	7·14	5·88	15
16	Diseases of the Genito-Urinary System	—	0·22	0·04	0·09	—	25·00	7·14	11·76	16
17	Diseases of the Musculo-Skeletal System	—	0·31	—	—	—	25·00	—	—	17
18	Diseases of the Skin	—	—	—	0·06	—	—	—	2·94	18
19	All Other Diseases	—	—	—	—	—	—	—	—	19
20	*Total Deaths from Diseases*	0·12	0·07	0·08	0·11	100	100	100	100	20
	Injuries									
21	Enemy Action	—	—	—	—	—	—	—	—	21
22	Non-Enemy Action	—	—	0·28	0·09	—	—	100	100	22
23	Not Specified	—	—	—	—	—	—	—	—	23
24	*Total Deaths from Injuries*	—	—	0·19	0·06	—	—	100	100	24
25	*Total Deaths*	0·12	0·07	0·10	0·11	—	—	—	—	25

TABLE 16

United Kingdom, 1939
Admissions to Hospitals. British Troops, Male
Annual Rates per 1,000 Strength

Sources: A.Fs. A. 31 (Jan. 1–Sept. 2)
Hollerith Tabulations (Sept. 3–Dec. 31)

CAUSES	Rates	CAUSES	Rates
Common Cold	11·72	Diseases of the Circulatory System—Others	2·37
Diphtheria	0·38	Diseases of the Blood and Blood-forming Organs	1·18
Dysentery	0·10	Diseases of the Ductless or Endocrine Glands	0·13
Enteric Group of Fevers	0·00	Diseases of the Breast	0·02
Influenza	12·53	Diseases of the Respiratory System—Larynx and Trachea	1·10
		Diseases of the Respiratory System—Bronchi and Bronchioles	8·83
Malaria	0·84	Diseases of the Respiratory System—Others	2·83
Measles	1·11		
Meningococcal Infection	0·28	Diseases of the Teeth and Gums	1·72
Mumps	0·68	Diseases of the Digestive System—Inflammation of the Tonsils	22·12
Pneumonia	2·53	Diseases of the Digestive System—Inflammation of the Pharynx	9·43
		Diseases of the Digestive System—Inflammation of the Stomach	3·03
P.U.O.	0·04	Diseases of the Digestive System—Gastric Ulcer	1·99
Rheumatic Fever	1·66	Diseases of the Digestive System—Duodenal Ulcer	1·45
Scarlet Fever	1·19	Diseases of the Digestive System—Liver	0·26
Tuberculosis—Pulmonary	0·98	Diseases of the Digestive System—Others	24·26
Tuberculosis—Others	0·33		
		Diseases due to Disorders of Nutrition or Metabolism	0·24
Venereal Diseases—Gonorrhoea	6·13	Diseases of the Genito-Urinary System	6·98
Venereal Diseases—Soft Chancre	0·31	Diseases of the Musculo-Skeletal System	10·47
Venereal Diseases—Syphilis	0·84	Diseases of the Areolar Tissue	16·83
Venereal Diseases—Others	0·33		
Other Diseases due to Infection	14·05	Diseases of the Skin	19·81
		All Other Diseases	5·13
Scabies	8·17		
Other Diseases due to Infestation by Metazoan Parasites	0·27	*Total Admissions for Diseases*	226·46
Diseases of the Nervous System	3·11		
Mental Diseases	2·51	Injuries—N.E.A.	30·13
		Injuries—E.A.	0·00
Diseases of the Eye	2·82		
Diseases of the Ear and Nose	11·98	*Total Admissions for Injuries*	30·13
Diseases of the Circulatory System—Valvular Diseases of the Heart	0·46		
Diseases of the Circulatory System—Disordered Action of the Heart	0·92	*Total Admissions*	256·59

CHAPTER II

FRANCE, 1939–40

On September 3, 1939, His Majesty's Government declared war on Germany. Nine days later the first contingent of the British Expeditionary Force landed in France. Germany invaded Holland, Belgium and Luxemburg on May 10, 1940 and less than four weeks later the British Expeditionary Force was being evacuated, mainly through Dunkirk.

Statistics which follow are the most accurate available of admissions to hospitals in France, of personnel of the B.E.F., for the seven months October 1939 to April 1940. The normal routine monthly returns (A.F. A.31) from Military Hospitals setting forth crude numbers of admissions by diseases, together with particulars of deaths, etc., are not available. There are, however, two other sources from which much of this information is obtainable.

The first is a record of admissions maintained at the Medical Directorate of Headquarters, B.E.F. In it are given precise details of admissions to hospitals for some seventeen diseases and disease groups. From the particular detail with which the record is permeated and because of the nature of these specific diseases, it is not unreasonable to infer that the data recorded were extracted from Hygiene Reports submitted to the Director of Hygiene.

This record is deficient (at least, in so far as present purposes are concerned) in that data relating to many diseases do not appear, figures relating to injuries are not included, and there is but little information in it regarding deaths. There is, however, much valuable information contained therein relating to admissions on account of the seventeen diseases before mentioned, particularly where, in the case of certain diseases, full particulars (i.e. number, rank, name, unit, and date of admission) of patients are quoted. This is of especial value as it enables a form of control to be exercised on the other available source of statistics.

This is, of course, the tabulations produced by the Hollerith section of the War Office from cards punched with data obtained from Hospital Record Cards (A.Fs. I.1220). It is a truism that the accuracy of the information, both as regards quantity and quality, contained in the tabulations is dependent entirely upon the accuracy of the information fed into the tabulating machine. That is to say, if the punched cards are deficient in quantity and if the information contained in the remainder is erroneous, then the final product will certainly be not more precise.

The limitations of the production of Army Medical Statistics *via* punched card machinery during the war have already been discussed and efforts made to evaluate the accuracy of tabulations produced for certain commands. As stated before, one cause of inaccuracy, and which was probably by far the largest factor, was the loss of primary records due, mainly, to enemy action. That many cards were so lost during the campaign in France cannot be doubted. Indeed, the loss was undeniably considerable when the Germans overran that country. An examination of admissions to hospitals recorded in both sources of information reveals serious discrepancies over the whole period under review. Expressed as a percentage of those quoted in B.E.F. records, admissions recorded in the Hollerith tabulations were

1939		1940	
October	58 per cent.	January	56 per cent.
November	54 per cent.	February	54 per cent.
December	58 per cent.	March	56 per cent.
		April	54 per cent.

That for the seven months ended April 1940 was fifty-five per cent.

From this, and assuming the B.E.F. figures are correct, it would appear that

(a) Of the A.Fs. I.1220 received in the War Office, only fifty-five per cent. were coded.

or

(b) Forty-five per cent. of A.Fs. I.1220 were not received in the War Office for coding.

As far as (a) is concerned, the 'Guide to Procedure' for the Medical File (of punched cards) issued by the Hollerith Section of the War Office categorically states that 'there was no percentage coding prior to September 1944'. It can only be assumed, then, that

(a) a very considerable leakage of A.Fs. I.1220 occurred,

(b) A.Fs. I.1220 received in the War Office were (unofficially) not all coded,

(c) the discrepancy was a combination of both these factors

or

(d) the B.E.F. record is faulty.

To some degree, an evaluation of the accuracy of the Hollerith tabulations can be made. That this is possible is due to the fortunate inclusion in the B.E.F. record of personal particulars of patients admitted for two causes. There is no question of the inaccuracy of these rolls and, if diagnoses are faulty, it can, by virtue of the peculiarity of the circumstances under which patients for at least one of the two causes were admitted, affect the issue but little. Details are:

		Cause 1	Cause 2
(a)	Admission as enumerated in Hollerith Tabulations .	142	30
(b)	Admissions as enumerated in B.E.F. records . .	317	41
(c)	(a) expressed as a percentage of (b)	68	73

Admissions due to these two causes admittedly are a small sample of the total for all causes. It is possible, as hinted above, that some final diagnoses differed from those recorded in the B.E.F. record but, if this were so, it would be to a limited extent only and the percentage deficiency of approximately thirty would tend to gravitate towards the overall deficiency of forty-five per cent.

On balance it does appear that the B.E.F. records are more accurate than the punched card tabulations. In view of this, statistics of admissions to hospitals which follow are those computed from the former. Monthly admission rates per 1,000 strength are presented in Table 17, and these are followed by relative and comparative rates in Tables 18 and 19 respectively. For the record, relative rates of admissions based on the Hollerith tabulations are included as Table 20.

Other statistics presented in this section are medical transfers from France to England. Such transfers did not necessarily imply invaliding from the Army. They may have been made for a variety of reasons, including the necessity of obtaining more specialised treatment than was available in military hospitals in France, and compassionate grounds. Such statistics are given in Tables 21 and 22. Figures were obtained from War Office records which were based on nominal rolls received at ports of disembarkation.

ADMISSIONS

Admissions to hospitals ranged from 42 per 1,000 in October to a peak rate of 61 in January, following which they declined to 37 in April. They were equivalent to an annual rate of 568 per 1,000. The high rate in January, which was almost entirely due to increased admissions on account of Influenza and 'other diseases of the Respiratory System', was half as much again as the rate recorded in October. The lowest rate, occurring in April, was nine-tenths that for October and three-fifths the peak rate in January.

Of the diseases and disease groups recorded in the tabulations, the highest admission rate was due to other diseases of the RESPIRATORY SYSTEM. In four months there was a dramatic increase in admissions, the rate in January being seventeen times that in October when 0·7 per 1,000 was registered. In November the rate was 2·9, in the following month it doubled to 6·0 while in January it increased to the peak rate of 12·2. A decline to 5·3 per 1,000 followed in February and by April the rate had fallen to 2·1. The average rate was 4·5 per 1,000, being equivalent to ten per cent. of all admissions.

Next in numerical order of importance came SCABIES which claimed an average rate of 3·3 per 1,000, some seven per cent. of all admissions. Except in December, when they abated to 2·4, admissions increased each month from 2·6 per 1,000 in October to 4·5 in April, an increase of seventy-five per cent.

Admission rates on account of VENEREAL DISEASES were extremely steady, having a range of only 0·3, i.e. from 2·23 per 1,000 in both January and April to 2·53 in December. This group accounted for five per cent. of all admissions. INFLUENZA was responsible for a rise in the admission rate of 1·5 in December to slightly under 8 per 1,000 in the following month. In February, admissions had subsided to 1·7 and by April they were at under 0·5. The rate for TONSILLITIS in October (0·9 per 1,000) was doubled by January but subsequent admissions declined until April, when the rate was just over 1 per 1,000.

The rates for PULMONARY TUBERCULOSIS exhibited no particular trend, but were rather erratic over the months, ranging from 0·06 in January and April to 0·12 in February. Admissions for RUBELLA were comparatively high in February and March at 4 and 3 respectively before declining to 0·5 in April. The average rate for RHEUMATIC FEVER for the five months December to April was under 0·04 per 1,000. In November there were no recorded admissions, but in October, the first month after the initial landing of the force, the rate was surprisingly high at 0·25 per 1,000.

CEREBRO-SPINAL FEVER provided rates which, although never more than 0·5 per 1,000, were considerably higher during the last four months than in the first three. In the latter, the average monthly rate was less than 0·02 per 1,000, but in the succeeding four months it rose to 0·30 with a peak of slightly under 0·5 in March. Admissions on account of IMPETIGO, which accounted for two per cent. of all admissions in October and April, were highest in October and November at over 0·8 per 1,000. They declined to 0·5 by February but climbed to 0·7 by April.

Rates for DIARRHOEA, after declining from 0·32 in October to 0·15 in November, thereafter remained fairly constant. Figures are not available for MEASLES until February 1940, when the rate was 0·33 per 1,000. In each of the two months which followed the comparatively low rate of 0·04 was recorded.

MEDICAL EVACUATIONS TO THE UNITED KINGDOM

Tables 21 and 22 record evacuations to the United Kingdom on medical grounds. It has already been mentioned that these movements of the sick did not necessarily imply discharge from the Army for medical reasons. This was particularly so in May and June when, consequent on the rapid advance of the German Army, evacuations were exceptionally numerous and many patients who, in the preceding months, would have recuperated in France, were sent home.

During the last quarter of 1939 evacuations did not reach 1,000 in any one month, while the monthly average was under 800. From January 1940, transfers to the United Kingdom increased each month (except in March when they were 200 less than in February). Evacuations in April were over twice those in January and nearly five times the number recorded for October. That the increasing *tempo* of evacuations exceeded that of the build-up of the force is seen in the following comparative table where, in October, both the size of the force and the number of evacuations are represented by 100.

		Size of Force	Number of Evacuations
1939	October	100	100
	November	121	133
	December	129	89
1940	January	142	183
	February	177	240
	March	191	209
	April	222	469

Note: No reliable strength figures are available for May and June

Up to, and including April 1940, evacuations due to disease accounted for between eighty and ninety per cent. of all evacuations. In May and June they dropped to between thirty and forty per cent. Throughout the nine months, slightly over one half of the cases evacuated were because of disease. The average composition of these evacuations was:

20 per cent. and over	Diseases of the Digestive System
15 to 19 per cent.	NIL
10 to 14 per cent.	Diseases of the Bones, Joints, etc. Diseases of the Skin
5 to 9 per cent.	Diseases of the Nervous System Diseases of the Respiratory System Mental Disorders
1 to 4 per cent.	Diseases of the Urinary System Diseases of the Ear Diseases of the Eye Venereal Disease Tuberculosis

	Pneumonia
	Diseases of the Generative System
	Meningococcal Infection
Under 1 per cent.	All others

Nearly fifty per cent. of evacuations were on account of injury. No cases of injury due to Enemy Action were evacuated before February. In May the number was over seven thousand, but in the next month they had declined by nearly one half. Evacuations for N.E.A. injuries, which totalled less than one half those caused by enemy action, increased from just over 100 in October to 500 in April, 1,750 in May, and 1,450 in June.

TABLE 17

B.E.F. France, 1939–40
Causes of Admissions to Hospitals, British Troops
Monthly Rates per 1,000 Strength

Source: Medical Headquarters, B.E.F. Records

	CAUSES	1939 Oct.	1939 Nov.	1939 Dec.	1940 Jan.	1940 Feb.	1940 Mar.	1940 Apr.	
1	Cerebro-Spinal Fever	0·02	0·01	0·02	0·20	0·30	0·47	0·23	1
2	Diarrhoea	0·32	0·15	0·14	0·11	0·12	0·15	0·10	2
3	Diphtheria	0·02	0·06	0·04	0·03	0·03	0·04	0·02	3
4	Dysentery	0·03	0·05	0·01	0·02	0·03	0·01	0·01	4
5	Enteric Group of Fevers	0·02	0·02	—	0·01	—	0·01	0·00	5
6	Impetigo	0·85	0·86	0·60	0·57	0·47	0·61	0·73	6
7	Influenza	0·62	0·70	1·45	7·91	1·68	0·51	0·37	7
8	Measles	N.A.	N.A.	N.A.	N.A.	0·33	0·04	0·04	8
9	Pneumonia	0·22	0·15	0·14	0·52	0·28	0·16	0·12	9
10	Rheumatic Fever	0·25	—	0·04	0·02	0·06	0·04	0·02	10
11	Rubella	N.A.	N.A.	N.A.	N.A.	4·32	3·07	0·50	11
12	Scabies	2·59	2·77	2·37	2·78	4·04	4·09	4·53	12
13	Scarlet Fever	N.A.	N.A.	N.A.	N.A.	0·19	0·08	0·04	13
14	Tonsillitis	0·94	1·74	1·57	1·91	1·08	1·35	1·23	14
15	Tuberculosis (Pulmonary)	0·08	0·10	0·08	0·06	0·12	0·07	0·06	15
16	Other Diseases of the Respiratory System	0·70	2·90	6·00	12·19	5·34	2·37	2·13	16
17	Venereal Disease:								17
18	Gonorrhoea	1·65	2·01	2·07	1·75	1·50	1·75	1·43	18
19	Syphilis	0·13	0·22	0·10	0·09	0·10	0·08	0·02	19
20	Chancroid	0·02	0·02	0·07	0·01	0·01	0·02	0·10	20
21	N.Y.D. and Other V.D.	0·60	0·25	0·29	0·38	0·71	0·65	0·67	21
22	Total V.D.	2·40	2·50	2·53	2·23	2·32	2·50	2·23	22
23	All Other Causes	32·90	33·80	29·07	32·34	34·87	30·69	24·30	23
24	*Total Admissions*	41·95	45·81	44·06	60·88	55·58	46·26	36·66	24

N.A. — Information not available. Included in 'All Other Causes'.

TABLE 18

B.E.F. France, 1939–40
Causes of Admissions to Hospitals, British Troops
Relative Rates

Source: Medical Headquarters, B.E.F. Records

	CAUSES	1939			1940				
		Oct.	Nov.	Dec.	Jan.	Feb.	Mar.	Apr.	
1	Cerebro-Spinal Fever	0·05	0·02	0·05	0·33	0·54	1·02	0·63	1
2	Diarrhoea	0·76	0·33	0·32	0·18	0·22	0·32	0·27	2
3	Diphtheria	0·05	0·13	0·09	0·05	0·05	0·09	0·05	3
4	Dysentery	0·07	0·11	0·02	0·03	0·05	0·02	0·03	4
5	Enteric Group of Fevers	0·05	0·04	—	0·01	—	0·02	0·01	5
6	Impetigo	2·02	1·88	1·36	0·93	0·85	1·32	1·99	6
7	Influenza	1·48	1·53	3·29	12·99	3·02	1·10	1·01	7
8	Measles	N.A.	N.A.	N.A.	N.A.	0·59	0·09	0·11	8
9	Pneumonia	0·52	0·33	0·32	0·85	0·50	0·35	0·33	9
10	Rheumatic Fever	0·59	—	0·09	0·03	0·11	0·09	0·05	10
11	Rubella	N.A.	N.A.	N.A.	N.A.	7·77	6·64	1·36	11
12	Scabies	6·17	6·04	5·38	4·36	7·27	8·84	12·36	12
13	Scarlet Fever	N.A.	N.A.	N.A.	N.A.	0·34	0·17	0·11	13
14	Tonsillitis	2·24	3·80	3·56	3·14	1·94	2·92	3·36	14
15	Tuberculosis (Pulmonary)	0·19	0·22	0·18	0·10	0·22	0·15	0·16	15
16	Other Diseases of the Respiratory System	1·67	6·33	13·62	20·02	9·61	5·12	5·81	16
17	Venereal Diseases	5·72	5·46	5·74	3·66	4·17	5·40	6·08	17
18	All Other Causes	78·42	73·78	65·98	53·12	62·74	66·34	66·28	18
19	*Total Admissions*	100	100	100	100	100	100	100	19

N.A. = Information not available. Included in 'All Other Causes'.

TABLE 19

B.E.F. France, 1939–40
Causes of Admissions to Hospitals, British Troops
Comparative Rates

Source: Medical Headquarters, B.E.F. Records.

	CAUSES	1939			1940				
		Oct.	Nov.	Dec.	Jan.	Feb.	Mar.	Apr.	
1	Cerebro-Spinal Fever	100	50	100	1,000	1,500	2,350	1,150	1
2	Diarrhoea	100	47	44	34	38	47	31	2
3	Diphtheria	100	300	200	150	150	200	100	3
4	Dysentery	100	167	33	67	100	33	33	4
5	Enteric Group of Fevers	100	100	—	50	—	50	16	5
6	Impetigo	100	101	71	67	55	72	86	6
7	Influenza	100	113	234	1,276	271	82	60	7
8	Measles	N.A.	N.A.	N.A.	N.A.	100	12	12	8
9	Pneumonia	100	68	64	236	127	73	55	9
10	Rheumatic Fever	100	—	16	8	24	16	8	10
11	Rubella	N.A.	N.A.	N.A.	N.A.	100	71	12	11
12	Scabies	100	107	92	107	156	158	175	12
13	Scarlet Fever	N.A.	N.A.	N.A.	N.A.	100	42	21	13
14	Tonsillitis	100	185	167	203	115	144	131	14
15	Tuberculosis (Pulmonary)	100	125	100	75	150	88	75	15
16	Other Diseases of the Respiratory System	100	414	857	1,741	763	339	304	16
17	Venereal Diseases	100	104	105	93	97	105	93	17
18	All Other Causes	100	103	88	98	106	93	74	18
19	*Total Admissions*	100	109	105	145	132	110	87	19

N.A. = Information not available. Included in 'All Other Causes'.

TABLE 20

B.E.F. France, 1939–40
Causes of Admissions to Hospitals British Troops
Relative Rates

Source: Hollerith Tabulations

	CAUSES	1939			1940				Averages	
		Oct.	Nov.	Dec.	Jan.	Feb.	Mar.	Apr.		
1	Common Cold	1·71	0·90	3·93	9·16	3·18	1·18	0·72	3·43	1
2	Diphtheria	—	0·03	0·09	0·04	0·06	0·09	0·03	0·05	2
3	Dysentery	—	—	0·05	0·02	0·01	0·05	0·02	0·02	3
4	Enteric Fever	0·06	—	0·07	0·04	—	0·05	—	0·03	4
5	Influenza	1·24	1·33	3·60	11·80	2·58	0·72	0·34	3·71	5
6	Jaundice, Catarrhal	0·32	0·72	0·37	0·35	0·49	0·76	0·65	0·53	6
7	Malaria	0·19	0·13	0·07	0·05	0·04	0·03	—	0·06	7
8	Measles	—	—	0·12	0·17	0·70	0·17	0·13	0·22	8
9	Meningococcal Infection	—	—	0·09	0·20	1·01	1·28	0·77	0·57	9
10	Mumps	—	0·05	0·05	0·07	0·34	0·43	0·08	0·17	10
11	Pneumonia	0·98	0·59	0·42	1·05	1·12	0·70	0·73	0·84	11
12	Rheumatic Fever	0·29	0·36	0·37	0·30	0·26	0·28	0·49	0·33	12
13	Scarlet Fever	0·03	0·08	0·21	0·18	0·55	0·52	0·11	0·28	13
14	Tuberculosis—Pulmonary	0·44	0·46	0·35	0·32	0·67	0·80	0·59	0·53	14
15	Tuberculosis—Other Types	0·25	0·15	0·07	0·04	0·03	0·14	0·11	0·10	15
16	Venereal Disease—Gonorrhoea	4·88	3·30	3·11	2·63	2·24	2·94	2·05	2·82	16
17	Venereal Disease—Syphilis	0·89	1·82	1·36	0·54	0·55	0·40	0·51	0·76	17
18	Venereal Disease—Soft Chancre	0·10	0·18	0·33	0·11	0·28	0·14	0·13	0·18	18
19	Venereal Disease—Other Types and Unspecified	0·10	0·05	—	0·16	0·28	0·54	0·55	0·28	19
20	Total V.D.	5·96	5·34	4·79	3·44	3·35	4·02	3·24	4·03	20
21	Rubella	—	—	0·12	1·96	11·70	4·60	0·56	3·40	21
22	P.U.O.	—	0·03	0·12	—	0·03	0·05	0·03	0·03	22
23	Other Infectious Diseases	0·48	0·46	0·47	0·32	0·73	1·42	0·98	0·72	23
24	Scabies	2·50	3·84	3·09	3·18	3·47	3·46	4·71	3·52	24
25	Other Infestations	0·32	0·46	0·33	0·17	0·28	0·17	0·15	0·24	25

TABLE 20—*Continued*

B.E.F. France, 1939–40
Causes of Admissions to Hospitals, British Troops
Relative Rates

Source: Hollerith Tabulations

	CAUSES	1939			1940				Averages	
		Oct.	Nov.	Dec.	Jan.	Feb.	Mar.	Apr.		
26	Diseases of the Nervous System	1·93	1·87	1·73	1·41	2·24	2·74	3·27	2·19	26
27	Mental Disorders	1·30	2·59	2·81	1·49	1·89	2·68	2·83	2·20	27
28	Diseases of the Eye	1·68	2·82	1·57	1·27	1·44	1·84	1·70	1·68	28
29	Diseases of the Ear, Nose and Throat	5·19	8·27	11·43	13·28	10·36	10·12	9·96	10·35	29
30	Diseases of the Cardio-Vascular System	3·04	3·84	3·67	1·81	2·34	2·49	2·91	2·70	30
31	Diseases of the Blood and Blood-forming Organs	0·41	0·72	0·35	0·38	0·36	0·58	0·69	0·49	31
32	Diseases of the Endocrine System	0·06	0·18	0·07	0·05	0·14	0·17	0·06	0·10	32
33	Diseases of the Breast	—	—	0·02	—	0·03	0·07	0·05	0·03	33
34	Diseases of the Respiratory System	7·73	7·81	11·87	15·09	10·64	6·01	6·14	9·71	34
35	Diseases of the Mouth, Teeth and Gums	0·67	1·23	1·05	0·54	0·70	0·89	1·00	0·83	35
36	Diseases of the Digestive System	24·23	18·74	14·49	8·92	11·44	14·83	14·79	14·09	36
37	Disorders of Nutrition and Metabolism	0·13	0·08	0·02	0·06	0·11	0·10	0·21	0·10	37
38	Diseases of the Genito-Urinary System	4·09	4·25	2·69	2·27	2·80	3·73	3·72	3·22	38
39	Diseases of the Musculo-Skeletal System	9·85	10·85	9·02	6·24	8·44	11·44	11·69	9·41	39
40	Diseases of the Areolar Tissue	5·13	4·14	3·53	2·80	2·91	3·33	4·54	3·54	40
41	Diseases of the Skin	4·43	5·71	3·67	2·92	3·33	5·14	6·70	4·43	41
42	Poisons	0·06	0·03	0·09	0·11	0·15	0·07	0·11	0·10	42
43	Other Diseases	3·39	3·15	4·07	2·86	3·63	4·50	5·19	3·84	43
44	*Total Admissions for Diseases*	88·09	90·79	90·93	94·38	93·55	91·65	90·06	91·86	44
45	Injuries—Head	1·11	0·44	0·56	0·28	0·34	0·46	0·36	0·44	45
46	Injuries—Fractures (other than to the head)	4·05	3·30	3·81	2·11	2·44	3·15	3·59	3·03	46
47	Injuries—Burns	0·60	0·33	0·63	0·38	0·35	0·40	0·46	0·43	47
48	Injuries—Others	6·15	5·14	4·07	2·85	3·33	4·34	5·53	4·23	48
49	*Total Admissions for Injuries*	11·91	9·21	9·07	5·62	6·45	8·35	9·94	8·14	49
50	*Total Admissions*	100	100	100	100	100	100	100	100	50

TABLE 21

France, 1939–40
Medical Evacuations to the United Kingdom
Crude Figures

Source: Embarkation Returns

CAUSES	1939			1940						
	Oct.	Nov.	Dec.	Jan.	Feb.	Mar.	Apr.	May	June	Totals
Diphtheria	—	—	—	—	—	—	1	3	—	4
Dysentery	—	—	—	1	2	—	1	6	1	11
Erysipelas	—	—	—	—	—	—	—	3	—	3
Influenza	—	2	—	3	1	—	2	8	7	23
Malaria	—	1	—	1	—	—	—	10	3	15
Meningococcal Infection	—	—	—	—	8	37	58	73	51	227
Mumps	—	—	—	—	—	—	—	6	1	7
Pneumonia	3	15	9	15	48	37	36	66	45	274
P.U.O.	—	—	—	1	—	—	4	15	2	22
Rheumatic Fever	2	2	8	17	20	16	22	41	11	139
Scarlet Fever	—	—	—	—	—	—	—	4	8	12
Tuberculosis—Pulmonary	3	32	21	26	45	38	45	30	15	255
Tuberculosis—Other Forms	1	4	2	6	2	5	6	7	2	35
Venereal Diseases—Gonorrhoea	—	—	—	—	—	5	—	139	91	235
Venereal Diseases—Syphilis	—	—	—	—	—	—	—	—	18	18
Other V.D.	—	—	—	—	—	—	—	17	61	78
Other Diseases due to Infection	9	14	4	8	7	4	12	23	11	92
Scabies	—	—	—	—	—	—	27	35	21	83
Other Diseases due to Infestations by Metazoan Parasites	—	—	—	—	1	—	2	7	—	10
Diseases of the Nervous System	60	35	42	61	83	118	204	742	186	1,531
Mental Diseases	21	47	62	80	75	91	137	266	277	1,056
Diseases of the Eye	13	33	19	28	31	31	81	111	31	378
Diseases of the Ear and Nose	23	45	12	43	92	80	150	168	53	666
Diseases of the Blood and Blood-forming Organs	12	8	8	4	10	17	19	24	20	122

TABLE 21—*Continued*

France, 1939–40
Medical Evacuations to the United Kingdom
Crude Figures

Source: Embarkation Returns

CAUSES	1939			1940						
	Oct.	Nov.	Dec.	Jan.	Feb.	Mar.	Apr.	May	June	Totals
Diseases of the Circulatory System										
Valvular Diseases of the Heart	7	11	8	12	16	20	16	22	5	117
Disordered Action of the Heart	4	16	19	57	36	16	18	8	6	180
Other Diseases	22	32	26	21	20	64	132	150	60	527
Diseases of the Ductless or Endocrine Glands	1	2	5	4	4	12	8	12	3	51
Diseases of the Respiratory System										
Larynx and Trachea	2	1	—	1	2	3	4	3	5	21
Bronchi and Bronchioles	38	60	64	163	177	120	196	200	85	1,103
Lung (other than T.B. and Pneumonia)	4	11	9	17	13	13	16	25	5	113
Other Diseases	6	14	11	8	20	19	40	64	32	214
Diseases of the Digestive System										
Inflammation of the Tonsils	2	3	1	3	10	3	42	79	35	178
Inflammation of the Pharynx	—	—	—	—	—	1	5	9	8	23
Liver	—	—	—	3	3	3	34	43	11	97
Other Diseases	246	277	109	249	349	281	604	889	420	3,424
Diseases of the Teeth and Gums	1	3	—	—	—	—	2	9	7	22
Disorders of Nutrition or Metabolism	3	—	—	1	3	6	2	9	1	25
Diseases of the Generative System	3	8	1	5	12	7	56	126	57	275
Diseases of the Bones, Joints and Muscles, etc.	48	100	56	138	198	172	401	529	216	1,858
Diseases of the Skin	21	24	7	43	102	58	349	787	231	1,622
Diseases of the Urinary System	30	14	10	14	32	30	88	89	40	347
Tumours and Cysts	3	7	6	11	10	16	27	32	15	127
Poisons	—	—	—	—	—	2	3	11	6	22
Other Diseases	24	22	38	47	52	40	28	338	485	1,074
Total Diseases	612	843	557	1,091	1,484	1,365	2,878	5,238	2,648	16,716
Injuries—N.E.A.	115	122	88	240	254	151	509	1,751	1,450	4,680
Injuries—E.A.	—	—	—	—	9	7	19	7,155	3,829	11,019
Total Injuries	115	122	88	240	263	158	528	8,906	5,279	15,699
Total Evacuations	727	965	645	1,331	1,747	1,523	3,406	14,144	7,927	32,415

TABLE 22

British Expeditionary Force, France, 1939–40
Medical Evacuations to the United Kingdom
Percentages of Total Monthly Evacuations

Source: Embarkation Returns

	CAUSES	1939			1940							
		Oct.	Nov.	Dec.	Jan.	Feb.	Mar.	Apr.	May	Jun.	Totals	
1	Diphtheria	—	—	—	—	—	—	0·03	0·02	—	0·01	1
2	Dysentery	—	—	—	0·08	0·11	—	0·03	0·04	0·01	0·03	2
3	Erysipelas	—	—	—	—	—	—	—	0·02	—	0·01	3
4	Influenza	—	0·21	—	0·23	0·06	—	0·06	0·06	0·09	0·07	4
5	Malaria	—	0·10	—	0·08	—	—	—	0·07	0·04	0·05	5
6	Meningococcal Infection	—	—	—	—	0·46	2·43	1·70	0·52	0·64	0·70	6
7	Mumps	—	—	—	—	—	—	—	0·04	0·01	0·02	7
8	Pneumonia	0·41	1·55	1·40	1·13	2·75	2·43	1·06	0·47	0·57	0·85	8
9	Pyrexia of Uncertain Origin	—	—	—	0·08	—	—	0·12	0·11	0·03	0·07	9
10	Rheumatic Fever	0·28	0·21	1·24	1·28	1·14	1·05	0·65	0·29	0·14	0·43	10
11	Scarlet Fever	—	—	—	—	—	—	—	0·03	0·10	0·04	11
12	Tuberculosis—Pulmonary	0·41	3·32	3·26	1·95	2·58	2·58	1·32	0·21	0·19	0·79	12
13	Tuberculosis—Other	0·14	0·41	0·31	0·45	0·11	0·33	0·18	0·05	0·03	0·11	13
14	Venereal Diseases—Gonorrhoea	—	—	—	—	—	0·33	—	0·98	1·15	0·72	14
15	Venereal Diseases—Syphilis	—	—	—	—	—	—	—	—	0·23	0·06	15
16	Venereal Diseases—Other	—	—	—	—	—	—	—	0·12	0·77	0·24	16
17	Other Diseases due to Infection	1·24	1·45	0·62	0·60	0·40	0·26	0·35	0·16	0·14	0·28	17
18	Diseases due to Infestation by Metazoan Parasites: Scabies	—	—	—	—	—	—	0·79	0·25	0·26	0·26	18
19	Other Diseases	—	—	—	—	0·06	—	0·06	0·05	—	0·03	19
20	Diseases of the Nervous System	8·25	3·63	6·51	4·58	4·75	7·75	5·99	5·25	2·35	4·72	20
21	Mental Diseases	2·89	4·87	9·61	6·01	4·29	5·98	4·02	1·88	3·49	3·26	21
22	Diseases of the Eye	1·79	3·42	2·95	2·10	1·77	2·04	2·38	0·78	0·39	1·17	22
23	Diseases of the Ear and Nose	3·16	4·66	1·86	3·23	5·27	5·25	4·40	1·19	0·67	2·05	23
24	Diseases of the Blood and Blood-forming Organs	1·65	0·83	1·24	0·30	0·57	1·12	0·56	0·17	0·25	0·38	24

TABLE 22—*Continued*

British Expeditionary Force, France, 1939–40
Medical Evacuations to the United Kingdom
Percentages of Total Monthly Evacuations

Source: Embarkation Returns

	CAUSES	1939			1940							
		Oct.	Nov.	Dec.	Jan.	Feb.	Mar.	Apr.	Apr.	Jun.	Totals	
	Diseases of the Circulatory System											
25	Valvular Diseases of the Heart	0·96	1·14	1·24	0·90	0·92	1·31	0·47	0·16	0·06	0·36	25
26	Disordered Action of the Heart	0·55	1·66	2·95	4·28	2·06	1·05	0·53	0·06	0·08	0·56	26
27	Other Diseases	3·03	3·32	4·03	1·58	1·14	4·20	3·88	1·06	0·76	1·63	27
28	Ductless or Endocrine Glands	0·14	0·21	0·78	1·30	0·23	0·79	0·23	0·08	0·04	0·16	28
	Diseases of the Respiratory System											
29	Larynx and Trachea	0·28	0·10	—	0·08	0·11	0·20	0·12	0·02	0·06	0·06	29
30	Bronchi and Bronchioles	5·23	6·21	9·92	12·25	10·13	7·88	5·75	1·41	1·07	3·40	30
31	Lung (Other than T.B. and Pneumonia)	0·55	1·14	1·40	1·28	0·74	0·85	0·47	0·18	0·06	0·35	31
32	Other Diseases	0·83	1·45	1·71	0·60	1·14	1·25	1·17	0·45	0·40	0·66	32
	Diseases of the Digestive System											
33	Inflamation of Tonsils	0·28	0·31	0·16	0·23	0·57	0·20	1·23	0·56	0·44	0·55	33
34	Inflammation of Pharynx	—	—	—	—	—	0·07	0·15	0·06	0·10	0·07	34
35	Liver	—	—	—	0·23	0·17	0·20	1·00	0·30	0·14	0·30	35
36	Other Diseases	33·84	28·70	16·90	18·71	19·98	18·45	17·73	6·29	5·30	10·56	36
37	Diseases of the Teeth and Gums	0·14	0·31	—	—	—	—	0·06	0·06	0·09	0·07	37
38	Disorders of Nutrition or Metabolism	0·41	—	—	0·08	0·17	0·39	0·06	0·06	0·01	0·08	38
39	Diseases of the Generative System	0·41	0·83	0·16	0·38	0·69	0·46	1·64	0·89	0·72	0·85	39
40	Diseases of the Bones, Joints, Muscles, Fasciae and Bursae	6·60	10·38	8·68	10·37	11·33	11·29	11·77	3·74	2·72	5·73	40
41	Diseases of the Skin	2·89	2·49	1·09	3·23	5·84	3·81	10·25	5·56	2·91	5·00	41
42	Diseases of the Urinary System	4·13	1·45	1·55	1·05	1·83	1·97	2·58	0·63	0·50	1·07	42
43	Tumours and Cysts	0·41	0·73	0·93	0·82	0·57	1·05	0·78	0·23	0·19	0·39	43
44	Poisons	—	—	—	—	—	0·13	0·09	0·08	0·08	0·07	44
45	Other Diseases	3·30	2·28	5·89	3·53	2·98	2·63	0·82	2·39	6·12	3·31	45
46	*Total Diseases*	84·18	87·36	86·36	81·97	84·95	89·63	84·50	37·03	33·40	51·57	46
47	Injuries—N.E.A.	15·82	12·64	13·64	18·03	14·54	9·91	14·94	12·38	18·29	14·43	47
48	Injuries—E.A.	—	—	—	—	0·52	0·45	0·56	50·59	48·30	33·99	48
49	*Total Injuries*	15·82	12·64	13·64	18·03	15·05	10·37	15·50	62·97	66·60	48·43	49
50	*Total Evacuations*	100	100	100	100	100	100	100	100	100	100	50

CHAPTER III

North-West Europe
1944 and 1945

DATA REGARDING British patients treated in medical units in North-West Europe have been assembled from various sources. In preparing the tabulations which follow, difficulty was experienced initially, due to there being no regular statistical returns in existence, either in the War Office or at Headquarters in Germany. These records did not appear to have been available when the 'Statistical Report on the Health of the Army, 1943–45' was written, for in that Report only statistics relating to wounds and injuries in Normandy during June and July, 1944, and the rates of Venereal Diseases from February 1945 to February 1946, are recorded.

Recourse was, therefore, made to other, albeit less satisfactory, sources. Tabulations were produced by the Hollerith section of the War Office. These gave information of certain cases admitted to hospital. As related elsewhere the man-power situation obtaining during the war, and for some time subsequently, precluded the coding of all Army Forms I.1220 received in the War Office, and, in so far as North-West Europe was concerned, a ten per cent. sample was taken, commencing with admissions which occurred on or after September 1, 1944. A hundred per cent. coding of admissions occurring before that date was made. The sample was taken by extracting all A.Fs. I.1220, the army number of which ended with the digit 5. These were coded and cards punched.

Other sources from which statistics were obtained were some monthly Hygiene Reports, Army Forms A.35 (Report of Notifiable Diseases) and V.D. returns, all hereinafter designated Hygiene Reports.

It is known that the cards stored by the Hollerith section of the War Office for the war years are deficient, due to losses of A.Fs. I.1220 in transit, a non-rendition of forms, leakages from E.M.S. hospitals, etc., of which mention has already been made. Indeed, an assessment was made in 1945, when nominal rolls of wounded evacuated from Normandy in June and July were used as a control. It was discovered, in this case, that the actual percentage of these evacuations for which A.Fs. I.1220 were coded was 6·9, instead of the expected ten per cent.

By using statistics extracted from the Hygiene Reports as a control, it is possible to assess with some degree of accuracy the present deficiency during the eleven months of 1945 for which both sets of figures are available. The following is the result of the comparison:

Hollerith Sample of A.Fs. I.1220 (alleged to be ten per cent.)	13,381
Admissions disclosed by Hygiene Reports	166,678
Percentage of Hygiene Reports Admissions represented by sample of A.Fs. I.1220	8·0

An explanation of the difference between this percentage and the lower (6·9) obtained on the previous occasion is that it was acknowledged at the time that A.Fs. I.1220 were incomplete due to very long term cases still being in hospital. It can be assumed, therefore, that the overall deficiency in the coding of these medical documents from North-West Europe is in the region of twenty per cent.

It is interesting to compare admissions for some individual diseases shown in the Hygiene Reports with the figures given in the Hollerith Tabulations and assess the percentage of A.Fs. I.1220 coded. Here, the following situation results.

	Hygiene Reports	Hollerith Tabulations	Percentages of A.Fs. I.1220 coded
Bronchitis	1,902	203	10·6
Influenza	2,200	8	3·6
Rheumatic Fever	68	17	25·0
Psychiatric Disorders	5,359	570	10·6
All Injuries	43,602	2,788	6·4
All Diseases	123,097	10,593	8·6
All Admissions	166,678	13,381	8·0

Assuming the statistics extracted from the Hygiene Reports are correct, of the items shown above, Bronchitis and Psychiatric Disorders were ten per cent. coded. Influenza and Injuries and All Diseases were less than ten per cent. and Rheumatic Fever more than ten per cent. The high percentage of Rheumatic Fever occasions no surprise having in view the comparatively small number of admissions. What is surprising is the relatively small percentage of coded cases of Influenza. It is possible that some of these cases, initially diagnosed and included in the Hygiene Reports as Influenza, were finally diagnosed as Common Cold, Bronchitis, etc., but the number cannot be very high.

It cannot, however, be assumed that all the statistics extracted from the Hygiene Reports are, in fact, correct. These reports were compiled from statistical and other information produced, initially, by medical units. There is no doubt that the following data are substantially correct:

(i) Total Admissions for Diseases.

(ii) Total Admissions for Injuries.

(iii) Total Admissions.

As regards individual diseases, however, changes in diagnoses are fairly common. On admission to a medical unit, a patient is provisionally diagnosed. This diagnosis is entered on his records and may subsequently be amended when a firm diagnosis is made. If the firm diagnosis was not made before the statistical returns are sent, it follows that the provisional diagnosis was included in the Hygiene Report. It is doubtful whether all amendments to provisional diagnoses were notified, or, if they were, amendments made to Hygiene Reports. In one theatre, it is known that amendments to returns were not made, if indeed they were received at General Headquarters, until after the cessation of hostilities.

A comparison of the disease rate (hospital admissions only) for 1945 with that in 1946 reveals that the latter is greater. This is undoubtedly chiefly due to the figure for 1946 including all cases of Venereal Diseases whether or not they were treated in hospital. It is understood that the majority of these patients were treated in other types of medical units. If it is adjusted accordingly, the rate for 1945 will exceed that for 1946.

Landings on the Normandy beaches began in June 1944, and statistics prepared from the Hollerith tabulations have been produced from July 1944. Because monthly strengths figures of British Troops operating in North-West Europe were not maintained at the appropriate branch of the War Office, monthly rates of admissions could not be calculated. Quarterly strengths were, however, available. From these mean strengths were calculated and equivalent annual rates for each quarter computed. Such admission rates for the main diseases and disease groups are included in Table 23. Therein, also, are similar rates of admissions for injuries, sub-divided as to whether or not they were caused by enemy action and 'cause not known'. In this section, too, admissions for certain disease and disease groups are analysed.

Hygiene Reports cover information from February 1945 to December 1945. For February, March and April, statistics relating to admissions to hospital of injuries and certain diseases only, are available. From May, in addition, are rates of admissions to all medical units on account of other diseases. Mean monthly rates are available from these returns. The strengths on which these were based differ only slightly from the mean quarterly strengths used in computing rates based on Hollerith tabulations. Here again, analyses of some disease and disease groups are included. Monthly rates are calculated here per 100,000 strength.

This is contrary to the usual practice obtaining for other tabulations herein, where rates are quoted at per 1,000 strength. This deviation was prompted by the fact that monthly admissions for some diseases were so few, and is permissible because of the large population at risk. Had rates been based on 1,000 strength, such admissions would be shown as '0·00' per 1,000 strength. By calculating them at 100,000 strength, a few admissions on account of, in many cases, important diseases are brought out in their true perspective and trends shown.

ADMISSIONS

Rates of admissions to hospital based on tabulations produced by the Hollerith Section of the War Office are given in Table 23. These are equivalent annual rates based on admissions for the six quarters from July 1944 to December 1945.

The disease rates recorded for the first two quarters were lower than those for the remainder of the period. This was not entirely unexpected as the Army which invaded France was a highly selected one, probably the fittest, physically, which has ever left England. No doubt, with the passage of time, it became diluted with troops who were less fit and this, to some extent, might explain the increase in admissions during 1945. The increase was also partly due to the rising incidence of admissions on account of venereal diseases. The lowest recorded rate of admissions for diseases was 127 per 1,000 in the last quarter of 1944. The highest was in the last quarter of 1945 at 176 per 1,000. Rates did not increase in each quarter for, in 1945, the first quarter produced a rate of 174, which was slightly lower than that for the final quarter. In the second quarter of that year it fell to 150 and rose in the penultimate quarter to 157.

As anticipated, the highest rate of admissions for injuries occurred during the first stages of the invasion. A rate of 132 per 1,000 for all types of injuries in the first quarter was succeeded, finally, by 57 in the quarter which saw the end of the fighting in Europe. In the last quarter, when all injuries were of the N.E.A. classification, the rate of admissions was 22.

The quarter July to September, 1944 also saw the peak rate for all admissions at 263 per 1,000. This was followed by the lowest recorded rate of 178. For the first quarter of 1945 a rate of 245 was reported. This was succeeded by rates of 207, 179 and 196 per 1,000.

DISEASES OF THE DIGESTIVE SYSTEM

Among individual diseases and disease groups, the highest number of admissions over the eighteen months under review was recorded by Diseases of the Digestive System. Apart from the first quarter, when the E.A.R. was 30, rates varied slightly between 15 and 20 per 1,000. Expressed as percentages of total admissions for diseases, the peak rate in the first quarter represented twenty-three per cent. and the lowest in the first quarter, nine per cent. The E.A.R. for 1945 was 18 per 1,000, some eleven per cent. of disease admissions. A breakdown of admissions for this system is given below.

North-West Europe, 1944–45
Admissions to Hospitals for Diseases of the Digestive System
E.A.Rs. per 1,000 Strength and Relative Rates

Source: Hollerith Tabulations

	1944		1945				1945
	QUARTER						
	1st	2nd	3rd	4th	5th	6th	Equivalent Annua Rates
1. *Equivalent Annual Rates*	July–Sept.	Oct.–Dec.	Jan.–Mar.	Apr.–June	July–Sept.	Oct.–Dec.	
Gastric Ulcers	0·03	0·22	0·27	0·05	—	0·13	0·11
Duodenal Ulcers	0·13	0·22	1·09	0·79	0·16	0·32	0·59
Peptic Ulcers, Unspecified	0·01	—	—	0·05	—	0·06	0·03
Perforation of Ulcer	0·02	0·06	—	0·05	0·06	0·04	0·04
Dyspepsia and Gastritis	2·75	3·26	3·66	2·52	2·51	2·34	2·76
Hernia	3·34	4·38	3·71	3·68	4·47	4·93	4·20
Haemorrhoids	2·84	2·81	2·46	3·26	2·02	2·08	2·46
Appendicitis	5·91	6·80	6·77	6·35	6·65	3·12	5·72
Other Causes	14·94	1·40	2·29	1·73	1·53	2·21	1·94
Totals	29·97	19·15	20·25	18·48	17·39	15·25	17·84
Percentages of total admissions for diseases	23	15	12	12	11	9	11
2. *Relative Rates*							
Gastric Ulcers	0·10	1·15	1·33	0·27	—	0·85	0·62
Duodenal Ulcers	0·43	1·15	5·38	4·27	0·92	2·10	3·31
Peptic Ulcers, Unspecified	0·03	—	—	0·27	—	0·39	0·17
Perforation of Ulcer	0·07	0·31	—	0·27	0·29	0·39	0·22
Dyspepsia and Gastritis	9·18	17·02	18·07	13·64	14·43	15·34	15·46
Hernia	11·14	22·87	18·32	19·91	25·70	32·33	23·53
Haemorrhoids	9·48	14·67	12·15	17·64	11·62	13·64	13·78
Appendicitis	19·72	33·51	33·43	34·36	38·24	20·46	32·04
Other Causes	49·85	7·31	11·31	9·36	8·80	14·49	10·87
Totals	100	100	100	100	100	100	100

Numerically, the most important contributory cause was APPENDICITIS. Rates of admission except for the first and last quarters are notable for their slight variation of from 5·9 to 6·8 per 1,000. In the last quarter the rate fell by fifty per cent. to 3·1. When admissions for appendicitis are expressed as a percentage of the total admissions for the disease group, in the first and last quarters they represent twenty per cent. and during the others between thirty-three and thirty-eight per cent. In 1945 as a whole, the rate was 5·7 per 1,000 which represented thirty-two per cent. of the total admissions for Diseases of the Digestive System.

Next in importance to appendicitis were HERNIAS. Admissions ranged from 3·3 per 1,000 in the first quarter to 4·9 in the last and were eleven and thirty-two per cent. of all admissions for the Group. The Equivalent Annual Rate for 1945 was 4·2, twenty-four per cent. of the total.

DYSPEPSIA and GASTRITIS which, in 1945, recorded an E.A.R. of 2·8 per 1,000 showed a variation in admissions of 1·3 over the six quarters. Rates increased from 2·8 in the first quarter to 3·7 in the third, then decreased each quarter to 2·3 in the last. Admissions for the first quarter were nearly ten per cent. of the total for the group; in the third quarter, they were eighteen and in the last, fifteen per cent. The average for 1945 was fifteen per cent of the total.

Rates of admission on account of HAEMORRHOIDS were 2·8 in the first quarter. They were at their peak of 3·3 in the fourth and fell to 2·1 in the last quarter. The E.A.R. for 1945 was 2·5 per 1,000, approximately fourteen per cent. of the total admissions for the group.

ULCERS contributed an E.A.R. of 0·77 per 1,000 in 1945; of these approximately four-fifths were DUODENAL, one-fifth GASTRIC, with a very few unspecified. Throughout the eighteen months, the highest rate of admissions occurred in the first quarter of 1945 and the lowest in the third quarter of the same year. Rates ranged from 0·19 to 1·36 and were slightly under five per cent. of the total admissions for the group. An analysis of Perforated Ulcers reveals that, in the first quarter, the rates of Gastric to Duodenal Ulcers were as 2 : 1; in the second and fifth, all were Gastric, and in the fourth and sixth quarters all were Duodenal Ulcers.

The rate of admissions of 14·94 per 1,000 during the first quarter against 'Other Causes' calls for comment. This high rate was due to an outbreak of enteritis in August 1944. It rapidly subsided and, in September, admissions on this account were only slightly above normal.

DISEASES OF THE EAR, NOSE AND THROAT

Next to Diseases of the Digestive System in numerical importance came Diseases of the Ear, Nose and Throat. The trend of admissions was contrary to that registered by Diseases of the Digestive System, admission rates for which, on the whole, decreased over the period.

Admissions for Diseases of the Ear, Nose and Throat increased from 7 per 1,000 in the first quarter to 23 in the last, an increase of over two hundred per cent. In 1945, the E.A.R. was 21 which represented nearly thirteen per cent. of the total disease admissions for that year. Over the whole period of eighteen months, the percentage of admissions for disease was only slightly lower at under twelve.

Below is an analysis of admissions for diseases of the Ear, Nose and Throat.

North-West Europe, 1944–45
Admissions to Hospitals for Diseases of the Ear, Nose and Throat
Equivalent Annual Rates per 1,000 Strength and Relative Rates

Source: Hollerith Tabulations

	1944		1945				1945
	QUARTER						Equivalent Annual Rates
	1st	2nd	3rd	4th	5th	6th	
1. *Equivalent Annual Rates*	July–Sept.	Oct.–Dec.	Jan.–Mar.	April–June	July–Sept.	Oct.–Dec.	
Otitis Media	1·85	2·41	2·18	1·94	1·20	1·78	1·76
Tonsillitis	3·20	6·01	14·15	13·70	13·20	16·23	14·32
Other Diseases	2·11	3·82	5·68	4·78	4·55	5·32	5·08
Totals	7·16	12·24	22·01	20·42	18·98	23·30	21·18
Percentages of total admissions for diseases	5	10	13	14	12	11	13
2. *Relative Rates*							
Otitis Media	25·84	19·69	9·90	9·50	6·32	7·71	8·32
Tonsillitis	44·69	49·10	64·29	67·09	69·55	69·66	67·67
Other Diseases	29·47	31·21	25·81	23·41	24·13	22·83	24·01
Totals	100	100	100	100	100	100	100

TONSILLITIS caused admissions which, on the average, were over sixty per cent. of the total for this disease group. Rates increased from 3 in the first quarter to 16 per 1,000 in the last and represented from forty-five to seventy per cent. of group admissions. The Equivalent Annual Rate for 1945 was 14 per 1,000.

The rate for OTITIS MEDIA increased in the second quarter from 1·85 to 2·41 and then decreased to a final rate of 1·78 per 1,000. The E.A.R. for 1945 was 1·76 per 1,000, some eight per cent. of the total admissions for the group.

VENEREAL DISEASES

An analysis of admissions to hospitals on account of Venereal Diseases follows. It is stressed that these figures relate to those treated in hospital only, for the majority received treatment in other medical units.

North-West Europe, 1944–45
Admissions to Hospitals for Venereal Diseases
E.A.Rs. per 1,000 Strength and Relative Rates

Source: Hollerith Tabulations

	1944		1945				1945
	QUARTER						Equivalent Annual Rates
	1st	2nd	3rd	4th	5th	6th	
1. *Equivalent Annual Rates*	July–Sept.	Oct.–Dec.	Jan.–Mar.	Apr.–June	July–Sept.	Oct.–Dec.	
Gonorrhoea . .	1·17	7·64	9·18	6·09	11·18	10·52	9·24
Syphilis . . .	0·81	1·40	2·24	1·63	7·14	11·23	5·56
Soft Chancre . .	0·02	—	0·22	0·11	0·11	0·26	0·18
Other Causes . .	0·13	0·73	2·18	2·05	3·82	3·70	2·94
Totals . .	2·13	9·77	13·82	9·88	22·26	25·71	17·92
Percentages of total admissions for diseases . . .	2	8	8	7	14	15	11
2. *Relative Rates*							
Gonorrhoea .	54·93	78·20	66·43	61·64	50·25	40·92	51·56
Syphilis . .	38·03	14·33	16·21	16·50	32·09	43·68	31·03
Soft Chancre .	0·94	—	1·59	1·11	0·49	1·01	1·00
Other Causes .	6·10	7·47	15·77	20·75	17·17	14·39	16·41
Totals . . .	100	100	100	100	100	100	100

As might be expected, the rate of admissions for this group of diseases was lowest in the first quarter at 2 per 1,000. Admissions increased to 26 in the last quarter. In the second and fourth quarters, the rate was slightly under 10 per 1,000, in the third quarter it was 14, with 22 and 26 in the last two quarters. Expressed as a percentage of the total admissions for diseases, admissions for Venereal Diseases were two per cent. in the first quarter, 8, 8 and 7 respectively for the next three and, for the two final quarters 14 and 15 per cent. The E.A.R. for 1945 was 18 per 1,000, some eleven per cent. of the total admissions for diseases.

Of the individual diseases of this group, GONORRHOEA caused most admissions at rates which rose from 1 to 8 in the second quarter, and to a peak of 11 per 1,000 in the last two quarters. This represented a variation of from forty-one to seventy-eight per cent. of the total admissions for Venereal Disease. The E.A.R. for 1945 was 9 per 1,000 which was slightly over one half that for the whole group.

The rate for SYPHILIS was also comparatively low in the first quarter at slightly under 1 per 1,000. It increased to 2·2 by the third quarter and fell to 1·6 in the fourth increasing considerably to 7 and 11 in the two final quarters. The rates were equal to from fourteen to forty per cent. of the total admissions for Venereal Diseases. It is of interest to note the high rates of Syphilis in the last two quarters as compared with those for Gonorrhoea. Indeed, in the last quarter, admissions for Syphilis were forty-four per cent. of the group as compared with forty-one per cent. for Gonorrhoea. The reason for this, of course, is that a considerable number of cases of Gonorrhoea were treated in other medical units. The Equivalent Annual Rate for 1945 was 5·6 per 1,000, which represented slightly under one-third the total rate for the group.

Admissions for SOFT CHANCRE were extremely few, ranging from a rate of 0·02 in the first quarter to 0·26 in the last. There were no admissions from this cause during the last quarter of 1944. The E.A.R. of 0·18 per 1,000 in 1945 was one per cent. of the total for the group.

DISEASES OF THE SKIN

Admissions for Diseases of the Skin accounted for eight to twelve per cent. of the total admissions for diseases. Rates increased from 10 per 1,000 in the opening quarter to 18 in the first six months of 1945 and then declined to 14 in the final half year. The E.A.R. for 1945 was 16 per 1,000 representing slightly under ten per cent. of the disease total. The following is a breakdown of admissions for this group.

North-West Europe, 1944–45
Admissions to Hospitals for Diseases of the Skin
E.A.Rs. per 1,000 Strength and Relative Rates

Source: Hollerith Tabulations

	1944		1945				1945
	QUARTER						Equivalent Annual Rates
	1st	2nd	3rd	4th	5th	6th	
1. *Equivalent Annual Rates*	July–Sept.	Oct.–Dec.	Jan.–Mar.	Apr.–June	July–Sept.	Oct.–Dec.	
Boils . . .	1·51	1·80	1·80	1·94	1·91	1·56	1·80
Carbuncles . .	1·26	0·95	0·98	0·73	0·76	0·78	0·81
Dermatitis . .	1·85	3·71	5·35	5·93	4·14	4·22	4·92
Eczema . . .	0·77	0·67	1·04	0·73	0·71	0·52	0·75
Impetigo . . .	2·70	3·26	3·71	2·99	1·25	1·62	2·42
Warts . . .	0·16	0·90	1·31	1·57	1·53	1·36	1·44
Other Diseases . .	2·20	2·02	3·55	3·57	2·94	3·70	3·41
Totals . .	10·45	13·31	17·75	17·48	13·25	13·76	15·56
Percentages of total admissions for diseases . .	8	10	10	12	8	8	9

North-West Europe, 1944–45
Admissions to Hospitals for Diseases of the Skin
E.A.Rs. per 1,000 Strength and Relative Rates

Source: Hollerith Tabulations

	1944		1945				1945
	QUARTER						Equivalent Annual Rates
	1st	2nd	3rd	4th	5th	6th	
2. *Relative Rates*	July–Sept.	Oct.–Dec.	Jan.–Mar.	Apr.–June	July–Sept.	Oct.–Dec.	
Boils	14·48	13·50	10·15	11·11	14·40	11·32	11·59
Carbuncles	12·01	7·17	5·54	4·20	5·76	5·66	5·21
Dermatitis	17·73	27·85	30·15	33·93	31·28	30·66	31·63
Eczema	7·34	5·06	5·85	4·20	5·35	3·77	4·85
Impetigo	25·84	24·47	20·92	17·12	9·47	11·79	15·54
Warts	1·56	6·75	7·38	9·01	11·52	9·91	9 25
Other diseases	21·04	15·19	20·00	20·42	22·22	26·89	21·92
Totals	100	100	100	100	100	100	100

Of individual diseases, DERMATITIS caused most admissions. Rates varied from 1·85 per 1,000 in the first quarter to a peak of 5·93 in the fourth and declined to 4·22 in the last quarter. These admissions represented eighteen, thirty-four and thirty-one per cent. of the respective quarterly admissions of the group. The E.A.R. for 1945 was 4·92 equal to thirty-two per cent. of the group admissions.

Admissions for IMPETIGO commenced at 2·7 per 1,000, rose to 3·7 in the third quarter and declined to 1·6 in the final period. As percentages of total admissions for skin diseases, they were twenty-six, twenty-one, and twelve respectively. The Equivalent Annual Rate for 1945 was 2·4, nearly sixteen per cent. of the group total.

Rates for BOILS were very steady, ranging from 1·5 in the initial quarter to a peak of 1·9 in the fourth and fifth quarters. In the final period the rate was 1·6 per 1,000. Admissions were, on the average, slightly under twelve per cent. of the total for Skin Diseases. In 1945 the E.A.R. was 1·8 per 1,000.

Admissions for WARTS during the first quarter were comparatively low at 0·16 per 1,000. They increased to 0·9 in the second quarter and to 1·3 in the third. This was followed by 1·6, 1·5 and, finally, 1·4 per 1,000. The E.A.R. for 1945 was 1·44 which represented nine per cent. of the total admissions for this group.

Rates for CARBUNCLES varied from 1·26 in the first quarter to 0·73 in the fourth. The E.A.R., at 0·81 per 1,000, represented five per cent. of the group.

ECZEMA was responsible for admission rates which ranged from 1·04 in the third quarter to exactly one half in the last. In 1945 the E.A.R. of 0·75 was slightly under five per cent. of the total for the group.

'Others' at 3 per 1,000 represented a large number of individual diseases, admissions for which were too few for rates to be calculated.

DISEASES OF THE MUSCULO-SKELETAL SYSTEM

Admissions on account of this group of diseases varied little during the six quarters under review. The lowest rate was 10 per 1,000 (in the last quarter) and the highest 14 (in the third quarter). These rates represented six and eight per cent. of the total admissions for disease during those quarters. The Equivalent Annual Rate for 1945 was 12 per 1,000 equal to some seven per cent. of all disease admissions.

The following is a breakdown of this group to component diseases.

North-West Europe, 1944–45
Admissions to Hospitals for Diseases of the Musculo-Skeletal System
E.A.Rs. per 1,000 Strength and Relative Rates

Source: Hollerith Tabulations

	1944		1945				1945
	QUARTER						Equivalent Annual Rates
	1st	2nd	3rd	4th	5th	6th	
1. *Equivalent Annual Rates*	July–Sept.	Oct.–Dec.	Jan.–Mar.	Apr.–June	July–Sept.	Oct.–Dec.	
Disease of the Joints:							
Synovitis	1·62	1·48	1·81	1·68	1·15	1·04	1·42
Arthritis	0·34	0·38	0·49	0·68	0·44	0·20	0·45
I.D.K.*	1·85	1·53	1·26	2·73	2·62	2·14	2·19
Others	0·45	0·71	0·60	0·26	0·44	0·20	0·38
Diseases of the Bone	0·23	0·44	0·33	0·32	0·44	0·20	0·32
Diseases of the Spine	0·07	0·27	0·22	0·21	0·16	0·13	0·18
Diseases of the Muscle	0·02	—	0·16	0·11	0·05	0·07	0·10
Diseases of Fasciae, Tendons, Tendon Sheaths and Bursae:							
Bursitis	0·87	0·17	0·88	0·32	0·60	0·52	0·58
Others	0·12	0·38	0·27	0·58	0·22	0·65	0·43
Diseases and Deformities of the Limbs:							
Ingrowing Toenails	0·18	0·38	0·16	0·05	0·33	0·20	0·18
Infected Fingers	1·80	2·03	2·80	2·05	1·75	2·40	2·25
Others	0·08	0·38	0·44	0·15	0·27	0·39	0·31
Rheumatic Conditions:†							
Non-Articular	3·17	3·13	3·73	3·10	2·29	1·62	2·69
Articular	0·26	0·49	0·99	0·58	0·65	0·65	0·72
Totals	11·07	11·80	14·15	12·81	11·40	10·39	12·19
Percentages of total admissions for diseases	8	9	8	9	7	6	7

North-West Europe, 1944–45
Admissions to Hospitals for Diseases of the Musculo-Skeletal System
E.A.Rs. per 1,000 Strength and Relative Rates (contd.)

Source: Hollerith Tabulations

2. *Relative Rates*	1944 1st July–Sept.	1944 2nd Oct.–Dec.	1945 3rd Jan.–Mar.	1945 4th Apr.–June	1945 5th July–Sept.	1945 6th Oct.–Dec.	1945 Equivalent Annual Rates
Diseases of the Joints:							
Synovitis	14·66	12·56	12·79	13·11	10·05	10·00	11·49
Arthritis	3·07	3·26	3·47	5·33	3·83	1·88	3·63
I.D.K.*	16·75	13·02	8·91	21·31	22·97	20·63	18·46
Others	4·11	6·05	4·26	2·05	3·83	1·88	3·01
Diseases of the Bone	2·09	3·72	2·33	2·46	3·83	1·88	2·63
Diseases of the Spine	0·61	2·33	1·55	1·64	1·44	1·25	1·47
Diseases of the Muscles	0·18	—	1·16	0·82	0·48	0·63	0·77
Diseases of Fasciae, Tendons, Tendon Sheaths and Bursae:							
Bursitis	7·85	1·40	6·20	2·46	5·26	5·00	4·73
Others	1·04	3·26	1·94	4·51	1·91	6·25	3·65
Diseases and Deformities of the Limbs:							
Ingrowing Toenails	1·66	3·26	1·16	0·41	2·87	1·88	1·58
Infected Fingers	16·26	17·21	19·77	15·98	15·31	23·13	18·55
Others	0·74	3·26	3·10	1·23	2·39	3·75	2·62
Rheumatic Conditions:†							
Non-Articular	28·65	26·51	26·36	24·18	20·10	15·63	21·57
Articular	2·33	4·19	6·98	4·51	5·74	6·25	5·87
Totals	100	100	100	100	100	100	100

* I.D.K. includes: Internal derangement of knee and other joints. Subluxation of intra-articular cartilage. Rupture of intra-articular cartilage. Ruptured crucial ligament of knee, and Loose body.

† Rheumatic Conditions excludes Rheumatic Fever.

The highest rate of admissions was caused by Diseases of the JOINTS which recorded an Equivalent Annual Rate in 1945 of under 5 per 1,000 which represented over one-third the total for the group. Of these diseases, nearly one-half were attributable to I.D.K., the admission rates for which varied from 1·26 to 2·73 per 1,000. SYNOVITIS, which accounted for one-quarter of the admissions for diseases of the Joints was responsible for rates ranging from 1·04 to 1·81 per 1,000. The rates for ARTHRITIS were lower from 0·20 to 0·68 per 1,000.

RHEUMATIC CONDITIONS accounted for the next highest rates of admissions with an E.A.R. in 1945 of 3·4. Rates fluctuated between 2·3 in the last quarter to 4·7 per 1,000 in the third, representing from twenty-two to thirty-three per cent. of the total admissions for the group. By far the greater number of these admissions were due to the non-articular type of rheumatism, which was responsible for rates ranging from 1·6 to 3·7 per 1,000. The E.A.R. was 2·69 as against that for the articular type at 0·72.

Next in numerical importance were Diseases and Deformities of the LIMBS, admissions for which ranged from 2·06 in the first quarter to a peak of 3·40 in the third and to 2·99 in the final quarter. These represented nineteen, twenty-four, and twenty-eight per cent. respectively of the total admissions for the group. Of these admissions, four-fifths were due to Infected Fingers and nearly ten per cent. to Ingrowing Toenails. The E.A.R. for 1945 was 2·74 per 1,000, and twenty-three per cent. of the group admissions.

More than one-half of the admissions on account of Diseases of the FASCIAE, TENDONS, TENDON SHEATH and BURSAE were for BURSITIS. Admissions for this sub-group varied over the six quarters from 0·6 per 1,000 in the second quarter to 1·2 in the last. The E.A.R. in 1945 was slightly over 1 per 1,000 representing some eight per cent. of the total admissions for diseases of the Musculo-Skeletal System.

The remaining diseases of the group each of which contributed admission rates at less than 0·5 per 1,000 were Diseases of the BONE, at 0·32. Diseases of the SPINE at 0·18 and Diseases of the MUSCLE at 0·1 per 1,000 strength.

DISEASES OF THE GENITO-URINARY SYSTEM

The rates of admission for this group of diseases increased steadily quarter by quarter from 2·9 per 1,000 initially to a final rate of 17·2, representing from two to ten per cent. of the total admissions for diseases. The Equivalent Annual Rate for 1945 was slightly under 12 per 1,000, being some seven per cent. of the admissions for disease.

The following is an analysis of this group.

North-West Europe, 1944–45
Admissions to Hospitals for Diseases of the Genito-Urinary System
E.A.Rs. per 1,000 Strength and Relative Rates

Source: Hollerith Tabulations

	1944		1945				1945
	QUARTER						Equivalent Annual Rates
	1st	2nd	3rd	4th	5th	6th	
1. *Equivalent Annual Rates*	July–Sept.	Oct.–Dec.	Jan.–Mar.	Apr.–June	July–Sept.	Oct.–Dec.	
Pyelitis	0·23	0·17	0·38	0·32	0·35	0·46	0·32
Renal Colic	0·18	0·17	0·22	0·32	0·24	0·29	0·20
Other Diseases of the Kidney	0·18	0·28	0·27	0·26	0·38	0·48	0·33
Cystitis	0·18	0·39	0·55	0·42	0·50	0·65	0·45
Urethritis N.V.	0·19	2·19	2·46	3·22	4·54	6·83	4·69
Other Diseases of the Urethra	0·17	0·06	0·11	0·11	0·24	0·34	0·23
Urinary Disorders	0·54	0·51	0·55	0·58	0·79	0·98	0·68
Balanitis N.V.	0·11	0·67	1·04	1·06	1·27	1·86	1·28
Varicocele	0·06	0·17	0·05	0·26	0·13	0·15	0·10
Hydrocele	0·14	—	0·16	0·11	0·25	0·38	0·26
Orchitis N.V.	0·06	0·11	0·05	0·11	0·11	0·13	0·09
Epididymitis N.V.	0·46	0·73	0·93	0·85	0·15	1·53	1·05
Other Diseases	0·40	1·12	1·81	1·73	2·16	3·12	2·14
Totals	2·90	6·57	8·58	9·35	12·11	17·20	11·82
Percentages of total admissions for diseases	2	5	5	6	8	10	7
2. *Relative Rates*							
Pyelitis	7·96	2·57	4·46	3·40	1·81	1·89	2·71
Renal Colic	6·09	2·57	2·55	3·40	0·90	0·75	1·70
Other Diseases of the Kidney	6·32	4·27	3·18	2·82	4·05	1·51	2·80
Cystitis	6·32	5·98	6·37	4·52	3·15	2·26	3·80
Urethritis N.V.	6·56	33·33	28·66	34·46	41·44	48·30	39·68
Other Diseases of the Urethra	5·85	0·85	1·27	1·13	2·25	2·64	1·95
Urinary Disorders	18·50	7·69	6·37	6·21	4·50	6·04	5·75
Balanitis N.V.	3·75	10·26	12·10	11·30	12·16	8·68	10·83
Varicocele	2·11	2·57	0·64	2·82	0·45	—	0·85
Hydrocele	4·68	—	1·91	1·13	1·81	3·40	2·19
Orchitis N.V.	2·11	1·71	0·64	1·13	0·90	0·38	0·76
Epididymitis N.V.	15·93	11·11	10·83	9·04	7·21	9·06	8·88
Other Diseases	13·82	17·09	21·02	18·64	19·37	15·09	18·10
Totals	100	100	100	100	100	100	100

Diseases of the KIDNEY accounted for admissions at an Equivalent Annual Rate in 1945 of 0·85 per 1,000 which represented some seven per cent. of the total admissions of the group. Over one-third were attributable to PYELITIS and one-quarter to RENAL COLIC.

After the first quarter when the rate was 0·18, admissions for CYSTITIS varied but little and ranged between 0·4 and 0·6 per 1,000. The E.A.R. in 1945 was 0·45 per 1,000, equal to just under four per cent. of group admissions.

Admissions for N.V. URETHRITIS increased quarterly from 0·2 per 1,000 in the first quarter to 6·8 in the last. The rate for 1945 was 4·7, some forty per cent. of the total admissions. Other Diseases of the URETHRA were responsible for comparatively few admissions at 0·23 per 1,000.

The rates of admissions on account of URINARY DISORDERS in the first four quarters were particularly stable ranging from 0·51 to 0·58 per 1,000. In the last two quarters they increased to 0·79 and 0·98. The E.A.R. for 1945 was 0·68.

Admissions for N.V. BALANITIS, like Urethritis, increased each quarter, although the rate of increase was not so pronounced. Rates were 0·11 in the first quarter, and 1·86 in the last. The 1945 rate of 1·28 per 1,000 was some eleven per cent. of the total admissions for the group.

The rates for VARICOCELE were comparatively low at 0·10 per 1,000 as were those for HYDROCELE at 0·26, N.V. ORCHITIS at 0·09 and N.V. EPIDIDYMITIS at 1·05.

MENTAL DISEASES

Admissions for Mental Diseases were highest in the first of the six quarters under review at 14 per 1,000. Rates decreased gradually until in the last quarter it was slightly over 4. These rates represented eleven and two per cent. respectively of all admissions on account of disease. The Equivalent Annual Rate for 1945 was 6·75 per 1,000, being four per cent. of the total disease admission rate.

An analysis of admissions for this group follows. It must be mentioned that in this, as well as in other tabulations in this sub-section, where no admissions are shown against any disease, it does not necessarily follow there were, in fact, no admissions for that particular disease, but that none were in the ten per cent. sample made for coding purposes, of which mention has already been made.

North-West Europe, 1944–45
Admissions to Hospitals for Mental Diseases
E.A.Rs. per 1,000 Strength and Relative Rates

Source: Hollerith Tabulations

	1944		1945				1945
	QUARTER						Equivalent Annual Rates
	1st	2nd	3rd	4th	5th	6th	
1. *Equivalent Annual Rates*	July–Sept.	Oct.–Dec.	Jan.–Mar.	Apr.–June	July–Sept.	Oct.–Dec.	
Psychoses:							
Manic Depressive	0·17	0·06	0·06	0·21	0·32	0·19	0·19
Schizophrenia	0·21	0·16	0·27	0·53	0·27	0·38	0·36
Paranoid State	—	—	—	—	0·05	—	0·01
Others	0·07	—	—	—	—	—	—
Psychoneuroses:							
Anxiety State	10·80	7·71	9·06	3·83	2·59	2·40	4·48
Hysteria	2·38	1·90	1·92	0·63	0·59	0·71	0·96
Others	0·13	0·22	0·06	0·05	0·22	0·06	0·10
Psychopathic Personality	0·51	0·34	0·55	0·47	0·65	0·13	0·46
Mental Deficiency	0·21	0·22	0·10	0·16	0·27	0·13	0·17
Other Disorders	0·02	0·06	—	0·10	—	—	0·02
Totals	14·50	10·67	12·02	5·99	4·96	4·02	6·75
Percentages of total admissions for diseases	11	8	7	4	3	2	4
2. *Relative Rates*							
Psychoses:							
Manic Depressive	1·20	0·52	0·46	3·51	6·52	4·84	2·87
Schizophrenia	1·45	1·57	2·28	8·77	5·43	9·68	5·34
Paranoid State	—	—	—	—	1·09	—	0·20
Others	0·48	—	—	—	—	—	—
Psychoneuroses:							
Anxiety State	74·46	72·25	75·34	64·04	52·17	59·68	66·32
Hysteria	16·43	17·80	15·98	10·53	11·96	17·74	14·17
Others	0·92	2·09	0·46	0·88	4·35	1·61	1·44
Psychopathic Personality	3·52	3·14	4·57	7·89	13·04	3·23	6·78
Mental Deficiency	1·45	2·09	0·91	2·63	5·43	3·23	2·46
Other Disorders	0·10	0·52	—	1·75	—	—	0·41
Totals	100	100	100	100	100	100	100

By far the greatest number of admissions were caused by ANXIETY STATE. In the first quarter, admissions were at the high rate of 10·8 per 1,000. This figure was exceeded only by admissions for Malaria (13·8), Diseases of the Digestive System (30) and Diseases of the Musculo-Skeletal System (11). In the second quarter they had dropped to 7·7, but increased to 9·1 in the third. During the fourth quarter, which saw the last of the fighting in Europe, the rate had dropped to 3·8 and this was followed by further declines to 2·6 and 2·4. Admissions over the period represented a variation of from fifty-two to seventy-five per cent. of the total diseases for the group. The equivalent annual rate for 1945 was 4·5 per 1,000, some two-thirds the group total.

Admission rates for HYSTERIA were also highest in the first quarter at 2·38. They declined until by the last quarter the rate was 0·71. The E.A.R. for 1945 was 1 per 1,000, fourteen per cent. of the total for the whole group.

In all, admissions on account of PSYCHONEUROSES over the whole period were of the order of 7·5 per 1,000, some eighty-two per cent. of the total group admissions. During 1945 the rate was 5·5, representing seventy-two per cent. of group admissions. During the last two quarters of 1945, when active operations in North-West Europe had ceased, the rate of admissions were slightly over 3 per 1,000.

Following Anxiety State and Hysteria in numerical importance came admissions on account of PSYCHOPATHIC PERSONALITY. Admissions varied but little in the first five quarters from 0·34 to 0·65. In the last quarter the rate fell from 0·65 to 0·13 per 1,000. The E.A.R. in 1945 was 0·46, some seven per cent. of the total admissions for the group.

In the PSYCHOSES sub-group, most admissions were caused by SCHIZOPHRENIA with a range from 0·16 to 0·53 per 1,000. The 1945 rate was 0·36. Admissions for MANIC DEPRESSIVE state recorded an E.A.R. of 0·19 in 1945. There were few recorded admissions for PARANOID state or for Other Psychotic Diseases. This sub-group registered admissions in 1945 at a rate of 0·56 per 1,000, eight per cent. of the total admissions for Mental Diseases.

Admissions for MENTAL DEFICIENCY registered an E.A.R. of 0·17 in 1945, under three per cent. of total group admissions.

DISEASES OF THE AREOLAR TISSUE

Admissions for diseases of the Areolar Tissue increased from 6 per 1,000 in the first quarter to 10 in the fourth and declined to under 8 in the last quarter. These represented five, seven, and four per cent. respectively of the total admissions for diseases. The Equivalent Annual Rate in 1945 was 8 per 1,000, some five per cent. of all disease admissions.

Diseases of this group were coded under six headings. When the ten per cent. sample of Hollerith cards for North-West Europe was analysed it was found no admissions were recorded for Malignant Tumours and Cysts, Subcutaneous Emphysema or for Other Diseases. Figures for the three causes which registered admissions are as follows:

North-West Europe, 1944–45
Admissions for Diseases of the Areolar Tissue
E.A.Rs. per 1,000 Strength and Relative Rates

Source: Hollerith Tabulations

	1944		1945				1945
	QUARTER						Equivalent Annual Rates
	1st	2nd	3rd	4th	5th	6th	
1. Equivalent Annual Rates	July–Sept.	Oct.–Dec.	Jan.–Mar.	Apr.–June	July–Sept.	Oct.–Dec.	
Cellulitis	4·98	5·33	7·76	8·61	5·95	6·04	7·11
Tumours and Cysts: Benign and Unspecified	0·12	0·17	0·22	0·21	0·32	0·21	0·24
Abscesses: Unspecified	0·83	0·62	0·76	1·10	1·26	1·35	1·10
Totals	5·93	6·12	8·74	9·92	7·53	7·60	8·45
Percentages of total admissions for disease	5	5	5	7	5	4	5
2. Relative Rates							
Cellulitis	83·98	87·16	88·78	86·77	78·99	79·44	84·18
Tumours and Cysts: Benign and Unspecified	2·06	2·75	2·50	2·12	4·35	2·80	2·86
Abscesses: Unspecified	13·96	10·09	8·75	11·11	16·66	17·76	12·96
Totals	100	100	100	100	100	100	100

As was only to be expected, the greatest number of admissions was caused by CELLULITIS. Rates increased steadily from 5 per 1,000 in the first quarter to 9 in the fourth, and then declined to 6 in the last two quarters. As a percentage of total admissions for this group, they ranged from seventy-nine to eighty-nine per cent. The E.A.R. was 7 per 1,000, eighty-four per cent. of the annual admissions.

The rates of admission for Unspecified ABSCESS varied from 0·62 in the second quarter to a peak of 1·35 in the last. The E.A.R. of 1·1 was thirteen per cent. of the group total. Benign and Unspecified TUMOURS and CYSTS accounted for an admission rate of 0·24 per 1,000.

DISEASES OF THE MOUTH, TEETH AND GUMS

Admissions for this group of diseases increased nearly ten fold over the eighteen months under review. The rate in the first quarter was 1·35 per 1,000 while that in the last was 12·72. The largest increase was in the penultimate quarter when the rate rose from 4 to nearly 11 per 1,000. Admissions were from one to seven per cent. of those for all diseases. In 1945, the E.A.R. of 9·57 was recorded, some six per cent. of all disease admissions.

An analysis of these admissions follows:

North-West Europe, 1944–45
Admissions for Diseases of the Mouth, Teeth and Gums
E.A.Rs. per 1,000 Strength and Relative Rates

Source: Hollerith Tabulations

	1944		1945				1945
	QUARTER						Equivalent Annual Rates
	1st	2nd	3rd	4th	5th	6th	
1. *Equivalent Annual Rates*	July–Sept.	Oct.–Dec.	Jan.–Mar.	Apr.–June	July–Sept.	Oct.–Dec.	
Vincent's Angina	0·58	0·67	0·86	1·37	3·62	4·45	3·21
Other Diseases of the Mouth	0·05	0·06	0·31	0·26	0·51	0·31	0·45
Gingivitis	0·23	0·62	0·81	1·21	5·54	6·52	4·34
Other Diseases of the Gums	0·01	—	0·05	—	—	—	0·02
Diseases of the Teeth	0·48	0·78	0·92	1·26	1·18	1·44	1·55
Totals	1·35	2·13	2·95	4·10	10·85	12·72	9·57
Percentages of total admissions for diseases	1	2	2	3	7	7	6
2. *Relative Rates*							
Vincent's Angina	42·74	31·58	29·32	33·33	33·33	34·98	33·52
Other Diseases of the Mouth	4·03	2·63	10·34	6·41	4·69	2·46	4·70
Gingivitis	16·93	28·95	27·59	29·49	51·04	51·23	45·39
Other Diseases of the Gums	0·81	—	1·72	—	—	—	0·19
Diseases of the Teeth	35·49	36·84	31·03	30·77	10·94	11·33	16·20
Totals	100	100	100	100	100	100	100

Admissions for VINCENT'S ANGINA increased quarter by quarter from an initial rate of 0·58 per 1,000 to 4·45 in the final quarter. The largest rise in rates occurred in the penultimate quarter when admissions increased from 1·4 to 3·6 per 1,000. The 1945 rate was 3·2, approximately one-third of the total admissions for the group. Other Diseases of the Mouth recorded an E.A.R. of 0·5 per 1,000.

GINGIVITIS caused rates of admissions which, like Vincent's Angina, increased each quarter. The rate in the first quarter of 0·2 was followed by 0·6, 0·8 and 1·2. The ensuing quarter saw a four-fold rise to 5·5 per 1,000. In the final period, the rate was 6·5. Expressed as percentages of total admissions for this group, these rates represented a range of seventeen to fifty-one per cent. In 1945, the E.A.R. was 4.3, some forty-five per cent. of the group total.

Diseases of the TEETH also were responsible for rates which increased throughout the period, although the rises were not so spectacular as those for Gingivitis or for Vincent's Angina. Here, the admission rate for the last quarter was three times that of the first, 1·44 per 1,000 as against 0·48. In 1945, the rate was 1·55 per 1,000, some sixteen per cent. of the group total.

DISEASES OF THE RESPIRATORY SYSTEM

Admissions for this group of diseases recorded increases in the second and third quarters and thereafter a decline. Rates were 2·2 per 1,000, 5·9 and 7·4, followed by 4·4, 3·3 and 3·1, representing from slightly under two to nearly five per cent. of all admissions for diseases. The Equivalent Annual Rate for 1945 was 4·5, some two and a half per cent. of disease admissions.

Hereunder is an analysis of admissions for this group:

North-West Europe, 1944–45
Admissions for Diseases of the Respiratory System
E.A.Rs. per 1,000 Strength and Relative Rates

Source: Hollerith Tabulations

	1944		1945				1945
	QUARTER						Equivalent Annual Rates
	1st	2nd	3rd	4th	5th	6th	
1. *Equivalent Annual Rate*	July–Sept.	Oct.–Dec.	Jan.–Mar.	Apr.–June	July–Sept.	Oct.–Dec.	
Bronchitis:							
Acute	0·47	1·55	2·09	0·87	0·62	0·59	1·04
Chronic	0·51	1·91	2·16	1·18	0·90	0·78	1·24
Unspecified	0·59	1·37	2·09	1·63	0·44	0·59	1·20
Pleurisy	0·37	0·28	0·33	0·26	0·49	0·39	0·37
Other Diseases	0·27	0·79	0·71	0·47	0·82	0·71	0·68
Totals	2·21	5·90	7·38	4·41	3·27	3·05	4·53
Percentages of total admissions for diseases	2	5	4	3	2	2	3
2. *Relative Rates*							
Bronchitis:							
Acute	21·27	26·27	28·32	19·72	18·96	19·28	22·96
Chronic	23·08	32·37	29·27	26·76	27·52	25·49	27·37
Unspecified	26·70	23·22	28·32	36·96	13·46	19·28	26·49
Pleurisy	16·74	4·75	4·47	5·90	14·98	12·75	8·17
Other Diseases	12·21	13·39	9·62	10·66	25·08	23·20	15·01
Totals	100	100	100	100	100	100	100

By far the greatest number of admissions was caused by BRONCHITIS. Admissions commenced at 1·6 per 1,000, increased to 4·8 and 6·3, then declined to 3·7 and 2·0 in the final two quarters. The Equivalent Annual Rate of 3·5 per 1,000 was slightly over three-quarters the total for the group. Chronic Bronchitis accounted for thirty-five per cent. of all admissions for Bronchitis, and Acute Bronchitis for some thirty per cent. 'Unspecified' Bronchitis, thirty per cent. of all Bronchitis admissions, were other types of Bronchitis together with, possibly, some acute and chronic cases.

Admissions for PLEURISY varied from 0·26 per 1,000 in the quarter April to June, 1945, to 0·49 in the subsequent quarter. This disease recorded an E.A.R. of 0·37 per 1,000, some eight per cent. of all admissions for the group.

Admissions for OTHER DISEASES of the Respiratory System were 0·68 per 1,000, just fifteen per cent. of the group total.

DISEASES OF THE EYE

This group of diseases accounted for admissions at a rate of 2·5 per 1,000 in 1945. During the period under review, rates rose from 1·9 in the first quarter to a peak of 4 in the third and declined to 1·9 in the final quarter. Admissions for this group are analysed in the following table.

North-West Europe, 1944–45
Admissions for Diseases of the Eye
Equivalent Annual Rates per 1,000 Strength and Relative Rates

Source: Hollerith Tabulations

	1944		1945				1945
	QUARTER						Equivalent Annual Rates
	1st	2nd	3rd	4th	5th	6th	
1. *Equivalent Annual Rates*	July–Sept.	Oct.–Dec.	Jan.–Mar.	Apr.–June	July–Sept.	Oct.–Dec.	
Conjunctivitis	0·67	1·18	1·25	0·71	0·82	0·58	0·84
Keratitis	0·70	0·73	1·25	0·99	0·44	0·58	0·82
Iritis	0·05	0·28	0·34	0·38	0·05	0·07	0·21
Blepharitis	0·06	0·11	0·17	0·16	—	0·20	0·13
Others	0·43	0·62	1·03	0·44	0·22	0·45	0·53
Totals	1·91	2·92	4·04	2·68	1·53	1·88	2·53
2. *Relative Rates*							
Conjunctivitis	34·93	40·38	30·99	26·53	53·57	31·03	33·33
Keratitis	36·99	25·00	30·99	36·73	28·57	31·03	32·20
Iritis	2·40	9·62	8·45	14·29	3·57	3·45	8·48
Blepharitis	3·08	3·85	4·22	6·12	—	10·34	5·09
Others	22·60	21·15	25·35	16·33	14·29	24·15	20·90
Totals	100	100	100	100	100	100	100

CONJUNCTIVITIS and KERATITIS, with annual rates of 0·8 per 1,000 in 1945, together accounted for two-thirds of the admissions of this group. In both cases the highest rate of 1·25 occurred in the third quarter and the lowest in the final period. Admissions for IRITIS increased from 0·05 per 1,000 in the first quarter to 0·38 in the fourth, declining eventually to 0·07. The annual rate was 0·21. There were no admissions in the fifth quarter for BLEPHARITIS which recorded an annual rate of 0·13 per 1,000.

DISEASES OF THE NERVOUS SYSTEM

Admissions for this group of diseases increased by fifty per cent. from the first quarter to the third (2 to 3 per 1,000), then declined until by the sixth quarter, the rate was slightly less than that of the first. The Equivalent Annual Rate for 1945 was 2·5 per 1,000.

An analysis of these admissions is given below.

North-West Europe, 1944–45
Admissions to Hospitals for Diseases of the Nervous System
Equivalent Annual Rates per 1,000 Strength and Relative Rates

Sources: Hollerith Tabulations

	1944		1945				1945
	QUARTER						Equivalent Annual Rates
	1st	2nd	3rd	4th	5th	6th	
1. *Equivalent Annual Rates*	July–Sept.	Oct.–Dec.	Jan.–Mar.	Apr.–June	July–Sept.	Oct.–Dec.	
Sciatica	0·64	1·06	1·00	1·02	0·89	0·58	0·87
Other Neuritis	0·16	0·34	0·39	0·17	0·11	0·19	0·22
Migraine	0·18	0·22	0·11	0·28	0·06	0·07	0·13
Other Diseases of uncertain Pathology	0·02	0·06	0·11	0·06	0·17	0·07	0·10
Effort Syndrome	0·18	0·06	0·28	0·17	0·17	—	0·16
Diseases of the Cerebral Meninges	0·12	0·06	—	—	0·11	0·19	0·08
Diseases of the Brain	0·11	0·22	0·06	0·06	—	—	0·03
Epilepsy	0·05	0·22	0·06	0·17	0·17	0·13	0·13
Disorders of the Cranial Nerves	0·35	0·34	0·72	0·80	0·45	0·40	0·59
Other Diseases	0·15	—	0·22	0·11	0·22	0·19	0·18
Totals	1·96	2·58	2·95	2·84	2·34	1·82	2·49
2. *Relative Rates*							
Sciatica	32·69	41·31	33·96	36·00	38·10	32·14	35·26
Other Neuritis	8·08	13·04	13·21	6·00	4·76	10·71	8·67
Migraine	9·23	8·70	3·77	10·00	2·38	3·58	5·20
Other Diseases of uncertain Pathology	1·16	2·17	3·77	2·00	7·14	3·58	3·58

North-West Europe, 1944–45
Admissions to Hospitals for Diseases of the Nervous System
Equivalent Annual Rates per 1,000 Strength and Relative Rates

Source: Hollerith Tabulations

	1944		1945				1945
	QUARTER						Equivalent Annual Rates
	1st	2nd	3rd	4th	5th	6th	
2. *Relative Rates—cont.*	July–Sept.	Oct.–Dec.	Jan.–Mar.	Apr.–June	July–Sept.	Oct.–Dec.	
Effort Syndrome	9·23	2·17	9·43	6·00	7·14	—	6·36
Diseases of the Cerebral Meninges	6·15	2·17	—	—	4·76	10·71	2·89
Diseases of the Brain	5·77	8·70	1·89	2·00	—	—	1·16
Epilepsy	2·69	8·70	1·89	6·00	7·14	7·14	5·20
Disorders of the Cranial Nerves	17·69	13·04	24·53	28·00	19·05	21·43	23·70
Other Diseases	7·31	—	7·55	4·00	9·53	10·71	7·51
Totals	100	100	100	100	100	100	100

More than one-third of the admissions of this group of diseases were due to SCIATICA, which recorded an Equivalent Annual Rate of 0·87 per 1,000 in 1945. Rates were lowest in the first and last quarters. Other admissions for NEURITIS were one-fourth those for Sciatica.

Disorders of the CRANIAL NERVES followed Sciatica in numerical importance with an E.A.R. in 1945 of 0·59 per 1,000, nearly one-quarter of the total admissions for this group. Admissions for MIGRAINE which were lower in the two final quarters, after the cessation of active operations, had an E.A.R. of 0·13, some five per cent. of the group total.

There were no recorded admissions for EFFORT SYNDROME in the last quarter. During the other periods rates ranged from 0·06 to 0·28. Admissions on account of Diseases of the CEREBRAL MENINGES registered an Equivalent Annual Rate of 0·08, and those for Diseases of the BRAIN, 0·03. The E.A.R. of 0·13 per 1,000 in 1945 for EPILEPSY was five per cent. the total admissions for this group.

DISEASES OF THE CARDIO-VASCULAR SYSTEM

This group of diseases accounted for admission rates ranging from 1·4 in the first quarter to 3·3 per 1,000 in the last. In 1945 the Equivalent Annual Rate at 3 per 1,000, represented nearly two per cent. of all admissions for disease. Admissions analysed according to Valvular Disease of the Heart, Varicose Veins, and Other Diseases of the System are as under.

North-West Europe, 1944–45
Admissions to Hospitals for Diseases of the Cardio-Vascular System
E.A.Rs. per 1,000 Strength and Relative Rates

Source: Hollerith Tabulations

	1944		1945				1945
	QUARTER						Equivalent Annual Rates
	1st	2nd	3rd	4th	5th	6th	
1. *Equivalent Annual Rates*	July–Sept.	Oct.–Dec.	Jan.–Mar.	Apr.–June	July–Sept.	Oct.–Dec.	
Valvular Disease of the Heart	0·01	0·06	0·05	—	0·05	—	0·03
Varicose Veins	0·66	1·40	1·86	1·84	2·13	2·47	2·07
Other Diseases	0·73	1·07	1·20	0·95	0·82	0·84	0·95
Totals	1·40	2·53	3·11	2·79	3·00	3·31	3·05
Percentages of total admissions for diseases	1	2	2	2	2	2	2
2. *Relative Rates*							
Valvular Disease of the Heart	0·72	2·37	1·61	—	1·67	—	0·98
Varicose Veins	47·14	55·34	59·81	65·95	71·00	74·62	67·87
Other Diseases	52·14	42·29	38·58	34·05	27·33	25·38	31·15
Totals	100	100	100	100	100	100	100

VARICOSE VEINS were responsible for rates which increased from 0·66 per 1,000 in the first quarter to 2·47 in the last. The rate for 1945 was 2·07, nearly seventy per cent. of the total for the group. There were very few admissions for VALVULAR DISEASE of the HEART which, in 1945, registered a rate of 0·03 per 1,000. There were no recorded admissions in the second and last quarters of this year.

Of admissions for other diseases, less than one-third were caused by Diseases of the VEINS, other than Varicose Veins. The remainder were on account of a wide variety of diseases comprising the balance of the group.

PNEUMONIA

Admissions for Pneumonia were 0·6 in the first quarter. They rose to 2 in the second and to a peak of 4 in the third (January to March). Thereafter they varied but little at 2·6, 1·8 and 2·2 per 1,000. The Equivalent Annual Rate in 1945 was 2·7. An analysis of admissions for this disease is given below.

North-West Europe, 1944–45
Admissions to Hospitals for Pneumonia
E.A.Rs. per 1,000 Strength and Relative Rates

Source: Hollerith Tabulations

	1944		1945				1945
	QUARTER						Equivalent Annual Rates
	1st	2nd	3rd	4th	5th	6th	
1. *Equivalent Annual Rates*	July–Sept.–	Oct.–Dec.	Jan.–Mar.	Apr.–June	July–Sept.	Oct.–Dec.	
Acute Primary and Lobar	0·40	1·01	0·98	0·53	0·44	1·30	0·81
Broncho-Pneumonia	0·04	0·34	1·04	0·26	0·49	0·13	0·48
Atypical Pneumonia	0·04	0·39	1·37	0·84	0·54	0·52	0·82
Other Types and Unspecified	0·16	0·28	0·71	1·00	0·38	0·32	0·60
Totals	0·64	2·02	4·10	2·63	1·85	2·27	2·71
2. *Relative Rates*							
Acute Primary and Lobar	62·07	50·00	24·00	20·00	23·53	57·14	29·89
Broncho-Pneumonia	6·90	16·67	25·34	10·00	26·47	5·71	17·71
Atypical Pneumonia	6·90	19·44	33·33	32·00	29·41	22·86	30·26
Other Types and Unspecified	24·13	13·89	17·33	38·00	20·59	14·29	22·14
Totals	100	100	100	100	100	100	100

The E.A.Rs. for 1945 for ACUTE PRIMARY and LOBAR Pneumonia and ATYPICAL Pneumonia differed very slightly at 0·81 and 0·82 per 1,000 respectively. Where, however, admissions for the former tended to increase (0·98 to 1·30), those for the latter decreased (1·37 to 0·52). These diseases were each responsible for approximately thirty per cent. of all group admissions. Admissions for BRONCHO-PNEUMONIA with an E.A.R. of 0·48 also tended to decline from 1·04 in the first quarter of 1945 to 0·13 in the last.

DIPHTHERIA

The lowest rate of admissions for Diphtheria occurred during the first quarter of the period under review. An initial rate of 0·08 per 1,000 increased to 2·08 in the second quarter and to 5·03 in the third. The three closing quarters recorded rates of 1·47, 1·42 and 1·95 respectively. The large increase in admissions in the second and third quarters commenced in December 1944, rose to a peak in the following month, and declined in February and March. By April admissions were at a normal rate. Comparative monthly admissions with November represented as 100 were:

December .	. 183	January .	. 300
February .	. 266	March .	. 200
	April .	. 83	

The Equivalent Annual Rate for 1945 was 2·47 per 1,000.

Diphtheria was normally diagnosed, and coded, under the following classifications: Laryngeal, Faucial, Nasal, Cutaneous, Paralysis and Gravis. A large number of cases were, however, diagnosed as Diphtheria without classification. These are shown in the analyses below as unclassified Diphtheria. There were no recorded cases of Laryngeal Diphtheria in the sample of Army Forms I.1220 coded.

North-West Europe, 1944–45
Admissions to Hospitals for Diphtheria
E.A.Rs. per 1,000 Strength and Relative Rates

Source: Hollerith Tabulations

	1944		1945				1945
	QUARTER						Equivalent Annual Rates
	1st	2nd	3rd	4th	5th	6th	
1. *Equivalent Annual Rates*	July–Sept.	Oct.–Dec.	Jan.–Mar.	Apr.–June	July–Sept.	Oct.–Dec.	
Faucial . . .	0·04	0·79	2·70	0·79	0·50	1·18	1·29
Nasal . . .	—	0·05	—	0·05	—	0·06	0·03
Cutaneous . .	—	—	—	—	—	0·06	0·02
Paralysis . . .	0·02	—	0·12	0·05	0·17	0·06	0·10
Gravis . . .	—	—	0·06	—	—	—	0·01
Diphtheria Unclassified . .	0·02	1·24	2·15	0·58	0·75	0·59	1·02
Totals . .	0·08	2·08	5·03	1·47	1·42	1·95	2·47
2. *Relative Rates*							
Faucial . .	46·15	37·84	53·66	53·57	35·29	60·00	52·23
Nasal . .	—	2·70	—	3·57	—	3·33	1·21
Cutaneous .	—	—	—	—	—	3·33	0·81
Paralysis . .	23·08	—	2·44	3·57	11·77	3·33	4·05
Gravis . .	—	—	1·22	—	—	—	0·40
Diphtheria Unclassified . .	30·77	59·46	42·68	39·29	52·94	30·00	41·30
Totals . .	100	100	100	100	100	100	100

With an E.A.R. of 1·29, Faucial Diphtheria was responsible for more admissions than any other class. An initial rate of 0·04 was followed in the second quarter by one of 0·79. This was succeeded by the peak rate of 2·70 then 0·79, 0·50, and, finally, 1·18 per 1,000. There were comparatively few admissions for other types of Diphtheria. Unclassified cases commenced at a rate of 0·02, reached 2·15 in the third quarter and thereafter declined to a final rate of 0·59. Admissions for Faucial Diphtheria were one-half the group total and those for unclassified Diphtheria, forty-one per cent.

OTHER DISEASES

COMMON COLD recorded an annual rate of slightly under 3 per 1,000. Admissions were lowest in the first quarter at 0·9 and highest in the third and last quarters at 3·3 and 3·9 respectively. INFLUENZA registered the highest rate at 0·27 in the third quarter. Rates varied but little between 0·11 and 0·27 per 1,000.

Admissions for SCABIES commenced with a low rate of 0·18 per 1,000 and closed at 1·6, with an E.A.R. of 1·4.

MALARIA recorded a rate of 1·19 in 1945. Apart from the first quarter of the period under review, admissions ranged from 0·8 to 1·6 per 1,000. During the first quarter, however, an admission rate of 13·8 was recorded. An analysis of these admissions indicates that most cases occurred in August, one-eighth less in July and one-half the August total in September. Admissions in June were only slightly less than those in July. Comparative admissions were:

July . .	100
August . .	117
September. .	60

Those admitted were diagnosed Benign Tertian, Sub-Tertian or Malaria (unspecified). No cases of Quartan Malaria were recorded in this quarter, but one was admitted in June. Comparative admissions were:

	July	*August*	*September*
Benign Tertian . .	39·40	66·67	77·27
Sub-Tertian . . .	0·54	0·35	—
Malaria (unspecified) .	60·06	32·98	22·73
	100·00	100·00	100·00

Diseases of the BLOOD and BLOOD-FORMING ORGANS caused admissions at an average rate in 1945 of 1 per 1,000 and DYSENTERY at 0·86. The latter, however, recorded the comparatively high rate of 4.3 in the first quarter. Admissions for P.U.O. were 0·7, and RHEUMATIC FEVER and MUMPS, 0·3 per 1,000. All other diseases produced admissions at lower rates.

INJURIES

Admissions to hospitals on account of injuries were classified, as in other theatres, according to whether they were received in action against the enemy (E.A. injuries) or otherwise (N.E.A. injuries). Many Army Forms I.1220 on being received in the War Office were found to be unclassified and are noted in the relevant tabulations in this section as 'Cause not known'.

As would be expected, the largest number of admissions for injuries were recorded during the first quarter of the period when the rate was 132 per 1,000. This was followed by the comparatively low rate of 51. In the third quarter it rose to 71 and then declined to 57 (fighting ceased early in May). Rates thereafter were 22 per 1,000 for both quarters.

Analyses of these injuries are presented in Tables 24 and 25. Of the four periods under review during which active operations were in progress, i.e. July 1944 to June 1945, admissions for injuries caused through enemy action were greater than those not so caused, except in the quarter April to June 1945. The former registered rates which began at 97 per 1,000, fell to 26, increased to 43, and finally declined to 25. Rates for N.E.A. injuries were comparatively constant. ranging from 23 to 29 per 1,000, being 26, 23, 26 and 29 respectively. The equivalent annual rates were 48 per 1,000 for E.A. Injuries and 26 for N.E.A. Injuries.

Comparative rates for these classes of injuries were:

	1944		1945		E.A.R.
	July–Sept.	Oct.–Dec.	Jan.–Mar.	Apr.–June	
Enemy Action	78·60	53·10	62·42	45·92	64·67
Non-Enemy Action	21·40	46·90	37·58	54·08	35·33
	100	100	100	100	100
Enemy Action	100	26	44	26	
Non-Enemy Action	100	85	97	110	

Disregarding those injuries, the cause of which is not known, admissions in the first quarter for those caused through Enemy Action were nearly eighty per cent. of all injuries. This rate declined until, in the last quarter, it was forty-six per cent. Injuries not due to Enemy Action increased from twenty-one per cent. in the first quarter to fifty-four per cent. in the quarter ended June 30, 1945. Enemy Action Injuries accounted for sixty-five per cent. of the Equivalent Annual Rate and N.E.A. Injuries some thirty-five per cent.

When admissions for the first quarter are taken as the base for comparison, those E.A. Injuries in the second and fourth quarters were one quarter, and those in the third quarter under one half those in the initial period. With N.E.A. Injuries, admissions in the second quarter were eighty-five, in the third ninety-seven, and in the fourth quarter, one hundred and ten per cent. of those in the first quarter. It must be remembered, of course, that active warfare ceased in the early days of May and that had fighting continued, admissions for E.A. Injuries might well have equalled, or even surpassed, those in the previous quarter.

Enemy Action Injuries

Admissions for HEAD INJURIES at slightly under 4 per 1,000 in the first quarter, were followed by rates of 1·6 in the second and fourth and 2·8 in the third. In the last three quarters, admissions were equivalent to between six and seven per cent. of the total for E.A. Injuries. In the first quarter they were four per cent.

FRACTURES at sites other than the head were responsible for rates which fluctuated between fourteen and four per 1,000. In spite of this, expressed as a percentage of all E.A. admissions, the range was but one per cent. from 14·23 to 15·42.

Admissions for BURNS varied little, from 0·8 in the first two quarters to 0·5 in the fourth. They were, in the first quarter, less than one per cent. of all E.A. Injuries, three per cent. in the second quarter and, in the third and fourth quarters, somewhat less than two per cent.

OLD INJURIES caused admission rates which varied little during the year. The range was from 0·11 to 0·16. In the last two quarters of 1945, however, admissions increased to 0·4 per 1,000.

Non-Enemy Action Injuries

Admissions for HEAD INJURIES ranged from 1 to 2·5 per 1,000, and increased and declined in alternate quarters. The lowest rate occurred in the first quarter and the highest in the second and sixth. They were equivalent to from four to thirteen per cent. of all N.E.A. Injuries.

FRACTURES at sites other than the head produced rates highest in the fourth quarter at 10 per 1,000 and lowest in the following quarter at 7. Expressed as percentages of all N.E.A. Injuries, admissions for Fractures ranged from thirty-three in the second quarter to thirty-eight per cent. in the last.

Admissions for BURNS increased from 2 per 1,000 in the first quarter to 3 in the third. In the fourth period the rate was 2·6, following which it declined to 0·9 and 0·5 in the final quarters. They were equivalent, in the first four quarters, to between seven and eleven per cent. of all admissions for N.E.A. Injuries.

OLD INJURIES accounted for rates which were slightly higher than those caused by Enemy Action. Rates ranged from 0·22 to 0·49 per 1,000.

Injuries—Cause not known

These were between five and ten per cent. of all admissions for injuries, at rates commencing at 8 and declining to slightly over 2 per 1,000. They contained a comparatively large percentage of admissions for Burns and for Old Injuries.

If these injuries are proportionately allocated to E.A. and N.E.A. Injuries according to the numbers admitted for those classes, the results are as below.

All Injuries

North-West Europe, 1944–45
Admissions to Hospitals for Injuries
(Adjustment of Tables 24 and 25)
Equivalent Annual Rates per 1,000 Strength and Relative Rates

Source: Hollerith Tabulations

	1944		1945			
	QUARTER					
	1st	2nd	3rd	4th	5th	6th
1. *Equivalent Annual Rates*	July–Sept.	Oct.–Dec.	Jan.–Mar.	Apr.–June	July–Sept.	Oct.–Dec.
Enemy Action:						
Head Injuries	4·20	1·72	2·96	1·68	—	—
Fractures (Other Sites)	14·76	3·84	6·54	4·06	0·06	—
Burns	0·84	0·83	0·69	0·50	—	—
Old Injuries	0·13	0·12	0·17	0·12	0·48	0·43
Other Injuries	83·75	20·37	33·96	20·00	0·24	0·07
Totals	103·68	26·88	44·32	26·36	0·78	0·50
Non-Enemy Action:						
Head Injuries	1·09	2·60	1·43	2·40	1·57	2·69
Fractures (Other Sites)	10·11	7·94	9·56	10·75	8·15	9·09
Burns	2·11	2·60	3·07	2·74	0·96	0·58
Old Injuries	0·28	0·23	0·51	0·39	0·30	0·45
Other Injuries	14·64	10·36	12·12	14·77	10·55	8·59
Totals	28·23	23·73	26·69	31·05	21·53	21·40
2. *Relative Rates*						
Enemy Action:						
Head Injuries	4·05	6·40	6·68	6·37	—	—
Fractures (Other Sites)	14·24	14·29	14·76	15·40	7·69	—
Burns	0·81	3·09	1·56	1·90	—	—
Old Injuries	0·12	0·44	0·38	0·46	61·54	86·00
Other Injuries	80·78	75·78	76·62	75·87	30·77	14·00
Totals	100	100	100	100	100	100
Non-Enemy Action:						
Head Injuries	3·86	10·96	5·36	7·73	7·29	6·86
Fractures (Other Sites)	35·81	33·46	35·82	34·62	37·85	34·97
Burns	7·48	10·96	11·50	8·82	4·46	9·57
Old Injuries	0·99	0·97	1·91	1·26	1·40	1·28
Other Injuries	51·86	43·65	43·41	47·57	49·00	47·30
Totals	100	100	100	100	100	100

Based on the above, Equivalent Annual Rates for the year ended June 30, 1945 (by which date active operations had ceased), are presented below.

North-West Europe, 1944–45
Admissions to Hospitals for Injuries for the year ended June 30, 1945
Equivalent Annual Rates per 1,000 Strength and Relative Rates

Source: Hollerith Tabulations

	Enemy Action Injuries		Non-Enemy Action Injuries		All Injuries	
	Equivalent Annual Rates	Relative Rates	Equivalent Annual Rates	Relative Rates	Equivalent Annual Rates	Relative Rates
Head Injuries	2·64	5·25	1·88	6·86	4·52	5·81
Fractures (Other Sites)	7·30	14·51	9·59	34·97	16·89	21·73
Burns	0·72	1·43	2·63	9·59	3·35	4·31
Old Injuries	0·13	0·26	0·35	1·28	0·48	0·62
Other Injuries	39·52	78·55	12·97	47·30	52·49	67·53
Totals	50·31	100	27·42	100	77·73	100

Admissions for all injuries recorded a rate of 78 per 1,000. Of these, two-thirds were sustained in action. One in every five injuries was a fracture, other than of the head. Admissions for Head Injuries were approximately one-third of those for fractures and slightly more than one-half were sustained in action. Casualties for Burns were higher among N.E.A. Injuries, being nearly four times the E.A. rate. Admissions for N.E.A. Old Injuries, although comparatively small, were nearly three times those of the other class.

ADMISSIONS TO ALL MEDICAL UNITS

Table 27 records admissions to all medical units for certain diseases. These statistics were obtained from monthly Hygiene reports, but only those from May to December 1945 are available. Mean Monthly Rates (M.M.Rs.) are given in the tabulation, together with an Equivalent Annual Rate for that year. Rates are based on 100,000 strength instead of the conventional 1,000 in order that the graduations of admissions, especially in respect of some rarer diseases, may be appreciated. As an example, M.M.Rs. of admissions for Cerebro-Spinal Fever are given in the table as 1·14, 1·06, 0·26, 0·54, 0·28, 0·28 and 0·34. Had they been calculated per 1,000 strength, rates would have been shown as 0·01, 0·01, 0·00, 0·01, 0·00, 0·00 and 0·00.

At first sight, it may be considered that the rates in this table should be greater than, or at least equivalent to those in Table 23, which records admissions to hospitals only. In point of fact, however, some rates are lower. This may be due to either or both of the following reasons:

(a) The statistics in Table 23 were built from a ten per cent. sample of A.F. I.1220, the sample comprising cards on which the Army number of the patient ended in the digit 5. It may be that, in the rarer disease, such cards may have been more frequent than the average warranted.

(b) Table 27 represents information for only the last eight months of 1945. Equivalent Annual Rates based on those months would necessarily be low if admissions during the period January to April were higher than the average. This is exemplified in Diphtheria and Jaundice for which admission rates in the quarter January to March 1945 were higher than those of the three ensuing quarters.

VENEREAL DISEASES

Of the diseases enumerated in Table 27, admissions for Venereal Diseases were by far the more numerous, with an Equivalent Annual Rate of 9,139 per 100,000 (91·39 per 1,000). Admissions rose from 280 in May to a peak of 1,010 in August, subsiding to 820 in December. An analysis of admissions for this group are given below.

URETHRITIS was responsible for eighty-five per cent. of the group admissions at monthly rates which ranged from 230 per 100,000 in May to a peak of 875 in August. Subsequently, a decline occurred and the rate fell to 655. The Equivalent Annual Rate was 7,721 per 100,000

North-West Europe, 1945
Admissions to all Medical Units for Venereal Diseases
Mean Monthly, Annual, Relative and Comparative Rates

Source: Hygiene Reports. *Rates per 100,000 Strength*

1. *Mean Monthly and Annual Rates*	Mean Monthly Rates, 1945								Annual Rates
	May	June	July	Aug.	Sept.	Oct.	Nov.	Dec.	
Syphilis									
(*a*) Early	23·47	30·70	52·56	91·01	97·03	88·93	97·00	100·16	871·29
(*b*) Late	0·27	2·38	0·69	0·14	0·75	0·30	0·69	1·62	10·26
Urethritis									
(*a*) Smear positive for Gc	140·68	266·37	534·77	630·79	642·88	582·84	565·68	553·34	5,876·02
(*b*) Smear negative for Gc	72·81	101·50	156·72	175·06	141·13	114·68	96·31	80·13	1,407·51
(*c*) Smear not reported	16·67	21·87	61·72	69·57	37·23	36·98	25·41	22·20	437·47
Chancroid	0·67	0·56	1·11	1·42	1·20	2·25	1·37	2·53	16·67
Other Venereal Diseases	24·54	21·59	46·60	43·30	40·37	56·44	51·85	61·90	519·89
Totals	279·11	444·97	854·17	1,011·29	960·59	882·42	838·31	821·88	9,139·11

2. *Relative Rates*

Syphilis									
(*a*) Early	8·41	6·90	6·15	9·00	10·10	10·08	11·57	12·19	9·53
(*b*) Late	0·10	0·54	0·08	0·01	0·08	0·03	0·08	0·19	0·11
Urethritis									
(*a*) Smear positive for Gc	50·40	59·86	62·61	62·37	66·93	66·05	67·48	67·33	64·30
(*b*) Smear negative for Gc	26·09	22·81	18·35	17·32	14·69	13·00	11·49	9·75	15·40
(*c*) Smear not reported	5·97	4·91	7·23	6·88	3·88	4·19	3·03	2·70	4·79
Chancroid	0·24	0·13	0·13	0·14	0·12	0·25	0·16	0·31	0·18
Other Venerea Diseases	8·79	4·85	5·45	4·28	4·20	6·40	6·19	7·53	5·69
Totals	100	100	100	100	100	100	100	100	100

3. *Comparative Rates* (*May = 100*)

Syphilis								
(*a*) Early	100	131	224	388	413	379	413	427
(*b*) Late	100	881	256	52	278	111	256	600
Urethritis								
(*a*) Smear positive for Gc	100	189	380	448	457	414	402	393
(*b*) Smear negative for Gc	100	139	215	240	194	158	132	110
(*c*) Smear not reported	100	131	370	417	223	222	152	133
Chancroid	100	84	166	212	179	336	204	378
Other Venereal Diseases	100	88	190	176	165	230	211	252
Totals	100	159	306	362	344	316	300	294

(77 per 1,000). Throughout the eight months, the percentage of Urethritis to all admissions in the group was fairly constant, with a range of 80 to 88. Positive smears were four times negative smears and those unreported as either positive or negative were some five per cent. of all cases.

SYPHILIS recorded an E.A.R. of 880 per 100,000 (8·8 per 1,000). This was slightly less than ten per cent. of all admissions for the group. The trend of these admissions was somewhat different to that of Urethritis, the rates for which increased until August and then declined. Admissions for Syphilis, however, except for a slight decrease in October, consistently recorded increases each month from 23 in May to 100 in December.

The rate for CHANCROID was comparatively low at 17 per 100,000 with a monthly range of 0·56 to 2·53 and a trend similar to that for Syphilis. Admissions for Other Venereal Diseases with an annual rate of 520 per 100,000 ranged from 22 to 62.

SCABIES

Next in order of numerical importance were admissions for Scabies. Here, rates are available for eleven months. The equivalent annual rate was 6,927 per 100,000 (69 per 1,000). Admissions in February at a rate of 360 increased to 400 in March, then declined to 280 in June. From July, which recorded a rate of 320, increases were registered each month until a rate of 1,200 was reached in November. This was followed by a slight decrease to 1,080 in December.

Mean Monthly rates, with Relative and Comparative Rates are given below.

North-West Europe, 1945
Admissions to All Medical Units for Scabies
Mean Monthly, Relative and Comparative Rates

Source: Hygiene Reports. *M.M.Rs. per 100,000 Strength*

Month	Mean Monthly Rate	Relative Rate	Comparative Rate
1945			
February	358	5·64	100
March	401	6·31	112
April	329	5·18	92
May	313	4·93	87
June	284	4·47	79
July	324	5·10	91
August	387	6·09	108
September	726	11·43	203
October	951	14·98	266
November	1199	18·88	335
December	1079	16·99	301
	E.A.R. 6927	100	

Admissions were highest in the last four months of the year when they were two to three times those in February, and comprised over sixty per cent. of the total for the eleven months. The highest monthly rate of 1,199 per 100,000 occurred in November. This was slightly under twenty per cent. of all admissions, over three times the rate for February, and over four times the lowest rate. Admissions were lowest in June, when admissions were four per cent. of the total and eighty per cent. of those in February.

DYSENTERY

The equivalent annual rate for this disease was 2,068 per 100,000 (21 per 1,000). Mean Monthly rates ranged from 290 to 160 during the period May to September and from 84 to 71 during October to December. An analysis of these admissions follows on page 219.

The admission rate in May was 260 per 100,000 (2·6 per 1,000). In June it fell to 187 then increased to 294 before declining to 248 in August. It decreased by one-third during September to 159. A sharp decline to 84 in October was followed by rates of 71 and 77 in the two following months.

North-West Europe, 1945
Admissions to All Medical Units for Dysentery
Mean Monthly, Equivalent Annual and Comparative Rates

Source: Hygiene Reports. *M.M.Rs. and E.A.Rs. per 100,000 Strength*

1. *Relative Rates*	May	June	July	Aug.	Sept.	Oct.	Nov.	Dec.	E.A.R.
Dysentery:									
Protozoal (Confirmed) .	0·25	—	0·53	0·40	0·28	1·13	—	0·17	4·14
Bacillary (Confirmed) .	1·77	0·93	7·36	10·63	4·11	2·27	1·14	1·03	43·86
Clinical (including Gastro-Enteritis)	258·12	186·17	285·62	236·49	154·16	80·47	69·62	75·86	2,019·76
Totals . .	260·14	187·10	293·51	247·52	158·55	83·87	70·76	77·06	2,067·76

2. *Comparative Rates*	May	June	July	Aug.	Sept.	Oct.	Nov.	Dec.
Protozoal .	100	—	212	160	112	452	—	68
Bacillary .	100	53	416	601	232	128	64	58
Clinical .	100	72	111	92	60	31	27	29
Totals . .	100	72	113	95	61	32	27	30

CLINICAL Dysentery (which included Gastro-Enteritis) was responsible for nearly ninety-eight per cent. of all Dysentery cases. These naturally followed the total admission trend of the group. Admissions for BACILLARY Dysentery, which were some two per cent. of all cases in the group, ranged from 0·93 in June to a peak of 10·63 in August. There were very few cases of confirmed PROTOZOAL Dysentery, those recorded being only one-fifth per cent. of all Dysentery cases.

JAUNDICE

The Equivalent Annual Rate of admissions for Jaundice in 1945 was 614 per 100,000 strength (6·14 per 1,000). Admissions, rates of which ranged from 41 in July to a peak of 67 in November are analysed below.

North-West Europe, 1945
Admissions to All Medical Units for Jaundice
Mean Monthly, Equivalent Annual and Comparative Rates

Source: Hygiene Reports. *M.M.Rs. and E.A.Rs. per 100,000 Strength*

1. *Infective Hepatitis, 1945*	Mean Monthly Rates	Comparative Rates
May	45·11	100
June	46·61	103
July	40·60	90
August	43·45	96
September	57·24	127
October	62·76	139
November	66·84	148
December	45·72	101
Equivalent Annual Rate per 100,000		612·49

2. *Post-Arsphenamine*
   1 admission in May, 2 in July and 2 in October.
3. *Leptospirosis*
   1 admission in October.

Admissions on account of POST-ARSPHENAMINE and LEPTOSPIROSIS were extremely few. Those for INFECTIVE HEPATITIS varied only slightly during the period May to August with rates which ranged from 41 to 46 per 100,000. In September, admissions increased to 57. This was followed by further increases to 63 and 67, but by December the rate declined to 46, only slightly above the rate in May.

DIPHTHERIA

Statistics relating to Diphtheria are available in respect of Faucial and Cutaneous. There were very few admissions for the latter cause; indeed they were less than two per cent. of the total. Monthly rates are given below.

North-West Europe, 1945
Admissions to All Medical Units for Diphtheria
Mean Monthly, Equivalent Annual and Comparative Rates

Source: Hygiene Reports. *M.M.Rs. and E.A.Rs. per 100,000 Strength*

1. *Mean Monthly and Equivalent Annual Rates*	May	June	July	Aug.	Sept.	Oct.	Nov.	Dec.	E.A.R.
Diphtheria:									
Faucial	18·57	11·42	11·04	7·53	16·01	13·74	22·72	18·67	179·55
Cutaneous	0·25	0·13	—	0·27	0·28	0·28	0·49	0·34	3·06
Totals	18·82	11·55	11·04	7·80	16·29	14·02	23·21	19·01	182·61
2. *Comparative Rates*									
Diphtheria	100	61	59	41	87	74	123	101	

Rates of admissions declined by over fifty per cent. from 19 per 100,000 in May to 8 in August. A rate of 16 in September increased to 23 in November and ended at 19, very slightly above the rate in May. The Equivalent Annual Rate was 183 per 100,000 (1·8 per 1,000).

MALARIA

Statistics in the Hygiene Reports for admissions on account of MALARIA were broken down to three components, Benign Tertian, Malignant Tertian and Clinical and Other Types. They were further split as to whether or not the Malaria was Indigenous. Analyses are given below.

Malaria recorded an Equivalent Annual Rate of 111 per 100,000 (1·11 per 1,000) in 1945. Monthly rates varied little during the period May to August and were in the range of 11 to 14. Rates during the last four months also showed little variation but were lower at from 5 to 7.

North-West Europe, 1945
Admissions to All Medical Units for Malaria
Mean Monthly, Equivalent Annual and Comparative Rates

Source: Hygiene Reports. *M.M.Rs. and E.A.Rs. per 100,000 Strength*

	May	June	July	Aug.	Sept.	Oct.	Nov.	Dec.	E.A.R.
1. *M.M.Rs. and E.A.Rs.*									
Indigenous:									
B.T.	—	0·40	0·66	1·08	1·70	0·85	0·49	0·86	9·06
M.T.	—	—	—	—	—	—	—	—	—
Clinical and Others	0·13	—	0·26	—	0·71	0·57	0·16	1·20	4·55
Total Indigenous	0·13	0·40	0·92	1·08	2·41	1·42	0·65	2·06	13·61
Non-Indigenous:									
B.T.	7·58	4·91	6·17	4·71	2·69	1·98	1·96	1·88	47·82
M.T.	0·13	—	0·13	0·27	—	—	—	—	0·79
Clinical and Others	3·54	5·31	6·96	6·05	2·27	3·54	2·29	2·23	48·28
Total Non-Indigenous	11·25	10·22	13·26	11·03	4·96	5·52	4·25	4·11	96·89
Total Malaria	11·38	10·62	14·18	12·11	7·37	6·94	4·90	6·17	110·50
2. *Relative Rates*									
Indigenous:									
B.T.	—	3·77	4·66	8·92	23·07	12·25	10·00	13·94	8·20
M.T.	—	—	—	—	—	—	—	—	—
Clinical and Others	1·14	—	1·83	—	9·63	8·21	3·27	19·45	4·12
Total Indigenous	1·14	3·77	6·49	8·92	32·70	20·46	13·27	33·39	12·32
Non-Indigenous:									
B.T.	66·61	46·23	43·51	38·89	36·50	28·53	40·00	30·47	43·28
M.T.	1·14	—	0·92	2·23	—	—	—	—	0·71
Clinical and Others	31·11	50·00	49·08	49·96	30·80	51·01	46·73	36·14	43·69
Total Non-Indigenous	98·86	96·23	93·51	91·08	67·30	79·54	86·73	66·61	87·68
Total Malaria	100	100	100	100	100	100	100	100	100
3. *Comparative Rates*									
Malaria:									
B.T.	100	70	90	76	58	37	32	36	
M.T.	100	—	100	208	—	—	—	—	
Clinical and Others	100	145	197	165	81	112	67	93	
Total Malaria	100	93	125	106	65	61	43	54	

Over the whole period, admissions on account of INDIGENOUS Malaria were one-eighth of the total of the group, but monthly percentages varied considerably from one in May to thirty in September and December. Rates increased from 0·13 per 100,000 in May to 2·4 in September, declined to 0·65 in November and ended with a rise to 2·06 in December. The Equivalent Annual Rate was 13·6. There were no recorded admissions for Malignant Tertian Malaria. Admissions for Benign Tertian Malaria were double those for Clinical and Other Types and ranged from 0·4 in June to 1·7 in September. There were no cases in May. Rates for Clinical Malaria ranged from 0·13 in May to 1·20 in December. No admissions were reported during June or August.

Admissions for NON-INDIGENOUS Malaria commenced at 11 in May, increased to 13 in July and steadily declined to 4 in December. The Equivalent Annual Rate was 97. Cases of Benign Tertian Malaria, which recorded an E.A.R. of 48, decreased from 7·6 in May to 2 in December. Rates for Clinical Malaria increased from 3·5 in May to 7 in July before declining eventually to 2·2 in December. Equivalent Annual Rates for Benign Tertian and Clinical admissions were almost equal at 47·8 and 48·3 respectively and were each approximately forty-three per cent. of all admissions for Malaria. There were very few cases of the Malignant Tertian type, and then only in May, July and August.

Compared with those in May, admissions for all Benign Tertian Malaria fell by thirty per cent. in June before increasing to ninety per cent. in July. Following this, there was a decline, until by December they were under forty per cent. of the May admissions. Rates for Clinical Malaria increased to slightly under double that in May, then decreased to under seventy per cent. in November. Admissions in December were ninety per cent. of those in May.

PNEUMONIA

Monthly rates of admissions for Pneumonia declined from 6 in May to 3 in September and October and increased to 8 in December. The Equivalent Annual Rate was 52 per 100,000 (0·5 per 1,000). These admissions are analysed below.

North-West Europe, 1945
Admissions to All Medical Units for Pneumonia
Mean Monthly, Equivalent Annual, Relative and Comparative Rates

Source: Hygiene Reports. *M.M.Rs. and E.A.Rs. per 100,000 Strength*

1. *M.M.Rs. and E.A.Rs.*	May	June	July	Aug.	Sept.	Oct.	Nov.	Dec.	E.A.R.
Pneumonia:									
Lobar	3·03	1·99	1·05	1·88	1·28	2·27	2·94	7·02	32·19
Virus (primary atypical)	2·40	1·59	0·79	0·94	0·99	0·14	0·49	0·68	12·03
Others (including Influenzal)	0·88	0·66	1·05	0·40	0·57	0·43	0·82	0·51	7·98
Totals	6·31	4·24	2·89	3·22	2·84	2·84	4·25	8·21	52·20
2. *Relative Rates*									
Pneumonia:									
Lobar	48·02	46·93	36·33	58·39	45·07	79·93	69·18	85·51	61·67
Virus	38·03	37·50	27·34	29·19	34·86	4·93	11·53	8·28	23·05
Others	13·95	15·57	36·33	12·42	20·07	15·14	19·29	6·21	15·28
Totals	100	100	100	100	100	100	100	100	100
3. *Comparative Rates*									
Pneumonia:									
Lobar	100	66	35	62	42	75	97	232	
Virus	100	66	33	39	41	6	20	28	
Others	100	75	119	45	65	49	93	58	
Totals	100	67	46	51	45	45	67	130	

LOBAR Pneumonia accounted for nearly two-thirds the total admissions for the group. Rates declined from 3 per 100,000 (·03 per 1,000) in May to 1 in July and then increased monthly to 3 in November. During the following month, admissions more than doubled to 7. The highest rate of admissions in respect of VIRUS Pneumonia occurred in May at 2·4 and the lowest in October at 0.14. In December (when the highest rate for Lobar Pneumonia was recorded), the rate was 0·68, slightly above one-half the average rate of admission for the period. OTHER TYPES produced rates which increased and decreased in alternate months. The range exhibited was from 0·4 to 1·05. These rates occurred in August and July respectively. The Equivalent Annual Rate of 8 per 100,000 was some fifteen per cent. of the total admissions for the group.

TUBERCULOSIS

Admissions for Tuberculosis varied but little during the eight months under review. The range of rates was from slightly under 3 in the first four months to 4 in September. The Equivalent Annual Rate was 39 per 100,000 (0·39 per 1,000). The majority of cases were of the PULMONARY type. OTHERS were six per cent. of the total. An analysis of these admissions are given below.

North-West Europe, 1945
Admissions to All Medical Units for Tuberculosis
Mean Monthly, Equivalent Annual and Comparative Rates

Source: Hygiene Reports. *M.M.Rs. and E.A.Rs. per 100,000 Strength*

1. *M.M.Rs. and E.A.Rs.*	May	June	July	Aug.	Sept.	Oct.	Nov.	Dec.	E.A.R.
Tuberculosis:									
Pulmonary .	2·40	2·26	2·76	2·56	4·11	3·68	3·60	3·25	36·93
Other types .	0·51	0·53	0·13	0·13	—	0·14	—	0·17	2·42
Totals . .	2·91	2·79	2·89	2·69	4·11	3·82	3·60	3·42	39·35
2. *Comparative Rates*									
Tuberculosis:									
Pulmonary .	100	94	115	107	171	153	150	135	
Other types .	100	104	25	25	—	27	—	33	
Totals . .	100	96	99	92	141	131	124	118	

SCARLET FEVER, MEASLES, MUMPS, CHICKEN POX AND RUBELLA

Equivalent Annual Rates for these diseases ranged from 7 per 100,000 in the case of Rubella to 20 for Scarlet Fever. Admissions are analysed below.

North-West Europe, 1945
Admissions to All Medical Units for
Scarlet Fever, Measles, Mumps, Chicken Pox and Rubella
Mean Monthly, Equivalent Annual and Comparative Rates

Source: Hygiene Reports. *M.M.Rs. and E.A.Rs. per 100,000 Strength*

1. *M.M.Rs. and E.A.Rs.*	May	June	July	Aug.	Sept.	Oct.	Nov.	Dec.	E.A.R.
Scarlet Fever	2·65	1·46	2·10	1·48	0·99	1·42	1·31	1·88	19·93
Measles	3·54	0·80	1·05	0·40	0·57	0·14	0·49	3·08	15·11
Mumps	2·53	1·20	1·18	0·27	1·13	1·28	1·47	0·68	14·61
Chicken Pox	1·14	0·80	0·92	0·94	0·57	0·71	0·65	2·91	12·96
Rubella	1·77	1·06	0·13	0·54	0·43	0·85	—	—	7·17

2. *Comparative Rates*	May	June	July	Aug.	Sept.	Oct.	Nov.	Dec.
Scarlet Fever	100	55	79	56	37	54	49	71
Measles	100	23	30	11	16	4	14	87
Mumps	100	47	47	11	45	51	58	27
Chicken Pox	100	70	81	82	50	62	57	255
Rubella	100	60	7	31	24	48	—	—

Apart from Chicken Pox, the highest rates of admission occurred in May. Most admissions on account of CHICKEN POX were in December, when the rate was two-and-a-half times that for May. During the period June to November, admissions for MEASLES were less than one-third those in May, but in December rose to nearly ninety per cent. There were no recorded cases of RUBELLA in November or December. The Equivalent Annual Rate for Measles at 15 was three-quarters of that for Scarlet Fever. The rate for Mumps was slightly less at 14, Chicken pox was 13 and Rubella 7.

ENTERIC GROUP OF FEVERS

This group was responsible for admissions at an Equivalent Annual Rate of 8 per 100,000 (0·08 per 1,000) analysed as under.

North-West Europe, 1945
Admissions to All Medical Units for Enteric Group of Fevers
Mean Monthly, Equivalent Annual, Relative and Comparative Rates

Source: Hygiene Reports. *M.M.Rs. and E.A.Rs. per 100,000 Strength*

1. *M.M.Rs. and E.A.Rs.*	May	June	July	Aug.	Sept.	Oct.	Nov.	Dec.	E.A.R.
Enteric Group of Fevers									
Typhoid	0·51	0·13	0·26	0·81	0·43	0·28	0·16	0·17	4·13
Paratyphoid	—	0·13	0·13	0·13	0·28	0·28	—	—	1·43
Clinical and Others	0·25	0·27	0·26	—	0·43	0·43	—	—	2·46
Totals	0·76	0·53	0·65	0·94	1·14	0·99	0·16	0·17	8·02

2. *Relative Rates*

Typhoid . .	67	25	40	86	38	28	100	100	51
Paratyphoid . .	—	25	20	14	24	28	—	—	18
Clinical and Others	33	50	40	—	38	44	—	—	31
Totals . .	100	100	100	100	100	100	100	100	100

3. *Comparative Rates*

Typhoid . .	100	25	51	159	84	55	31	33
Paratyphoid . .	—	100	100	100	215	215	—	—
Clinical and Others	100	108	104	—	172	172	—	—
Totals . .	100	70	86	124	150	130	21	22

Admission rates commenced in May at 0·76, declined to 0·53 in June, rose to 1·14 in September and fell to 0·16 in November and December. TYPHOID accounted for one half, and PARATYPHOID less than twenty per cent. of all admissions for this group. There were no cases of Paratyphoid in May, November or December.

OTHER DISEASES

(a) CEREBRO-SPINAL FEVER, with an Equivalent Annual Rate of 5·9 per 100,000.

(b) POLIOMYELITIS, which recorded rates (apart from September when there were no admissions) in the range 0·17 (December) to 0·67 (August), with an E.A.R. of 4 per 100.000.

(c) TYPHUS FEVER, with admissions in May, June and August only. The E.A.R. was 1·01 per 100,000.

(d) ENCEPHALITIS, which registered low rates of admission in May and September only.

TABLE 23

North-West Europe, 1944–45. Admissions to Hospitals (Quarterly). British Troops
Equivalent Annual Rates per 1,000 Strength

Source: Hollerith Tabulations

	CAUSES	1944		1945				
		July–Sept.	Oct.–Dec.	Jan.–Mar.	Apr.–June	July–Sept.	Oct.–Dec.	
1	Common Cold	0·94	2·36	3·28	2·36	1·96	3·90	1
2	Diphtheria	0·08	2·08	5·03	1·47	1·42	1·95	2
3	Dysentery	4·30	0·45	1·09	0·74	1·42	0·19	3
4	Enteric Group of Fevers	0·21	—	—	0·21	0·11	—	4
5	Influenza	0·19	0·17	0·27	0·11	0·05	0·13	5
6	Jaundice, Catarrhal	1·44	1·85	5·79	4·04	4·53	5·52	6
7	Malaria	13·81	1·63	1·20	1·63	1·09	0·84	7
8	Measles	0·03	—	0·05	0·32	0·16	0·19	8
9	Meningococcal Infection	0·03	0·06	—	0·11	—	0·06	9
10	Mumps	0·12	0·17	0·49	0·42	0·11	0·19	10
11	Pneumonia	0·64	2·02	4·10	2·63	1·85	2·27	11
12	Rheumatic Fever	0·15	0·28	0·49	0·16	0·22	0·39	12
13	Scarlet Fever	0·03	0·06	0·16	0·26	0·05	0·26	13
14	Tuberculosis—Pulmonary	0·38	0·17	—	0·11	—	0·06	14
15	Tuberculosis—Other	0·08	—	—	—	—	—	15
16	Venereal Diseases	2·13	9·77	13·82	9·88	22·26	25·71	16
17	Pyrexia of Unknown Origin	0·94	0·45	0·55	0·68	1·25	0·45	17
18	Other Infectious Diseases	1·28	1·40	2·51	1·16	2·18	2·66	18
19	Scabies	0·18	0·62	1·42	1·05	1·31	1·62	19
20	Other Diseases due to Infestation by Metazoan Parasites	0·28	0·22	0·11	0·32	0·27	0·32	20
21	Diseases of the Nervous System	1·96	2·58	2·95	2·84	2·34	1·82	21
22	Mental Diseases	14·50	10·67	12·02	5·99	4·96	4·02	22
23	Diseases of the Eye	1·91	2·92	4·04	2·68	1·53	1·88	23
24	Diseases of the Ear, Nose and Throat	7·16	12·24	22·01	20·42	18·98	23·30	24
25	Diseases of the Cardio-Vascular System	1·40	2·53	3·11	2·79	3·00	3·31	25
26	Diseases of the Blood and Blood-forming Organs	0·97	1·24	0·93	1·21	0·71	1·10	26
27	Diseases of the Endocrine System	0·27	—	0·05	0·26	0·11	0·19	27
28	Diseases of the Breast	0·09	0·06	0·11	0·16	0·33	0·06	28
29	Diseases of the Respiratory System	2·21	5·90	7·38	4·41	3·27	3·05	29
30	Diseases of the Mouth, Teeth and Gums	1·35	2·13	2·95	4·10	10·85	12·72	30
31	Diseases of the Digestive System	29·97	19·15	20·25	18·48	17·39	15·25	31

32	Diseases due to Disorders of Nutrition and Metabolism	0·12	0·06	0·22	0·42	0·71	1·30	32
33	Diseases of the Genito-Urinary System	2·90	6·57	8·58	9·35	12·11	17·20	33
34	Diseases of the Muscular System	11·07	11·80	14·15	12·81	11·40	10·39	34
35	Diseases of the Areolar Tissue	5·93	6·12	8·74	9·92	7·53	7·60	35
36	Diseases of the Skin	10·45	13·31	17·75	17·48	13·25	13·76	36
3	Poisons	0·05	0·17	0·27	0·16	—	0·26	37
38	All Other Diseases	11·40	6·12	7·70	8·72	8·45	12·02	38
39	*Total Admissions for Diseases*	130·99	127·37	173·59	149·80	157·18	175·93	39
40	Injuries—E.A.	97·14	25·51	42·55	24·84	0·71	0·45	40
41	Injuries—N.E.A.	26·45	22·53	25·62	29·25	19·47	19·09	41
42	Injuries—Cause Not Known	8·32	2·58	2·84	3·32	2·13	2·36	42
43	*Total Admissions for Injuries*	131·91	50·62	71·01	57·41	22·31	21·91	43
44	*Total Admissions*	262·92	177·98	244·60	207·23	179·49	195·96	44

TABLE 24

North-West Europe, 1944–45
Admissions to Hospitals through Injury
Equivalent Annual Rates per 1,000 Strength

Source: Hollerith Tabulations

	1944		1945			
	QUARTERS					
	1st	2nd	3rd	4th	5th	6th
	July–Sept.	Oct.–Dec.	Jan.–Mar.	Apr.–June	July–Sept.	Oct.–Dec.
1. *Enemy Action*						
Head Injuries	3·93	1·63	2·84	1·58	—	—
Fractures (Other Sites)	13·82	3·65	6·28	3·83	0·05	—
Burns	0·79	0·79	0·66	0·47	—	—
Old Injuries	0·12	0·11	0·16	0·11	0·44	0·39
Other Injuries	78·47	19·33	32·61	18·85	0·22	0·06
Totals	97·14	25·51	42·55	24·84	0·71	0·45
2. *Non-Enemy Action*						
Head Injuries	1·02	2·47	1·37	2·26	1·42	2·40
Fractures (Other Sites)	9·47	7·53	9·18	10·13	7·36	8·11
Burns	1·98	2·47	2·95	2·57	0·87	0·52
Old Injuries	0·26	0·22	0·49	0·37	0·27	0·39
Other Injuries	13·72	9·83	11·63	13·91	9·54	7·66
Totals	26·45	22·53	25·62	29·25	19·47	19·09
3. *Cause Not Known*						
Head Injuries	0·31	0·11	0·27	0·11	0·22	0·26
Fractures (Other Sites)	1·66	0·28	0·38	0·79	0·60	0·39
Burns	1·41	0·56	0·49	0·48	0·11	0·13
Old Injuries	0·25	0·62	0·38	0·26	0·16	0·64
Other Injuries	4·70	1·01	1·32	1·68	1·04	0·94
Totals	8·32	2·58	2·84	3·32	2·13	2·36
Total admissions through Injuries	131·91	50·62	71·01	57·41	22·31	21·91
Percentage of admissions for all Causes	50	28	29	28	12	11

TABLE 25

North-West Europe, 1944–45
Admissions to Hospitals through Injury
Relative Rates

Source: Hollerith Tabulations

	1944		1945			
	QUARTERS					
	1st	2nd	3rd	4th	5th	6th
	July–Sept.	Oct.–Dec.	Jan.–Mar.	Apr.–June	July–Sept.	Oct.–Dec.
1. *Enemy Action*						
Head Injuries	4·05	6·39	6·67	6·36	—	—
Fractures (Other Sites)	14·23	14·31	14·76	15·42	7·04	—
Burns	0·81	3·10	1·55	1·89	—	—
Old Injuries	0·12	0·43	0·38	0·44	61·97	86·36
Other Injuries	80·79	75·77	76·64	75·89	30·99	13·64
Totals	100	100	100	100	100	100
2. *Non-Enemy Action*						
Head Injuries	3·86	10·97	5·35	7·73	7·30	12·58
Fractures (Other Sites)	35·80	33·43	35·83	34·64	37·82	45·50
Burns	7·49	10·97	11·51	8·79	4·47	2·73
Old Injuries	0·98	0·98	1·92	1·27	1·39	2·04
Other Injuries	51·87	43·65	45·39	47·57	49·02	40·15
Totals	100	100	100	100	100	100
3. *Cause Not Known*						
Head Injuries	3·72	4·26	9·51	3·31	10·33	11·02
Fractures (Other Sites)	19·93	10·85	13·38	23·80	28·17	16·52
Burns	16·93	21·71	17·25	14·46	5·16	5·51
Old Injuries	3·00	24·03	13·38	7·83	7·51	27·12
Other Injuries	56·42	39·15	46·48	50·60	48·83	39·83
Totals	100	100	100	100	100	100

TABLE 26

North-West Europe, 1945. Admissions to Hospitals.
Mean Monthly and Equivalent Annual Rates per 1,000 Strength. British Troops, Male

Source: Monthly Hygiene Returns

CAUSES	Feb.	March	April	May	June	July	August	Sept.	Oct.	Nov.	Dec.	E.A.R.
Bronchitis:												
(a) Acute	31·19	23·74	16·54	16·93	8·10	9·46	11·30	8·36	11·76	11·28	12·84	176·18
(b) Chronic	14·44	12·87	40·36	6·44	4·65	5·52	4·04	3·54	3·97	4·74	4·28	114·38
Influenza	9·53	4·02	4·10	2·65	1·20	1·58	1·35	1·13	1·28	0·65	4·62	35·03
Impetigo	41·18	49·22	48·30	25·90	20·85	17·74	20·18	18·28	27·34	19·61	19·01	335·57
Otitis:												
(a) Media	25·20	28·03	19·98	16·68	11·55	19·44	18·83	12·75	16·01	14·54	11·30	211·97
(b) Externa	8·60	9·79	8·60	7·45	6·24	8·41	11·30	9·35	10·34	8·50	7·71	105·04
Peptic Ulcer:												
(a) Gastric	6·91	5·50	7·41	5·69	7·70	4·20	5·38	5·10	5·53	6·70	3·25	69·13
(b) Duodenal	13·37	7·91	3·70	6·06	4·65	5·91	2·69	3·83	3·97	3·92	2·40	63·72
Rheumatic Fever	1·23	2·01	2·12	1·14	—	0·13	0·40	0·28	0·57	1·31	0·34	10·40
Psychiatric Disorders:												
(a) Psychoses	8·91	9·52	19·58	8·72	7·97	3·68	7·13	5·53	6·23	6·37	3·94	95·54
(b) Psychoneuroses (including Psychopathic Personality)	203·75	163·34	84·42	35·25	25·10	31·40	18·97	26·64	22·53	14·71	19·18	703·95
(c) Mental Dullness and Deficiency	5·69	3·75	2·25	0·63	0·93	3·28	0·81	0·71	0·43	1·80	0·68	22·87
Effects of Cold	7·68	1·74	0·66	—	—	—	—	—	—	—	—	11·00
Total Admissions for Diseases	1,970·22	1,884·25	1,619·86	1,312·60	1,145·56	1,371·98	1,610·61	1,639·82	1,641·32	1,674·60	1,562·48	19,017·82
Injuries—N.E.A.	351·11	348·13	460·74	419·34	285·89	236·35	224·78	244·28	249·63	233·69	210·12	3,560·79
Injuries—E.A.	876·93	883·86	921·34	105·26	7·70	0·13	—	0·14	—	—	—	3,689·40*
Total Admissions	3,198·26	3,116·24	3,001·94	1,837·18	1,439·16	1,608·46	1,835·39	1,884·25	1,890·95	1,908·29	1,772·60	26,268·01

* Estimated

TABLE 27

North-West Europe, 1945. Admissions to All Medical Units for certain Diseases
Mean Monthly and Equivalent Annual Rates per 100,000 Strength. British Troops, Male

Source: Monthly Hygiene Reports and V.D. Returns

	CAUSES	May	June	July	August	Sept.	October	November	December	Equivalent Annual Rates	
1	Chicken Pox	1·14	0·80	0·92	0·94	0·57	0·71	0·65	2·91	12·96	1
2	Diphtheria	18·82	11·55	11·04	7·80	16·29	14·02	23·21	19·01	182·61	2
3	Encephalitis	0·13	—	—	—	0·14	—	—	—	0·41	3
4	Dysentery	260·14	187·10	293·51	247·52	158·55	83·87	70·76	77·06	2,067·76	4
5	Enteric Group of Fevers	0·76	0·53	0·65	0·94	1·14	0·99	0·16	0·17	8·02	5
6	Infective Hepatitis	45·11	46·61	40·60	43·45	57·24	62·76	66·84	45·72	612·49	6
7	Malaria	11·38	10·62	14·18	12·11	7·37	6·94	4·90	6·17	110·50	7
8	Measles	3·54	0·80	1·05	0·40	0·57	0·14	0·49	3·08	15·11	8
9	Cerebro-Spinal Fever	1·14	1·06	0·26	0·54	0·28	0·28	—	0·34	5·85	9
10	Mumps	2·53	1·20	1·18	0·27	1·13	1·28	1·47	0·68	14·61	10
11	Pneumonia	6·31	4·24	2·89	3·22	2·84	2·84	4·25	8·21	52·20	11
12	Poliomyelitis	0·25	0·40	0·26	0·67	—	0·43	0·49	0·17	4·01	12
13	Typhus Fever	0·13	0·27	—	0·27	—	—	—	—	1·01	13
14	Rubella	1·77	1·06	0·13	0·54	0·43	0·85	—	—	7·17	14
15	Scarlet Fever	2·65	1·46	2·10	1·48	0·99	1·42	1·31	1·88	19·93	15
16	Scabies*	312·58	283·50	323·85	387·01	725·61	950·50	1,198·87	1,079·21	6,927·19	16
17	Tuberculosis	2·91	2·79	2·89	2·69	4·11	3·82	3·60	3·42	39·35	17
18	Venereal Diseases	279·11	444·97	854·17	1,011·29	960·59	882·42	838·31	821·88	9,139·11	18

* M.M.Rs. for February, March and April were 358·49, 401·36 and 328·95.

CHAPTER IV

BRITISH NORTH AFRICAN and CENTRAL MEDITERRANEAN FORCES

STATISTICS FOR the British North African and Central Mediterranean Forces which appear in this section have been obtained from weekly reports of admissions to medical units, rendered through Districts to, and consolidated at, Medical Branch, General Headquarters. This is at variance with most other Commands where medical units compiled statistical returns, sometimes on a modified form of A.F. A.31, at monthly intervals, for submission to G.H.Q. The return used by B.N.A. and C.M.F. was peculiar to, and appears to have been devised for use solely within, that Command. Diseases individually reported differ somewhat from those reported in a comparable Command, i.e., Middle East Forces. The latter reported admissions for such diseases as Mumps, P.U.O., Effects of Heat, Measles, etc., whereas B.N.A. and C.M.F. did not. Similarly, admissions for Dermatophytosis, Pediculosis, Gas Gangrene, etc., appear in the returns for B.N.A. and C.M.F., but not in those for M.E.F. On the other hand, admissions for Dysentery, Enteric Fever, Jaundice and Malaria, which were common to returns in both Commands were broken down in the B.N.A. and C.M.F. returns. Indeed, Malaria was broken down not only to B.T., M.T. and Q., but also, under these headings, to Primary and Relapse. Incidentally, it is interesting to note that only in this Command was Malaria broken down to Primary and Relapse.

From the landings until mid-1945, only one significant change was made in the nature of the return. Until November 1943, medical statistics for all classes of Troops were reported under the blanket heading of 'All Troops', no distinction being made as to the ethnic composition of the Forces. From that month, however, admissions were listed under the different national entities. It was possible, therefore, from January 1944 to prepare separate morbidity tabulations for British, Canadian, New Zealand, Indian and African Troops as well as for 'All Troops'.

In mid-1945, this policy was changed. Instead of the weekly return of admissions to Medical Units being rendered, a monthly return was introduced. In the new return, the number of diseases to be reported was doubled, more information was required and the number of sheets in the return was increased from one to a minimum of six. The return became cumbersome. As an instance of the greater detail required, the weekly return required Venereal Disease to be broken down under five headings, Gonorrhoea, Syphilis, Chancroid, Lympho-granuloma and 'Other Forms', but the monthly return required figures under the headings Syphilis early, Syphilis late, Urethritis smear + ve GC, Urethritis smear − ve GC, Urethritis not tested, a similar three headings for Vaginitis or Cervicitis, Lympho-granuloma and Chancroid. Again, the weekly report required figures for Diphtheria, but the monthly return required this to be split under the headings Faucial, Laryngeal and Nasal, Cutaneous and Polyneuritis. In all, the new return contained over 100 items against 59 in the old.

At the same time, a regrouping of nationalities was made for statistical purposes. Where, during the previous eighteen months it had been possible to produce statistics separately for Canadian and New Zealand Troops, these were now bulked together under the heading 'Dominion Troops'. Again, African Troops were now placed under the heading of 'Colonial Troops', which included such diverse ethnic groups as Seychellois, Maltese, Cypriots, etc. The net result is that for 1945 figures can be given only for the first six months in respect of Canadian, New Zealand and African Troops.

The basic medical statistics required from a force overseas can be grouped under three headings:

(1) Admissions, by diagnoses, to medical units.

(2) Death, by causes, occurring in medical units.

(3) Invalids, by diagnoses, transferred to the United Kingdom or country of origin.

Although the returns reviewed above met the requirements of (1) they are lacking in detail regarding deaths and invalids. The only information available from the returns regarding deaths in medical units is the total number occurring from disease. Although this data is desirable, it is still more desirable to know the causes of such deaths, also the statistics relating to deaths from injuries, through Enemy Action and other causes. It is not possible, therefore, as in some other Commands, to prepare mortality tabulations for B.N.A. and C.M.F. The information obtainable from the returns with regard to invalids is even less than that for deaths. The only data available is the number of invalids recommended for transfer. What is required, here, is the number, by diagnoses, of invalids actually transferred to the United Kingdom (or other country) during each accounting period. Here again, it is impossible to prepare invaliding statistics for the Command.

Up to mid-1945, the returns were submitted weekly. These have been converted to a monthly basis, and mean monthly rates (M.M.R.) per 1,000 strength have been computed. In consolidating from the weekly returns, some months will contain 4 weeks (28 days) and others 5 weeks (35 days). Such figures have been adjusted to a month of fixed length, 30·5 days, almost exactly one twelfth of a calendar year. The annual rates were obtained by a summation of the twelve mean monthly rates.

The Force began landings in North West Africa on November 8, 1942 and reasonably accurate figures for admissions to Medical Units were available from early 1943. The tabulations which follow, therefore, commence from January 1, 1943 and those available before that date have been ignored as unreliable. As in most other sections, rates are shown per 1,000 strength. In some cases, mainly in 1943, weekly returns, although listing admissions, omit some District strengths. In such cases, admissions figures have been ignored. District strengths fluctuated so violently in 1943, that it was felt safer to ignore the available admission figures, rather than to attempt to 'average out' the rates. For this reason, the figures do not include all known admissions and any discrepancy in statistics between this and other volumes is thus partly explained. Apart from this, the tabulations here presented include all information reported on the returns relating to admissions.

With one exception, the figures given in this section relate to admissions to all medical units, be they General Hospitals, Casualty Clearing Stations, Field Ambulances, or other type of unit. Care had been taken administratively, to ensure that there were no 'double admissions', i.e. transfers between units being shown as admissions to both units. The inviolable rule was that cases diagnosed for the first time only were shown as admissions, irrespective of the fact that they might have been transferred, undiagnosed, from another unit. The exception referred to above was the figures for SCABIES. Here, *all* cases were reported, whether admitted to medical units or whether treatment was given in a unit medical centre or elsewhere.

Tables 28, 30 and 32 exhibit the causes of admission for All Troops during 1943, 1944 and 1945 with Tables 29, 31 and 33 showing the breakdown of certain diseases and disease groups for those years.

Diseases which displayed a striking seasonal swing had peak incidence during the periods noted:

Diphtheria . . . . November–January

Dysentery. . . . . June–October

Infective Hepatitis . . . . September–January

Malaria . . . . July–October (1943)
March–August (1944)

Pediculosis . . . . December–March

Sandfly Fever . . . . July–October

The incidence of the ENTERIC GROUP of Fevers did not show any particular trend in 1943, but in the following year admissions increased sharply from June to September.

Admissions for diseases as below, decreased in 1944 as compared with 1943.

Dermatophytosis............	from	19·9 to 9·0 per 1,000
Dysentery.................	from	29·1 to 11·5 per 1,000
Malaria....................	from	82·9 to 66·0 per 1,000
Pediculosis	from	48·9 to 16·3 per 1,000
Scabies....................	from	28·4 to 17·1 per 1,000
Diseases of the Digestive System	from	113·6 to 74·2 per 1,000

Diseases showing large increases in 1944 as compared with 1943 were:

Psychoneuroses..............	from	8·5 to 21·5 per 1,000
Venereal Diseases............	from	26·9 to 50·6 per 1,000

(The E.A.R. for 1945 was 63·7)

PRIMARY MALARIA showed a striking decrease of over fifty per cent. from 77·7 in 1943 to 35·3 per 1,000 in 1944. MALARIA RELAPSE, however, as might be expected, increased sharply from 5·3 in 1943 to 30·8 in 1944. Relapse occurred chiefly during the period March to June 1944, when the mean monthly rates were well over 3 per 1,000.

The annual morbidity rates do not vary greatly, being 564 in 1943, 552 in 1944 with an E.A.R. of 468 for 1945. MALARIA and VENEREAL DISEASES together accounted for one fifth of the total admissions for diseases in both 1943 and 1944. SCABIES, PEDICULOSIS, I.A.T. and DERMATOPHYTOSIS together accounted for a further quarter in 1943 and one seventh in 1944, while admissions for INFECTIVE HEPATITIS, PSYCHIATRIC DISORDERS and DYSENTERY together were one-eighth of the total in both years.

Tables 34 to 53 show the causes of admission to medical units during 1944, and, for the first six months of 1945 (with an equivalent annual rate) separately for Canadian, New Zealand, Indian and African Troops. Table 44 shows the causes of admission for British Troops for the whole of 1945. These tables indicate:

(a) a low rate for DIPHTHERIA among Indians and Africans.

(b) an extremely high rate for INFLUENZA among Canadians in 1944 (10·8 per 1,000 as compared with 3·5 for the next highest class of troops and an All Troops rate of 2·2).

(c) Canadian and New Zealand Troops were more prone to INFECTIVE HEPATITIS.

(d) Indian and African Troops were more prone to TUBERCULOSIS.

(e) there was very little difference in the rates for DYSENTERY between British and Indian Troops. This is contrary to the conclusion reached in the chapter dealing with the Army in India where the rates for British Other Ranks were from two to four times those for Indian Other Ranks.

(f) a comparatively low incidence for MALARIA among New Zealand, Indian and African Troops.

(g) British Troops were more prone to SANDFLY FEVER than were the other classes of troops.

(h) the rates for SCABIES were lowest among Indian and African Troops.

(i) Canadian Troops had the highest incidence of VENEREAL DISEASES in 1944, followed by Africans, British and New Zealanders, with Indians less than one third of the Canadian rate.

(j) PSYCHIATRIC DISORDERS were highest among Africans with Canadians a close second. Indians had the lowest rate, one quarter that of Africans.

(k) British Troops had a much higher incidence of PEDICULOSIS and SCABIES than any other class of Troops.

No attempt has been made to compare the 1918 admissions for certain diseases in Italy with the tabulations presented here. The Medical Statistics volume of the 'Official History of the Medical Services in the Great War' tabulates only four diseases, Dysentery, Malaria, Pneumonia and Venereal Diseases for all British Troops in Italy in 1918, although more detailed figures are available for such troops in the forward areas. As the data herein recorded included British Troops serving in areas other than Italy, a comparison with the 1918 records is not valid.

TABLE 28

British North African and Central Mediterranean Forces. All Troops. Causes of Admission to Medical Units, 1943
Mean Monthly and Annual Rates per 1,000 Strength

Source: B.N.A.F. and C.M.F. Weekly Health States

	CAUSES	Jan.	Feb.	Mar.	Apr.	May	June	July	Aug.	Sept.	Oct.	Nov.	Dec.	Annual	
1	Diphtheria	0·16	0·06	0·10	0·07	0·03	0·05	0·04	0·16	0·42	0·64	0·88	0·79	3·39	1
2	Dermatophytosis	0·09	0·06	0·60	1·08	1·13	1·30	1·54	4·38	4·48	1·96	1·39	0·95	19·86	2
3	Dysentery	0·89	0·64	0·47	0·44	3·58	7·21	3·96	2·49	3·51	2·44	1·78	1·72	29·12	3
4	Enteric Group of Fevers	0·04	0·05	0·02	0·01	0·03	0·01	0·03	0·03	0·07	0·04	0·06	0·10	0·48	4
5	Food Poisoning	—	—	0·01	—	—	—	—	—	—	—	0·01	0·02	0·03	5
6	Gas Gangrene	0·04	0·02	0·01	0·02	0·07	0·00	0·01	0·01	0·01	0·01	0·01	0·03	0·24	6
7	Helminthic Diseases	—	—	—	—	0·00	—	—	—	0·02	0·01	0·00	0·01	0·04	7
8	Influenza	0·08	0·05	0·11	0·08	0·01	0·03	0·01	—	0·00	0·04	0·14	0·17	0·70	8
9	Jaundice	1·92	0·61	0·40	0·20	0·14	0·24	0·90	1·30	4·54	8·76	10·16	7·90	36·04	9
10	Malaria	1·56	0·75	0·19	0·07	0·11	3·03	21·97	17·89	14·03	14·08	6·48	2·78	82·94	10
11	Meningitis—Meningococcal	0·03	0·02	0·01	—	0·03	0·01	0·01	0·01	0·01	0·01	0·01	0·01	0·15	11
12	Meningitis—Other Forms	0·01	—	—	0·01	—	0·00	0·02	0·02	0·04	0·01	0·01	0·01	0·12	12
13	Pediculosis	13·06	11·64	9·43	5·83	2·45	0·85	0·64	0·70	0·57	0·51	1·02	2·16	48·85	13
14	Pneumonia—Pneumococcal	0·18	0·02	0·06	0·05	0·02	0·04	0·03	0·01	0·03	0·05	0·06	0·06	0·60	14
15	Pneumonia—Other Forms	0·06	0·13	0·17	0·13	0·04	0·04	0·05	0·05	0·07	0·05	0·08	0·14	1·01	15
16	Poliomyelitis	—	—	—	—	—	0·01	—	—	—	—	0·03	0·01	0·04	16
17	Sandfly Fever	—	—	0·01	0·00	0·01	0·02	0·25	0·16	0·15	0·27	0·06	0·00	0·92	17
18	Scabies†	7·65	5·49	3·65	2·18	1·55	1·24	0·83	1·13	1·15	0·83	1·37	1·31	28·38	18
19	Smallpox	0·05	0·01	0·03	0·01	0·01	0·04	0·02	0·06	0·02	0·03	0·02	0·02	0·32	19
20	Tetanus	—	—	—	0·01	—	—	—	—	0·01	0·00	0·01	0·01	0·05	20
21	Tuberculosis—Pulmonary	0·08	0·03	0·01	0·03	0·06	0·04	0·05	0·07	0·08	0·05	0·01	0·01	0·52	21
22	Tuberculosis—Other Forms	0·02	0·01	0·01	0·01	0·00	—	0·00	0·01	0·01	0·00	0·02	0·02	0·10	22
23	Typhus	—	0·05	0·05	0·01	0·00	—	—	—	0·01	0·02	0·00	0·01	0·15	23
24	Undulant Fever	—	—	—	—	0·00	0·01	—	0·00	—	—	0·00	0·00	0·03	24
25	Venereal Diseases	2·50	1·73	1·50	1·07	0·81	1·04	1·22	1·58	1·78	3·57	4·61	5·52	26·94	25

TABLE 28—*Continued.*

British North African and Central Mediterranean Forces. All Troops. Causes of Admission to Medical Units, 1943
Mean Monthly and Annual Rates per 1,000 Strength

Source: B.N.A.F. and C.M.F. Weekly Health States

	CAUSES	Jan.	Feb.	Mar.	Apr.	May	June	July	Aug.	Sept.	Oct.	Nov.	Dec.	Annual	
26	Diseases of the Digestive System	Figures not available	3·30	3·00	4·74	13·82	14·94	11·50	10·35	13·39	10·99	10·96	7·10	113·58*	26
27	Diseases of the Respiratory System		3·60	2·47	2·25	1·92	1·93	2·56	3·46	4·29	3·83	4·43	3·73	37·60*	27
28	Diseases of the Nervous System		0·65	0·49	0·64	0·41	0·41	0·38	0·27	0·51	0·50	0·45	0·37	5·55*	28
29	Diseases of the Skin		2·47	2·31	2·26	1·70	1·90	2·53	2·78	4·23	3·81	4·33	0·34	34·53*	29
30	Psychoses		0·08	0·07	0·03	0·03	0·03	0·01	0·03	0·04	0·06	0·04	0·03	0·40*	30
31	Psychoneuroses (including Exhaustion)		0·60	1·28	0·71	0·58	0·35	0·42	0·27	0·62	0·95	0·51	1·55	8·54*	31
32	I.A.T.		2·68	2·86	2·70	2·13	2·55	3·82	4·84	6·83	5·63	5·32	3·90	47·19*	32
33	*Total Admissions for Diseases*		29·25	20·98	23·71	30·34	47·84	59·30	58·80	71·84	66·25	61·78	46·82	563·91*	33
34	Injuries—Enemy Action		3·39	6·14	15·98	5·97	0·13	0·50	0·94	1·67	6·37	4·81	9·43	60·36*	34
35	Injuries—Non-Enemy Action		6·13	7·57	8·33	6·99	6·82	6·30	4·95	6·53	5·12	5·47	4·54	75·01*	35
36	*Total Admissions for Injuries*		9·52	13·71	24·31	12·96	6·95	6·80	5·89	8·20	11·49	10·28	13·98	135·37*	36
37	*Total Admissions*		38·77	34·69	48·02	43·31	54·79	66·10	64·69	80·03	77·74	72·06	60·80	699·28*	37

* Equivalent Annual Rates.
† Includes cases treated outside Medical Units.

TABLE 29

British North African and Central Mediterranean Forces. All Troops. Causes of Admission to Medical Units, 1943
Breakdown of Certain Diseases as Shown in Table 28. Mean Monthly and Annual Rates per 1,000 Strength

Source: B.N.A.F. and C.M.F. Weekly Health States

	CAUSES	Jan.	Feb.	Mar.	Apr.	May	June	July	Aug.	Sept.	Oct.	Nov.	Dec.	Annual	
	Dysentery														
1	Protozoal	—	0·01	—	0·02	—	0·00	—	0·04	0·03	0·04	0·05	0·02	0·20	1
2	Bacillary	0·79	0·26	0·14	0·19	1·52	3·06	1·90	0·82	1·32	0·88	0·50	1·14	12·51	2
3	Clinical	0·10	0·37	0·33	0·23	2·06	4·15	2·06	1·64	2·16	1·52	1·22	0·55	16·41	3
4	*Totals*	0·89	0·64	0·47	0·44	3·58	7·21	3·96	2·49	3·51	2·44	1·78	1·72	29·12	4
	Enteric Group of Fevers														
5	Typhoid	0·02	0·03	0·01	0·00	0·01	0·01	0·02	0·01	0·05	0·03	0·04	0·04	0·27	5
6	Para A.	0·01	0·01	—	—	—	—	—	—	0·00	—	—	—	0·02	6
7	Para B.	—	0·01	—	0·00	0·00	—	—	0·00	0·01	0·00	0·00	0·00	0·04	7
8	Para C	—	—	—	—	0·00	—	—	—	—	—	—	—	0·00	8
9	Clinical	0·01	—	0·01	0·01	0·01	0·01	0·01	0·01	0·01	0·01	0·02	0·06	0·15	9
10	*Totals*	0·04	0·05	0·02	0·01	0·03	0·01	0·03	0·03	0·07	0·04	0·06	0·10	0·48	10
	Jaundice														
11	Infective Hepatitis	0·92	0·57	0·37	0·18	0·07	0·14	0·53	1·11	3·92	8·57	9·98	7·75	34·10	11
12	Leptospirosis	—	—	—	—	0·01	—	—	—	0·01	0·01	0·01	—	0·03	12
13	Post-Arsphenamine	—	0·02	0·03	0·02	0·02	0·04	0·06	0·05	0·04	0·01	0·01	0·01	0·29	13
14	Other Forms	—	0·02	—	0·01	0·04	0·06	0·30	0·14	0·57	0·18	0·17	0·14	1·62	14
15	*Totals*	0·92	0·61	0·40	0·20	0·14	0·24	0·90	1·30	4·54	8·76	10·16	7·90	36·04	15
	Malaria														
16	Primary B.T.	1·14	0·40	0·06	0·01	0·03	1·77	10·38	6·78	4·05	3·59	1·88	0·84	30·93	16
17	Primary Q.	—	0·01	—	—	0·00	0·01	0·08	0·03	0·02	0·03	0·01	0·02	0·20	17
18	Primary M.T.	0·28	0·10	—	0·01	0·01	0·41	3·24	2·22	1·63	1·75	1·11	0·34	11·10	18
19	Primary Clinical	0·14	0·14	0·10	0·02	0·04	0·77	8·07	8·29	7·40	7·36	2·40	0·74	35·47	19
20	*Total Primary*	1·55	0·65	0·15	0·04	0·09	2·96	21·77	17·32	13·10	12·73	5·41	1·94	77·69	20
21	Relapse B.T.	—	0·05	0·01	0·02	0·02	0·05	0·10	0·27	0·36	0·49	0·32	0·41	2·10	21
22	Relapse Q.	—	—	0·01	—	—	—	0·00	—	0·01	0·01	0·01	0·00	0·04	22
23	Relapse M.T.	—	0·02	0·01	—	—	0·01	0·02	0·15	0·20	0·35	0·49	0·28	1·53	23
24	Relapse Clinical	0·02	0·02	0·01	0·01	0·00	0·01	0·08	0·16	0·37	0·50	0·25	0·16	1·59	24
25	*Total Relapse*	0·02	0·10	0·03	0·03	0·03	0·08	0·21	0·57	0·93	1·34	1·07	0·85	5·25	25
26	*Total Malaria*	1·56	0·75	0·19	0·07	0·11	3·03	21·97	17·89	14·03	14·08	6·48	2·78	82·94	26

TABLE 29—*Continued*

British North African and Central Mediterranean Forces. All Troops. Causes of Admission to Medical Units, 1943
Breakdown of Certain Diseases as Shown in Table 28. Mean Monthly and Annual Rates per 1,000 Strength

Source: B.N.A.F. and C.M.F. Weekly Health States

	CAUSES	Jan.	Feb.	Mar.	Apr.	May	June	July	Aug.	Sept.	Oct.	Nov.	Dec.	Annual	
	Pediculosis														
27	Capitas	0·07	0·06	0·10	0·07	0·05	0·02	0·00	0·03	0·01	0·01	0·02	0·02	0·45	27
28	Corporis	8·90	8·82	7·56	4·39	1·81	0·29	0·17	0·11	0·15	0·09	0·31	1·12	33·72	28
29	Pubis	4·09	2·77	1·78	1·37	0·60	0·54	0·46	0·55	0·41	0·40	0·69	1·02	14·68	29
30	*Totals*	13·06	11·64	9·43	5·83	2·45	0·85	0·64	0·70	0·57	0·51	1·02	2·16	48·85	30
	Venereal Diseases														
31	Gonorrhoea	1·74	0·71	0·61	0·52	0·42	0·61	0·62	0·74	0·77	1·40	1·60	1·86	11·61	31
32	Syphilis	0·38	0·21	0·23	0·09	0·06	0·10	0·10	0·11	0·14	0·18	0·16	0·23	1·97	32
33	Chancroid	0·28	0·17	0·11	0·09	0·06	0·10	0·14	0·28	0·28	0·29	0·75	0·58	3·03	33
34	Lympho-granuloma	—	0·01	—	—	—	—	—	—	0·00	0·01	—	0·00	0·02	34
35	Other Forms	0·09	0·64	0·50	0·38	0·27	0·29	0·37	0·46	0·59	1·70	2·12	2·85	10·30	35
	Totals	2·50	1·73	1·50	1·07	0·81	1·04	1·22	1·58	1·78	3·57	4·61	5·52	26·94	36

TABLE 30

British North African and Central Mediterranean Forces. All Troops. Causes of Admission to Medical Units, 1944
Mean Monthly and Annual Rates per 1,000 Strength

Source: B.N.A.F. and C.M.F., Weekly Health States

	Causes	Jan.	Feb.	Mar.	Apr.	May	June	July	Aug.	Sept.	Oct.	Nov.	Dec.	Annual	
1	Diphtheria	0·81	0·68	0·72	0·38	0·23	0·18	0·18	0·17	0·19	0·32	0·47	0·59	4·91	1
2	Dermatophytosis	0·69	0·69	0·70	0·68	0·53	0·76	0·68	0·77	0·76	0·64	0·47	0·59	7·95	2
3	Dysentery	0·45	0·31	0·36	0·22	0·37	1·73	2·38	1·59	1·45	1·36	0·80	0·49	11·52	3
4	Enteric Group of Fevers	0·04	0·05	0·03	0·02	0·04	0·14	0·19	0·14	0·19	0·10	0·08	0·04	1·05	4
5	Food Poisoning	0·05	0·00	0·02	0·01	0·01	0·16	0·00	0·05	0·02	0·00	0·12	0·01	0·44	5
6	Gas Gangrene	0·02	0·08	0·04	0·01	0·01	0·02	0·01	0·01	0·03	0·02	0·01	0·02	0·27	6
7	Helminthic Diseases	0·02	0·01	0·02	0·02	0·08	0·06	0·09	0·10	0·05	0·03	0·03	0·04	0·56	7
8	Influenza	0·22	0·41	0·62	0·41	0·13	0·07	0·02	0·01	0·03	0·15	0·10	0·08	2·24	8
9	Jaundice	3·76	2·74	2·11	1·34	0·92	1·09	1·58	2·29	4·25	4·84	4·39	3·62	32·93	9
10	Malaria	2·33	3·58	7·58	8·29	6·99	7·31	7·36	7·32	5·91	4·06	2·94	2·34	66·01	10
11	Meningitis—Meningococcal	0·00	0·00	0·01	0·00	0·00	0·00	0·01	0·00	0·01	0·00	0·01	0·01	0·06	11
12	Meningitis—Other Forms	0·00	0·00	0·00	0·01	0·02	0·01	0·01	0·04	0·03	0·01	0·01	0·01	0·16	12
13	Pediculosis	1·97	1·86	2·69	1·57	1·04	0·73	0·69	0·68	0·65	0·97	1·50	1·99	16·33	13
14	Pneumonia—Pneumococcal	0·07	0·12	0·28	0·26	0·18	0·23	0·20	0·08	0·06	0·07	0·10	0·16	1·81	14
15	Pneumonia—Other Forms	0·13	0·11	0·15	0·15	0·16	0·17	0·14	0·10	0·12	0·14	0·13	0·21	1·70	15
16	Poliomyelitis	0·01	—	0·01	—	—	0·01	0·01	0·01	0·01	0·01	0·01	0·00	0·06	16
17	Sandfly Fever	0·00	—	0·00	0·00	0·01	0·08	0·38	0·67	0·77	0·08	0·01	0·00	2·00	17
18	Scabies†	1·35	1·45	1·85	1·33	1·17	1·15	1·01	1·02	0·98	1·26	1·79	2·73	17·08	18
19	Smallpox	0·02	0·01	0·02	0·03	0·00	0·02	0·02	—	—	—	0·00	0·00	0·12	19
20	Tetanus	—	—	0·00	0·00	0·00	—	—	—	0·00	0·00	0·01	0·00	0·02	20
21	Tuberculosis—Pulmonary	0·02	0·02	0·04	0·05	0·04	0·06	0·07	0·06	0·07	0·06	0·08	0·11	0·66	21
22	Tuberculosis—Other Forms	0·00	—	0·00	0·01	0·00	0·01	0·00	0·00	0·01	0·00	0·01	0·01	0·06	22
23	Typhus	0·01	0·01	0·01	0·00	0·00	0·00	—	0·00	—	—	—	—	0·03	23
24	Undulant Fever	0·00	0·00	0·00	—	0·00	0·01	0·00	0·00	0·00	0·00	0·01	0·01	0·04	24
25	Venereal Disease	4·03	3·63	4·51	3·78	3·42	5·12	5·07	3·85	3·77	3·45	4·44	5·55	50·63	25
26	Diseases of the Digestive System	5·56	4·79	5·47	4·01	3·95	9·45	10·23	7·47	6·98	5·36	5·10	5·87	74·24	26
27	Diseases of the Respiratory ,,	3·40	4·01	4·87	3·09	2·08	2·66	2·59	2·00	2·03	2·53	2·94	3·95	36·15	27
28	Diseases of the Nervous ,,	0·27	0·40	0·39	0·26	0·34	0·45	0·51	0·38	0·44	0·29	0·34	0·52	4·59	28
29	Diseases of the Skin	3·24	3·56	3·75	2·64	2·47	2·76	2·74	2·49	2·64	2·21	2·78	3·25	34·32	29
30	Psychoses	0·04	0·10	0·17	0·05	0·15	0·21	0·21	0·60	0·08	0·11	0·04	0·11	1·32	30
31	Psychoneuroses (including Exhaustion)	1·44	2·22	1·62	0·78	2·75	2·23	2·23	1·09	2·75	1·50	1·32	1·55	21·47	31
32	I.A.T.	3·50	3·08	3·28	2·25	2·30	3·03	3·12	2·97	4·14	3·77	3·54	4·04	39·01	32
33	*Total Admissions for Diseases*	39·74	39·19	50·63	41·06	40·04	56·33	57·58	48·76	51·52	40·48	41·89	44·97	552·19	33
34	Injuries—Enemy Action	7·16	10·06	9·27	3·70	16·75	15·48	13·85	7·23	16·48	7·72	3·39	8·44	117·92	34
35	Injuries—Non-Enemy Action	4·11	2·99	2·61	3·57	4·44	8·32	6·72	5·05	5·10	3·68	3·91	4·81	55·31	35
36	*Total Admissions for Injuries*	11·27	13·05	11·88	7·27	20·59	23·80	20·57	11·28	21·58	11·40	7·30	13·25	173·22	36
37	*Total Admissions*	51·01	52·24	62·51	48·33	60·62	80·13	78·15	60·04	73·10	51·88	49·19	58·22	725·41	37

† Includes cases treated outside Medical Units.

TABLE 31

British North African and Central Mediterranean Forces. All Troops. Causes of Admission to Medical Units, 1944
Breakdown of Certain Diseases Shown in Table 30

Source: B.N.A.F. and C.M.F. Weekly Health States

	Causes	Jan.	Feb.	Mar.	Apr.	May	June	July	Aug.	Sept.	Oct.	Nov.	Dec.	Annual	
	Dysentery														
1	Protozoal	0·02	0·03	0·04	0·04	0·04	0·06	0·08	0·06	0·09	0·12	0·17	0·14	0·88	1
2	Bacillary	0·10	0·06	0·09	0·03	0·09	0·61	0·79	0·56	0·62	0·51	0·27	0·12	3·85	2
3	Clinical	0·34	0·22	0·23	0·15	0·25	1·06	1·51	0·98	0·74	0·72	0·36	0·23	6·79	3
	Totals	0·45	0·31	0·36	0·22	0·37	1·73	2·38	1·59	1·45	1·36	0·80	0·49	11·52	4
4	*Enteric Group of Fevers*														
5	Typhoid	0·02	0·03	0·01	0·01	0·01	0·02	0·01	0·03	0·03	0·04	0·03	0·02	0·24	5
6	Para A	0·00	0·00	—	—	—	—	0·00	—	0·00	0·00	0·00	0·00	0·02	6
7	Para B	0·01	0·00	0·01	0·00	—	0·01	0·01	0·01	0·01	0·01	0·00	0·01	0·07	7
8	Para C	0·00	0·00	—	—	—	—	—	0·00	0·00	0·00	—	—	0·01	8
9	Clinical	0·01	0·01	0·01	0·01	0·02	0·12	0·18	0·10	0·15	0·05	0·04	0·01	0·71	9
	Totals	0·04	0·05	0·03	0·02	0·04	0·14	0·19	0·14	0·19	0·10	0·08	0·04	1·05	10
	Jaundice														
11	Infective Hepatitis	3·74	2·71	2·08	1·33	0·86	1·02	1·51	2·24	4·16	4·79	4·31	3·54	32·28	11
12	Leptospirosis	—	0·01	—	—	0·01	0·01	0·01	0·01	0·03	0·01	0·01	0·00	0·10	12
13	Post Arsphenamine	0·01	0·01	0·03	0·01	0·05	0·06	0·06	0·04	0·05	0·05	0·08	0·08	0·52	13
14	Other Forms	0·02	0·01	—	—	0·00	0·00	—	—	—	—	—	—	0·03	14
	Totals	3·76	2·74	2·11	1·34	0·92	1·09	1·58	2·29	4·25	4·84	4·39	3·62	32·93	15
	Malaria														
16	Primary B.T.	0·70	1·13	3·20	3·83	3·13	3·08	3·89	3·40	2·58	1·45	0·95	0·60	27·92	16
17	Primary Q.	0·03	0·01	0·03	0·01	0·00	0·00	—	—	0·00	0·01	0·01	—	0·09	17
18	Primary M.T.	0·17	0·24	0·14	0·12	0·07	0·04	0·11	0·12	0·09	0·11	0·04	0·04	1·29	18
19	Primary Clinical	0·28	0·22	0·48	0·61	0·42	0·69	0·57	1·33	0·68	0·35	0·22	0·12	5·96	19
	Total Primary	1·17	1·60	3·85	4·56	3·62	3·81	4·56	4·85	3·36	1·91	1·22	0·76	35·26	20
21	Relapse B.T.	0·71	1·48	3·29	3·37	3·16	3·24	2·61	2·25	2·33	2·00	1·59	1·47	27·49	21
22	Relapse Q.	0·01	0·00	0·01	0·01	0·00	—	—	—	—	—	0·01	—	0·04	22
23	Relapse M.T.	0·29	0·25	0·15	0·16	0·07	0·04	0·04	0·02	0·04	0·04	0·02	0·05	1·16	23
24	Relapse Clinical	0·15	0·25	0·28	0·19	0·14	0·22	0·16	0·20	0·18	0·12	0·10	0·07	2·06	24
	Total Relapse	1·16	1·98	3·74	3·74	3·37	3·50	2·80	2·47	2·55	2·16	1·72	1·58	30·75	25
	Total Malaria	2·33	3·58	7·58	8·29	6·99	7·31	7·36	7·32	5·91	4·06	2·94	2·34	66·01	26

	Pediculosis														
27	Capitas	0·01	0·01	0·06	0·07	0·19	0·11	0·12	0·13	0·06	0·08	0·03	0·13	0·98	27
28	Corporis	1·08	1·08	1·69	0·74	0·36	0·11	0·10	0·07	0·07	0·17	0·37	0·31	6·14	28
29	Pubis	0·88	0·77	0·93	0·76	0·49	0·52	0·47	0·48	0·53	0·73	1·11	1·56	9·21	29
	Totals	1·97	1·86	2·69	1·57	1·04	0·73	0·69	0·68	0·65	0·97	1·50	1·99	16·33	30
	Venereal Diseases														
31	Gonorrhoea	1·54	1·49	2·24	2·10	1·73	2·73	2·58	2·07	2·05	1·75	2·55	2·89	25·71	31
32	Syphilis	0·21	0·23	0·32	0·24	0·28	0·27	0·32	0·30	0·31	0·30	0·34	0·53	3·67	32
33	Chancroid	0·26	0·80	0·81	0·58	0·71	1·23	1·16	0·83	0·82	0·76	0·81	1·01	9·78	33
34	Lympho-granuloma	0·00	0·01	0·01	0·03	0·00	0·00	0·03	0·01	0·06	0·00	—	0·00	0·16	34
35	Other Forms	2·02	1·10	1·13	0·82	0·70	0·89	0·98	0·65	0·54	0·64	0·73	1·12	11·31	35
	Totals	4·03	3·63	4·51	3·78	3·42	5·12	5·07	3·85	3·77	3·45	4·44	5·55	50·63	36

TABLE 32

British North African and Central Mediterranean Forces. All Troops. Causes of Admission to Medical Units, 1945
Mean Monthly Rates (Jan. to June) and Equivalent Annual Rates per 1,000 Strength

Source: B.N.A.F. and C.M.F. Weekly Health States

	CAUSES	Jan.	Feb.	Mar.	Apr.	May	June	E.A.R.	
1	Diphtheria	0·58	0·42	0·25	0·15	0·12	0·07	3·19	1
2	Dermatophytosis	0·34	0·53	0·66	1·02	1·69	1·99	12·45	2
3	Dysentery	0·38	0·25	0·20	0·21	0·42	0·84	4·59	3
4	Enteric Group of Fevers	0·02	0·01	0·01	0·01	0·01	0·03	0·15	4
5	Food Poisoning	0·09	0·01	0·01	0·02	0·01	0·05	0·39	5
6	Gas Gangrene	0·01	—	0·00	0·01	—	—	0·05	6
7	Helminthic Diseases	0·04	0·03	0·02	0·03	0·04	0·03	0·39	7
8	Influenza	0·08	0·04	0·11	0·02	0·02	0·00	0·54	8
9	Jaundice	1·60	1·18	0·92	0·73	0·71	0·84	11·98	9
10	Malaria	1·30	1·25	1·49	1·78	2·27	2·24	20·67	10
11	Meningitis	0·01	0·03	0·02	0·01	0·01	0·02	0·20	11
12	Pediculosis	2·47	2·72	2·34	1·91	1·98	1·91	26·66	12
13	Pneumonia	0·43	0·64	1·14	1·38	0·76	0·37	9·46	13
14	Poliomyelitis	0·00	0·00	0·00	0·00	0·01	0·02	0·09	14
15	Sandfly Fever	—	—	0·00	—	0·41	2·15	5·13	15
16	Scabies	3·06	3·29	3·07	2·79	2·89	3·08	36·35	16
17	Smallpox	0·03	0·00	0·00	0·00	0·00	0·00	0·09	17
18	Tetanus	0·00	—	—	—	0·00	—	0·01	18
19	Tuberculosis—Pulmonary	0·07	0·14	0·11	0·09	0·11	0·09	1·21	19
20	Tuberculosis—Other Forms	0·01	0·01	0·01	0·01	0·02	0·01	0·12	20
21	Typhus	—	—	—	—	—	0·01	0·01	21
22	Undulant Fever	0·00	0·00	0·01	0·01	0·00	0·01	0·07	22
23	Venereal Diseases	5·45	5·75	5·19	4·80	5·13	5·58	63·77	23
24	Diseases of the Digestive System	4·49	3·79	3·57	3·47	3·94	4·28	47·10	24
25	Diseases of the Respiratory System	4·55	3·90	3·49	2·30	2·04	2·11	36·78	25
26	Diseases of the Nervous System	0·32	0·28	0·21	2·29	0·23	0·21	3·07	26
27	Diseases of the Skin	3·05	3·04	2·94	2·51	2·65	2·39	33·16	27
28	Psychoses	0·11	0·05	0·07	0·07	0·08	0·09	0·94	28
29	Psychoneuroses (including Exhaustion)	1·09	0·53	0·51	0·89	0·49	0·32	7·64	29
30	I.A.T.	4·27	2·75	2·65	2·36	2·44	2·94	34·82	30
31	*Total Admissions for Diseases*	42·29	37·96	36·32	34·42	37·89	44·92	467·58	31
32	Injuries—Enemy Action	3·45	1·26	1·52	8·56	0·28	—	30·17	32
33	Injuries—Non-Enemy Action	4·88	4·39	5·23	5·60	6·36	5·66	64·21	33
34	*Total Admissions for Injuries*	8·33	5·65	6·76	14·16	6·64	5·66	94·38	34
35	*Total Admissions*	50·62	43·61	43·08	48·58	44·53	50·58	561·96	35

TABLE 33

British North African and Central Mediterranean Forces. All Troops. Causes of Admission to Medical Units, 1945
Mean Monthly Rates (Jan. to June) and Equivalent Annual Rates per 1,000 Strength. Breakdown of Certain Diseases Shown in Table 32

Source: B.N.A.F. and C.M.F. Weekly Health States

	CAUSES	Jan.	Feb.	Mar.	Apr.	May	June	E.A.R.	
	Dysentery								
1	Protozoal	0·13	0·08	0·10	0·05	0·08	0·11	1·07	1
2	Bacillary and B.E.	0·09	0·04	0·04	0·05	0·18	0·37	1·55	2
3	Clinical and I.E.	0·16	0·13	0·06	0·10	0·16	0·37	1·97	3
4	*Totals*	0·38	0·25	0·20	0·21	0·42	0·84	4·59	4
	Enteric Group of Fevers								
5	Typhoid	0·01	0·01	0·00	0·00	0·00	0·00	0·08	5
6	Para A	—	0·00	—	—	0·00	—	0·01	6
7	Para B	0·01	0·00	—	0·00	—	0·00	0·03	7
8	Para C	—	—	—	—	—	—	—	8
9	Clinical	0·00	0·00	0·00	0·00	0·00	0·01	0·04	9
10	*Totals*	0·02	0·01	0·01	0·01	0·01	0·03	0·15	10
	Jaundice								
11	Infective Hepatitis	1·57	1·15	0·89	0·70	0·70	0·83	11·67	11
12	Leptospirosis	—	0·01	0·00	—	—	0·00	0·02	12
13	Post-Arsphenamine	0·04	0·03	0·03	0·03	0·01	0·01	0·29	13
14	*Totals*	1·60	1·18	0·92	0·73	0·71	0·84	11·98	14
	Malaria								
15	Primary B.T.	0·27	0·24	0·40	0·53	0·74	0·92	7·18	15
16	Primary Q.	0·00	0·00	0·00	—	0·00	0·00	0·02	16
17	Primary M.T.	0·01	0·01	0·01	0·00	0·05	0·02	0·19	17
18	Primary Clinical	0·08	0·07	0·06	0·10	0·14	0·12	1·16	18
19	*Total Primary*	0·36	0·32	0·47	0·63	0·93	1·06	7·55	19
20	Relapse B.T.	0·88	0·87	0·95	1·06	1·24	1·09	12·20	20
21	Relapse Q.	—	0·00	—	0·00	0·00	0·01	0·03	21
22	Relapse M.T.	0·01	0·01	0·01	0·01	0·01	0·01	0·12	22
23	Relapse Clinical	0·05	0·05	0·06	0·07	0·09	0·08	0·77	23
24	*Total Relapse*	0·94	0·93	1·02	1·14	1·35	1·18	13·12	24
25	*Total Malaria*	1·30	1·25	1·49	1·78	2·27	2·24	20·67	25

TABLE 33—*Continued*

British North African and Central Mediterranean Forces. All Troops. Causes of Admission to Medical Units, 1945
Mean Monthly Rates (Jan. to June) and Equivalent Annual Rates per 1,000 Strength. Breakdown of Certain Diseases Shown in Table 32

Source: B.N.A.F. and C.M.F. Weekly Health States

	CAUSES	Jan.	Feb.	Mar.	Apr.	May	June	E.A.R.	
	Pediculosis								
26	Capitas	0·23	0·09	0·08	0·03	0·03	0·06	1·04	26
27	Corporis	0·35	0·48	0·36	0·45	0·27	0·09	4·00	27
28	Pubis	1·89	2·16	1·91	1·43	1·67	1·77	21·66	28
29	*Totals*	2·47	2·72	2·34	1·91	1·97	1·91	26·66	29
	Venereal Diseases								
30	Gonorrhoea	2·93	3·09	2·62	2·59	2·97	3·40	35·19	30
31	Syphilis	0·55	0·65	0·47	0·47	0·44	0·68	6·53	31
32	Chancroid	0·93	1·00	0·85	0·81	0·98	0·74	10·62	32
33	Lympho-granuloma	0·01	—	0·00	—	0·00	—	0·02	33
34	Other Forms	1·03	1·02	1·23	0·93	0·74	0·76	11·41	34
35	*Totals*	5·45	5·75	5·19	4·80	5·13	5·58	63·77	35

TABLE 34

British North African and Central Mediterranean Forces. British Troops. Causes of Admission to Medical Units, 1944
Mean Monthly and Annual Rates per 1,000 Strength

Source: B.N.A.F. and C.M.F. Weekly Health States

	CAUSES	Jan.	Feb.	Mar.	Apr.	May	June	July	Aug.	Sept.	Oct.	Nov.	Dec.	Annual	
1	Diphtheria	0·97	0·81	0·68	0·43	0·26	0·16	0·20	0·18	0·18	0·38	0·50	0·40	5·15	1
2	Dermatophytosis	0·84	0·87	0·74	0·91	0·73	0·71	0·88	1·02	0·83	0·79	0·64	0·64	9·59	2
3	Dysentery	0·42	0·35	0·29	0·25	0·40	1·44	2·78	1·77	1·38	1·56	0·89	0·41	11·93	3
4	Enteric Group of Fevers	0·05	0·05	0·03	0·02	0·02	0·05	0·09	0·08	0·10	0·08	0·07	0·03	0·66	4
5	Food Poisoning	0·06	0·00	0·02	0·01	0·01	0·14	0·00	0·07	0·01	0·00	0·17	0·00	0·50	5
6	Gas Gangrene	0·01	0·09	0·03	0·01	0·02	0·02	0·01	0·01	0·03	0·02	0·01	0·01	0·27	6
7	Helminthic Diseases	0·01	0·01	0·02	0·01	0·02	0·01	0·01	0·07	0·03	0·01	0·01	0·02	0·21	7
8	Influenza	0·21	0·23	0·32	0·12	0·02	0·02	0·01	0·00	0·02	0·15	0·08	0·01	1·19	8
9	Jaundice	3·88	2·58	1·39	1·19	0·96	0·84	1·07	1·37	2·52	3·63	3·53	2·55	25·50	9
10	Malaria	2·80	4·48	7·79	9·99	8·97	7·25	8·74	9·20	5·87	4·96	3·78	2·38	76·21	10
11	Meningitis—Meningococcal	0·00	0·00	0·00	0·00	0·00	—	0·01	0·00	0·00	0·00	0·00	0·01	0·04	11
12	Meningitis—Other Forms	0·00	0·00	0·00	0·01	0·03	0·01	0·01	0·02	0·03	0·00	0·01	0·01	0·14	12
13	Pediculosis	2·25	2·31	2·77	2·08	1·29	0·79	0·94	0·87	0·71	1·30	2·02	1·99	19·31	13
14	Pneumonia—Pneumococcal	0·06	0·14	0·27	0·30	0·20	0·28	0·24	0·07	0·05	0·08	0·10	0·09	1·82	14
15	Pneumonia—Other Forms	0·15	0·11	0·14	0·20	0·19	0·16	0·16	0·11	0·11	0·15	0·14	0·16	1·79	15
16	Poliomyelitis	0·01	—	0·01	—	—	0·00	0·01	0·01	0·01	0·01	0·01	0·01	0·07	16
17	Sandfly Fever	0·00	—	0·00	0·00	0·01	0·09	0·52	0·90	0·80	0·10	0·02	0·00	2·45	17
18	Scabies	1·58	1·70	1·78	1·66	1·44	1·10	1·28	1·16	0·96	1·58	2·26	2·44	18·92	18
19	Smallpox	0·02	0·01	0·02	0·04	0·00	0·02	—	—	—	—	0·00	0·00	0·12	19
20	Tetanus	—	—	0·00	0·00	—	—	—	—	0·00	0·00	0·00	0·00	0·02	20
21	Trench Foot	0·04	0·00	0·01	—	0·02	—	—	—	—	—	0·08	0·20	0·35	21
22	Tuberculosis—Pulmonary	0·03	0·02	0·04	0·05	0·04	0·05	0·09	0·06	0·06	0·05	0·07	0·04	0·60	22
23	Tuberculosis—Other Forms	0·00	—	0·00	0·01	0·01	0·00	—	0·00	0·01	0·00	0·01	0·01	0·05	23
24	Typhus	0·01	0·01	0·01	0·00	0·00	—	0·00	—	—	—	—	—	0·03	24
25	Undulant Fever	0·00	0·00	0·00	—	0·00	0·01	0·00	0·00	0·00	0·00	0·01	0·01	0·04	25
26	Venereal Diseases	4·52	4·44	4·19	4·65	4·09	4·16	4·34	4·22	3·36	3·63	4·60	4·45	50·64	26
27	Diseases of the Digestive System	5·71	4·67	4·31	4·27	3·99	6·78	9·25	6·28	5·18	4·97	4·88	3·85	64·13	27
28	Diseases of the Respiratory System	3·65	3·91	3·65	2·82	1·79	1·87	2·26	1·89	1·65	2·45	2·95	2·92	31·81	28
29	Diseases of the Nervous System	0·24	0·35	0·26	0·22	0·30	0·27	0·44	0·29	0·27	0·25	0·20	0·24	3·32	29
30	Diseases of the Skin	3·65	3·66	3·22	2·95	2·69	2·32	2·80	2·49	2·14	2·24	2·80	2·57	33·52	30
31	Psychoses	0·05	0·09	0·18	0·07	0·16	0·20	0·26	0·07	0·07	0·13	0·03	0·06	1·34	31
32	Psychoneuroses (including Exhaustion)	1·51	2·73	1·19	0·80	3·08	2·14	2·58	1·22	2·27	1·58	1·61	1·12	21·82	32
33	I.A.T.	3·94	3·34	2·74	2·42	2·37	2·45	2·95	3·01	3·22	3·74	3·90	3·39	37·47	33
34	*Total Admissions for Diseases*	43·51	41·75	42·48	43·87	42·07	46·30	58·37	49·29	40·90	39·84	42·51	35·70	526·59	34
35	Injuries—Battle Casualties	7·01	10·11	5·61	3·59	12·25	12·35	11·68	4·12	10·39	5·37	3·73	4·84	91·04	35
36	Injuries—Accidental	3·96	2·44	1·42	2·98	3·43	4·84	4·50	3·54	3·16	2·67	3·12	3·01	39·06	36
37	Injuries—Self-Inflicted	0·02	0·02	0·03	0·02	0·01	0·01	0·02	0·02	0·02	0·02	0·01	0·02	0·21	37
38	Injuries—Burns	0·36	0·43	0·46	0·53	0·57	0·84	0·81	0·53	0·49	0·36	0·41	0·45	6·23	38
39	*Total Admissions for Injuries*	11·36	13·00	7·51	7·12	16·26	18·04	17·00	8·20	14·05	8·41	7·26	8·32	136·54	39
40	*Total Admissions*	54·87	54·75	50·00	51·00	58·33	64·34	75·37	57·49	54·95	48·26	49·77	44·02	663·13	40

TABLE 35

British North African and Central Mediterranean Forces. British Troops. Causes of Admission to Medical Units, 1944
Breakdown of Certain Diseases Shown in Table 34. Mean Monthly and Annual Rates per 1,000 Strength

Source: B.N.A.F. and C.M.F. Weekly Health States

	CAUSES	Jan.	Feb.	Mar.	Apr.	May	June	July	Aug.	Sept.	Oct.	Nov.	Dec.	Annual	
	Dysentery														
1	Protozoal	0·02	0·03	0·04	0·05	0·04	0·04	0·10	0·06	0·09	0·11	0·15	0·11	0·85	1
2	Bacillary and B.E.	0·10	0·08	0·07	0·04	0·12	0·53	0·93	0·63	0·59	0·61	0·35	0·10	4·14	2
3	Clinical and I.E.	0·31	0·24	0·18	0·16	0·24	0·87	1·75	1·08	0·70	0·84	0·39	0·19	6·94	3
4	*Totals*	0·42	0·35	0·29	0·25	0·40	1·44	2·78	1·77	1·38	1·56	0·89	0·41	11·93	4
	Enteric Group of Fevers														
5	Typhoid	0·02	0·04	0·01	0·01	0·02	0·01	0·01	0·03	0·03	0·03	0·04	0·02	0·25	5
6	Para A	0·00	0·00	—	—	—	—	0·00	—	0·00	—	0·00	0·00	0·02	6
7	Para B	0·01	0·00	0·01	0·00	—	0·01	0·01	0·01	0·01	0·01	0·01	0·01	0·07	7
8	Para C	—	0·00	—	—	—	—	—	0·00	—	—	—	—	0·00	8
9	Clinical	0·02	0·01	0·01	0·01	0·00	0·03	0·07	0·03	0·06	0·04	0·03	0·01	0·32	9
10	*Totals*	0·05	0·05	0·03	0·02	0·02	0·05	0·09	0·08	0·10	0·08	0·07	0·03	0·66	10
	Jaundice														
11	Infective Hepatitis	3·84	2·54	1·35	1·17	0·87	0·77	0·98	1·32	2·43	3·57	3·42	2·47	24·74	11
12	Leptospirosis	—	0·01	—	—	0·01	0·01	0·01	0·01	0·04	0·00	0·01	0·00	0·09	12
13	Post-Arsphenamine	0·01	0·02	0·03	0·02	0·08	0·06	0·09	0·04	0·05	0·06	0·10	0·08	0·63	13
14	Other Forms	0·02	0·01	—	—	0·01	—	—	—	—	—	—	—	0·04	14
15	*Totals*	3·88	2·58	1·39	1·19	0·96	0·84	1·07	1·37	2·52	3·63	3·53	2·55	25·50	15
	Malaria														
16	Primary B.T.	0·88	1·43	3·26	4·41	3·91	3·01	4·21	4·15	2·54	1·69	1·14	0·55	31·18	16
17	Primary Q.	0·03	0·01	0·03	0·01	0·00	0·00	—	—	0·00	0·01	0·01	—	0·11	17
18	Primary M.T.	0·20	0·31	0·14	0·13	0·09	0·04	0·14	0·16	0·10	0·10	0·04	0·03	1·48	18
19	Primary Clinical	0·28	0·27	0·38	0·59	0·48	0·57	0·65	1·74	0·66	0·38	0·27	0·10	6·36	19
20	*Total Primary*	1·39	2·02	3·82	5·14	4·48	3·63	4·99	6·05	3·30	2·18	1·46	0·68	39·13	20
21	Relapse B.T.	0·88	1·87	3·52	4·38	4·23	3·39	3·48	2·88	2·37	2·60	2·13	1·59	33·31	21
22	Relapse Q.	0·01	0·00	0·01	0·02	0·00	—	—	—	—	—	0·01	—	0·05	22
23	Relapse M.T.	0·35	0·32	0·16	0·21	0·10	0·04	0·05	0·03	0·05	0·05	0·03	0·03	1·41	23
24	Relapse Clinical	0·17	0·27	0·28	0·25	0·17	0·19	0·22	0·25	0·17	0·14	0·14	0·08	2·32	24
	Total Relapse	1·40	2·47	3·98	4·85	4·50	3·62	3·75	3·16	2·59	2·78	2·32	1·70	37·10	25
26	*Total Malaria*	2·80	4·48	7·79	9·99	8·97	7·25	8·74	9·20	5·87	4·96	3·78	2·38	76·21	26

	Pediculosis														
27	Capitas	0·01	0·01	0·07	0·09	0·13	0·11	0·16	0·14	0·06	0·10	0·02	0·03	0·93	27
28	Corporis	1·22	1·32	1·73	0·98	0·51	0·12	0·14	0·10	0·08	0·20	0·52	0·33	7·24	28
29	Pubis	1·02	0·97	0·98	1·01	0·66	0·55	0·65	0·63	0·57	0·99	1·48	1·63	11·14	29
30	*Totals*	2·25	2·31	2·77	2·08	1·29	0·79	0·94	0·87	0·71	1·30	2·02	1·99	19·31	30
	Venereal Diseases														
31	Gonorrhoea	1·63	1·79	2·03	2·46	2·09	2·30	2·30	2·29	1·83	1·93	2·71	2·52	25·90	31
32	Syphilis	0·21	0·27	0·32	0·30	0·36	0·21	0·34	0·30	0·25	0·32	0·31	0·47	3·65	32
33	Chancroid	0·30	1·01	0·69	0·76	0·79	0·96	0·93	0·93	0·77	0·82	0·88	0·83	9·66	33
34	Lympho-granuloma	0·00	0·01	0·01	0·05	0·00	0·00	0·04	0·01	—	—	—	0·01	0·12	34
35	Other Forms	2·37	1·37	1·15	1·08	0·85	0·68	0·74	0·69	0·52	0·55	0·70	0·62	11·30	35
36	*Totals*	4·52	4·44	4·19	4·65	4·09	4·16	4·34	4·22	3·36	3·63	4·60	4·45	50·64	36

TABLE 36

British North African and Central Mediterranean Forces. Canadian Troops. Causes of Admission to Medical Units, 1944

Mean Monthly and Annual Rates per 1,000 Strength

Source: B.N.A.F. and C.M.F. Weekly Health States

	CAUSES	Jan.	Feb.	Mar.	Apr.	May	June	July	Aug.	Sept.	Oct.	Nov.	Dec.	Annual	
1	Diphtheria	0·58	0·61	0·61	0·54	0·39	0·23	0·35	0·41	0·15	0·30	1·25	0·35	5·77	1
2	Dermatophytosis	0·24	0·02	0·13	0·07	0·13	0·10	0·04	0·09	0·07	0·49	0·27	0·04	1·67	2
3	Dysentery	1·34	0·40	0·34	0·13	0·37	1·08	1·98	1·62	0·54	0·75	0·52	0·33	9·38	3
4	Enteric Group	0·21	—	0·01	0·04	0·07	0·78	1·33	0·94	0·02	0·54	0·34	0·03	5·31	4
5	Food Poisoning	—	—	—	—	—	0·29	—	—	0·01	—	—	—	0·30	5
6	Gas Gangrene	0·12	0·02	0·01	—	—	—	—	—	0·01	—	—	0·01	0·18	6
7	Helminthic Diseases	0·06	—	—	—	0·05	0·01	0·12	0·03	0·07	0·04	0·07	0·06	0·52	7
8	Influenza	0·91	2·95	1·59	2·84	1·04	0·33	0·11	0·02	0·07	0·24	0·29	0·37	10·75	8
9	Jaundice	10·50	6·83	4·73	2·94	1·34	1·80	4·86	7·97	12·02	16·56	16·41	9·41	95·37	9
10	Malaria	1·58	0·82	2·64	7·87	5·51	5·69	9·56	6·57	4·38	4·18	2·70	2·05	53·56	10
11	Meningitis—Meningococcal	—	—	—	—	—	—	0·02	—	—	—	—	0·01	0·03	11
12	Meningitis—Other Forms	—	0·02	—	0·01	0·04	—	0·02	0·07	—	0·04	—	—	0·20	12
13	Pediculosis	0·94	0·19	0·48	0·08	0·22	0·04	0·04	0·38	0·03	0·02	0·25	1·28	3·94	13
14	Pneumonia—Pneumococcal	0·12	0·11	0·10	0·13	0·24	0·03	0·02	0·07	0·04	0·10	0·18	0·41	1·54	14
15	Pneumonia—Other Forms	—	0·23	0·14	0·54	0·17	0·12	0·14	0·17	0·01	0·05	0·09	0·23	1·89	15
16	Sandfly Fever	—	—	—	—	—	—	0·09	0·15	0·11	—	—	—	0·35	16
17	Scabies	0·88	1·20	0·82	0·67	0·89	0·23	0·26	1·24	0·22	0·28	1·14	3·86	11·68	17
18	Tuberculosis—Pulmonary	—	—	0·02	0·03	0·01	—	—	0·05	—	0·02	0·06	0·03	0·22	18
19	Tuberculosis—Other Forms	—	—	—	—	—	0·03	—	—	—	—	0·02	—	0·05	19
20	Trench Foot	—	—	—	—	—	—	—	—	—	—	—	0·26	0·26	20
21	Venereal Diseases	6·22	0·99	2·95	2·51	2·49	7·81	15·60	6·28	3·09	5·47	9·08	10·08	72·57	21
22	Diseases of the Digestive System	12·33	10·14	7·11	5·07	4·17	18·78	26·32	18·89	13·04	10·70	8·47	7·58	142·58	22
23	Diseases of the Respiratory System	4·16	7·13	5·78	5·55	3·22	4·69	8·09	4·17	2·49	3·94	5·00	5·67	59·88	23
24	Diseases of the Nervous System	1·12	0·89	0·70	0·35	0·40	0·83	0·88	0·85	0·68	0·50	1·61	0·89	9·71	24
25	Diseases of the Skin	3·52	4·47	3·53	2·55	2·05	2·38	4·44	4·19	4·03	3·92	4·74	3·76	43·57	25
26	Psychoses	—	0·04	0·06	0·04	0·12	0·11	0·23	0·03	0·01	0·04	0·05	0·07	0·80	26
27	Psychoneuroses (Including Exhaustion)	3·83	0·65	1·77	1·44	4·34	0·99	2·53	0·87	5·54	3·16	0·85	4·52	30·48	27
28	I.A.T.	3·01	2·93	2·75	2·63	2·32	3·34	3·97	3·93	6·56	6·88	6·17	5·92	50·41	28
29	*Total Admissions for Diseases*	60·99	51·99	53·72	58·72	48·84	73·13	102·91	80·70	79·93	79·40	78·09	63·06	831·50	29
30	Injuries—Enemy Action	15·30	9·72	5·44	3·95	40·31	10·74	4·65	2·71	44·15	14·15	1·56	26·57	179·23	30
31	Injuries—Accidental	4·22	1·71	1·63	4·17	4·50	9·86	9·02	7·43	5·64	5·31	6·15	5·17	64·80	31
32	Injuries—Self Inflicted	0·73	0·44	0·16	0·06	0·26	0·18	0·05	0·05	0·13	0·12	0·07	0·16	2·40	32
33	Injuries—Burns	1·37	1·08	1·01	0·79	1·19	1·63	2·90	1·23	1·02	0·63	0·60	0·58	14·00	33
34	*Total Admissions for Injuries*	21·62	12·95	8·24	8·96	46·25	22·40	16·62	11·41	50·93	20·21	8·38	32·48	260·43	34
35	*Total Admissions*	82·61	64·94	61·96	67·68	95·09	95·53	119·52	92·11	130·86	99·61	86·47	95·54	1,091·93	35

TABLE 37

British North African and Central Mediterranean Forces. Canadian Troops. Causes of Admission to Medical Units, 1944
Detailed Breakdown of Certain Diseases Shown in Table 36. Mean Monthly and Annual Rates per 1,000 Strength

Source: B.N.A.F. and C.M.F. Weekly Health States

	CAUSES	Jan.	Feb.	Mar.	Apr.	May	June	July	Aug.	Sept.	Oct.	Nov.	Dec.	Annual	
	Dysentery														
1	Protozoal	—	0·02	—	0·01	0·01	0·03	0·02	0·03	0·03	0·14	0·24	0·07	0·60	1
2	Bacillary and B.E.	0·03	—	0·08	—	0·01	0·10	0·46	0·17	0·25	0·30	0·02	0·06	1·46	2
3	Clinical and I.E.	1·31	0·38	0·26	0·11	0·34	0·96	1·51	1·41	0·26	0·31	0·27	0·20	7·32	3
4	*Totals*	1·34	0·40	0·34	0·13	0·37	1·08	1·98	1·62	0·54	0·75	0·52	0·33	9·38	4
	Enteric Group of Fevers														
5	Typhoid	—	—	0·01	—	—	—	—	0·07	0·01	0·23	0·02	—	0·34	5
6	Para A	—	—	—	—	—	—	—	—	—	0·02	—	—	0·02	6
7	Para B	0·03	—	—	—	—	—	0·02	0·03	—	—	—	—	0·08	7
8	Para C	—	—	—	—	—	—	—	0·02	0·01	0·02	—	—	0·05	8
9	Clinical	0·18	—	—	0·04	0·07	0·78	1·32	0·82	1·00	0·28	0·33	0·03	4·83	9
10	*Totals*	0·21	—	0·01	0·04	0·07	0·78	1·33	0·94	1·02	0·54	0·34	0·03	5·31	10
	Jaundice														
11	Infective Hepatitis	10·50	6·83	4·72	2·92	1·34	1·80	4·86	7·97	12·00	16·53	16·41	9·37	95·26	11
12	Leptospirosis	—	—	—	—	—	—	—	—	—	0·02	—	—	0·02	12
13	Post-Arsphenamine	—	—	0·01	0·01	—	—	—	—	0.01	0·02	—	0·04	0·10	13
14	Other Forms	—	—	—	—	—	—	—	—	—	—	—	—	—	14
15	*Totals*	10·50	6·83	4·73	2·94	1·34	1·80	4·86	7·97	10·02	16·56	16·41	9·41	95·37	15
	Malaria														
16	Primary B.T.	0·15	0·08	1·46	4·86	3·22	2·71	7·55	4·00	2·04	1·96	1·32	0·96	30·32	16
17	Primary Q.	—	—	—	—	—	—	—	—	—	—	—	—	—	17
18	Primary M.T.	0·15	0·02	0·05	0·19	0·05	—	—	0·07	—	0·05	0·04	0·07	0·69	18
19	Primary Clinical	0·85	0·13	0·85	1·51	0·70	1·45	0·98	0·83	0·80	0·82	0·31	0·32	9·56	19
20	*Total Primary*	1·15	0·23	2·36	6·56	3·98	4·16	8·53	4·90	2·85	2·83	1·66	1·36	40·57	20
21	Relapse B.T.	0·03	0·11	0·15	1·21	1·37	1·12	1·00	1·57	1·33	1·13	0·98	0·52	10·50	21
22	Relapse Q.	—	—	—	—	—	—	—	—	—	—	—	—	—	22
23	Relapse M.T.	0·09	0·02	—	0·04	—	—	—	—	—	0·02	—	0·11	0·28	23
24	Relapse Clinical	0·30	0·46	0·14	0·06	0·17	0·41	0·04	0·10	0·20	0·21	0·05	0·05	2·20	24
25	*Total Relapse*	0·43	0·59	0·28	1·31	1·54	1·53	1·04	1·67	1·53	1·35	1·03	0·69	12·98	25
26	*Total Malaria*	1·58	0·82	2·64	7·87	5·51	5·69	9·56	6·57	4·38	4·18	2·70	2·05	53·56	26

TABLE 37—*Continued*

British North African and Central Mediterranean Forces. Canadian Troops. Causes of Admission to Medical Units, 1944
Detailed Breakdown of Certain Diseases Shown in Table 36. Mean Monthly and Annual Rates per 1,000 Strength

Source: B.N.A.F. and C.M.F. Weekly Health States

	CAUSES	Jan.	Feb.	Mar.	Apr.	May	June	July	Aug.	Sept.	Oct.	Nov.	Dec.	Annual	
	Pediculosis														
27	Capitas	—	—	—	0·03	0·22	0·03	0·04	0·32	0·03	—	0·18	1·05	1·89	27
28	Corporis	0·03	0·06	0·36	0·01	—	—	—	—	—	—	—	—	0·47	28
29	Pubis	0·91	0·13	0·11	0·05	—	0·01	—	0·05	—	0·02	0·07	0·23	1·57	29
30	*Totals*	0·94	0·19	0·48	0·08	0·22	0·04	0·04	0·38	0·03	0·02	0·25	1·28	3·94	30
	Venereal Diseases														
31	Gonorrhoea	4·16	0·76	2·53	2·15	1·55	4·24	7·65	2·96	1·52	1·89	4·92	3·61	37·94	31
32	Syphilis	0·82	0·13	0·10	0·10	0·17	0·51	0·65	0·55	0·58	0·52	0·58	0·27	4·96	32
33	Chancroid	0·27	0·02	0·01	0·10	0·42	1·66	2·88	1·33	0·58	0·69	1·19	1·33	10·48	33
34	Lympho-granuloma	—	—	—	—	—	—	0·04	—	0·08	0·04	—	—	0·15	34
35	Other Forms	0·97	0·08	0·31	0·17	0·35	1·41	4·39	1·45	0·33	2·33	2·39	4·86	19·03	35
36	*Totals*	6·22	0·99	2·95	2·51	2·49	7·81	15·60	6·28	3·09	5·47	9·08	10·08	72·57	36

TABLE 38

British North African and Central Mediterranean Forces. New Zealand Troops. Causes of Admission to Medical Units, 1944
Mean Monthly and Annual Rates per 1,000 Strength

Source: B.N.A.F. and C.M.F. Weekly Health States

	CAUSES	Jan.	Feb.	Mar.	April	May	June	July	Aug.	Sept.	Oct.	Nov.	Dec.	Annual	
1	Diphtheria	0·19	0·07	0·15	0·06	0·04	0·21	0·05	0·05	0·04	0·97	0·51	2·20	4·54	1
2	Dermatophytosis	—	—	—	—	—	—	0·10	—	—	0·20	—	0·94	1·25	2
3	Dysentery	2·12	0·37	0·44	0·26	0·35	4·52	1·93	1·39	0·50	2·76	2·17	1·22	18·02	3
4	Enteric Group of Fevers	0·10	0·29	—	—	0·14	0·21	0·05	—	0·04	—	—	0·36	1·19	4
5	Gas Gangrene	—	—	0·10	—	—	0·04	—	0·15	—	0·31	—	0·18	0·78	5
6	Helminthic Diseases	—	0·15	0·05	0·13	0·07	0·13	0·10	—	0·17	0·41	0·86	0·40	2·46	6
7	Influenza	—	0·37	0·05	0·19	0·14	0·08	0·05	0·05	0·13	0·41	0·40	0·67	2·54	7
8	Jaundice	4·63	8·36	4·27	2·38	1·09	2·01	8·60	16·34	22·01	33·11	22·55	8·79	134·14	8
9	Meningitis—Meningococcal	—	—	—	—	—	0·04	—	0·05	—	—	—	—	0·09	9
10	Meningitis—Other Forms	—	—	—	—	—	0·04	—	0·55	0·08	0·05	—	0·05	0·77	10
11	Malaria	0·10	0·07	—	0·06	0·28	0·55	2·55	1·19	0·21	0·56	0·46	0·22	6·25	11
12	Pediculosis	0·39	0·81	0·54	0·65	0·14	0·38	0·31	0·84	0·17	0·87	2·62	2·33	10·03	12
13	Pneumonia—Pneumococcal	0·48	0·15	0·20	1·03	0·21	0·46	0·56	0·54	0·17	0·20	0·51	0·18	4·70	13
14	Pneumonia—Other Forms	—	0·07	0·05	—	0·18	—	0·26	—	—	0·92	0·57	0·81	2·85	14
15	Poliomyelitis	—	—	—	—	—	—	—	0·10	—	—	—	—	0·10	15
16	Sandfly Fever	—	—	—	—	—	—	—	—	0·13	0·15	—	—	0·28	16
17	Scabies	0·10	0·22	0·49	0·13	0·56	0·92	1·32	0·50	0·59	1·18	2·79	2·96	11·75	17
18	Tuberculosis Pulmonary	—	—	—	—	0·07	0·04	—	—	—	0·05	0·06	0·05	0·27	18
19	Venereal Diseases	0·10	1·39	0·20	0·64	4·01	7·32	8·76	1·68	2·44	3·78	4·16	4·35	38·82	19
20	Diseases of the Digestive System	11·28	7·41	6·82	5·80	9·74	21·64	17·41	24·41	17·56	21·51	28·15	12·91	184·73	20
21	Diseases of the Respiratory System	6·27	8·00	6·77	5·99	7·00	4·94	3·00	3·86	2·73	6·54	4·44	7·53	67·07	21
22	Diseases of the Nervous System	0·29	1·47	0·98	1·68	1·37	1·72	2·14	0·59	1·47	0·87	1·25	2·11	15·93	22
23	Diseases of the Skin	2·41	3·23	2·70	3·09	3·41	5·23	5·65	4·60	4·03	5·26	9·46	8·87	57·96	23
24	Psychoses	—	—	—	—	0·11	0·25	0·05	0·05	0·04	0·10	0·06	0·05	0·70	24
25	Psychoneuroses (including Exhaustion)	0·48	2·13	8·00	0·32	1·13	0·84	1·38	2·72	1·30	1·48	0·57	1·48	21·82	25
26	I.A.T.	4·05	6·09	5·05	2·51	3·55	4·56	6·67	6·39	6·89	7·46	6·50	7·40	67·11	26
27	*Total Admissions for Diseases*	36·17	66·68	59·75	34·73	59·02	72·86	82·58	91·69	77·70	81·14	90·47	72·12	824·91	27
28	Injuries—Battle Casualties	8·29	17·75	39·54	3·48	11·89	19·96	33·76	34·56	19·70	17·88	2·85	19·36	229·02	28
29	Injuries—Accidental	3·67	8·95	5·69	4·70	8·20	13·31	17·46	11·19	10·25	7·77	10·60	5·69	107·47	29
30	Injuries—Self Inflicted	—	—	0·10	—	—	—	—	—	—	—	—	—	0·10	30
31	Injuries—Burns	1·45	1·91	1·03	0·64	2·67	2·80	2·19	2·77	0·76	1·12	0·91	0·67	18·93	31
32	*Total Admissions for Injuries*	13·41	28·61	46·36	8·83	22·76	36·08	53·40	48·52	30·70	26·77	14·36	25·73	355·51	32
33	*Total Admissions*	49·57	95·29	106·10	43·56	81·78	108·94	135·99	140·20	108·41	107·91	104·83	97·84	1,180·42	33

TABLE 39

British North African and Central Mediterranean Forces. New Zealand Troops, 1944

Detailed Breakdown of Certain Disease Groups Shown in Table 38. Mean Monthly and Annual Rates per 1,000 Strength

Source: B.N.A.F. and C.M.F. Weekly Health States

	CAUSES	Jan.	Feb.	Mar.	Apr.	May	June	July	Aug.	Sept.	Oct.	Nov.	Dec.	Annual	
	Dysentery														
1	Protozoal	—	—	—	—	—	0·21	—	0·10	0·04	0·92	0·91	0·67	2·85	1
2	Bacillary and B.E.	0·77	—	0·15	0·13	—	1·34	0·31	0·40	0·21	0·41	0·80	0·40	4·91	2
3	Clinical and I.E.	1·35	0·37	0·29	0·13	0·35	2·97	1·63	0·90	0·25	1·43	0·46	0·13	10·26	3
4	*Totals*	2·12	0·37	0·44	0·26	0·35	4·52	1·93	1·39	0·50	2·76	2·17	1·22	18·02	4
	Enteric Group of Fevers														
5	Typhoid	—	—	—	—	—	0·21	0·05	—	—	—	—	0·22	0·48	5
6	Para A	—	—	—	—	—	—	—	—	—	—	—	0·05	0·05	6
7	Para B	—	—	—	—	—	—	—	—	—	—	—	0·09	0·09	7
8	Para C	0·10	—	—	—	—	—	—	—	—	—	—	—	0·10	8
9	Clinical	—	0·29	—	—	0·14	—	—	—	0·04	—	—	—	0·48	9
10	*Totals*	0·10	0·29	—	—	0·14	0·21	0·05	—	0·04	—	—	0·36	1·19	10
	Jaundice														
11	Infective Hepatitis	4·63	8·36	4·27	2·38	1·09	2·01	8·60	16·34	22·01	33·06	22·55	8·79	134·09	11
12	Leptospirosis	—	—	—	—	—	—	—	—	—	—	—	—	—	12
13	Post-Arsphenamine	—	—	—	—	—	—	—	—	—	0·05	—	—	0·05	13
14	Other Forms	—	—	—	—	—	—	—	—	—	—	—	—	—	14
15	*Totals*	4·63	8·36	4·27	2·38	1·09	2·01	8·60	16·34	22·01	33·11	22·55	8·79	134·14	15
	Malaria														
16	Primary B.T.	—	—	—	—	0·14	0·13	2·29	1·04	0·17	0·26	0·11	0·18	4·31	16
17	Primary Q.	—	—	—	—	—	—	—	—	—	—	—	—	—	17
18	Primary M.T.	—	—	—	—	—	—	—	—	—	—	—	—	—	18
19	Primary Clinical	0·10	—	—	0·06	0·11	0·04	0·05	0·10	0·04	0·05	0·11	0·05	0·71	19
20	*Total Primary*	0·10	—	—	0·06	0·25	0·17	2·34	1·14	0·21	0·31	0·23	0·22	5·02	20
21	Relapse B.T.	—	—	—	—	0·04	0·38	0·20	0·05	—	0·20	0·23	—	1·10	21
22	Relapse Q.	—	—	—	—	—	—	—	—	—	—	—	—	—	22
23	Relapse M.T.	—	—	—	—	—	—	—	—	—	—	—	—	—	23
24	Relapse Clinical	—	0·07	—	—	—	—	—	—	—	0·05	—	—	0·12	24
25	*Total Relapse*	—	0·07	—	—	0·04	0·38	0·20	0·05	—	0·26	0·23	—	1·22	25
26	*Total Malaria*	0·10	0·07	—	0·06	0·28	0·55	2·55	1·19	0·21	0·56	0·46	0·22	6·25	26

	Pediculosis														
27	Capitas	—	—	—	—	—	—	—	0·05	—	0·05	—	—	0·10	27
28	Corporis	—	0·59	0·20	0·26	0·04	—	—	—	—	0·66	0·17	0·36	2·27	28
29	Pubis	0·39	0·22	0·34	0·39	0·11	0·38	0·31	0·79	0·17	0·15	2·45	1·97	7·66	29
30	*Totals*	0·39	0·81	0·54	0·65	0·14	0·38	0·31	0·84	0·17	0·87	2·62	2·33	10·03	30
	Venereal Diseases														
31	Gonorrhoea	—	0·51	0·10	0·45	1·37	2·97	3·00	0·59	0·97	1·58	1·99	2·33	15·88	31
32	Syphilis	—	—	0·10	0·13	—	0·17	0·20	0·25	0·13	0·36	0·46	0·09	1·88	32
33	Chancroid	—	0·07	—	—	1·72	2·34	4·74	0·35	0·63	0·82	0·51	0·58	11·77	33
34	Lympho-granuloma	—	—	—	—	—	—	—	0·09	—	—	—	—	0·09	34
35	Others	0·10	0·81	—	0·07	0·91	1·84	0·82	0·40	0·71	1·02	1·20	1·35	9·21	35
36	*Totals*	0·10	1·39	0·20	0·64	4·01	7·32	8·76	1·68	2·44	3·78	4·16	4·35	38·82	36

TABLE 40

British North African and Central Mediterranean Forces. Indian Troops. Causes of Admission to Medical Units, 1944
Mean Monthly and Annual Rates per 1,000 Strength

Source: B.N.A.F. and C.M.F. Weekly Health States

	CAUSES	Jan.	Feb.	Mar.	Apr.	May	June	July	Aug.	Sept.	Oct.	Nov.	Dec.	Annual	
1	Diphtheria	0·05	—	0·03	0·07	—	—	—	—	0·02	—	0·03	0·03	0·23	1
2	Dermatophytosis	—	0·12	—	—	—	0·74	0·49	0·32	0·10	0·47	0·13	0·03	2·39	2
3	Dysentery	0·46	0·12	0·55	0·39	0·53	1·13	1·87	1·76	1·49	1·27	0·68	0·36	10·59	3
4	Enteric Group	—	0·08	—	—	0·09	—	—	—	0·02	0·02	—	—	0·21	4
5	Gas Gangrene	—	0·04	0·03	0·04	0·02	—	0·03	0·02	—	—	—	0·04	0·22	5
6	Food Poisoning	—	—	—	—	—	—	—	—	—	—	—	0·03	0·03	6
7	Helminthic Diseases	0·26	—	0·09	0·32	0·93	0·76	1·16	0·79	0·14	0·14	0·02	0·06	4·63	7
8	Influenza	—	—	1·93	0·04	—	—	—	—	—	—	—	0·01	1·98	8
9	Jaundice	1·07	0·73	0·78	1·81	0·92	0·64	1·00	1·10	0·76	1·18	1·48	1·39	12·87	9
10	Malaria	0·61	0·53	0·78	1·20	0·90	0·92	1·81	1·81	1·49	2·11	0·88	0·38	13·42	10
11	Meningitis—Meningococcal	—	—	0·17	—	—	—	0·03	—	—	—	0·05	—	0·25	11
12	Meningitis—Other Types	—	—	—	—	—	—	—	—	—	0·04	0·02	—	0·06	12
13	Pediculosis	3·66	0·82	0·89	0·25	1·60	—	0·11	0·05	0·02	0·08	0·13	0·37	7·96	13
14	Pneumonia—Pneumococcal	—	0·08	0·12	—	0·09	0·09	0·14	0·15	0·09	0·06	0·05	0·16	1·01	14
15	Pneumonia—Other Types	0·05	—	0·03	—	0·02	0·09	—	0·02	0·15	0·06	0·05	0·10	0·58	15
16	Sandfly Fever	—	—	—	—	—	—	—	0·10	0·22	0·04	0·02	—	0·37	16
17	Scabies	0·97	0·73	1·47	0·74	0·53	1·26	0·62	1·07	0·81	0·87	0·63	1·00	10·71	17
18	Tuberculosis—Pulmonary	—	0·08	—	0·18	0·09	0·16	0·05	0·07	0·14	0·18	0·17	0·59	1·72	18
19	Tuberculosis—Other Types	—	—	—	—	—	—	0·05	—	0·02	—	—	0·03	0·10	19
20	Trench Foot	—	—	—	—	—	—	—	—	—	—	0·02	0·34	0·35	20
21	Venereal Diseases	2·64	1·18	0·81	1·06	1·27	2·21	2·60	1·91	1·39	1·20	1·83	3·07	21·16	21
22	Diseases of the Digestive System	4·83	5·34	5·34	3·54	4·60	4·02	6·93	6·84	4·18	3·76	2·57	12·33	64·27	22
23	Diseases of the Respiratory System	4·93	6·03	8·88	5·38	2·94	3·38	1·73	2·08	2·08	2·93	3·44	4·22	48·02	23
24	Diseases of the Nervous System	0·51	0·73	0·40	0·25	0·56	0·62	0·38	0·90	0·41	0·32	0·35	1·21	6·63	24
25	Diseases of the Skin	2·80	2·36	3·81	2·23	3·26	2·51	2·41	2·78	1·56	1·77	1·99	2·42	29·89	25
26	Psychoses	0·10	0·73	—	—	0·32	0·12	0·03	0·02	0·02	0·16	0·06	0·51	2·07	26
27	Psychoneuroses (including Exhaustion)	0·86	0·04	0·52	0·39	0·88	1·01	0·22	0·39	0·58	0·35	0·52	0·18	5·94	27
28	I.A.T.	3·86	3·01	3·69	2·41	3·65	3·59	3·49	3·37	3·11	3·43	2·29	2·51	38·41	28
29	*Total Admissions for Diseases*	34·12	29·93	37·49	28·10	41·47	41·66	44·73	43·41	31·26	32·95	28·34	32·76	426·20	29
30	Injuries—Enemy Action	19·47	26·51	38·18	10·03	41·98	22·20	49·08	28·54	26·96	26·27	6·44	11·18	308·85	30
31	Injuries—Accidental	5·85	4·81	2·65	5·42	7·74	11·97	12·83	9·62	5·20	7·09	3·90	4·74	76·22	31
32	Injuries—Self Inflicted	0·10	0·01	0·55	0·04	—	—	0·14	—	0·39	—	0·05	0·93	2·80	32
33	Injuries—Burns	1·02	0·94	1·18	0·85	0·53	1·56	1·16	0·98	0·34	0·51	0·30	0·80	10·17	33
34	*Total Admissions for Injuries*	26·44	32·87	42·56	18·33	50·25	35·73	63·21	39·14	32·89	33·87	10·69	17·65	403·63	34
35	*Total Admissions*	60·56	62·80	80·05	46·43	91·72	77·39	107·94	82·55	64·15	66·82	39·03	50·41	829·83	35

TABLE 41

British North African and Central Mediterranean Forces. Indian Troops. Causes of Admission to Medical Units, 1944
Detailed Breakdown of Certain Diseases Shown in Table 40. Mean Monthly and Annual Rates per 1,000 Strength

Source: B.N.A.F. and C.M.F. Weekly Health States

	CAUSES	Jan.	Feb.	Mar.	Apr.	May	June	July	Aug.	Sept.	Oct.	Nov.	Dec.	Annual	
	Dysentery														
1	Protozoal	—	0·04	0·03	0·04	0·07	0·09	—	0·02	0·07	0·12	0·22	0·04	0·74	1
2	Bacillary and B.E.	0·41	0·08	0·17	—	0·02	0·41	0·79	0·83	0·63	0·35	0·08	0·08	0·86	2
3	Clinical and I.E.	0·05	—	0·35	0·35	0·44	0·62	1·08	0·90	0·80	0·80	0·38	0·23	6·00	3
4	*Totals*	0·46	0·12	0·55	0·39	0·53	1·13	1·87	1·76	1·49	1·27	0·68	0·36	10·59	4
	Enteric Group of Fevers														
5	Typhoid	—	—	—	—	—	—	—	—	0·02	0·02	—	—	0·04	5
6	Para A	—	—	—	—	—	—	—	—	—	—	—	—	—	6
7	Para B	—	—	—	—	—	—	—	—	—	—	—	—	—	7
8	Para C	—	—	—	—	—	—	—	—	—	—	—	—	—	8
9	Clinical	—	0·08	—	—	0·09	—	—	—	—	—	—	—	0·17	9
10	*Totals*	—	0·08	—	—	0·09	—	—	—	0·02	0·02	—	—	0·21	10
	Jaundice														
11	Infective Hepatitis	1·07	0·73	0·78	1·81	0·83	0·62	0·95	0·93	0·71	1·14	1·47	1·35	12·38	11
12	Leptospirosis	—	—	—	—	0·09	0·02	0·05	0·10	0·02	0·02	—	—	0·30	12
13	Post-Arsphenamine	—	—	—	—	—	—	—	0·07	0·03	0·02	0·02	0·04	0·19	13
14	Other Forms	—	—	—	—	—	—	—	—	—	—	—	—	—	14
15	*Totals*	1·07	0·73	0·78	1·81	0·92	0·64	1·00	1·10	0·76	1·18	1·48	1·39	12·87	15
	Malaria														
16	Primary B.T.	0·15	0·12	—	0·74	0·25	0·46	0·95	0·81	0·80	0·95	0·54	0·13	5·89	16
17	Primary Q.	—	—	—	—	—	—	—	—	—	—	—	—	—	17
18	Primary M.T.	—	—	0·03	—	0·02	—	0·03	0·02	0·02	0·34	0·05	0·01	0·52	18
19	Primary Clinical	0·10	0·12	0·12	—	0·09	0·05	0·14	0·15	0·03	0·12	0·06	0·01	0·99	19
20	*Total Primary*	0·26	0·24	0·14	0·74	0·37	0·51	1·11	0·98	0·85	1·40	0·65	0·16	7·39	20
21	Relapse B.T.	0·20	0·29	0·52	0·43	0·46	0·41	0·70	0·71	0·61	0·69	0·19	0·16	5·36	21
22	Relapse Q.	—	—	—	—	—	—	—	—	—	—	—	—	—	22
23	Relapse M.T.	0·05	—	—	—	—	—	—	0·02	—	—	0·03	0·07	0·18	23
24	Relapse Clinical	0·10	—	0·12	0·04	0·07	—	—	0·10	0·03	0·02	0·02	—	0·49	24
25	*Total Relapse*	0·36	0·29	0·63	0·46	0·53	0·41	0·70	0·83	0·64	0·71	0·24	0·23	6·03	25
26	*Total Malaria*	0·61	0·53	0·78	1·20	0·90	0·92	1·81	1·81	1·49	2·11	0·88	0·38	13·42	26

TABLE 41—*Continued*

British North African and Central Mediterranean Forces. Indian Troops. Causes of Admission to Medical Units, 1944
Detailed Breakdown of Certain Diseases Shown in Table 40. Mean Monthly and Annual Rates per 1,000 Strength

Source: B.N.A.F. and C.M.F. Weekly Health States

	CAUSES	Jan.	Feb.	Mar.	Apr.	May	June	July	Aug.	Sept.	Oct.	Nov.	Dec.	Annual	
	Pediculosis														
27	Capitas	0·05	—	—	—	1·16	—	—	0·02	—	—	—	0·01	1·25	27
28	Corporis	3·36	0·82	0·78	0·25	0·09	—	—	—	—	0·04	—	0·10	5·43	28
29	Pubis	0·25	—	0·12	—	0·35	—	0·11	0·02	0·02	0·04	0·13	0·25	1·28	29
30	*Totals*	3·66	0·82	0·89	0·25	1·60	—	0·11	0·05	0·02	0·08	0·13	0·37	7·96	30
	Venereal Diseases														
31	Gonorrhoea	0·56	0·45	0·26	0·67	0·39	0·64	1·38	1·07	0·78	0·47	0·92	1·21	8·81	31
32	Syphilis	—	0·22	0·29	0·18	0·21	0·12	0·08	0·29	0·17	0·06	0·46	0·51	2·60	32
33	Chancroid	—	0·20	—	0·04	0·42	0·97	1·03	0·49	0·22	0·28	0·16	0·79	4·58	33
34	Lympho-granuloma	—	—	—	—	—	—	—	—	—	—	—	—	—	34
35	Other Forms	2·09	0·29	0·26	0·18	0·25	0·48	0·11	0·05	0·22	0·39	0·30	0·56	5·18	35
36	*Totals*	2·64	1·18	0·81	1·06	1·27	2·21	2·60	1·90	1·39	1·20	1·83	3·07	21·16	36

TABLE 42

British North African and Central Mediterranean Forces. African Troops. Causes of Admission to Medical Units, 1944
Mean Monthly and Estimated Annual Rates per 1,000 Strength

Source: B.N.A.F. and C.M.F. Weekly Health States

	CAUSES	June	July	Aug.	Sept.	Oct.	Nov.	Dec.	E.A.R.	
1	Diphtheria	—	—	0·11	0·15	0·11	0·27	0·12	1·31	1
2	Dermatophytosis	2·20	1·04	0·47	—	0·19	0·03	0·05	6·81	2
3	Dysentery	1·19	2·38	1·53	0·73	0·98	0·83	0·54	14·02	3
4	Enteric Group of Fevers	0·13	—	—	—	—	0·03	—	0·27	4
5	Food Poisoning	—	—	—	0·34	—	—	0·03	0·63	5
6	Gas Gangrene	—	—	—	—	0·04	—	—	0·07	6
7	Helminthic Diseases	0·06	—	—	—	—	—	—	0·10	7
8	Influenza	0·25	0·06	—	—	0·45	0·18	1·93	3·48	8
9	Jaundice	0·63	0·55	1·90	2·56	2·46	1·84	1·95	20·37	9
10	Malaria	1·25	5·00	2·00	1·83	1·36	0·92	0·54	22·13	10
11	Meningitis—Meningococcal	—	—	—	0·08	—	—	0·07	0·26	11
12	Meningitis—Other Forms	—	—	—	—	—	0·03	—	0·05	12
13	Pediculosis	—	0·18	0·05	0·23	0·30	0·30	0·52	2·72	13
14	Pneumonia—Pneumococcal	0·13	0·06	—	0·04	0·04	0·06	0·30	1·06	14
15	Pneumonia—Other Forms	0·19	0·06	0·05	0·04	0·23	0·21	0·15	1·58	15
16	Sandfly Fever	—	0·12	0·42	0·46	—	—	—	1·72	16
17	Scabies	0·13	0·24	0·37	0·34	0·57	0·51	1·09	5·55	17
18	Tuberculosis—Pulmonary	0·06	—	0·16	0·08	0·30	0·21	0·17	1·68	18
19	Tuberculosis—Other Forms	—	—	—	0·04	0·24	0·03	0·03	0·22	19
20	Trench Foot	—	—	—	—	—	0·06	2·34	4·12	20
21	Venereal Diseases	1·93	3·33	4·85	7·53	7·83	7·48	5·38	65·77	21
22	Diseases of the Digestive System	4·20	8·10	6·43	5·88	5·79	5·11	4·22	68·11	22
23	Diseases of the Respiratory System	1·00	1·04	1·58	1·80	3·37	3·21	4·34	28·00	23
24	Diseases of the Nervous System	0·38	0·55	1·00	1·57	0·76	0·56	0·91	9·81	24
25	Diseases of the Skin	1·25	0·79	1·74	2·25	1·85	2·29	2·81	22·27	25
26	Psychoses	—	0·06	0·05	0·34	0·08	0·21	0·12	1·48	26
27	Psychoneuroses (including Exhaustion)	3·26	6·76	1·21	2·45	2·16	1·96	1·48	33·05	27
28	I.A.T.	1·07	8·47	2·90	4·78	4·73	2·73	2·57	46·69	28
29	*Total Admissions for Diseases*	24·77	49·60	42·78	63·81	54·45	49·66	46·88	568·90	29
30	Injuries—Enemy Action	34·12	38·39	9·38	6·50	18·58	1·87	0·94	188·16	30
31	Injuries—Accidental	12·10	10·48	9·96	9·32	8·44	7·01	6·66	109·67	31
32	Injuries—Self Inflicted	—	—	0·16	0·23	—	0·03	—	0·72	32
33	Injuries—Burns	0·82	1·16	0·79	0·54	0·72	0·42	0·74	8·87	33
34	*Total Admissions for Injuries*	47·04	50·02	20·28	16·58	27·74	9·33	8·34	307·41	34
35	*Total Admissions*	71·81	99·17	63·06	80·39	82·19	58·98	55·22	876·45	35

TABLE 43

British North African and Central Mediterranean Forces. African Troops. Causes of Admission to Medical Units, 1944
Breakdown of Certain Diseases Shown in Table 42. Mean Monthly and Estimated Annual Rates per 1,000 Strength

Source: B.N.A.F. and C.M.F. Weekly Health States

	CAUSES	June	July	Aug.	Sept.	Oct.	Nov.	Dec.	E.A.R.	
	Dysentery									
1	Protozoal	—	0·31	0·16	0·04	0·08	0·27	0·25	1·87	1
2	Bacillary and B.E.	0·56	1·28	1·00	0·27	0·38	0·12	0·07	6·31	2
3	Clinical and I.E.	0·63	0·79	0·37	0·42	0·53	0·45	0·22	5·84	3
	Totals	1·19	2·38	1·53	0·73	0·98	0·83	0·54	14·02	4
	Enteric Group of Fevers									
5	Typhoid	—	—	—	—	—	0·03	—	0·05	5
6	Para A	—	—	—	—	—	—	—	—	6
7	Para B	—	—	—	—	—	—	—	—	7
8	Para C	—	—	—	—	—	—	—	—	8
9	Clinical	0·13	—	—	—	—	—	—	0·21	9
	Totals	0·13	—	—	—	—	0·03	—	0·27	10
	Jaundice									
11	Infective Hepatitis	0·50	0·55	1·84	2·56	2·42	1·78	1·83	19·69	11
12	Leptospirosis	—	—	—	—	—	—	—	—	12
13	Post-Arsphenamine	—	—	0·05	—	0·04	0·06	0·12	0·47	13
14	Other Forms	0·13	—	—	—	—	—	—	0·21	14
	Totals	0·63	0·55	1·90	2·56	2·46	1·84	1·95	20·37	15
	Malaria									
16	Primary B.T.	0·56	2·99	0·69	0·99	0·53	0·39	0·12	10·74	16
17	Primary Q.	—	—	—	—	—	—	—	—	17
18	Primary M.T.	0·13	0·31	0·11	0·08	0·19	0·12	0·15	1·83	18
19	Primary Clinical	—	0·49	0·37	0·08	0·23	0·03	0·03	2·08	19
20	*Total Primary*	0·69	3·78	1·16	1·15	0·95	0·54	0·30	14·65	20
21	Relapse B.T.	0·38	1·10	0·79	0·61	0·38	0·39	0·22	6·62	21
22	Relapse Q.	—	—	—	—	—	—	—	—	22
23	Relapse M.T.	0·19	0·06	—	—	—	—	0·03	0·47	23
24	Relapse Clinical	—	0·06	0·05	0·08	0·04	—	—	0·39	24
25	*Total Relapse*	0·56	1·22	0·84	0·69	0·42	0·39	0·25	7·48	25
26	*Total Malaria*	1·25	5·00	2·00	1·83	1·36	0·92	0·54	22·13	26

	Pediculosis									
27	Capitas	—	0·06	—	—	0·08	0·03	—	0·29	27
28	Corporis	—	—	—	—	0·08	0·06	0·03	0·27	28
29	Pubis	—	0·12	0·05	0·23	0·15	0·21	0·49	2·16	29
30	*Totals*	—	0·18	0·05	0·23	0·30	0·30	0·52	2·72	30
	Venereal Diseases									
31	Gonorrhoea	0·69	2·01	3·48	4·66	4·39	4·10	2·84	37·99	31
32	Syphilis	0·25	0·49	0·42	0·34	0·53	0·86	0·77	6·27	32
33	Chancroid	0·75	0·37	0·53	1·03	2·20	2·02	1·31	14·06	33
34	Lympho-granuloma	—	—	—	—	—	—	—	0·07	34
35	Other Forms	0·25	0·49	0·42	1·49	0·68	0·51	0·47	7·38	35
39	*Totals*	1·95	3·35	4·85	7·53	7·83	7·48	5·38	65·77	36

TABLE 44

British North African and Central Mediterranean Forces. British Troops. Causes of Admission to Medical Units, 1945
Mean Monthly and Annual Rates per 1,000 Strength

Source: B.N.A.F. and C.M.F. Weekly Health States (Jan.–June) and Monthly States (July–Dec.)

	CAUSES	Jan.	Feb.	Mar.	Apr.	May	June	July	Aug.	Sept.	Oct.	Nov.	Dec.	Annual	
1	Diphtheria	0·46	0·37	0·25	0·17	0·13	0·08	0·08	0·09	0·12	0·16	0·15	0·15	2·21	1
2	Dermatophytosis	0·37	0·62	0·81	1·27	2·02	2·40	N.A.	N.A.	N.A.	N.A.	N.A.	N.A.	14·97*	2
3	Dysentery	0·35	0·23	0·18	0·19	0·39	0·93	0·40	0·33	0·27	0·20	0·16	0·13	3·75	3
4	Enteric Group of Fevers	0·02	0·01	0·01	0·01	0·00	0·03	0·03	0·02	0·04	0·03	0·01	0·01	0·21	4
5	Food Poisoning	0·11	0·01	0·01	0·02	0·02	0·07	0·15	0·17	—	0·01	—	0·01	0·59	5
6	Gas Gangrene	0·01	—	—	0·00	—	—	N.A.	N.A.	N.A.	N.A.	N.A.	N.A.	0·02*	6
7	Helminthic Disease	0·02	0·01	0·02	0·02	0·01	0·01	0·02	0·01	0·01	0·02	0·01	0·01	0·17	7
8	Influenza	0·02	0·02	0·05	0·00	0·00	—	0·03	0·02	0·01	0·01	0·01	0·05	0·23	8
9	Jaundice	1·41	1·14	0·93	0·79	0·76	0·87	1·07	1·54	1·97	1·54	1·28	1·07	14·36	9
10	Malaria	1·55	1·42	1·75	2·16	2·61	2·60	2·70	1·53	1·02	0·62	0·37	0·37	18·70	10
11	Meningitis	0·01	0·02	0·01	0·00	0·01	0·03	0·01	0·01	0·00	—	0·00	—	0·12*	11
12	Pediculosis†	2·84	3·13	2·78	2·11	2·25	2·35	N.A.	N.A.	N.A.	N.A.	N.A.	N.A.	30·91	12
13	Pneumonia	0·36	0·58	1·30	1·60	0·86	0·43	0·31	0·18	0·15	0·23	0·38	0·49	6·88	13
14	Poliomyelitis	0·01	0·00	0·00	0·00	0·01	0·03	0·07	0·03	0·03	0·02	0·02	0·01	0·22	14
15	Sandfly Fever	—	—	0·00	—	0·49	2·72	3·00	1·26	0·37	0·02	0·01	—	7·86	15
16	Scabies†	3·02	3·53	3·56	3·21	3·15	3·49	N.A.	N.A.	N.A.	N.A.	N.A.	N.A.	39·90*	16
17	Smallpox	0·01	0·00	0·00	0·00	0·00	0·01	0·02	—	—	—	—	—	0·04	17
18	Tetanus	—	—	—	—	—	—	—	—	—	—	0·00	—	0·00	18
19	Tuberculosis—Pulmonary	0·05	0·07	0·07	0·04	0·07	0·05	0·13	0·11	0·07	0·02	0·03	0·04	0·75	19
20	Tuberculosis—Other Forms	0·01	0·00	0·01	0·01	0·01	0·00	0·00	0·01	0·01	0·01	0·01	0·01	0·08	20
21	Typhus	—	—	—	—	—	0·01	0·00	—	—	—	—	—	0·01	21
22	Undulant Fever	0·00	0·00	0·01	0·01	0·00	0·00	N.A.	N.A.	N.A.	N.A.	N.A.	N.A.	0·05*	22
23	Venereal Diseases	5·18	5·40	5·20	4·90	4·74	4·76	5·34	7·09	6·18	6·96	7·44	7·98	71·17	23
24	Diseases of the Digestive System	4·14	3·51	3·36	3·22	3·87	4·23	N.A.	N.A.	N.A.	N.A.	N.A.	N.A.	38·35	24
25	Diseases of the Respiratory System	4·13	3·18	3·13	2·18	1·91	2·08	N.A.	N.A.	N.A.	N.A.	N.A.	N.A.	36·72	25
26	Diseases of the Nervous System	0·27	0·25	0·18	0·19	0·16	0·18	N.A.	N.A.	N.A.	N.A.	N.A.	N.A.	1·46	26
27	Diseases of the Skin	2·85	2·89	2·88	2·52	2·48	2·20	N.A.	N.A.	N.A.	N.A.	N.A.	N.A.	31·65*	27
28	Psychoses	0·07	0·05	0·04	0·02	0·06	0·09	0·11	0·16	0·10	0·13	0·14	0·12	1·09	28
29	Psychoneuroses (including Exhaustion)	0·91	0·45	0·53	1·01	0·46	0·33	0·52	0·36	0·35	0·27	0·47	0·60	6·25	29
30	I.A.T.	4·03	2·63	2·73	2·39	2·46	3·07	3·56	3·83	3·39	3·51	3·32	3·22	39·14	30
31	*Total Admissions for Diseases*	39·80	36·87	35·11	33·69	36·47	44·22	43·90	38·91	32·26	29·35	30·01	32·57	433·16	31
32	Injuries—Enemy Action	2·42	0·62	0·98	4·67	0·13	—	0·08	0·01	0·01	0·02	0·01	0·00	8·95	32
33	Injuries—Non-enemy Action	4·48	3·97	4·59	4·90	5·81	5·03	5·62	4·49	3·32	3·06	3·42	3·81	52·51	33
34	*Total Admissions for Injuries*	6·90	4·59	5·57	9·57	5·94	5·03	5·70	5·00	3·33	3·08	3·43	3·82	61·46	34
35	*Total Admissions*	46·71	41·46	40·68	43·26	42·41	49·25	49·60	43·41	35·60	32·43	33·44	36·38	494·62	35

† Includes cases treated outside Medical Units.
* Equivalent Annual Rates.
N.A. No figures available.

TABLE 45

British North African and Central Mediterranean Forces. British Troops. Causes of Admission to Medical Units, 1945
Breakdown of Certain Diseases Shown in Table 44. Mean Monthly and Annual Rates per 1,000 Strength

Source: B.N.A.F. and C.M.F. Weekly Health States (Jan.–June) and Monthly States (July–Dec.)

	CAUSES	Jan.	Feb.	Mar.	Apr.	May	June	July	Aug.	Sept.	Oct.	Nov.	Dec.	Annual	
	Dysentery														
1	Protozoal	0·10	0·06	0·07	0·04	0·04	0·08	0·01	0·03	0·04	0·02	0·06	—	0·55	1
2	Bacillary and B.E.	0·09	0·03	0·04	0·05	0·17	0·43	0·35	0·25	0·18	0·15	0·04	0·06	1·85	2
3	Clinical and I.E.	0·17	0·13	0·07	0·10	0·17	0·42	0·04	0·05	0·05	0·03	0·05	0·07	1·35	3
4	*Totals*	0·35	0·23	0·18	0·19	0·39	0·93	0·40	0·33	0·27	0·20	0·16	0·13	3·75	4
	Enteric Group of Fevers														
5	Typhoid	0·01	0·01	0·00	0·00	0·00	0·02	0·02	0·01	0·02	0·02	0·01	0·01	0·13	5
6	Para A	—	0·00	—	—	0·00	—	}						}	6
7	Para B	0·01	0·00	—	0·00	—	0·01	0·1	0·00	0·02	0·01	0·00	—	0·06	7
8	Para C	—	—	—	—	—	—	}						}	8
9	Clinical	0·00	0·00	0·00	0·00	—	0·01	0·00	0·01	—	0·00	—	—	0·03	9
10	*Totals*	0·02	0·01	0·01	0·01	0·00	0·03	0·03	0·02	0·04	0·03	0·01	0·01	0·21	10
	Jaundice														
11	Infective Hepatitis	1·36	1·10	0·89	0·75	0·74	0·85	1·06	1·54	1·96	1·53	1·28	1·07	14·14	11
12	Leptospirosis	—	0·01	0·00	—	—	0·00	0·00	—	0·00	0·00	—	—	0·02	12
13	Post-Arsphenamine	0·05	0·03	0·03	0·04	0·02	0·01	0·01	0·00	0·01	—	—	—	0·20	13
14	*Totals*	1·41	1·14	0·93	0·79	0·76	0·87	1·07	1·54	1·97	1·54	1·28	1·07	14·36	14
	Malaria														
15	Primary B.T.	0·28	0·25	0·49	0·65	0·84	1·06	1·06	0·60	0·40	0·14	0·06	0·10	5·93	15
16	Primary Q.	0·00	0·00	0·00	—	—	0·00	0·01	0·01	—	—	0·00	0·00	0·04	16
17	Primary M.T.	0·01	0·01	0·01	0·00	0·05	0·03	0·05	0·06	0·05	0·07	0·01	0·00	0·34	17
18	Primary Clinical	0·08	0·07	0·06	0·12	0·16	0·14	0·20	0·08	0·06	0·04	0·02	0·02	1·04	18
19	*Total Primary*	0·37	0·33	0·56	0·77	1·05	1·23	1·32	0·76	0·51	0·24	0·09	0·12	7·34	19
20	Relapse B.T.	1·11	1·03	1·12	1·29	1·44	1·27	1·30	0·70	0·45	0·36	0·25	0·24	10·55	20
21	Relapse Q.	—	0·00	—	0·00	0·00	0·01	0·00	—	—	—	—	—	0·02	21
22	Relapse M.T.	0·01	0·01	0·02	0·01	0·01	0·01	0·02	0·03	0·02	0·01	0·01	—	0·15	22
23	Relapse Clinical	0·06	0·05	0·06	0·09	0·10	0·09	0·07	0·04	0·04	0·01	0·02	0·01	0·64	23
24	*Total Relapse*	1·18	1·10	1·20	1·39	1·55	1·37	1·39	0·77	0·51	0·38	0·28	0·25	11·36	24
25	*Total Malaria*	1·55	1·42	1·75	2·16	2·61	2·60	2·70	1·53	1·02	0·62	0·37	0·37	18·70	25

TABLE 45—*Continued*

British North African and Central Mediterranean Forces. British Troops. Causes of Admission to Medical Units, 1945
Breakdown of Certain Diseases Shown in Table 44. Mean Monthly and Annual Rates per 1,000 Strength

Source: B.N.A.F. and C.M.F. Weekly Health States (Jan.–June) and Monthly States (July–Dec.)

	CAUSES	Jan.	Feb.	Mar.	Apr.	May	June	July	Aug.	Sept.	Oct.	Nov.	Dec.	Annual	
	Pediculosis†														
26	Capitas	0·05	0·04	0·10	0·04	0·03	0·07	N.A.	N.A.	N.A.	N.A.	N.A.	N.A.	0·65*	26
27	Corporis	0·44	0·48	0·32	0·34	0·17	0·10	N.A.	N.A.	N.A.	N.A.	N.A.	N.A.	3·68*	27
28	Pubis	2·35	2·60	2·37	1·74	2·05	2·17	N.A.	N.A.	N.A.	N.A.	N.A.	N.A.	26·59*	28
29	*Totals*	2·84	3·13	2·78	2·11	2·25	2·35	N.A.	N.A.	N.A.	N.A.	N.A.	N.A.	30·91*	29
	Venereal Diseases														
30	Gonorrhoea	2·97	2·99	2·68	2·78	2·87	3·05	3·98	5·66	5·10	5·64	6·05	6·51	50·26	30
31	Syphilis	0·54	0·59	0·45	0·45	0·43	0·68	0·65	0·72	0·56	0·58	0·67	0·81	7·13	31
32	Chancroid	0·98	1·01	0·79	0·76	0·73	0·56	0·70	0·71	0·50	0·74	0·72	0·65	8·85	32
33	Lympho-granuloma	0·01	—	0·00	—	0·00	—	—	—	0·03	—	—	0·01	0·04	33
34	Other Forms	0·69	0·82	1·28	0·91	0·71	0·48	—	—	—	—	—	—	4·88	34
35	*Totals*	5·18	5·40	5·20	4·90	4·74	4·76	5·34	7·09	6·18	6·96	7·44	7·98	71·17	35

† Includes cases treated outside Medical Units
* Equivalent Annual Rates.
N.A. No figures available.

TABLE 46

British North African and Central Mediterranean Forces. Canadian Troops. Causes of Admission to Medical Units, 1945
Mean Monthly Rates (Jan. to June) and Equivalent Annual Rates per 1,000 Strength

Source: B.N.A.F. and C.M.F. Weekly Health States

	CAUSES	Jan.	Feb.	Mar.	Apr.	May	June	E.A.R.	
1	Diphtheria	2·08	1·62	0·92	—	0·97	—	11·18	1
2	Dermatophytosis	0·35	0·55	0·21	2·05	0·97	0·78	8·28	2
3	Dysentery	0·49	0·40	0·49	—	—	—	2·77	3
4	Influenza	0·58	0·15	0·14	—	—	—	1·75	4
5	Jaundice	3·21	2·42	2·62	0·68	—	—	17·86	5
6	Malaria	1·04	1·77	1·77	1·03	0·97	—	13·16	6
7	Meningitis	—	0·09	0·14	—	—	—	0·47	7
8	Pediculosis	2·75	1·68	2·40	—	0·97	—	15·62	8
9	Pneumonia	0·53	1·84	2·26	1·71	0·97	—	14·61	9
10	Scabies	7·09	5·26	6·29	6·16	2·42	0·78	56·02	10
11	Tuberculosis	0·02	0·15	—	—	—	0·78	1·90	11
12	Venereal Diseases	11·17	17·47	22·91	14·37	15·99	14·78	193·38	12
13	Diseases of the Digestive System	8·24	10·71	14·21	3·42	0·97	1·56	78·22	13
14	Diseases of the Respiratory System	6·14	7·28	11·31	3·08	—	—	55·63	14
15	Diseases of the Nervous System	0·37	0·52	0·21	—	—	—	2·21	15
16	Diseases of the Skin	4·04	4·28	7·21	3·76	4·84	—	48·29	16
17	Psychoses	0·04	0·31	—	0·34	—	—	1·37	17
18	Psychoneuroses (including Exhaustion)	2·98	1·90	0·64	1·03	—	—	13·09	18
19	I.A.T.	6·25	4·25	3·89	2·05	—	—	32·88	19
20	*Total Admissions for Diseases*	59·73	58·15	79·20	56·47	34·39	19·45	614·77	20
21	Injuries—Enemy Action	11·61	5·57	1·56	—	—	—	37·47	21
22	Injuries—Non-Enemy Action	6·21	7·37	11·67	9·58	5·81	—	81·29	22
23	*Total Admissions for Injuries*	17·82	12·94	13·23	9·58	5·81	—	118·76	23
24	*Total Admissions*	77·55	71·09	92·43	66·05	40·20	19·45	733·53	24

During the period under review the following cases were reported:
Enteric Group; Clinical, 1 case. Food Poisoning, 2 cases. Gas Gangrene, 3 cases. Helminthiasis, 4 cases. Post-Arsphenamine Jaundice, 1 case.
There were no reported cases of:
Poliomyelitis, Sandfly Fever, Smallpox, Tetanus, Trench Foot, Typhus, Undulant Fever.

TABLE 47

British North African and Central Mediterranean Forces. Canadian Troops. Causes of Admission to Medical Units, 1945
Breakdown of Certain Diseases Shown in Table 46. Mean Monthly Rates (Jan. to June) and Equivalent Annual Rates per 1,000 Strength

Source: B.N.A.F. and C.M.F. Weekly Health States

	CAUSES	Jan.	Feb.	Mar.	Apr.	May	June	E.A.R.	
	Dysentery								
1	Protozoal	0·35	0·28	0·35	—	—	—	1·96	1
2	Bacillary and B.E.	0·05	0·06	0·14	—	—	—	0·51	2
3	Clinical and I.E.	0·09	0·06	—	—	—	—	0·30	3
4	*Totals*	0·49	0·40	0·49	—	—	—	2·77	4
	Malaria								
5	Primary B.T.	0·49	0·61	0·50	—	—	—	3·20	5
6	Primary Q.	—	—	—	—	—	—	—	6
7	Primary M.T.	—	—	—	—	—	—	—	7
8	Primary Clinical	0·23	0·34	0·14	—	—	—	1·41	8
9	*Total Primary*	0·72	0·95	0·64	—	—	—	4·61	9
10	Relapse B.T.	0·28	0·80	1·13	1·03	0·97	—	8·41	10
11	Relapse Q.	—	—	—	—	—	—	—	11
12	Relapse M.T.	—	—	—	—	—	—	—	12
13	Relapse Clinical	0·04	0·03	—	—	—	—	0·13	13
14	*Total Relapse*	0·32	0·83	1·13	1·03	0·97	—	8·54	14
15	*Total Malaria*	1·04	1·77	1·77	1·03	0·97	—	13·16	15
	Pediculosis								
16	Capitas	2·36	1·19	0·28	—	—	—	7·68	16
17	Corporis	0·07	0·03	0·21	—	—	—	0·63	17
18	Pubis	0·32	0·46	1·91	—	0·97	—	7·31	18
19	*Totals*	2·75	1·68	2·40	—	0·97	—	15·62	19
	Venereal Diseases								
20	Gonorrhoea	4·98	8·93	13·01	6·16	8·24	7·00	96·63	20
21	Syphilis	0·87	1·74	1·91	1·37	2·42	2·33	21·29	21
22	Chancroid	0·70	1·59	4·24	3·76	3·39	3·89	35·17	22
23	Lympho-granuloma	—	—	—	—	0·97	—	1·94	23
24	Other Forms	4·62	5·20	3·75	3·08	0·97	1·56	38·35	24
25	*Totals*	11·17	17·47	22·91	14·37	15·99	14·78	193·38	25

TABLE 48

British North African and Central Mediterranean Forces. New Zealand Troops. Causes of Admission to Medical Units, 1945
Mean Monthly Rates (Jan. to June) and Equivalent Annual Rates per 1,000 Strength

Source: B.N.A.F. and C.M.F. Weekly Health States

	CAUSES	Jan.	Feb.	Mar.	Apr.	May	June	E.A.R.	
1	Diphtheria	1·76	1·26	1·34	0·22	0·45	0·12	10·31	1
2	Dermatophytosis	0·57	0·69	0·53	0·39	1·05	1·16	8·77	2
3	Dysentery	1·31	0·92	0·62	1·11	1·91	1·04	13·82	3
4	Enteric Group of Fevers	One case	—	—	—	One case	—	0·20	4
5	Food Poisoning	—	—	—	—	—	—	—	5
6	Gas Gangrene	—	—	—	0·28	—	—	0·55	6
7	Helminthic Diseases	0·51	0·40	0·09	0·06	0·09	0·12	2·53	7
8	Influenza	0·06	0·06	1·16	0·22	0·27	—	3·53	8
9	Jaundice*	4·44	3·50	1·69	0·78	0·73	0·93	24·12	9
10	Malaria	0·11	—	0·62	0·50	0·68	0·99	5·81	10
11	Meningitis	—	0·06	—	0·06	—	—	0·22	11
12	Pediculosis	2·16	1·21	1·16	1·94	0·95	0·58	15·99	12
13	Pneumonia	0·91	1·09	1·47	1·71	1·09	0·23	13·12	13
14	Poliomyelitis	—	—	—	—	—	—	—	14
15	Sandfly Fever	—	—	—	—	0·09	0·06	0·30	15
16	Scabies	3·24	3·90	3·52	3·05	6·77	4·29	49·53	16
17	Smallpox	—	—	—	—	—	—	—	17
18	Tetanus	—	—	—	—	—	—	—	18
19	Tuberculosis—Pulmonary	0·06	0·17	0·13	0·06	0·14	0·17	1·46	19
20	Tuberculosis—Other Forms	—	—	—	0·06	—	0·06	0·23	20
21	Typhus	—	—	—	—	—	—	—	21
22	Undulant Fever	0·11	—	—	—	—	—	0·23	22
23	Venereal Diseases	4·44	5·28	5·03	5·60	14·03	22·31	113·37	23
24	Diseases of the Digestive System	9·11	5·97	7·48	7·98	7·40	5·45	86·75	24
25	Diseases of the Respiratory System	6·09	8·15	6·50	3·27	3·77	2·61	60·76	25
26	Diseases of the Nervous System	0·85	0·80	0·18	2·22	0·77	0·52	10·69	26
27	Diseases of the Skin	6·60	6·71	5·96	3·32	7·63	7·48	75·42	27
28	Psychoses	—	0·06	0·09	—	0·05	—	0·38	28
29	Psychoneuroses (including Exhaustion)	0·85	—	0·27	1·00	0·41	0·06	5·17	29
30	I.A.T.	6·83	5·45	4·27	4·38	4·13	3·89	57·89	30
31	*Total Admissions for Diseases*	63·97	55·14	49·94	51·95	58·14	61·78	681·82	31
32	Injuries—Enemy Action	5·01	5·05	1·07	57·05	3·18	—	142·70	32
33	Injuries—Non-Enemy Action	9·16	8·66	12·99	11·24	12·63	9·39	128·16	33
34	*Total Admissions for Injuries*	14·17	13·71	14·06	68·29	15·81	9·39	270·86	34
35	*Total Admissions*	78·14	68·85	64·00	120·24	73·94	71·16	952·68	35

* Infective Hepatitis only. No other cases of Jaundice recorded.

TABLE 49

British North African and Central Mediterranean Forces. New Zealand Troops. Causes of Admission to Medical Units, 1945
Breakdown of Certain Diseases Shown in Table 48. Mean Monthly Rates (Jan. to June) and Equivalent Annual Rates per 1,000 Strength

Source: B.N.A.F. and C.M.F. Weekly Health States

	CAUSES	Jan.	Feb.	Mar.	Apr.	May	June	E.A.R.	
	Dysentery								
1	Protozoal	0·85	0·34	0·49	0·50	0·82	0·52	7·05	1
2	Bacillary and B.E.	0·34	0·23	0·04	0·28	0·77	0·30	3·87	2
3	Clinical and I.E.	0·11	0·34	0·09	0·33	0·32	0·23	2·86	3
	Totals	1·31	0·91	0·62	1·11	1·91	1·04	13·82	4
4	*Malaria*								
5	Primary B.T.	0·06	—	0·27	0·22	0·41	0·70	3·30	5
6	Primary Q.	—	—	—	—	—	—	—	6
7	Primary M.T.	—	—	—	—	—	—	—	7
8	Primary Clinical	—	—	—	0·11	—	0·17	0·57	8
9	*Total Primary*	0·06	—	0·27	0·33	0·41	0·87	3·87	9
..									
10	Relapse B.T.	0·06	—	0·36	0·11	0·18	0·12	1·64	10
11	Relapse Q.	—	—	—	0·06	—	—	0·11	11
12	Relapse M.T.	—	—	—	—	—	—	—	12
13	Relapse Clinical	—	—	—	—	0·09	—	0·18	13
14	*Total Relapse*	0·06	—	0·36	0·17	0·27	0·12	1·94	14
15	*Total Malaria*	0·11	—	0·62	0·50	0·68	0·99	5·81	15
	Pediculosis								
16	Capitas	—	—	—	—	—	—	—	16
17	Corporis	0·06	—	—	0·67	0·23	—	1·90	17
18	Pubis	2·11	1·21	1·16	1·27	0·73	0·58	14·10	18
19	*Totals*	2·16	1·21	1·16	1·94	0·95	0·58	15·99	19
	Venereal Diseases								
20	Gonorrhoea	1·76	2·98	2·09	2·55	7·86	12·29	59·06	20
21	Syphilis	0·57	0·29	0·31	—	0·09	0·23	29·80	21
22	Chancroid	0·74	0·92	0·94	1·11	3·23	1·97	17·79	22
23	Lympho-granuloma	—	—	—	—	—	—	—	23
24	Other Forms	1·37	1·09	1·69	1·94	2·86	7·82	33·54	24
25	*Totals*	4·44	5·28	5·03	5·60	14·03	22·31	113·37	25

TABLE 50

British North African and Central Mediterranean Forces. Indian Troops. Causes of Admission to Medical Units, 1945
Mean Monthly and Annual Rates per 1,000 Strength

Source: B.N.A.F. and C.M.F. Weekly Health States (Jan.–June) and Monthly States (July–Dec.)

	CAUSES	Jan.	Feb.	Mar.	Apr.	May	June	July	Aug.	Sept.	Oct.	Nov.	Dec.	Annual	
1	Diphtheria	0·04	0·05	0·02	0·05	0·01	—	—	0·02	0·02	—	—	—	0·20	1
2	Dermatophytosis	0·05	0·02	0·08	0·09	0·40	0·37	N.A.	N.A.	N.A.	N.A.	N.A.	N.A.	2·03*	2
3	Dysentery	0·26	0·10	0·21	0·20	0·22	0·44	0·40	0·22	0·23	0·22	0·09	0·42	3·00	3
4	Enteric Group of Fevers	—	—	0·02	—	0·03	—	—	—	—	—	—	—	0·05	4
5	Food Poisoning	—	—	—	—	—	0·02	0·06	0·02	—	—	—	—	0·09	5
6	Gas Gangrene	—	—	0·02	0·02	—	—	N.A.	N.A.	N.A.	N.A.	N.A.	N.A.	0·08*	6
7	Helminthic Diseases	0·09	0·09	0·01	0·06	0·11	0·09	0·71	0·67	0·18	0·40	0·20	0·56	3·16	7
8	Influenza	—	—	0·33	0·02	—	—	0·02	0·02	—	—	—	—	0·38	8
9	Jaundice	1·36	0·61	0·78	0·60	0·75	0·65	0·56	0·75	0·57	0·84	1·34	1·49	10·29	9
10	Malaria	0·28	0·51	0·75	0·43	1·32	0·95	1·06	1·09	0·57	0·45	0·32	0·74	8·47	10
11	Meningitis	—	—	0·02	0·02	—	—	—	—	—	—	—	—	0·04	11
12	Pediculosis†	0·21	1·22	1·11	1·46	1·56	0·25	N.A.	N.A.	N.A.	N.A.	N.A.	N.A.	11·61*	12
13	Pneumonia	0·78	0·44	0·28	0·29	0·15	0·11	0·12	0·33	0·08	0·15	0·23	0·14	3·09	13
14	Poliomyelitis	—	—	—	—	—	—	0·02	—	—	—	—	—	0·02	14
15	Sandfly Fever	—	—	—	—	0·18	0·05	0·69	0·02	0·49	0·11	—	—	1·54	15
16	Scabies	0·58	1·38	0·82	0·88	1·06	0·90	0·72	0·76	0·34	0·33	0·58	0·37	8·72	16
17	Smallpox	0·32	—	0·01	—	—	—	0·06	—	—	—	—	—	0·39	17
18	Tetanus	0·02	—	—	—	0·04	—	—	—	—	—	—	—	0·06	18
19	Tuberculosis—Pulmonary	0·28	0·53	0·41	0·38	0·11	0·33	0·32	0·02	0·16	0·18	0·18	0·28	3·19	19
20	Tuberculosis—Other Forms	0·02	0·03	0·01	0·05	0·01	—	0·02	—	0·03	0·02	—	—	0·20	20
21	Typhus	—	—	—	—	—	—	—	—	—	—	—	—	—	21
22	Undulant Fever	—	—	0·02	0·02	0·03	—	N.A.	N.A.	N.A.	N.A.	N.A.	N.A.	0·13*	22
23	Venereal Diseases	2·89	3·11	2·60	2·21	2·53	3·37	5·13	8·97	7·58	8·90	12·18	7·11	66·57	23
24	Diseases of the Digestive System	3·03	2·39	3·26	3·95	4·01	5·29	}N.A.	N.A.	N.A.	N.A.	N.A.	N.A.	{43·86*	24
25	Diseases of the Respiratory System	6·61	7·22	5·40	3·22	2·86	2·81							{56·22*	25
26	Diseases of the Nervous System	0·37	0·26	0·35	0·47	0·57	0·46	}N.A.	N.A.	N.A.	N.A.	N.A.	N.A.	{4·94*	26
27	Diseases of the Skin	2·52	2·62	2·57	2·38	2·22	1·92							{28·43*	27
28	Psychoses	0·04	0·05	0·09	0·08	0·07	0·11	0·19	0·22	0·08	0·20	0·41	0·05	1·57	28
29	Psychoneuroses (including Exhaustion)	0·46	0·41	0·32	0·20	0·69	0·26	0·69	0·27	0·21	0·24	0·15	0·14	4·03	29
30	I.A.T.	4·39	2·87	2·52	2·38	2·46	2·20	3·75	4·41	1·80	1·91	2·80	2·37	33·85	30
31	*Total Admissions for Diseases*	39·02	31·74	39·52	37·90	39·62	43·54	33·70	42·76	26·90	26·51	33·56	29·97	424·72	31
32	Injuries—Enemy Action	4·99	3·79	6·63	21·42	0·46	—	—	0·17	—	—	—	—	37·45	32
33	Injuries—Non-Enemy Action	4·46	4·11	6·22	7·35	6·75	8·05	7·04	7·35	4·01	4·23	6·58	6·32	72·51	33
34	*Total Admissions for Injuries*	9·44	7·90	12·85	28·77	7·25	8·05	7·04	7·52	4·01	4·23	6·58	6·32	109·96	34
35	*Total Admissions*	48·46	39·63	52·37	66·68	46·87	51·59	40·73	50·28	30·91	30·74	40·14	36·29	534·68	35

† Includes cases treated outside Medical Units.
* Equivalent Annual Rates.
N.A. No figures available.

TABLE 51

British North African and Central Mediterranean Forces. Indian Troops. Causes of Admission to Medical Units, 1945
Breakdown of Certain Diseases Shown in Table 50. Mean Monthly and Annual Rates per 1,000 Strength

Source: B.N.A.F. and C.M.F. Weekly Health States (Jan.–June) and Monthly States (July–Dec.)

	CAUSES	Jan.	Feb.	Mar.	Apr.	May	June	July	Aug.	Sept.	Oct.	Nov.	Dec.	Annual	
	Dysentery														
1	Protozoal	0·18	0·05	0·09	—	0·14	0·11	—	0·03	0·05	0·02	0·03	—	0·69	1
2	Bacillary and B.E.	0·02	—	0·06	0·05	0·04	0·16	0·37	0·16	0·18	0·15	—	0·09	1·26	2
3	Clinical and I.E.	0·07	0·05	0·06	0·15	0·04	0·18	0·03	0·03	—	0·05	0·06	0·33	1·05	3
4	*Totals*	0·26	0·10	0·21	0·20	0·22	0·44	0·40	0·22	0·23	0·22	0·09	0·42	3·00	4
	Jaundice														
5	Infective Hepatitis	1·34	0·59	0·78	0·55	0·75	0·65	0·54	0·75	0·57	0·84	1·34	1·49	10·19	5
6	Leptospirosis	—	—	—	—	—	—	0·02	—	—	—	—	—	0·02	6
7	Post-Arsphenamine	0·02	0·02	—	0·05	—	—	—	—	—	—	—	—	0·08	7
8	*Totals*	1·36	0·61	0·78	0·60	0·75	0·65	0·56	0·75	0·57	0·84	1·34	1·49	10·29	8
	Malaria														
9	Primary B.T.	0·11	0·15	0·10	0·11	0·46	0·48	0·26	0·37	0·16	0·13	0·15	0·33	2·80	9
10	Primary Q.	—	—	0·01	—	—	—	—	—	—	—	0·06	0·05	0·12	10
11	Primary M.T.	—	0·02	—	—	0·08	0·02	0·07	0·08	0·15	0·29	—	—	0·71	11
12	Primary Clinical	—	0·05	0·07	0·03	0·08	0·05	0·13	0·17	0·03	0·02	—	0·05	0·69	12
13	*Total Primary*	0·11	0·22	0·18	0·14	0·62	0·55	0·47	0·62	0·34	0·44	0·20	0·42	4·31	13
14	Relapse B.T.	0·16	0·22	0·51	0·27	0·61	0·35	0·40	0·41	0·20	0·02	0·12	0·09	3·35	14
15	Relapse Q.	—	—	—	—	—	—	—	—	—	—	—	0·14	0·14	15
16	Relapse M.T.	0·02	—	0·01	0·02	0·03	0·02	0·09	—	0·02	—	—	—	0·20	16
17	Relapse Clinical	—	0·07	0·05	—	0·06	0·04	0·10	0·06	0·02	—	—	0·09	0·48	17
18	*Total Relapse*	0·18	0·29	0·56	0·29	0·69	0·40	0·59	0·47	0·23	0·02	0·12	0·33	4·16	18
19	*Total Malaria*	0·28	0·51	0·75	0·43	1·32	0·95	1·06	1·09	0·57	0·45	0·32	0·74	8·47	19
	Pediculosis†														
20	Capitas	—	—	0·01	—	0·01	—	N.A.	N.A.	N.A.	N.A.	N.A.	N.A.	0·05*	20
21	Corporis	0·04	1·02	1·01	1·42	1·26	0·07	N.A.	N.A.	N.A.	N.A.	N.A.	N.A.	9·63*	21
22	Pubis	0·18	0·20	0·08	0·05	0·28	0·18	N.A.	N.A.	N.A.	N.A.	N.A.	N.A.	1·92*	22
	Totals	0·21	1·22	1·11	1·46	1·56	0·25	N.A.	N.A.	N.A.	N.A.	N.A.	N.A.	11·61*	23
	Venereal Disease														
24	Gonorrhoea	1·23	1·17	0·93	0·82	0·90	1·35	2·54	4·04	3·19	3·94	6·23	3·53	29·90	24
25	Syphilis	0·44	0·61	0·39	0·44	0·46	0·69	1·06	1·62	0·80	0·91	1·69	2·74	11·85	25
26	Chancroid	0·58	0·76	0·63	0·38	0·85	1·09	1·53	3·31	3·52	4·05	4·25	0·84	21·79	26
27	Lympho-granuloma	0·02	—	—	—	—	—	—	—	0·07	—	—	—	0·08	27
28	Other forms	0·62	0·56	0·64	0·56	0·32	0·25	—	—	—	—	—	—	2·95	28
	Totals	2·89	3·11	2·60	2·21	2·53	3·37	5·13	8·97	7·58	8·90	12·18	7·11	66·57	29

† Includes cases treated outside Medical Units.
* Equivalent Annual Rates.
N.A. No figures available.

TABLE 52

British North African and Central Mediterranean Forces. African Troops. Causes of Admission to Medical Units, 1945
Mean Monthly Rates (Jan. to June) and Equivalent Annual Rates per 1,000 Strength

Source: B.N.A.F. and C.M.F. Weekly Health States

	CAUSES	Jan.	Feb.	Mar.	Apr.	May	June	E.A.R.	
1	Diphtheria	0·12	0·19	0·03	0·09	0·05	0·02	1·01	1
2	Dermatophytosis	0·15	0·13	0·16	0·09	0·50	0·19	2·46	2
3	Dysentery	0·32	0·38	0·16	0·07	0·38	0·46	3·54	3
4	Enteric Group of Fevers	0·03	0·03	—	—	—	—	0·11	4
5	Food Poisoning	—	0·08	—	—	—	—	0·16	5
6	Gas Gangrene	—	—	—	0·02	—	—	0·04	6
7	Helminthic Diseases	0·03	0·05	0·02	0·18	0·18	0·10	1·11	7
8	Influenza	0·21	0·24	0·06	0·16	0·05	0·05	1·43	8
9	Jaundice	0·80	0·54	0·38	0·36	0·25	0·80	6·20	9
10	Malaria	0·26	0·27	0·28	0·36	1·04	0·90	6·22	10
11	Meningitis	0·03	0·08	0·08	0·09	0·02	—	0·58	11
12	Pediculosis	0·41	1·23	0·37	0·52	0·29	0·24	6·13	12
13	Pneumonia	0·53	0·51	0·50	0·54	0·43	0·17	5·37	13
	Poliomyelitis	—	—	—	—	—	—	—	14
15	Sandfly Fever	—	—	—	—	0·04	0·10	0·27	15
16	Scabies	1·09	0·99	0·70	0·94	1·29	1·29	12·59	16
17	Smallpox	—	—	—	—	—	—	—	17
18	Tetanus	—	—	—	—	—	—	—	18
19	Tuberculosis—Pulmonary	0·15	0·46	0·06	0·22	0·43	0·12	2·87	19
20	Tuberculosis—Other Forms	—	0·05	—	—	0·05	0·05	0·31	20
21	Typhus	—	—	—	—	—	—	—	21
22	Undulant Fever	—	—	—	—	—	0·05	0·10	22
23	Venereal Diseases	4·77	4·61	4·72	6·61	8·17	9·89	77·55	23
24	Diseases of the Digestive System	3·65	2·74	2·41	3·63	3·24	3·10	37·54	24
25	Diseases of the Respiratory System	4·12	3·62	2·51	1·75	1·58	1·29	14·86	25
26	Diseases of the Nervous System	0·56	0·27	0·25	0·25	0·25	0·12	3·40	26
27	Diseases of the Skin	3·48	2·95	1·99	2·17	2·81	2·93	32·67	27
28	Psychoses	1·12	0·08	0·15	0·52	0·32	0·21	4·81	28
29	Psychoneuroses (including Exhaustion)	1·86	0·86	0·58	0·58	0·56	0·39	9·64	29
30	I.A.T.	3·21	1·66	1·26	1·17	1·72	2·18	22·41	30
31	*Total Admissions for Diseases*	45·12	36·83	29·78	28·29	41·18	47·90	458·19	31
32	Injuries—Enemy Action	2·12	0·56	0·07	10·93	0·34	—	28·06	32
33	Injuries—Non-Enemy Action	7·01	5·82	5·93	7·73	8·47	7·66	75·23	33
34	*Total Admissions for Injuries*	9·13	6·38	6·00	18·66	8·81	7·66	113·29	34
35	*Total Admissions*	54·25	43·21	35·78	46·95	49·99	55·56	571·48	35

TABLE 53

British North African and Central Mediterranean Forces. African Troops. Causes of Admission to Medical Units, 1945
Breakdown of Certain Diseases Shown in Table 52. Mean Monthly Rates (Jan. to June) and Equivalent Annual Rates per 1,000 Strength

Source: B.N.A.F. and C.M.F. Weekly Health States

	CAUSES	Jan.	Feb.	Mar.	Apr.	May	June	E.A.R.	
	Dysentery								
1	Protozoal	0·06	0·05	0·09	0·07	0·09	0·19	1·11	1
2	Bacillary and B.E.	0·15	0·11	0·05	—	0·22	0·07	1·17	2
3	Clinical and I.E.	0·12	0·22	0·03	—	0·07	0·19	1·26	3
4	*Totals*	0·32	0·38	0·16	0·07	0·38	0·46	3·54	4
	Jaundice								
5	Infective Hepatitis	0·80	0·54	0·36	0·36	0·25	0·80	6·19	5
6	Leptospirosis	—	—	—	—	—	—	—	6
7	Post-Arsphenamine	—	—	0·02	—	—	—	0·02	7
8	*Totals*	0·80	0·54	0·38	0·36	0·25	0·80	6·20	8
	Malaria								
9	Primary B.T.	0·09	0·08	0·05	0·05	0·25	0·12	1·26	9
10	Primary Q.	—	—	—	—	0·02	—	0·04	10
11	Primary M.T.	0·09	—	0·02	—	0·04	—	0·28	11
12	Primary Clinical	0·03	0·03	0·03	0·02	0·07	0·02	0·41	12
13	*Total Primary*	0·21	0·11	0·09	0·07	0·38	0·14	1·99	13
14	Relapse B.T.	0·06	0·11	0·12	0·27	0·66	0·66	3·74	14
15	Relapse Q.	—	—	—	—	—	—	—	15
16	Relapse M.T.	—	0·05	—	—	—	—	0·11	16
17	Relapse Clinical	—	—	0·07	0·02	—	0·10	0·39	17
18	*Total Relapse*	0·06	0·16	0·19	0·29	0·66	0·75	4·24	18
19	*Total Malaria*	0·26	0·27	0·28	0·36	1·04	0·90	6·22	19
	Pediculosis								
20	Capitas	—	—	—	0·05	0·04	—	0·16	20
21	Corporis	0·12	0·16	0·05	0·13	0·02	—	0·95	21
22	Pubis	0·30	1·07	0·33	0·34	0·23	0·24	5·01	22
23	*Totals*	0·41	1·23	0·37	0·52	0·29	0·24	6·13	23
	Venereal Diseases								
24	Gonorrhoea	2·45	2·41	2·29	2·98	4·39	6·11	41·25	24
25	Syphilis	0·41	0·70	0·54	0·85	0·60	0·85	7·87	25
26	Chancroid	1·30	0·75	1·01	1·66	2·44	1·48	17·26	26
27	Lympho-granuloma	—	—	—	—	—	—	—	27
28	Other Forms	0·62	0·75	0·89	1·12	0·75	1·45	11·17	28
29	*Totals*	4·77	4·61	4·72	6·61	8·17	9·89	77·55	29

CHAPTER V

MIDDLE EAST FORCE

THAT PORTION of the British Army stationed in the Middle East before the war consisted of Regular Units in Egypt, the Sudan, Palestine and Cyprus. Soldiers were posted to the area for a period of five years.

After the outbreak of war, the Command was re-inforced, not only from Britain but also by Dominion and Colonial Units from India, Australia, New Zealand, South Africa and East and West Africa. In addition, there was a considerable amount of volunteer local recruitment chiefly among Maltese, Cypriots and Palestinian Jews.

In January 1942, the Persia and Iraq Command (P.A.I.C.) was absorbed by the Middle East Force, but in October of that year it was divorced from M.E.F. and once more became a separate entity. Subsequently, in February 1945, it was again absorbed. Similarly, in March 1942, troops in Malta came under the administration of M.E.F. until May 1943. Aden also came under the control of the Command in 1943 and remained so at the end of 1945.

Before the war, hospitals rendered monthly statistical morbidity returns on Army Form A.31. This return showed, *inter alia*, crude figures of admissions and deaths by diseases. Returns were consolidated at Command Headquarters and forwarded to the War Office. Hospital Record Cards (Army Forms I.1220) which were maintained for each patient and which included a summary of the case notes were forwarded direct to the War Office by individual hospitals.

During the course of the war, a Medical Statistical Section was established at the headquarters of the Officer i/c 2nd Echelon (O2E). A.Fs. A.31 which, contrary to the practice in the United Kingdom where the compilation of these forms was abandoned, were still in use and were sent to that Section, as were A.Fs. I.1220. A.Fs. A.31 were consolidated at the Section under the component Commands of M.E.F. and further consolidated to produce medical statistics for the whole Force.

For each year from 1942, annual Medical Statistical Reports containing the consolidations were published by O2E and from A.Fs. I.1220 received from hospitals, several investigations were made which were published in the 'Statistical Report on the Health of the Army, 1943–45'. A.Fs. I.1220 were eventually transmitted to the War Office.

As might be expected, the statistics produced by the Medical Statistical Section at O2E were of a more detailed character than those obtainable from the consolidated A.Fs. A.31 received in the War Office.

In the ensuing tabulations, statistics for the years 1939 and 1940 were obtained from War Office records; those for 1941 from a report submitted to the War Office by Medical Branch, G.H.Q., M.E.F., while those for the years 1942–45 were extracted from the Annual Statistical Reports produced by O2E. From the information in the 1942–45 reports it has been possible to present data regarding the ethnic groups of which the Force was composed.

Two defects from which the reports suffered were that they did not report information regarding personnel invalided from the Command, neither are statistics available regarding admissions and deaths for Officers and Other Ranks separately.

As far as can be ascertained, there is no reason to doubt in any marked degree the accuracy of the statistics here presented. All sources are reliable and data for the years 1941–45 have been obtained from original documents. The reports show comparatively few undiagnosed cases at the end of each year and these have been included in 'all other diseases'.

The tabulations which follow show the rates per 1,000 strength of admissions to and deaths in HOSPITALS only. No low grade morbidity is included.

The following tables relating to admissions and deaths are presented:

Class of Personnel	Period Covered	Table Nos.	
		Admissions	Deaths
All Troops	1941–45	54	68
United Kingdom Troops	1939–45	55	69
Indian Troops	1941–45	59	70
Dominion Troops	1942	56	71
South African Troops	1943–45	57	72–74
New Zealand Troops	1943–45	58	72–74
British African Troops	1943–45	60	75
Other British Troops	1944–45	61	76
Women's Services	1942–45	62	77
All Other Troops	1942–45	63	78
All Troops By Commands	1942–45	64–67	79–82

The morbidity rates for All Troops (Table 54) show a steady decline throughout the years 1941 to 1945, from 585 per 1,000 in 1941 to 357 in 1945. Factors which may have affected this are:

(i) The rapid acclimatisation of Troops in the Command.

(ii) With the exception of a comparatively small number of local enlistments, newcomers to the Command were trained and somewhat accustomed to the rigours of Army life.

(iii) Troops sent to the Middle East were of at least a fairly high medical category. Those considered unfit for duty in a subtropical climate were retained at home.

(iv) Those who were invalided were evacuated from the Command and some subsequently retained in the Army in a low medical category. They were then possibly more susceptible to disease and became a medical liability of the country to which evacuated.

(v) The prompt effective measures taken by the Army medical authorities to prevent and control disease.

The admission rates for DYSENTERY may possibly be cited in exemplification of this last factor. If the annual mean strength of All Troops in 1941 is taken as 1,000 the relative strengths for the ensuing years with relevant admission rates for Dysentery may be shown as below.

Year	1941	1942	1943	1944	1945
Relative Strength . . .	1,000	1,937	1,696	1,080	1,108
Rates of Admission for Dysentery .	32	33	33	38	29

The admission rates for DIPHTHERIA showed a decline from 5 in 1941 to 0·5 in 1945. The rate for INFECTIVE HEPATITIS in 1945 was approximately half that in 1942.

MALARIA increased from 21 in 1941 to 34 in 1944 and fell to one half the latter rate in 1945. This trend in 1945 is noted in other Commands. SANDFLY FEVER declined steadily and remarkably from 36 in 1941 to 5 in 1945. Against this, however, PYREXIA OF UNKNOWN ORIGIN (P.U.O.) rose considerably. It is possible that, due to faulty diagnosis on the part of Medical Officers with no great experience in tropical diseases, many of the cases placed under this heading should have been allocated properly to some of the febrile diseases. The rates for P.U.O. were 1941—8, 1942—9, 1943—20, 1944—23, and 1945—18 per 1,000 strength.

Admissions on account of SCABIES declined from 14 in 1941 to 4 in 1945, as did diseases of the SKIN and I.A.T. from 63 to 43.

The rates for VENEREAL DISEASES dropped from 41 in 1942 to 23 in 1943, rose to 30 in 1944 and 39 in 1945.

Apart from 1942 when the rate was 3 per 1,000, admissions on account of EFFECTS OF HEAT remained steady at between 0·2 and 0·5.

Admissions for MENTAL DISEASES increased to 14 in 1942 from 7 in 1941, and declined steadily during the next three years to 6 in 1945. The rates for NERVOUS DISEASES fell from 14 in 1941 to 7 in 1942 and, finally, to 4 in 1945.

Admissions for INJURIES through ENEMY ACTION were 35 in 1941, 31 in 1942, 22 in 1943, 0·77 in 1944 and 0·06 in 1945. Rates for INJURIES not caused by enemy action (N.E.A.) declined some months after the conclusion of active operations. Figures for the years 1941 to 1945 were 49, 48, 49, 43 and 34 respectively.

Tables 55 to 60 record the rates of admissions to hospitals according to ethnic groups and Tables 61 to 63 those of Other British Troops, Women's Services and All Other Troops respectively. Table 56 relates to Dominion Troops (1942) which included those from Australia, New Zealand, and South Africa. Separate figures are available for the latter two classes from 1943 to 1945, while Australians, being very few in number, are included in 'Other British Troops'. All Other Troops include those of other nationalities, e.g. Poles, Cypriots, Palestinian Jews, etc., in the Command.

Comparison of Tables 55 to 60 discloses the following outstanding features:

(i) United Kingdom Troops were more prone to DIPHTHERIA, EFFECTS OF HEAT, TONSILLITIS and SKIN DISEASES.

(ii) Troops of the United Kingdom and New Zealand were more susceptible to INFECTIVE HEPATITIS but less prone to TUBERCULOSIS.

(iii) Indian Troops were less prone to DIPHTHERIA and PNEUMONIA but more prone to MALARIA and, especially, to EYE DISEASES.

(iv) Native African Troops were particularly prone to DYSENTERY, PNEUMONIA, SCHISTOSOMIASIS and BRONCHITIS but were conspicuously less prone to MALARIA.

(v) Indian and Native African Troops were less prone to INFECTIVE HEPATITIS, INFLUENZA, DISEASES OF THE EAR AND NOSE and, particularly, TONSILLITIS, but were more prone to MUMPS and TUBERCULOSIS.

(vi) South African Troops were less prone to DYSENTERY but more susceptible to MEASLES and TUBERCULOSIS.

(vii) South African and New Zealand Troops were more prone to INFLUENZA.

(viii) Troops of African domicile were more prone to VENEREAL DISEASES than were the other groups.

(ix) Troops of European Stock were more liable to MENTAL DISEASES than were non-European.

These indications are tabulated below:

Disease	Ethnic Group: Prone	Ethnic Group: Less Prone
Diphtheria	British	Indians
Dysentery	Native Africans	South Africans
Infective Hepatitis	British, New Zealanders	Indians, Native Africans
Influenza	South Africans, New Zealanders	Indians, Native Africans
Malaria	Indians	Native Africans
Measles	New Zealanders	—
Mumps	Indians, Native Africans	—
Pneumonia	Native Africans	Indians
Tuberculosis	South Africans, Native Africans	British, New Zealanders
Venereal Diseases	South Africans, Native Africans	—
Effects of Heat	British	—
Mental Diseases	European Stock	Non-European Stock
Bronchitis	Native Africans	—
Tonsillitis	British	Indians, Native Africans
Ear and Nose Diseases	—	Indians, Native Africans
Eye Diseases	Indians	—
Skin Diseases	British	—
Schistosomiasis	Native Africans	—

Tables 64 to 67 exhibit the rates per 1,000 strength of admissions to hospitals of All Troops by the various Commands within the framework of the Middle East Force. From these tables the following emerges.

(i) DIPHTHERIA was more prevalent in Egypt (1942, 1943) than elsewhere. The incidence of this disease decreased there from 3·5 in 1942 to 0·4 in 1945.

(ii) The highest rates of hospitalisation for DYSENTERY also occurred in Egypt.

(iii) MALARIA was more rife in the Sudan and Eritrea than in other Commands. There was a conspicuous fall in the incidence of this disease in 1945 in all areas, the most dramatic being in Sudan and Eritrea where the rates for 1943, 1944 and 1945 were 134, 98 and 27 respectively. It is interesting to note the continuous steady fall of Malaria cases in Cyprus from 43 in 1942, to 24 in 1943, 13 in 1944 and, finally, to 10 in 1945.

(iv) Extremely high rates for PNEUMONIA occurred in Cyrenaica in 1944 and 1945, the figures being 24 and 12 respectively as against the all M.E.F. rates of 6 and 4.

(v) SANDFLY FEVER accounted for numerous admissions to hospital in Cyprus and, apart from 1943, the rates were over twice as high as those in the Command next in order of high rates for this disease.

(vi) Admissions for SCABIES were also conspicuously much higher in Cyprus than elsewhere.

(vii) VENEREAL DISEASES increased over the years 1942–45 in Syria, where the admission rate in 1945 was four times that of 1942

(42 and 13 respectively), in Cyprus, where the 1945 rate was just over three times that of 1942 (135 and 43) and at Aden where the 1945 rate was slightly over four times that for 1942 (70 and 16).

(viii) While the admission rate for BRONCHITIS rose steadily in Syria from 5 in 1942 to 15 in 1945 and in Aden (from 6 to 22 in the same years), in all other Commands for which statistics are available for those years, the rates declined.

(ix) TONSILLITIS was more prevalent in the Sudan and Eritrea, followed by Cyprus with Egypt a close third. The lowest rate for this disease occurred in Aden.

(x) Diseases of the SKIN occurred more frequently in Aden, Cyprus and the Sudan and Eritrea.

Tables 68 to 82 show the causes and rates of deaths in military hospitals. Table 68 refers to All Troops, Tables 69 to 78 to the various classes of troops, while Tables 79 to 82 break down the data in Table 68 to the component Commands of M.E.F.

Apart from 1941, when the rate was 0·92 per 1,000, deaths of all troops from *disease* fluctuated only slightly, the highest rate being 1·69 and the lowest 1·28.

TUBERCULOSIS accounted for the largest number of deaths, rising from 0·03 in 1941 to a peak of 0·46 in 1944. The rate in 1945 was 0·41. The mortality rates for this disease were highest among Indian and Native African Troops. The relevant figures are:

Year	Indians	Native Africans	All Troops
1943	0·50	0·81	0·21
1944	1·14	1·41	0·46
1945	0·56	1·03	0·41

Other Diseases of the DIGESTIVE System were responsible for the next highest number of deaths, the rates being 0·11 in 1941, 0·19 in 1942, 0·14 in 1943 and 1944, and 0·11 in 1945.

Deaths from INJURIES not attributable to Enemy Action were from one third to one quarter of the total number of deaths from injuries and disease, the rates being:

	1941	1942	1943	1944	1945
Injuries–N.E.A.	0·77	1·02	0·74	0·69	0·48
Total Deaths	2·16	3·31	2·44	2·39	1·77
Percentages	35	31	30	29	27

Sum mary

Admissions to hospitals on account of disease steadily declined from one in every two persons in 1941 to one in every three in 1945.

The main causes of admission were DYSENTERY, MALARIA, P.U.O., VENEREAL DISEASES, diseases of the RESPIRATORY and DIGESTIVE SYSTEMS and diseases of the SKIN.

As in other malarious areas, the rates of admission for MALARIA showed a substantial reduction in 1945. The most striking and steady decline in admissions was in respect of SANDFLY FEVER, the rate for which in 1945 was one seventh that in 1941.

TABLE 54

Middle East Forces. Admissions to Hospital, 1941–45. All Troops

Annual Rates per 1,000 Strength

Source: Annual Report o.2.E., G.H.Q., M.E.F.

	CAUSES	1941	1942	1943	1944	1945	
1	Diphtheria	5·05	2·50	2·84	1·33	0·47	1
2	Dysentery	32·47	33·31	33·21	37·80	28·66	2
3	Enteric Group of Fevers	0·61	0·66	1·03	0·56	0·48	3
4	Infective Hepatitis	(i)	16·10	14·66	10·09	7·83	4
5	Influenza	9·37	3·37	1·92	2·33	0·66	5
6	Malaria	21·50	29·17	29·13	33·75	17·09	6
7	Measles	3·48	0·84	0·58	0·24	0·27	7
8	Meningococcal Infection	0·57	0·42	0·45	0·25	0·14	8
9	Mumps	7·04	3·92	2·50	2·15	1·47	9
10	Pneumonia	5·91	4·21	4·88	6·41	4·37	10
11	P.U.O.	8·05	8·61	20·44	23·10	18·15	11
12	Relapsing Fever	(i)	0·23	0·18	0·08	0·17	12
13	Rheumatic Fever	0·93	0·62	0·68	0·55	0·22	13
14	Sandfly Fever	35·80	21·48	14·60	6·50	4·87	14
15	Schistosomiasis	(i)	0·14	0·65	1·13	0·83	15
16	Scabies	13·83	13·55	8·30	5·83	4·13	16
17	Smallpox	0·03	0·16	0·16	0·50	0·06	17
18	Tuberculosis	1·28	1·77	1·94	2·85	2·77	18
19	Typhus Fever	(i)	0·56	0·29	0·06	0·05	19
20	Venereal Diseases—Gonorrhoea	13·95	7·98	N.A.	7·71	10·15	20
21	Venereal Diseases—Syphilis	3·11	3·71	N.A.	6·59	9·89	21
22	Venereal Diseases—Others	24·13	19·73	N.A.	16·22	19·31	22
23	Total V.D.	41·19	31·42	22·77	30·52	39·55	23
24	Effects of Heat	(i)	2·80	0·54	0·24	0·51	24
25	Mental Diseases—Psychoses	6.64	14·43	3·19	3·15	2·19	25
26	Mental Diseases—Psychoneuroses			9·20	7·72	3·95	26
27	Nervous Diseases	14·27	6·93	4·93	5·10	3·94	27
28	Valvular Disease of the Heart	0·69	0·38	0·77	0·98	0·42	28
29	Other Circulatory conditions	9·48	5·08	5·50	5·51	4·06	29
30	Inflammation of the Bronchi	14·24	12·39	13·50	16·51	11·29	30
31	Other Diseases of the Respiratory System	10·19	8·57	8·53	9·86	8·12	31
32	Inflammation of the Tonsils	32·65	22·88	22·70	20·68	16·08	32
33	Other Diseases of the Digestive System	99·54	79·11	54·86	52·79	41·84	33
34	Diseases of the Ear and Nose	23·08	14·87	15·87	15·01	11·42	34
35	Diseases of the Eye	12·48	11·95	9·90	9·26	7·26	35

36	Skin and I.A.T. (excl. Scabies)	63·06	50·47	56·65	49·21	42·61	36
37	All Other Diseases	111·58	102·68	74·49	73·86	72·25	37
38	*Total Admissions for Diseases*	585·01	505·57	441·85	435·89	356·97	38
39	Injuries—N.E.A.	48·88	48·00	48·72	42·61	33·53	39
40	Injuries—E.A.	35·32	31·10	22·47	0·77	0·06	40
41	*Total Admissions for Injuries*	84·20	79·10	71·19	43·38	33·59	41
42	*Total Admissions*	669·21	584·67	513·04	479·27	390·56	42

Note: (i) Any cases included in 'All Other Diseases'.

TABLE 55

Middle East Forces. Admissions to Hospital, 1939–45. United Kingdom Troops
Annual Rates per 1,000 Strength

Sources: 1939 and 1941 Consolidation A.Fs. A.31; 1940—Hollerith Tabulations from A.Fs. I.1220; 1942-45—Annual Report O2E M.E.F.

	CAUSES	1939	1940	1941	1942	1943	1944	1945	
1	Diphtheria	3·00	3·78	7·05	4·85	4·56	2·35	1·10	1
2	Dysentery	11·39	31·00	42·03	43·81	30·27	27·75	27·00	2
3	Enteric Group of Fevers	0·25	0·35	0·70	0·84	0·78	0·55	0·81	3
4	Infective Hepatitis—True	(i)	} 13·73	} (ii)	} 23·23	} 18·61	{ 12·56	11·00	4
5	Infected Hepatitis—Post-Arsphenamine	(i)					1·02	0·74	5
6	Influenza	3·51	7·10	3·02	3·10	1·28	1·40	0·75	6
7	Malaria	19·86	22·01	27·21	26·79	23·98	41·52	21·63	7
8	Measles	0·94	0·23	0·54	0·43	0·23	0·31	0·22	8
9	Meningococcal Infection	0·07	0·29	0·38	0·15	0·13	0·12	0·11	9
10	Mumps	0·18	0·51	0·64	1·10	0·43	0·21	0·40	10
11	Pneumonia	4·56	3·90	5·52	4·64	2·78	3·61	4·52	11
12	P.U.O.	0·33	0·77	10·84	11·52	28·15	29·18	27·09	12
13	Relapsing Fever	(i)	0·08	(i)	0·12	0·11	0·04	0·06	13
14	Rheumatic Fever	1·37	1·92	1·12	0·77	0·70	0·31	0·30	14
15	Sandfly Fever	26·12	31·20	40·85	35·05	18·86	9·52	5·10	15
16	Schistosomiasis	(i)	0·03	(i)	0·08	0·03	0·01	—	16
17	Smallpox	—	0·02	0·01	0·11	0·17	0·45	0·04	17
18	Tuberculosis	1·09	2·02	1·59	1·17	0·89	0·78	1·01	18
19	Typhus Fever	(i)	0·09	(i)	0·15	0·31	0·04	0·01	19
20	Scabies	4·23	13·72	21·85	16·70	6·38	2·98	1·79	20
21	Venereal Diseases—Gonorrhoea	30·24	22·46	15·97	8·53	} 15·92	4·34	7·22	21
22	Venereal Diseases—Syphilis	2·53	4·13	4·29	2·43		3·00	5·39	22
23	Venereal Diseases—Other	6·26	7·60	19·71	14·65		8·39	11·76	23
24	Total V.D.	39·03	34·19	39·97	25·61	15·92	15·73	24·37	24
25	Effects of Heat	(i)	1·49	(i)	5·38	0·78	0·23	1·23	25
26	Mental Diseases—Psychoses	} 1·81	} 5·76	} 6·65	} 20·03	{ 2·62	1·80	1·63	26
27	Mental Diseases—Psychoneuroses					11·33	8·30	4·98	27
28	Nervous Diseases	7·05	4·64	16·56	6·77	4·34	3·28	3·35	28
29	Valvular Disease of the Heart	0·11	0·48	0·96	0·23	0·22	0·23	0·21	29
30	Other Diseases of the Circulatory System	2·60	4·92	9·60	7·51	5·73	5·38	4·69	30
31	Inflammation of the Bronchi	10·53	11·70	17·81	12·31	9·81	9·46	6·87	31
32	Other Diseases of the Respiratory System	4·27	5·68	9·19	7·76	6·86	7·85	6·80	32
33	Inflammation of the Tonsils	41·20	38·99	46·78	38·64	31·64	28·16	27·47	33
34	Other Diseases of the Digestive System	68·36	86·39	123·64	91·73	52·67	46·60	45·19	34
35	Diseases of the Ear and Nose	21·34	19·17	24·67	18·02	16·21	16·26	16·16	35

36	Diseases of the Eye	4·49	6·08	14·14	10·23	6·97	5·92	6·14	36
37	Skin and I.A.T. (Excl. Scabies)	74·23	82·86	89·93	71·77	69·42	61·03	65·72	37
38	All Other Diseases	74·59	116·78	113·37	88·21	55·21	50·53	61·21	38
39	*Total Admissions for Diseases*	426·51	551·78	676·62	578·81	428·38	395·43	379·70	39
40	Injuries—N.E.A.	49·12	} 41·97	53·86	51·42	45·68	37·95	41·16	40
41	Injuries—E.A.	0·98		38·37	40·35	28·89	0·28	0·05	41
42	*Total Admissions for Injuries*	50·10	41·97	92·23	91·77	74·57	38·23	41·21	42
43	*Total Admissions*	476·61	593·75	768·85	670·57	502·95	433·70	420·88	43

Notes: (i) Any cases are included in 'All Other Diseases'. (ii) Included in 'Other Diseases of the Digestive System'.

TABLE 56

*Middle East Forces. Admissions to Hospital, 1942. Dominion Troops**
Annual rates per 1,000 Strength

Source: Annual Report O.2.E, G.H.Q., M.E.F.

	CAUSES OF ADMISSION		Rate per 1,000 Strength	
1	Diphtheria		2·14	1
2	Dysentery		30·43	2
3	Enteric Group of Fevers		0·50	3
4	Infective Hepatitis		28·40	4
5	Influenza		10·51	5
6	Malaria		22·20	6
7	Measles		1·37	7
8	Meningococcal Infection		0·73	8
9	Mumps		4·93	9
10	Pneumonia		5·86	10
11	P.U.O.		13·70	11
12	Relapsing Fever		0·43	12
13	Rheumatic Fever		0·99	13
14	Sandfly Fever		13·94	14
15	Schistosomiasis		0·47	15
16	Smallpox		—	16
17	Tuberculosis		2·07	17
18	Typhus Fever		0·11	18
19	Scabies		6·67	19
20	Venereal Diseases—Gonorrhoea	12·15		20
21	Venereal Diseases—Syphilis	4·60		21
22	Venereal Diseases—Other	29·19		22
23	Total Venereal Diseases		45·94	23
24	Effects of Heat		0·10	24
25	Mental Diseases		21·36	25
26	Nervous Diseases		14·49	26
27	Valvular Disease of the Heart		0·73	27
28	Other Diseases of the Circulatory System		10·07	28
29	Inflammation of the Bronchi		17·72	29
30	Other Diseases of the Respiratory System		17·30	30
31	Inflammation of the Tonsils		20·96	31
32	Other Diseases of the Digestive System		86·50	32
33	Diseases of the Ear and Nose		24·96	33
34	Diseases of the Eye		14·46	34
35	Skin and I.A.T. (excluding Scabies)		47·62	35
36	All Other Diseases		116·54	36
37	*Total Admissions for Diseases*		584·20	37
38	Injuries—N.E.A.		71·99	38
39	Injuries—E.A.		67·26	39
40	*Total Admissions for Injuries*		139·25	40
41	*Total Admissions*		723·45	41

* Dominion Troops consisted of Australian, New Zealand and South African Forces.

TABLE 57

Middle East Forces. Admissions to Hospital, 1943–45. South African Troops
Annual Rates per 1,000 Strength

Source: 2nd Echelon M.E.F. Annual Reports

	CAUSES	1943	1944	1945	
1	Diphtheria	0·35	0·92	0·18	1
2	Dysentery	17·16	22·35	11·14	2
3	Enteric Group of Fevers	0·39	0·40	0·14	3
4	Infective Hepatitis—True	} 5·64	4·36	4·48	4
5	Infective Hepatitis—Post-Arsphenamine		0·83	0·80	5
6	Influenza	5·13	6·50	1·64	6
7	Malaria	13·99	14·59	13·22	7
8	Measles	1·52	0·20	0·04	8
9	Meningococcal Infection	0·12	0·40	—	9
10	Mumps	2·39	0·56	0·66	10
11	Pneumonia	3·08	4·16	2·95	11
12	P.U.O.	13·85	21·26	17·99	12
13	Relapsing Fever	0·21	—	0·15	13
14	Rheumatic Fever	0·23	0·26	0·07	14
15	Sandfly Fever	17·73	4·32	2·37	15
16	Schistosomiasis	0·94	0·92	0·33	16
17	Smallpox	0·37	0·46	—	17
18	Tuberculosis	2·37	3·14	2·33	18
19	Typhus	0·05	0·13	0·44	19
20	Venereal Diseases—Syphilis	N.A.	13·43	13·44	20
21	Venereal Diseases—Gonorrhoea	N.A.	7·95	15·37	21
22	Venereal Diseases—Other Forms	N.A.	30·00	38·60	22
23	Total V.D.	35·15	51·38	67·41	23
24	Scabies	3·45	6·30	18·10	24
25	Effects of Heat	0·23	0·07	0·11	25
26	Mental Diseases—Psychoses	3·17	4·92	3·75	26
27	Mental Diseases—Psychoneuroses	11·22	14·00	4·66	27
28	Nervous Diseases	3·91	8·22	3·90	28
29	Valvular Disease of the Heart	0·62	0·73	0·33	29
30	Other Diseases of the Circulatory System	6·58	6·80	1·97	30
31	Inflammation of the Bronchi	12·28	16·93	8·99	31
32	Other Diseases of the Respiratory System	9·52	10·10	5·50	32
33	Inflammation of the Tonsils	13·78	16·64	12·64	33
34	Other Diseases of the Digestive System	42·39	45·02	29·24	34
35	Diseases of the Ear and Nose	16·98	19·38	13·55	35
36	Diseases of the Eye	7·59	7·46	5·10	36
37	Diseases of the Skin and I.A.T. (excl. Scabies)	38·90	43·97	32·08	37
38	All Other Diseases	82·55	106·98	93·41	38
39	*Total Diseases*	373·82	444·65	359·64	39
40	Injuries—E.A.	5·43	0·26	—	40
41	Injuries—N.E.A.	59·71	82·98	48·80	41
42	*Total Injuries*	65·14	83·24	48·80	42
43	*Total Admissions*	438·96	527·89	408·43	43

TABLE 58

Middle East Forces. Admissions to Hospital, 1943–45. New Zealand Troops
Annual Rates per 1,000 Strength

Source: 2nd Echelon M.E.F. Annual Reports

	CAUSES	1943	1944	1945	
1	Diphtheria	2·09	2·11	0·48	1
2	Dysentery	46·93	25·78	10·13	2
3	Enteric Group of Fevers	5·73	0·23	0·48	3
4	Infective Hepatitis—True	13·99 (4 and 5)	8·44	9·97	4
5	Infective Hepatitis—Post-Arsphenamine		2·11	0·64	5
6	Influenza	7·39	7·50	2·25	6
7	Malaria	14·99	16·87	7·72	7
8	Measles	0·30	—	0·32	8
9	Meningococcal Infection	0·22	0·23	0·16	9
10	Mumps	0·22	1·64	0·64	10
11	Pneumonia	13·25	8·20	3·86	11
12	P.U.O.	25·20	11·25	10·13	12
13	Relapsing Fever	0·39	—	—	13
14	Rheumatic Fever	0·22	1·17	—	14
15	Sandfly Fever	10·91	2·81	0·48	15
16	Schistosomiasis	—	—	—	16
17	Smallpox	0·09	0·47	—	17
18	Tuberculosis	0·91	1·87	1·93	18
19	Typhus	0·39	—	—	19
20	Venereal Diseases—Syphilis	N.A.	3·52	2·57	20
21	Venereal Diseases—Gonorrhoea	N.A.	6·09	10·78	21
22	Venereal Diseases—Other Forms	N.A.	7·50	11·10	22
23	Total V.D.	14·56	17·11	24·45	23
24	Scabies	4·43	8·91	16·09	24
25	Effects of Heat	0·61	0·70	—	25
26	Mental Diseases—Psychoses	1·65	4·92	2·57	26
27	Mental Diseases—Psychoneuroses	14·91	7·50	2·41	27
28	Nervous Diseases	7·13	3·05	1·45	28
29	Valvular Disease of the Heart	0·35	1·17	0·16	29
30	Other Diseases of the Circulatory System	4·69	6·09	2·25	30
31	Inflammation of the Bronchi	14·47	10·08	3·06	31
32	Other Diseases of the Respiratory System	9·00	5·86	6·59	32
33	Inflammation of the Tonsils	25·33	22·73	8·69	33
34	Other Diseases of the Digestive System	65·57	70·31	41·34	34
35	Diseases of the Ear and Nose	50·76	30·70	10·94	35
36	Diseases of the Eye	7·34	10·31	5·31	36
37	Diseases of the Skin and I.A.T. (excl. Scabies)	60·84	52·26	35·39	37
38	All Other Diseases	96·00	87·18	73·83	38
39	*Total Diseases*	520·86	429·58	283·73	39
40	Injuries—E.A.	70·62	3·98	—	40
41	Injuries—N.E.A.	69·40	60·23	46·49	41
42	*Total Injuries*	140·01	64·21	46·49	42
43	*Total Admissions*	660·87	493·79	330·22	43

TABLE 59

Middle East Forces. Admissions to Hospitals, 1941–45. Indian Troops. Annual Rates per 1,000 Strength

Source: 2nd Echelon M.E.F. Annual Reports

	CAUSES	1941	1942	1943	1944	1945	
1	Diphtheria	—	0·05	0·08	0·05	0·09	1
2	Dysentery	16·64	21·91	12·51	14·40	9·18	2
3	Enteric Group of Fevers	0·13	0·12	0·07	0·07	0·15	3
4	Infective Hepatitis—True	N.A.	3·00	5·64	9·81	5·15	4
5	Infective Hepatitis—Post-Arsphenamine				0·76	0·35	5
6	Influenza	0·37	0·27	0·07	0·79	0·21	6
7	Malaria	8·43	50·60	41·89	30·28	21·70	7
8	Measles	0·49	0·33	0·08	0·31	0·08	8
9	Meningococcal Infection	0·15	0·89	0·08	0·12	0·03	9
10	Mumps	13·37	7·76	4·37	5·81	1·53	10
11	Pneumonia	1·40	1·73	2·03	3·24	2·44	11
12	P.U.O.	1·12	2·03	1·66	5·00	4·33	12
13	Relapsing Fever	N.A.	0·42	0·41	0·19	0·25	13
14	Rheumatic Fever	0·41	0·29	0·21	0·31	0·08	14
15	Sandfly Fever	1·57	11·08	5·29	3·26	12·19	15
16	Schistosomiasis	N.A.	0·05	0·53	0·29	0·09	16
17	Smallpox	0·04	0·50	0·07	0·52	0·03	17
18	Tuberculosis	0·86	2·24	2·59	2·81	1·39	18
19	Typhus	N.A.	0·06	0·22	—	0·01	19
20	Venereal Diseases—Syphilis	4·41	5·11	20·85	6·69	11·77	20
21	Venereal Diseases—Gonorrhoea	4·60	3·73		4·40	7·02	21
22	Venereal Diseases—Other Forms	8·97	31·07		15·64	15·88	22
23	Total V.D.	17·98	39·91	20·85	26·73	34·67	23
24	Scabies	14·73	13·78	9·90	10·45	3·32	24
25	Effects of Heat	N.A.	1·80	0·18	0·07	0·32	25
26	Mental Diseases—Psychoses	0·95	4·20	2·43	2·50	1·06	26
27	Mental Diseases—Psychoneuroses			2·46	3·67	1·17	27
28	Nervous Diseases	2·84	3·18	3·64	4·62	3·19	28
29	Valvular Disease of the Heart	0·26	0·22	0·32	0·45	0·04	29
30	Other Diseases of the Circulatory System	3·65	1·76	2·46	4·98	1·44	30
31	Inflammation of the Bronchi	3·50	9·85	17·43	25·50	8·86	31
32	Other Diseases of the Respiratory System	7·24	8·72	7·81	12·19	7·84	32

TABLE 59—(*contd.*)

Middle East Forces. Admissions to Hospitals, 1941–45. Indian Troops. Annual Rates per 1,000 Strength

Source: 2nd Echelon M.E.F. Annual Reports

	CAUSES	1941	1942	1943	1944	1945	
33	Inflammation of the Tonsils	2·88	6·67	5·95	7·36	4·87	33
34	Other Diseases of the Digestive System	32·27	78·16	50·81	49·90	32·70	34
35	Diseases of the Ear and Nose	4·64	8·77	11·19	13·93	7·83	35
36	Diseases of the Eye	8·40	19·18	22·72	24·54	9·57	36
37	Diseases of the Skin and I.A.T. (excluding Scabies)	12·19	38·42	53·65	52·90	33·74	37
38	All Other Diseases	52·05	152·56	102·34	106·92	72·46	38
39	*Total Diseases*	208·54	490·66	391·96	424·71	282·36	39
40	Injuries—E.A.	39·51	9·43	17·58	5·55	0·09	40
41	Diseases—N.E.A.	23·13	46·30	59·67	63·61	30·72	41
42	*Total Injuries*	62·66	55·73	77·25	69·16	30·81	42
43	*Total Admissions*	271·16	546·39	469·21	493·87	313·17	43

TABLE 60

Middle East Forces
Admissions to Hospitals, 1943–45
British African Troops
Annual Rates per 1,000 Strength

Source: 2nd Echelon M.E.F. Annual Reports

	CAUSES	1943	1944	1945	
1	Diphtheria	1·55	0·07	0·16	1
2	Dysentery	106·20	117·14	91·50	2
3	Enteric Group of Fevers	0·67	0·34	0·32	3
4	Infective Hepatitis—True	} 3·84	3·02	1·97	4
5	Infective Hepatitis—Post-Arsphenamine		0·62	0·38	5
6	Influenza	1·43	1·32	0·16	6
7	Malaria	6·89	4·96	4·34	7
8	Measles	0·60	0·04	0·09	8
9	Meningococcal Infection	1·57	0·78	0·58	9
10	Mumps	7·51	4·44	1·56	10
11	Pneumonia	21·57	21·86	8·90	11
12	P.U.O.	12·15	12·38	22·19	12
13	Relapsing Fever	0·04	—	0·21	13
14	Rheumatic Fever	0·54	0·29	0·11	14
15	Sandfly Fever.	13·05	6·28	1·29	15
16	Schistosomiasis	3·38	3·48	3·39	16
17	Smallpox	0·23	0·51	0·16	17
18	Tuberculosis	3·75	6·25	2·18	18
19	Typhus	0·20	0·05	0·01	19
20	Venereal Diseases—Syphilis		14·74 }	19·87 }	20
21	Venereal Diseases—Gonorrhoea	} 38·39	10·65 }	14·87 }	21
22	Venereal Diseases—Other Forms		37·98 }	44·13 }	22
23	Total V.D.	38·39	63·37	78·87	23
24	Scabies	8·10	3·91	3·27	24
25	Effects of Heat	0·31	0·14	0·06	25
26	Mental Diseases—Psychoses	3·34	3·06	2·63	26
27	Mental Diseases—Psychoneuroses	3·32	3·78	3·60	27
28	Nervous Diseases	2·67	2·99	2·92	28
29	Valvular Disease of the Heart	0·69	1·09	0·41	29
30	Other Diseases of the Circulatory System	4·95	3·64	2·71	30
31	Inflammation of the Bronchi	21·35	24·54	21·17	31
32	Other Diseases of the Respiratory System	14·17	11·21	7·54	32
33	Inflammation of the Tonsils	5·45	5·22	5·79	33
34	Other Diseases of the Digestive System	54·47	51·78	43·55	34
35	Diseases of the Ear and Nose	9·44	10·20	6·34	35
36	Diseases of the Eye	8·00	8·84	8·50	36
37	Diseases of the Skin and I.A.T. (excl. Scabies)	30·77	30·44	27·05	37
38	All Other Diseases	83·86	78·02	75·40	38
39	*Total Diseases*	474·42	497·05	429·31	39
40	Injuries—E.A.	12·89	—	—	40
41	Injuries—N.E.A.	31·13	28·76	26·91	41
42	*Total Injuries*	44·02	28·76	26·91	42
43	*Total Admissions*	518·45	525·81	456·22	43

Note: The term 'British African' includes all native personnel from British Territories in Africa.

TABLE 61

Middle East Forces
Admissions to Hospitals, 1944–45
Other British Troops
Annual Rates per 1,000 Strength

Source: Annual Report O.2.E., G.H.Q., M.E.F.

	CAUSES	1944	1945	
1	Diphtheria	1·02	0·31	1
2	Dysentery	35·35	21·95	2
3	Enteric Group of Fevers	0·53	0·54	3
4	Infective Hepatitis	10·49	8·01	4
5	Influenza	2·43	1·11	5
6	Malaria	38·32	19·58	6
7	Measles	0·40	0·50	7
8	Meningococcal Infection	0·22	0·15	8
9	Mumps	6·02	2·30	9
10	Pneumonia	6·59	3·91	10
11	P.U.O.	35·09	26·78	11
12	Relapsing Fever	0·49	0·31	12
13	Rheumatic Fever	0·27	0·08	13
14	Sandfly Fever	7·26	1·23	14
15	Schistosomiasis	0·58	0·23	15
16	Scabies	23·27	9·77	16
17	Smallpox	1·28	0·19	17
18	Tuberculosis	2·12	2·76	18
19	Typhus Fever	—	0·11	19
20	Venereal Diseases—Gonorrhoea	29·12	25·67	20
21	Venereal Diseases—Syphilis	14·73	20·00	21
22	Venereal Diseases—Others	40·18	37·85	22
23	Total V.D.	84·03	83·52	23
24	Effects of Heat	0·40	0·27	24
25	Mental Diseases—Psychoses	9·51	4·56	25
26	Mental Diseases—Psychoneuroses	19·12	9·39	26
27	Nervous Diseases	6·68	3·33	27
28	Valvular Disease of the Heart	0·88	0·27	28
29	Other Circulatory Conditions	5·97	4·18	29
30	Inflamation of the Bronchi	28·63	14·71	30
31	Other Diseases of the Respiratory System	19·73	10·19	31
32	Inflammation of the Tonsils	39·60	29·85	32
33	Other Diseases of the Digestive System	106·19	59·92	33
34	Diseases of the Ear and Nose	20·00	14·09	34
35	Diseases of the Eye	18·05	12·03	35
36	Skin and I.A.T. (excluding Scabies)	77·70	57·43	36
37	All Other Diseases	115·13	89·85	37
38	*Total Admissions for Diseases*	723·16	493·40	38
39	Injuries—N.E.A.	60·13	40·04	39
40	Injuries—E.A.	0·09	0·31	40
41	*Total Admissions for Injuries*	60·22	40·35	41
42	*Total Admissions*	783·38	533·75	42

Note: The term 'Other British Troops' refers to all male personnel from British Territories outside Africa and not included in Tables 55 to 60.

TABLE 62

Middle East Forces
Admissions to Hospitals, 1942–45
Women's Services
Annual Rates per 1,000 Strength

Source: 2nd Echelon M.E.F. Annual Reports

	CAUSES	1942	1943	1944	1945	
1	Diphtheria	N.A.	4·55	2·56	1·64	1
2	Dysentery	54·28	37·71	30·24	30·84	2
3	Enteric Group of Fevers	N.A.	1·96	0·78	0·55	3
4	Infective Hepatitis—True	8·83	11·78	6·12	9·69	4
5	Infective Hepatitis—Post-Arsphenamine			0·44	0·41	5
6	Influenza	N.A.	10·85	8·56	2·59	6
7	Malaria	27·80	107·87	18·79	12·28	7
8	Measles	N.A.	3·00	0·78	0·96	8
9	Meningococcal Infection	N.A.	0·31	—	0·14	9
10	Mumps	N.A.	1·76	0·11	0·53	10
11	Pneumonia	N.A	3·82	3·56	2·59	11
12	P.U.O.	N.A.	29·14	29·24	24·70	12
13	Relapsing Fever	N.A.	0·41	0·33	0·27	13
14	Rheumatic Fever	N.A.	0·93	2·22	1·23	14
15	Sandfly Fever	60·24	26·45	5·11	1·36	15
16	Schistosomiasis	N.A.	—	0·11	—	16
17	Smallpox	N.A.	0·10	0·22	—	17
18	Tuberculosis	N.A.	1·86	4·00	5·46	18
19	Typhus	N.A.	0·21	0·11	0·14	19
20	Venereal Diseases—Syphilis	N.A.	1·24	—	—	20
21	Venereal Diseases—Gonorrhoea	N.A.		0·11	0·41	21
22	Venereal Diseases—Other Forms	N.A.		0·11	0·27	22
23	Total V.D.	N.A.	1·24	0·22	0·68	23
24	Scabies	3·09	3·93	3·11	2·73	24
25	Effects of Heat	N.A.	0·31	0·67	0·41	25
26	Mental Diseases—Psychoses	16·11	4·24	2·00	1·50	26
27	Mental Diseases—Psychoneuroses		9·92	9·45	6·55	27
28	Nervous Diseases	N.A.	12·19	10·56	10·37	28
29	Valvular Disease of the Heart	N.A.	1·86	1·78	3·00	29
30	Other Diseases of the Circulatory System	N.A.	8·78	10·34	14·19	30
31	Inflammation of the Bronchi	N.A.	16·43	13·23	12·55	31
32	Other Diseases of the Respiratory System	N.A.	15·91	15·57	16·10	32
33	Inflammation of the Tonsils	78·11	57·66	50·59	51·86	33
34	Other Diseases of the Digestive System	160·19	116·14	82·83	72·33	34
35	Diseases of the Ear and Nose	29·79	27·18	20·46	20·33	35
36	Diseases of the Eye	N.A.	5·79	4·34	5·59	36
37	Diseases of the Skin and I.A.T. (excluding Scabies)	89·14	61·38	48·59	43·67	37
38	All Other Diseases*	338·48	156·95	142·76	179·31	38
39	*Total Diseases*	866·06	742·61	529·80	536·57	39
40	Injuries—E.A.	1·10	1·35	—	—	40
41	Injuries—N.E.A.	39·72	35·75	24·57	22·93	41
42	*Total Injuries*	40·82	37·10	24·57	22·93	42
43	*Total Admissions*	906·88	779·71	554·37	559·50	43

* Includes diseases listed 'N.A.'

Note: The term 'Women's Services' includes all female personnel of all Forces in M.E.F.

TABLE 63

Middle East Forces
Admissions to Hospitals, 1942–45
All Other Troops
Annual Rates per 1,000 Strength

Source: Annual Reports O.2.E., G.H.Q., M.E.F

	CAUSES	1942	1943	1944	1945	
1	Diphtheria	N.A.	0·94	0·36	0·11	1
2	Dysentery	24·74	26·46	28·32	14·75	2
3	Enteric Group of Fevers	N.A.	2·04	1·08	0·49	3
4	Infective Hepatitis	5·28	18·58	7·53	3·04	4
5	Influenza	N.A.	2·62	3·65	0·21	5
6	Malaria	17·67	51·49	44·79	13·93	6
7	Measles	N.A.	1·67	0·09	0·60	7
8	Meningococcal Infections	N.A.	1·44	0·23	0·03	8
9	Mumps	N.A.	6·27	3·30	3·21	9
10	Pneumonia	N.A.	4·91	5·46	3·40	10
11	P.U.O.	N.A.	14·92	14·13	12·78	11
12	Relapsing Fever	N.A.	0·24	0·06	0·18	12
13	Rheumatic Fever	N.A.	1·34	1·47	0·23	13
14	Sandfly Fever	8·62	7·21	1·55	1·96	14
15	Schistosomiasis	N.A.	1·53	3·22	1·56	15
16	Scabies	12·38	17·26	6·97	2·17	16
17	Smallpox	N.A.	0·09	0·41	0·03	17
18	Tuberculosis	N.A.	4·23	5·82	2·81	18
19	Typhus Fever	N.A.	0·40	0·12	0·01	19
20	Venereal Diseases—Gonorrhoea	N.A.	N.A.	10·76 }	8·91 }	20
21	Venereal Diseases—Syphilis	N.A.	N.A.	5·91 }	4·99 }	21
22	Venereal Diseases—Other	N.A.	N.A.	11·30 }	7·14 }	22
23	Total V.D.	24·39	39·31	27·97	21·04	23
24	Effects of Heat	N.A.	0·28	0·35	0·11	24
25	Mental Diseases—Psychoses	}7·80	6·06	4·57	2·03	25
26	Mental Diseases—Psychoneuroses		8·53	5·26	2·51	26
27	Nervous Diseases	N.A.	8·66	9·39	2·67	27
28	Valvular Disease of the Heart	N.A.	3·14	3·16	0·20	28
29	Other Circulatory Conditions	N.A.	7·08	6·30	2·53	29
30	Inflammation of the Bronchi	N.A.	19·54	21·22	12·48	30
31	Other Diseases of the Respiratory System	N.A.	11·11	9·43	6·52	31
32	Inflammation of the Tonsils	6·53	15·11	12·00	10·68	32
33	Other Diseases of the Digestive System	40·93	65·33	54·13	35·89	33
34	Diseases of the Ear and Nose	6·28	13·46	11·13	7·17	34
35	Diseases of the Eye	N.A.	13·08	8·59	4·30	35
36	Skin and I.A.T. (excluding Scabies)	19·53	37·05	23·59	24·05	36
37	All Other Diseases	135·51*	101·47	79·74	57·24	37
38	*Total Admissions for Diseases*	296·87	512·87	405·40	240·87	38
39	Injuries—N.E.A.	24·21	53·93	33·44	21·74	39
40	Injuries—E.A.	6·71	8·78	0·30	0·06	40
41	*Total Admissions for Injuries*	30·91	62·71	33·74	21·80	41
42	*Total Admissions*	327·78	575·58	439·14	272·67	42

* Includes diseases listed 'N.A.' (except V.D.).

Note: The term 'All Other Troops' refers to all Dominion, Colonial and Allied male personnel (excluding U.S. personnel) not included in Tables 55 to 62.

TABLE 64

Middle East Forces. Admissions to Hospitals, 1942. All Troops. By Commands
Annual Rates per 1,000 Strength

Source: Annual Report O.2.E. M.E.F.

	CAUSES	Egypt and 8th Army	Palestine	Syria 9th Army	Cyprus 9th Army	Sudan	Eritrea	Malta (a) E.A.R.	Aden (b) E.A.R.	Persia and Iraq 10th Army E.A.R. (c)	Total M.E.F.	
1	Diphtheria	3·48	2·62	0·27	2·33	1·67	—	1·33	—	0·28	2·50	1
2	Dysentery	43·72	22·28	10·74	23·67	38·36	26·15	11·70	11·60	16·26	33·31	2
3	Enteric Group of Fevers	0·63	1·05	0·53	0·16	0·74	0·78	1·12	—	0·30	0·66	3
4	Infective Hepatitis	22·41	13·87	5·45	6·19	4·63	3·90	6·94	0·47	3·20	16·10	4
5	Influenza	4·71	3·06	1·75	2·93	0·74	—	—	—	0·29	3·37	5
6	Malaria	22·66	20·45	27·73	43·49	47·26	107·85	0·14	49·95	44·61	29·17	6
7	Measles	0·52	1·40	0·55	13·15	0·19	0·11	—	0·24	0·05	0·84	7
8	Meningococcal Infection	0·31	0·62	0·07	0·71	—	0·11	—	—	0·80	0·42	8
9	Mumps	4·00	7·31	1·25	8·52	1·11	8·12	0·07	3·31	1·70	3·92	9
10	Pneumonia	5·67	4·00	1·28	2·82	5·93	1·89	0·65	1·66	1·04	4·21	10
11	P.U.O.	9·72	14·76	7·49	7·87	13·53	3·78	0·82	1·89	0·64	8·61	11
12	Relapsing Fever	0·19	0·35	0·05	2·66	—	0·45	0·03	—	0·01	0·23	12
13	Rheumatic Fever	0·79	0·35	0·29	0·65	0·37	0·11	0·07	0·24	0·40	0·62	13
14	Sandfly Fever	13·52	27·09	39·63	86·93	38·00	0·22	7·58	—	20·71	21·48	14
15	Schistosomiasis	0·17	0·23	0·02	—	—	0·22	—	—	0·03	0·14	15
16	Scabies	14·37	17·46	4·73	33·50	4·26	7·01	21·79	2·13	5·67	13·55	16
17	Smallpox	0·01	0·01	0·25	—	—	—	—	—	0·73	0·16	17
18	Tuberculosis	1·66	2·53	0·52	1·31	3·34	0·67	1·02	3·79	1·90	1·77	18
19	Typhus Fever	0·10	0·17	0·04	0·11	—	0·78	—	—	2·58	0·56	19
20	Venereal Diseases—Gonorrhoea	6·54	17·98	5·29	28·40	22·24	20·92	3·47	4·50	1·67	7·98	20
21	Venereal Diseases—Soft Chancre	3·59	12·62	2·45	3·80	4·45	0·22	—	—	1·35	4·21	21
22	Venereal Diseases—Syphilis	4·43	3·48	0·84	10·04	7·41	26·82	0·65	0·71	0·28	3·71	22
23	Venereal Diseases—Other Forms	10·75	10·67	4·78	0·92	40·59	10·13	0·95	11·13	39·56	15·52	23
24	Total Venereal Diseases	25·31	44·75	13·36	43·16	74·69	58·09	5·07	16·34	42·86	31·42	24
25	Effects of Heat	0·13	0·07	—	—	5·37	0·56	—	—	14·98	2·80	25
26	Mental Diseases—Psychoses	} 20·50	15·09	1·24	5·21	8·71	1·78	3·09	0·95	2·51	14·43	26
27	Mental Diseases—Psychoneuroses											27
28	Nervous Diseases	8·54	9·91	2·48	6·35	8·15	5·68	2·79	3·55	1·09	6·93	28
29	Valvular Disease of the Heart	0·37	0·91	0·18	0·49	0·19	0·43	0·07	0·24	0·08	0·38	29
30	Other Diseases of the Circulatory System	6·02	7·38	1·86	5·97	8·71	3·34	2·38	0·71	1·26	5·08	30

TABLE 64—(*contd.*)

Middle East Forces. Admissions to Hospitals, 1942. All Troops. By Commands. Annual Rates per 1,000 Strength

Source: Annual Report O.2.E., M.E.F.

	CAUSES	Egypt and 8th Army	Palestine	Syria 9th Army	Cyprus 9th Army	Sudan	Eritrea	Malta (a) E.A.R.	Aden (b) E.A.R.	Persia and Iraq 10th Army E.A.R. (c)	Total M.E.F.	
31	Inflammation of the Bronchi	14·81	16·37	4·79	27·36	17·23	13·80	4·62	5·68	1·84	12·39	31
32	Other Diseases of the Respiratory System	9·26	13·01	2·71	5·22	9·82	4·45	2·01	3·08	6·10	8·57	32
33	Inflammation of the Tonsils	27·99	22·79	6·79	29·66	39·10	21·59	5·71	6·39	10·97	22·88	33
34	Other Diseases of the Digestive System	82·30	90·28	27·49	66·19	105·82	72·11	26·39	50·90	77·93	79·11	34
35	Diseases of the Ear and Nose	18·05	18·27	6·48	15·58	30·21	4·12	8·23	3·31	4·04	14·87	35
36	Diseases of the Eye	12·85	16·99	2·77	11·24	13·71	12·13	2·58	7·81	9·10	11·95	36
37	Skin and I.A.T. (excluding Scabies)	56·59	54·69	22·54	82·80	79·32	28·94	28·86	50·42	28·02	50·47	37
38	All Other Diseases	93·70	97·92	21·66	173·83	164·41	100·49	24·68	152·20	150·99	102·68	38
39	*Total Admissions for Diseases*	525·01	548·03	217·00	710·13	725·53	488·94	169·68	376·89	452·99	505·57	39
40	Injuries—N.E.A.	53·02	61·88	17·84	62·54	43·37	48·63	18·63	41·43	28·63	48·00	40
41	Injuries—E.A.	53·21	2·32	0·76	—	5·19	0·22	4·66	0·24	0·90	31·10	41
42	*Total Admissions for Injuries*	106·23	64·20	18·60	62·54	48·56	48·85	23·29	41·67	29·53	79·10	42
43	*Total Admissions*	631·24	612·23	235·60	772·60	774·09	537·79	192·97	418·56	482·52	584·67	43

(a) Equivalent Annual Rates based on admissions from June to December.
(b) Equivalent Annual Rates based on admissions from July to December.
(c) Equivalent Annual Rates based on admissions from January to August.

TABLE 65

Middle East Forces. Admissions to Hospitals, 1943. All Troops. By Commands
Annual Rates per 1,000 Strength

Source: Annual Report O.2.E., M.E.F.

	CAUSES	Egypt-Cyrenaica and Tripolitania	Palestine	Syria	Cyprus	Sudan and Eritrea	Malta	Aden	Total M.E.F.	
1	Diphtheria	3·43	1·68	1·52	1·25	2·61	1·37	—	2·84	1
2	Dysentery	38·06	27·37	20·43	8·37	20·85	20·37	17·49	33·21	2
3	Enteric Group of Fevers	1·23	0·77	0·37	0·25	1·40	0·81	—	1·03	3
4	Infective Hepatitis	16·26	10·11	13·89	11·12	8·82	10·87	3·78	14·66	4
5	Influenza	2·08	2·95	0·56	—	2·21	0·11	—	1·92	5
6	Malaria	20·24	61·69	49·14	24·44	134·52	4·19	43·33	29·13	6
7	Measles	0·43	0·83	0·29	1·31	0·20	—	12·29	0·58	7
8	Meningococcal Infection	0·44	0·13	0·03	0·44	0·20	0·04	11·82	0·45	8
9	Mumps	2·16	0·80	0·29	37·06	1·60	0·07	1·26	2·50	9
10	Pneumonia	5·83	3·10	2·90	2·50	2·21	1·83	2·36	4·88	10
11	P.U.O.	22·17	25·02	13·65	7·81	13·83	3·76	0·79	20·44	11
12	Relapsing Fever	0·14	0·26	0·13	1·56	0·20	—	0·16	0·18	12
13	Rheumatic Fever	0·60	1·04	0·51	0·44	1·00	1·34	0·16	0·68	13
14	Sandfly Fever	9·91	18·65	35·28	54·62	1·20	17·20	0·16	14·60	14
15	Schistosomiasis	0·74	0·81	0·19	—	0·60	—	0·47	0·65	15
16	Smallpox	0·20	0·07	0·08	—	0·20	—	—	0·16	16
17	Tuberculosis	1·78	3·13	1·05	2·12	3·01	1·97	3·31	1·94	17
18	Typhus	0·39	0·06	0·10	0·06	0·20	0·11	—	0·29	18
19	Venereal Diseases	19·22	26·93	33·86	57·43	64·76	11·64	47·27	22·77	19
20	Scabies	8·03	3·54	8·48	25·50	3·81	21·25	2·84	8·30	20
21	Effects of Heat	0·60	0·33	0·13	0·19	3·61	0·91	0·63	0·54	21
22	Mental Diseases—Psychoses	3·64	3·40	1·26	0·69	1·40	1·69	0·63	3·19	22
23	Mental Diseases—Psychoneuroses	10·57	8·57	4·47	3·69	5·21	4·68	0·47	9·20	23
24	Nervous Diseases	4·42	9·06	2·98	4·56	9·42	4·15	1·26	4·93	24
25	Valvular Disease of the Heart	0·43	2·85	0·59	0·12	0·60	0·35	0·16	0·77	25
26	Other Diseases of the Circulatory System	5·60	7·58	2·73	3·00	8·62	4·26	3·47	5·50	26
27	Inflammation of the Bronchi	13·25	15·65	11·67	12·62	13·83	13·40	20·48	13·50	27
28	Other Diseases of the Respiratory System	8·35	9·95	8·10	4·75	16·84	8·48	8·51	8·53	28
29	Inflammation of the Tonsils	24·66	21·75	15·42	21·94	35·89	10·69	9·14	22·70	29
30	Other Diseases of the Digestive System	54·85	69·72	34·97	55·43	71·77	43·83	64·12	54·86	30
31	Diseases of the Ear and Nose	16·01	17·30	12·84	14·19	15·44	17·03	14·97	15·87	31
32	Diseases of the Eye	9·29	12·62	10·45	13·75	6·21	6·05	19·69	9·90	32
33	Skin and I.A.T. (excluding Scabies)	59·07	47·61	48·31	82·31	50·32	50·41	69·48	56·65	33
34	All Other Diseases	69·02	98·27	77·65	90·24	95·63	54·11	131·56	74·49	34
35	*Total Admissions for Diseases*	433·10	513·63	414·29	543·78	598·24	316·96	492·04	441·85	35
36	Injuries—E.A.	31·95	2·43	0·91	1·81	0·80	0·53	—	48·72	36
37	Injuries—N.E.A.	47·30	53·78	46·14	78·56	44·91	44·64	53·57	22·47	37
38	*Total Admissions for Injuries*	79·25	56·21	47·05	80·37	45·71	45·17	53·57	71·19	38
39	*Total Admissions*	512·35	569·84	461·34	624·15	643·95	362·13	545·61	513·04	39

TABLE 66

Middle East Forces. Admissions to Hospitals, 1944. All Troops. By Commands
Rates per 1,000 Strength

Source: Annual Report O.2.E., M.E.F.

	CAUSES	Egypt	Cyrenaica	Tripolitania	Palestine	Syria	Cyprus	Sudan-Eritrea	Aden	Total M.E.F.	
1	Diphtheria	1·72	0·38	0·13	1·06	0·91	0·72	0·30	—	1·33	1
2	Dysentery	45·72	29·38	22·48	29·46	24·61	13·61	20·88	23·12	37·80	2
3	Enteric Group of Fevers	0·68	0·21	0·07	0·49	0·42	0·12	0·61	0·75	0·56	3
4	Infective Hepatitis—True	8·40	5·86	3·68	10·50	16·33	11·44	8·47	5·64	} 10·09	4
5	Infective Hepatitis—Post-Arsphenamine	0·97	0·62	0·07	0·90	0·69	0·96	0·30	—		5
6	Influenza	2·69	2·91	0·07	2·19	1·37	1·81	—	—	2·33	6
7	Malaria	35·33	5·54	4·68	40·36	36·90	12·65	98·03	57·71	33·75	7
8	Measles	0·25	—	—	0·29	0·32	0·60	—	—	0·24	8
9	Meningococcal Infection	0·23	0·97	0·13	0·08	0·22	—	—	0·56	0·25	9
10	Mumps	1·92	3·95	2·14	2·34	1·79	2·77	0·91	3·01	2·15	10
11	Pneumonia	5·96	24·29	6·22	3·88	2·96	2·77	3·03	5·83	6·41	11
12	P.U.O.	23·57	6·72	16·80	34·57	14·57	16·26	28·14	1·69	23·10	12
13	Relapsing Fever	0·03	0·10	—	0·05	0·05	0·96	—	1·88	0·08	13
14	Rheumatic Fever	0·68	0·59	0·40	0·25	0·54	0·48	0·30	—	0·55	14
15	Sandfly Fever	3·33	0·35	2·14	10·04	19·91	38·78	1·51	—	6·50	15
16	Schistosomiasis	1·27	1·32	2·21	0·88	0·66	0·12	—	0·19	1·13	16
17	Smallpox	0·76	0·14	—	0·18	0·12	—	—	—	0·50	17
18	Tuberculosis	3·41	1·52	1·20	2·91	1·20	1·57	1·21	2·26	2·85	18
19	Typhus Fever	0·07	—	—	0·08	0·05	—	—	—	0·06	19
20	Syphilis	6·68	7·21	4·08	4·99	8·35	10·12	7·56	10·90	7·71	20
21	Gonorrhoea	7·02	6·34	16·53	6·52	7·10	21·20	19·06	18·61	6·59	21
22	Other V.D.	18·30	3·98	4·42	12·22	17·19	37·82	21·18	33·27	16·22	22
23	Total V.D.	32·00	17·53	25·03	23·81	32·69	69·14	47·80	62·78	30·52	23
24	Scabies	6·18	8·97	2·74	2·63	7·69	15·54	3·33	2·82	5·83	24
25	Effects of Heat	0·24	0·80	0·07	0·04	0·02	1·32	1·51	—	0·24	25
26	Mental Diseases—Psychoses	4·26	1·07	1·74	1·59	1·86	1·45	6·35	—	3·15	26
27	Mental Diseases—Psychoneuroses	8·26	5·79	5·35	9·20	5·95	0·72	3·93	2·82	7·72	27
28	Nervous Diseases	5·41	3·74	4·08	5·14	4·26	6·14	13·01	—	5·10	28
29	Valvular Disease of the Heart	1·21	0·21	0·33	1·04	0·49	0·48	—	—	0·98	29

30	Other Diseases of the Circulatory System	5·79	2·88	6·42	6·23	3·57	4·46	15·73	2·82	5·51	30
31	Inflammation of the Bronchi	14·78	30·21	25·16	15·82	13·03	16·86	19·06	36·84	16·51	31
32	Other Diseases of the Respiratory System	8·97	7·80	7·70	11·70	12·66	18·43	15·73	3·01	9·86	32
33	Inflammation of the Tonsils	21·93	8·73	13·65	23·60	17·82	23·85	23·90	14·10	20·68	33
34	Other Diseases of the Digestive System	55·95	35·82	50·72	53·24	40·25	53·84	83·81	65·79	52·79	34
35	Diseases of the Ear and Nose	15·33	17·77	11·98	14·74	13·47	8·91	22·69	13·91	15·01	35
36	Diseases of the Eye	9·77	4·50	7·23	9·15	8·94	7·11	3·63	27·26	9·26	36
37	Skin and I.A.T.	49·25	36·73	35·80	51·16	54·04	45·77	45·39	92·67	49·21	37
38	All Other Diseases	76·42	68·95	69·73	72·75	58·42	75·64	91·98	110·15	73·86	38
39	*Total Admissions for Diseases*	452·69	336·35	330·16	442·28	398·70	455·26	561·58	537·59	435·89	39
40	Injuries—E.A.	1·11	0·17	—	0·43	0·12	0·84	0·30	—	42·61	40
41	Injuries—N.E.A.	40·50	38·70	49·79	43·70	51·76	54·44	32·98	46·43	0·77	41
42	*Total Admissions for Injuries*	41·61	38·87	49·79	44·13	51·88	55·28	33·28	46·43	43·38	42
43	*Total Admissions*	494·30	375·22	379·95	486·41	450·58	510·54	594·86	584·02	479·27	43

TABLE 67

Middle East Forces. Admissions to Hospitals, 1945. All Troops. By Commands
Annual Rates per 1,000 Strength

Source: Annual Report O.2.E., G.H.Q., M.E.F.

	CAUSES	Egypt	Palestine	Syria	Cyprus	Sudan and Eritrea	Aden	Cyrenaica	Tripolitania	Persia and Iraq	Total M.E.F.	
1	Diphtheria	0·39	1·19	0·38	0·41	0·22	0·22	0·28	0·10	0·19	0·47	1
2	Dysentery	36·48	22·97	19·17	7·72	16·42	13·32	23·50	21·60	17·77	28·66	2
3	Enteric Group of Fevers	0·47	0·89	0·38	—	0·22	0·22	0·37	—	0·29	0·48	3
4	Infective Hepatitis	5·86	10·38	9·62	8·54	7·20	9·39	4·64	9·08	5·38	7·83	4
5	Influenza	0·68	0·71	0·97	5·49	0·90	4·37	0·18	—	0·04	0·66	5
6	Malaria	12·30	26·69	22·74	9·55	26·76	41·48	2·62	2·62	26·05	17·09	6
7	Measles	0·15	0·14	0·38	—	0·22	—	2·62	—	0·11	0·27	7
8	Meningococcal Infection	0·19	0·18	0·03	0·41	—	—	0·09	0·10	0·03	0·14	8
9	Mumps	1·08	0·45	0·69	1·63	0·22	1·75	3·72	19·88	0·93	1·47	9
10	Pneumonia	3·80	4·92	3·25	6·10	2·47	4·80	11·73	11·40	2·89	4·37	10
11	P.U.O.	19·14	28·86	24·81	15·24	13·94	5·68	11·08	23·11	3·87	18·15	11
12	Relapsing Fever	0·19	0·04	—	0·20	—	0·22	0·41	0·10	0·27	0·17	12
13	Rheumatic Fever	0·20	0·29	0·31	0·61	0·22	—	0·32	0·61	0·06	0·22	13
14	Sandfly Fever	0·72	2·12	2·15	12·39	0·45	—	0·14	3·53	24·60	4·87	14
15	Schistosomiasis	0·72	0·39	0·55	0·20	0·22	—	3·36	8·07	0·09	0·83	15
16	Scabies	5·31	2·64	1·83	23·97	6·97	5·24	3·22	3·13	1·37	4·13	16
17	Smallpox	0·05	0·08	0·07	—	—	0·22	0·09	—	0·04	0·06	17
18	Tuberculosis	3·14	4·07	1·07	4·06	2·25	5·90	1·43	1·82	1·17	2·77	18
19	Typhus Fever	0·03	0·17	—	—	—	—	—	—	0·01	0·05	19
20	Venereal Diseases—Syphilis	9·96	8·40	9·90	24·99	10·34	14·63	7·73	8·17	10·59	9·89	20
21	Venereal Diseases—Gonorrhoea	7·33	12·12	15·78	44·90	26·76	24·89	12·09	18·27	9·14	10·15	21
22	Venereal Diseases—Other Forms	21·32	17·40	16·51	64·81	22·04	30·79	6·21	5·05	17·66	19·31	22
23	Total V.D.	38·61	37·92	42·19	134·70	59·14	70·31	26·03	31·49	37·39	39·35	23
24	Effects of Heat	0·11	0·20	0·03	—	1·35	0·44	0·05	0·10	2·56	0·51	24
25	Mental Diseases—Psychoses	3·07	1·59	2·04	4·47	2·02	0·22	1·66	0·71	0·23	2·19	25
26	Mental Diseases—Psychoneuroses	4·04	7·48	3·11	9·55	2·25	2·84	3·68	3·33	0·34	3·95	26
27	Nervous Diseases	3·86	4·89	7·72	2·03	9·89	—	4·23	2·62	1·76	3·94	27
28	Valvular Disease of the Heart	0·55	0·48	0·24	0·61	0·67	—	0·32	0·20	0·04	0·42	28
29	Other Diseases of the Circulatory System	4·35	6·16	2·15	7·92	8·77	2·18	3·40	5·45	1·30	4·06	29

30	Inflammation of the Bronchi	10·51	10·49	14·57	7·92	19·56	22·27	29·75	27·95	4·29	·29	30
31	Other Diseases of the Respiratory System	8·03	7·85	6·92	15·03	15·29	6·77	11·91	5·15	7·59	· 2	31
32	Inflammation of the Tonsils	17·69	22·46	13·50	21·54	19·79	16·59	10·71	14·73	6·37	16 8	32
33	Other Diseases of the Digestive System	38·83	46·11	48·49	37·38	63·41	73·36	43·09	50·26	40·25	41 4	33
34	Diseases of the Ear and Nose	11·01	13·12	13·12	14·43	15·52	15·28	15·36	13·93	8·04	11 2	34
35	Diseases of the Eye	6·95	8·83	11·14	11·38	2·70	20·52	5·52	5·85	4·94	7 6	35
36	Diseases of the Skin and I.A.T. (excluding Scabies)	37·53	58·86	50·77	55·47	28·56	87·55	33·71	58·94	37·31	42·61	36
37	All Other Diseases	68·38	77·70	83·37	92·24	87·70	93·67	76·20	75·18	69·78	72·25	37
38	*Total Admissions for Diseases*	344·42	411·32	387·76	511·19	415·30	504·81	335·42	401·04	307·36	356·98	38
39	Injuries—N.E.A.	29·35	43·22	51·60	74·16	27·88	40·61	38·58	49·75	23·50	33·53	39
40	Injuries—E.A.	0·03	0·21	—	1·42	—	—	—	—	—	0·06	40
41	*Total Admissions for Injuries*	29·38	43·43	51·60	75·58	27·88	40·61	38·58	49·75	23·50	33·59	41
42	*Total Admissions*	373·80	454·76	439·40	586·75	443·22	545·41	373·99	450·80	330·85	390·56	42

Table 68

Middle East Forces
Deaths in Hospital, 1941–45
All Troops
Annual Rates per 1,000 Strength

Source: Annual Reports O.2.E., G.H.Q., M.E.F.

	Causes	1941	1942	1943	1944	1945	
1	Diphtheria	0·04	0·05	0·02	0·01	—	1
2	Dysentery	0·06	0·10	0·03	0·02	0·02	2
3	Enteric Group of Fevers	0·04	0·09	0·13	0·06	0·04	3
4	Infective Hepatitis	N.A.	0·02	0·05	0·07	0·02	4
5	Influenza	—	0·00	0·00	—	—	5
6	Malaria	0·04	0·05	0·02	0·03	0·01	6
7	Measles	—	0·00	—	0·00	—	7
8	Meningococcal Infection	0·04	0·03	0·03	0·05	0·02	8
9	Pneumonia	0·07	0·10	0·09	0·10	0·04	9
10	P.U.O.	0·00	0·01	0·00	—	0·00	10
11	Relapsing Fever	—	0·00	—	0·00	—	11
12	Rheumatic Fever	0·00	—	0·00	—	—	12
13	Schistosomiasis	N.A.	—	—	0·01	—	13
14	Smallpox	0·00	0·01	0·03	0·03	0·00	14
15	Tuberculosis	0·03	0·12	0·21	0·46	0·41	15
16	Typhus Fever	N.A.	0·08	0·06	0·01	—	16
17	Venereal Diseases	—	0·01	0·00	0·00	0·00	17
18	Other Diseases due to Infection	0·10	0·07	—	—	—	18
19	Effects of Heat	N.A.	0·06	0·01	—	0·02	19
20	Mental Diseases—Psychoses	} 0·01	} 0·03	0·02	0·02	0·02	20
21	Mental Diseases—Psychoneuroses			0·01	0·00	0·00	21
22	Nervous Diseases	0·09	0·09	0·10	0·06	0·05	22
23	Valvular Disease of the Heart	0·00	0·01	0·04	0·08	0·05	23
24	Other Diseases of the Respiratory System	0·07	0·10	0·07	0·10	0·10	24
25	Inflammation of the Bronchi	0·00	0·01	0·01	0·02	0·00	25
26	Other Diseases of the Circulatory System	0·05	0·07	0·07	0·05	0·03	26
27	Inflammation of the Tonsils	0·00	—	0·00	—	0·00	27
28	Other Diseases of the Digestive System	0·11	0·19	0·14	0·14	0·11	28
29	Diseases of the Ear and Nose	0·01	0·01	0·02	0·01	0·00	29
30	Diseases of the Eye	—	0·00	—	—	0·00	30
31	Skin and I.A.T. (excluding Scabies)	0·02	0·01	0·01	0·00	0·02	31
32	All Other Diseases	0·13	0·37	0·31	0·35	0·28	32
33	*Total Deaths from Diseases*	0·92	1·70	1·48	1·69	1·28	33
34	Injuries—N.E.A.	0·77	1·02	0·74	0·69	0·48	34
35	Injuries—E.A.	0·47	0·60	0·22	0·02	0·01	35
36	*Total Deaths from Injuries*	1·24	1·62	0·96	0·70	0·49	36
37	*Total Deaths*	2·16	3·31	2·44	2·39	1·77	37

TABLE 69

Middle East Forces
Deaths in Hospital, 1941–45
United Kingdom Troops
Annual Rates per 1,000 Strength

Source: Annual Reports O.2.E., G.H.Q., M.E.F.

	CAUSES	1941	1942	1943	1944	1945	
1	Diphtheria	0·07	0·11	0·04	0·02	—	1
2	Dysentery	0·07	0·07	0·02	0·00	0·01	2
3	Enteric Group of Fevers	0·04	0·11	0·08	0·05	0·06	3
4	Infective Hepatitis	(a)	0·02	0·02	0·05	0·01	4
5	Influenza	—	—	—	—	—	5
6	Malaria	0·05	0·06	0·02	0·01	0·01	6
7	Measles	—	—	—	—	—	7
8	Meningococcal Infection	0·04	0·01	0·02	0·03	0·01	8
9	Mumps	—	—	—	—	—	9
10	Pneumonia	0·06	0·10	0·05	0·06	0·02	10
11	P.U.O.	—	—	0·00	—	—	11
12	Relapsing Fever	—	0·00	—	—	—	12
13	Rheumatic Fever	0·00	—	0·01	—	—	13
14	Sandfly Fever	—	—	—	—	—	14
15	Schistosomiasis	—	—	—	—	—	15
16	Smallpox	—	0·02	0·04	0·02	—	16
17	Tuberculosis	0·02	0·07	0·05	0·04	0·02	17
18	Typhus Fever	—	0·02	0·08	0·01	—	18
19	Scabies	—	—	—	—	—	19
20	Venereal Diseases	—	0·00	—	—	—	20
21	Other Diseases due to Infection	0·06	0·11	—	—	—	21
22	Effects of Heat	—	0·11	0·00	—	0·06	22
23	Mental Diseases—Psychoses	} 0·00	} 0·04	0·01	—	0·01	23
24	Mental Diseases—Psychoneuroses			0·01	—	—	24
25	Nervous Diseases	0·08	0·11	0·11	0·08	0·06	25
26	Valvular Disease of the Heart	0·00	0·01	0·01	0·02	0·04	26
27	Other Diseases of the Circulatory System	0·07	0·10	0·05	0·05	0·06	27
28	Inflammation of the Bronchi	0·00	0·01	0·01	0·01	—	28
29	Other Diseases of the Respiratory System	0·04	0·09	0·06	0·03	0·01	29
30	Inflammation of the Tonsils	0·01	—	—	—	0·01	30
31	Other Diseases of the Digestive System	0·12	0·23	0·11	0·09	0·12	31
32	Diseases of the Ear and Nose	0·02	0·01	0·02	0·01	—	32
33	Diseases of the Eye	—	0·00	—	—	—	33
34	Skin and I.A.T. (excluding Scabies)	0·02	0·02	0·01	—	—	34
35	All Other Diseases	0·14	0·30	0·19	0·19	0·11	35
36	*Total Deaths from Diseases*	0·93	1·73	1·03	0·81	0·64	36
37	Injuries—N.E.A.	0·96	1·16	0·63	0·55	0·46	37
38	Injuries—E.A.	0·46	0·85	0·31	0·01	—	38
39	*Total Deaths from Injuries*	1·42	2·01	0·94	0·56	0·46	39
40	*Total Deaths*	2·35	3·75	1·97	1·37	1·10	

(a) Included in 'All Other Diseases'.

TABLE 70

Middle East Forces
Deaths in Hospital, 1941–45
Indian Troops
Annual Rates per 1,000 Strength

Source: Annual Reports O.2.E., G.H.Q., M.E.F.

	CAUSES	1941	1942	1943	1944	1945	
1	Diphtheria	—	—	—	—	—	1
2	Dysentery	0·06	0·03	—	—	—	2
3	Enteric Group of Fevers	—	0·02	0·01	—	0·01	3
4	Infective Hepatitis	—	0·03	0·02	0·07	0·05	4
5	Influenza	—	—	—	—	—	5
6	Malaria	0·04	0·04	0·01	0·05	0·01	6
7	Measles	—	—	—	—	—	7
8	Meningococcal Infection	—	0·07	0·01	0·02	—	8
9	Mumps	—	—	—	—	—	9
10	Pneumonia	0·04	0·06	0·05	0·05	0·03	10
11	P.U.O.	0·04	0·01	—	—	—	11
12	Relapsing Fever	—	—	—	—	—	12
13	Rheumatic Fever	—	—	—	—	—	13
14	Schistosomiasis	—	—	—	—	—	14
15	Smallpox	0·02	0·01	—	—	—	15
16	Tuberculosis	0·06	0·13	0·50	1·14	0·56	16
17	Typhus Fever	—	—	0·01	—	0·01	17
18	Venereal Diseases	—	0·02	—	—	—	18
19	Effects of Heat	—	0·07	—	—	—	19
20	Mental Diseases	—	0·01	—	—	0·01	20
21	Nervous Diseases	0·04	0·03	0·06	—	0·04	21
22	Valvular Disease of the Heart	—	—	0·02	0·02	0·01	22
23	Other Diseases of the Circulatory System	0·02	0·05	0·04	0·07	0·08	23
24	Inflammation of the Bronchi	0·02	—	0·01	0·07	—	24
25	Other Diseases of the Respiratory System	0·04	0·07	0·05	0·10	0·02	25
26	Inflammation of the Tonsils	—	—	0·01	—	—	26
27	Other Diseases of the Digestive System	0·02	0·12	0·12	0·12	0·09	27
28	Diseases of the Ear and Nose	—	0·01	—	—	—	28
29	Diseases of the Eye	—	—	—	—	—	29
30	Skin and I.A.T. (excluding Scabies)	0·02	0·02	0·01	0·02	0·01	30
31	All Other Diseases	0·14	0·79	0·26	0·38	0·19	31
32	*Total Deaths from Diseases*	0·54	1·61	1·21	2·12	1·12	32
33	Injuries—N.E.A.	0·26	0·72	0·67	0·83	0·65	33
34	Injuries—E.A.	0·24	0·19	0·07	0·10	0·03	34
35	*Total Deaths from Injuries*	0·50	0·91	0·74	0·93	0·69	35
36	*Total Deaths*	1·05	2·52	1·95	3·05	1·81	36

TABLE 71

Middle East Forces
Deaths in Hospital, 1942
*Dominion Troops**
Annual Rates per 1,000 Strength

Source: Annual Reports O.2.E., G.H.Q., M.E.F.

	CAUSES	Rates per 1,000 Strength	
1	Diphtheria	0·02	1
2	Dysentery	0·02	2
3	Enteric Group of Fevers	0·02	3
4	Infective Hepatitis	0·02	4
5	Influenza	—	5
6	Malaria	—	6
7	Measles	0·02	7
8	Meningococcal Infection	0·04	8
9	Mumps	—	9
10	Pneumonia	0·14	10
11	P.U.O.	0·01	11
12	Relapsing Fever	—	12
13	Rheumatic Fever	—	13
14	Sandfly Fever	—	14
15	Schistosomiasis	—	15
16	Smallpox	—	16
17	Tuberculosis	0·10	17
18	Typhus Fever	0·01	18
19	Scabies	—	19
20	Venereal Diseases	—	20
21	Effects of Heat	—	21
22	Mental Diseases	0·02	22
23	Nervous Diseases	0·06	23
24	Valvular Disease of the Heart	0·02	24
25	Other Diseases of the Circulatory System	0·10	25
26	Inflammation of the Bronchi	0·01	26
27	Other Diseases of the Respiratory System	0·05	27
28	Inflammation of the Tonsils	—	28
29	Other Diseases of the Digestive System	0·19	29
30	Diseases of the Ear and Nose	—	30
31	Diseases of the Eye	—	31
32	Skin and I.A.T. (excluding Scabies)	0·01	32
33	All Other Diseases	0·21	33
34	*Total Deaths from Diseases*	1·06	34
35	Injuries—N.E.A.	1·05	35
36	Injuries—E.A.	1·04	36
37	*Total Deaths from Injuries*	2·10	37
38	*Total Deaths*	3·16	38

* Dominion Troops consisted of Australian, New Zealand and South African Forces

TABLE 72

Middle East Forces
Deaths in Hospital, 1943
New Zealand and South African Troops
Annual Rates per 1,000 Strength

Source: Annual Reports O.2.E., G.H.Q., M.E.F.

	CAUSES	Rates per 1,000 Strength	
1	Diphtheria	—	1
2	Dysentery	0·01	2
3	Enteric Group of Fevers	0·04	3
4	Infective Hepatitis	0·01	4
5	Influenza	—	5
6	Malaria	—	6
7	Measles	—	7
8	Meningococcal Infection	—	8
9	Mumps	—	9
10	Pneumonia	0·07	10
11	P.U.O.	0·01	11
12	Relapsing Fever	—	12
13	Rheumatic Fever	—	13
14	Sandfly Fever	—	14
15	Schistosomiasis	—	15
16	Scabies	—	16
17	Smallpox	0·03	17
18	Tuberculosis	0·17	18
19	Typhus Fever	0·04	19
20	Venereal Diseases	—	20
21	Effects of Heat	—	21
22	Mental Diseases—Psychoses	0·03	22
23	Mental Diseases—Psychoneuroses	—	23
24	Nervous Diseases	0·06	24
25	Valvular Disease of the Heart	0·01	25
26	Other Circulatory Conditions	0·07	26
27	Inflammation of the Bronchi	0·01	27
28	Other Diseases of the Respiratory System	0·01	28
29	Inflammation of the Tonsils	—	29
30	Other Diseases of the Digestive System	0·08	30
31	Diseases of the Ear and Nose	0·03	31
32	Diseases of the Eye	—	32
33	Skin and I.A.T. (excluding Scabies)	—	33
34	All Other Diseases	0·39	34
35	*Total Deaths from Diseases*	1·10	35
36	Injuries—N.E.A.	0·52	36
37	Injuries—E.A.	0·24	37
38	*Total Deaths from Injuries*	0·76	38
39	*Total Deaths*	1·86	39

TABLE 73

Middle East Forces
Deaths in Hospital, 1944–45
South African Troops
Annual Rates per 1,000 Strength

Source: Annual Reports O.2.E., G.H.Q., M.E.F.

	CAUSES	1944	1945	
1	Diphtheria	—	—	1
2	Dysentery	0·03	—	2
3	Enteric Group of Fevers	—	0·04	3
4	Infective Hepatitis	0·07	—	4
5	Influenza	—	—	5
6	Malaria	0·13	0·04	6
7	Measles	—	—	7
8	Meningococcal Infections	0·07	—	8
9	Mumps	—	—	9
10	Pneumonia	0·07	—	10
11	P.U.O.	—	—	11
12	Relapsing Fever	—	—	12
13	Rheumatic Fever	—	—	13
14	Sandfly Fever	—	—	14
15	Schistosomiasis	—	—	15
16	Scabies	—	—	16
17	Smallpox	0·03	—	17
18	Tuberculosis	0·26	0·22	18
19	Typhus Fever	—	—	19
20	Venereal Diseases	—	—	20
21	Effects of Heat	—	—	21
22	Mental Diseases—Psychoses	0·03	—	22
23	Mental Diseases—Psychoneuroses	—	—	23
24	Nervous Diseases	0·07	—	24
25	Valvular Disease of the Heart	0·03	0·04	25
26	Other Circulatory Conditions	0·23	0·04	26
27	Inflammation of the Bronchi	—	—	27
28	Other Diseases of the Respiratory System	0·07	—	28
29	Inflammation of the Tonsils	—	—	29
30	Other Diseases of the Digestive System	0·20	0·07	30
31	Diseases of the Ear and Nose	—	—	31
32	Diseases of the Eye	—	—	32
33	Skin and I.A.T. (excluding Scabies)	—	—	33
34	All Other Diseases	0·26	0·15	34
35	*Total deaths from Diseases*	1·55	0·58	35
36	Injuries—N.E.A.	0·63	0·51	36
37	Injuries—E.A.	—	—	37
38	*Total Deaths from Injuries*	0·63	0·51	38
39	*Total Deaths*	2·18	1·09	39

TABLE 74

Middle East Forces
Deaths in Hospital, 1944–45
New Zealand Troops
Annual Rates per 1,000 Strength

Source: Annual Reports O.2.E., G.H.Q., M.E.F.

	CAUSES	1944	1945	
1	Diphtheria	—	—	1
2	Dysentery	—	—	2
3	Enteric Group of Fevers	—	—	3
4	Infective Hepatitis	—	—	4
5	Influenza	—	—	5
6	Malaria	—	—	6
7	Measles	—	—	7
8	Meningococcal Infection	0·23	—	8
9	Mumps	—	—	9
10	Pneumonia	—	—	10
11	P.U.O.	—	—	11
12	Relapsing Fever	—	—	12
13	Rheumatic Fever	—	—	13
14	Sandfly Fever	—	—	14
15	Schistosomiasis	—	—	15
16	Scabies	—	—	16
17	Smallpox	—	—	17
18	Tuberculosis	—	—	18
19	Typhus Fever	—	—	19
20	Venereal Diseases	—	—	20
21	Effects of Heat	—	—	21
22	Mental Diseases—Psychoses	—	—	22
23	Mental Diseases—Psychoneuroses	—	—	23
24	Nervous Diseases	—	—	24
25	Valvular Disease of the Heart	—	—	25
26	Other Circulatory Conditions	—	—	26
27	Inflammation of the Bronchi	—	0·16	27
28	Other Diseases of the Respiratory System	—	—	28
29	Inflammation of the Tonsils	—	—	29
30	Other Diseases of the Digestive System	—	0·16	30
31	Diseases of the Ear and Nose	—	—	31
32	Diseases of the Eye	—	—	32
33	Skin and I.A.T. (excluding Scabies)	—	—	33
34	All Other Diseases	0·23	0·16	34
35	*Total Deaths from Diseases*	0·47	0·48	35
36	Injuries—N.E.A.	0·47	0·80	36
37	Injuries—E.A.	—	—	37
38	*Total Deaths from Injuries*	0·47	0·80	38
39	*Total Deaths*	0·94	1·29	39

TABLE 75

Middle East Forces
Deaths in Hospital, 1943–45
British African Troops
Annual Rates per 1,000 Strength

Source: Annual Reports O.2.E., G.H.Q., M.E.F.

	CAUSES	1943	1944	1945	
1	Diphtheria	—	—	—	1
2	Dysentery	0·04	0·07	0·06	2
3	Enteric Group of Fevers	0·18	0·07	0·03	3
4	Infective Hepatitis	0·04	0·05	0·05	4
5	Influenza	—	—	—	5
6	Malaria	0·04	0·02	0·02	6
7	Measles	—	0·02	—	7
8	Meningococcal Infection	0·16	0·13	0·14	8
9	Mumps	—	—	—	9
10	Pneumonia	0·45	0·24	0·09	10
11	P.U.O.	0·02	—	0·02	11
12	Relapsing Fever	—	—	—	12
13	Rheumatic Fever	—	—	—	13
14	Sandfly Fever	—	—	—	14
15	Schistosomiasis	—	0·05	—	15
16	Scabies	—	—	—	16
17	Smallpox	0·05	0·13	0·02	17
18	Tuberculosis	0·81	1·41	1·03	18
19	Typhus Fever	0·11	—	—	19
20	Venereal Diseases	—	0·02	—	20
21	Effects of Heat	0·02	—	—	21
22	Mental Diseases—Psychoses	0·04	0·05	0·06	22
23	Mental Diseases—Psychoneuroses	—	—	—	23
24	Nervous Diseases	0·22	0·09	0·06	24
25	Valvular Disease of the Heart	0·05	0·20	0·08	25
26	Other Circulatory Conditions	0·16	0·27	0·33	26
27	Inflammation of the Bronchi	—	0·04	0·02	27
28	Other Diseases of the Respiratory System	0·20	0·14	0·11	28
29	Inflammation of the Tonsils	—	—	—	29
30	Other Diseases of the Digestive System	0·32	0·20	0·21	30
31	Diseases of the Ear and Nose	0·02	—	—	31
32	Diseases of the Eye	—	—	—	32
33	Skin and I.A.T. (excl. Scabies)	—	0·02	0·02	33
34	All Other Diseases	0·63	0·85	0·76	34
35	*Total Deaths from Diseases*	3·56	4·07	3·09	35
36	Injuries—N.E.A.	0·45	0·54	0·33	36
37	Injuries—E.A.	0·02	—	—	37
38	*Total Deaths from Injuries*	0·47	0·54	0·33	38
39	*Total Deaths*	4·02	4·62	3·42	39

Note: The term 'British African' includes all native male personnel from British Territories in Africa.

11CMS

TABLE 76

Middle East Forces
Deaths in Hospital, 1944–45
Other British Troops
Annual Rates per 1,000 Strength

Source: Annual Reports O.2.E., G.H.Q., M.E.F.

	CAUSES	1944	1945	
1	Diphtheria	—	—	1
2	Dysentery	0·04	—	2
3	Enteric Group of Fevers	—	0·04	3
4	Infective Hepatitis	—	—	4
5	Influenza	—	—	5
6	Malaria	0·09	—	6
7	Measles	—	—	7
8	Meningococcal Infection	—	—	8
9	Mumps	—	—	9
10	Pneumonia	0·18	0·04	10
11	P.U.O.	—	—	11
12	Relapsing Fever	—	—	12
13	Rheumatic Fever	0·04	—	13
14	Sandfly Fever	—	—	14
15	Schistosomiasis	—	—	15
16	Scabies	—	—	16
17	Smallpox	—	—	17
18	Tuberculosis	0·31	0·11	18
19	Typhus Fever	—	—	19
20	Venereal Diseases	—	—	20
21	Effects of Heat	—	—	21
22	Mental Diseases	—	—	22
23	Nervous Diseases	0·04	0·08	23
24	Valvular Disease of the Heart	0·09	0·04	24
25	Other Circulatory Conditions	0·04	0·15	25
26	Inflammation of the Bronchi	—	—	26
27	Other Diseases of the Respiratory System	0·09	0·04	27
28	Inflammation of the Tonsils	—	—	28
29	Other Diseases of the Digestive System	0·18	0·11	29
30	Diseases of the Ear and Nose	—	—	30
31	Diseases of the Eye	—	—	31
32	Skin and I.A.T. (excl. Scabies)	—	0·11	32
33	All Other Diseases	0·53	0·31	33
34	*Total Deaths from Diseases*	1·64	1·03	34
35	Injuries—N.E.A.	0·84	0·34	35
36	Injuries—E.A.	—	—	36
37	*Total Deaths from Injuries*	0·84	0·34	37
38	*Total Deaths*	2·48	1·38	38

Note: The term 'Other British Troops' refers to all male personnel from British Territories outside Africa and not included in Tables 69 to 75.

Table 77

Middle East Forces
Deaths in Hospital, 1942-45
Women's Services
Annual Rates per 1,000 Strength

Source: Annual Reports O.2.E., G.H.Q., M.E.F.

	Causes	1942	1943	1944	1945	
1	Diphtheria	—	0·10	—	—	1
2	Dysentery	—	—	—	—	2
3	Enteric Group of Fevers	0·22	0·10	0·11	—	3
4	Infective Hepatitis	—	0·41	—	—	4
5	Influenza	—	—	—	—	5
6	Malaria	—	—	—	—	6
7	Measles	—	—	—	—	7
8	Meningococcal Infection	—	—	—	—	8
9	Mumps	—	—	—	—	9
10	Pneumonia	0·22	—	—	—	10
11	P.U.O.	—	—	—	—	11
12	Relapsing Fever	—	—	—	—	12
13	Rheumatic Fever	—	—	—	—	13
14	Sandfly Fever	—	—	—	—	14
15	Schistosomiasis	—	—	—	—	15
16	Scabies	—	—	—	—	16
17	Smallpox	—	—	—	—	17
18	Tuberculosis	—	—	—	0·14	18
19	Typhus Fever	—	—	—	—	19
20	Effects of Heat	—	—	—	—	20
21	Venereal Diseases	—	—	—	—	21
22	Mental Diseases—Psychoses	—	—	—	—	22
23	Mental Diseases—Psychoneuroses	—	—	—	—	23
24	Nervous Diseases	—	—	—	—	24
25	Valvular Disease of the Heart	—	—	—	0·27	25
26	Other Circulatory Conditions	—	0·10	0·11	—	26
27	Inflammation of the Bronchi	—	—	—	—	27
28	Other Diseases of the Respiratory System	—	—	—	—	28
29	Inflammation of the Tonsils	—	0·10	—	—	29
30	Other Diseases of the Digestive System	0·22	0·21	0·11	—	30
31	Diseases of the Ear and Nose	—	—	—	—	31
32	Diseases of the Eye	—	—	—	—	32
33	Skin and I.A.T. (excluding Scabies)	—	—	—	—	33
34	All Other Diseases	0·22	0·21	0·22	0·14	34
35	*Total Deaths from Diseases*	0·88	1·23	0·55	0·55	35
36	Injuries—N.E.A.	1·10	0·72	0·44	0·27	36
37	Injuries—E.A.	—	—	—	—	37
38	*Total Deaths from Injuries*	1·10	0·72	0·44	0·27	38
39	*Total Deaths*	1·98	1·96	1·00	0·82	39

Table 78

Middle East Forces
Deaths in Hospitals, 1943-45
All Other Troops
Annual Rates per 1,000 Strength

Source: Annual Reports O.2.E., G.H.Q., M.E.F.

	Causes	1942	1943	1944	1945	
1	Diphtheria	—	—	0·01	—	1
2	Dysentery	0·29	0·09	0·04	0·01	2
3	Enteric Group of Fevers	0·15	0·38	0·14	0·03	3
4	Infective Hepatitis	—	0·15	0·13	0·01	4
5	Influenza	0·02	*	—	—	5
6	Malaria	0·07	0·01	0·03	—	6
7	Measles	—	—	—	—	7
8	Meningococcal Infection	0·03	0·06	0·05	—	8
9	Mumps	—	—	—	—	9
10	Pneumonia	0·07	0·10	0·14	0·06	10
11	P.U.O.	0·01	*	—	—	11
12	Relapsing Fever	0·01	—	—	—	12
13	Rheumatic Fever	—	—	—	—	13
14	Sandfly Fever	—	—	—	—	14
15	Schistosomiasis	—	—	—	—	15
16	Scabies	—	—	—	—	16
17	Smallpox	—	0·01	0·03	—	17
18	Tuberculosis	0·24	0·27	0·68	0·65	18
19	Typhus Fever	0·36	0·07	0·01	—	19
20	Venereal Diseases	—	—	—	—	20
21	Effects of Heat	0·01	—	—	—	21
22	Mental Diseases—Psychoses	} 0·03	0·03	0·06	0·02	22
23	Mental Diseases—Psychoneuroses		*	0·01	—	23
24	Nervous Diseases	0·11	0·08	0·03	0·06	24
25	Valvular Disease of the Heart	—	0·18	0·19	0·10	25
26	Other Circulatory Conditions	0·08	0·12	0·10	0·06	26
27	Inflammation of the Bronchi	0·02	*	0·01	—	27
28	Other Diseases of the Respiratory System	0·05	0·10	0·03	0·03	28
29	Inflammation of the Tonsils	—	*	—	—	29
30	Other Diseases of the Digestive System	0·17	0·20	0·21	0·07	30
31	Diseases of the Ear and Nose	—	—	0·01	0·01	31
32	Diseases of the Eye	—	—	—	0·01	32
33	Skin and I.A.T. (excluding Scabies)	—	—	—	0·04	33
34	All Other Diseases	0·35	0·60	0·40	0·39	34
35	*Total Deaths from Diseases*	2·16	2·45	2·32	1·56	35
36	Injuries—N.E.A.	1·04	1·46	1·08	0·46	36
37	Injuries—E.A.	0·15	0·12	—	0·01	37
38	*Total Deaths from Injuries*	1·19	1·58	1·08	0·47	38
39	*Total Deaths*	3·35	4·03	3·40	2·03	39

* Any cases included in 'All Other Diseases'.

Note: The term 'All Other Troops' refers to all Dominion, Colonial and Allied male personnel (excluding U.S. personnel) not included in Tables 69 to 77.

Middle East Forces. Deaths in Hospitals, 1942. All Troops. By Commands
Rates per 1,000 Strength

Source: Annual Report O.2.E., M.E.F.

	CAUSES	Egypt and 8th Army	Pales-tine	Syria 9th Army	Cyprus 9th Army	Sudan	Eritrea	Malta (a) E.A.R.	Aden (b) E.A.R.	Persia and Iraq 10th Army (c) E.A.R.	Total M.E.F.	
1	Diphtheria	0·08	0·02	—	0·05	—	—	—	—	—	0·05	1
2	Dysentery	0·07	0·04	—	0·05	—	0·22	0·10	—	0·27	0·10	2
3	Enteric Group of Fevers	0·10	0·09	0·04	—	0·19	0·22	0·07	0·24	0·06	0·09	3
4	Infective Hepatitis	0·02	0·01	—	—	—	0·11	—	—	0·03	0·02	4
5	Influenza	—	—	—	—	—	—	—	—	0·02	0·00	5
6	Malaria	0·03	0·04	0·06	0·05	—	0·22	—	—	0·10	0·05	6
7	Measles	0·00	—	—	—	—	—	—	—	—	0·00	7
8	Meningococcal Infection	0·02	0·07	—	0·11	—	—	—	—	0·07	0·03	8
9	Mumps	—	—	—	—	—	—	—	—	—	—	9
10	Pneumonia	0·12	0·15	0·01	0·11	—	0·11	—	0·24	0·03	0·10	10
11	P.U.O.	0·00	—	—	—	—	—	—	—	0·01	0·01	11
12	Relapsing Fever	—	0·01	—	—	—	0·11	—	—	—	0·00	12
13	Rheumatic Fever	—	—	—	—	—	—	—	—	—	—	13
14	Sandfly Fever	—	—	—	—	—	—	—	—	—	—	14
15	Schistosomiasis	—	—	—	—	—	—	—	—	—	—	15
16	Scabies	—	—	—	—	—	—	—	—	—	—	16
17	Smallpox	—	—	0·05	—	—	—	—	—	0·04	0·01	17
18	Tuberculosis	0·10	0·22	0·07	—	—	—	0·07	0·24	0·18	0·12	18
19	Typhus Fever	0·01	0·01	—	—	—	—	—	—	0·42	0·08	19
20	Venereal Diseases	0·01	—	—	—	—	—	—	—	0·01	0·01	20
21	Effects of Heat	0·01	0·01	—	—	—	—	—	—	0·32	0·06	21
22	Mental Diseases—Psychoses	0·04	0·01	—	—	—	—	—	—	0·01	0·03	22
23	Mental Diseases—Psychoneuroses			—	—	—	—	—	—			23
24	Nervous Diseases	0·11	0·13	0·01	—	—	—	0·07	—	0·02	0·09	24
25	Valvular Disease of the Heart	0·00	0·02	—	0·05	—	—	—	—	—	0·01	25
26	Other Diseases of the Circulatory System	0·10	0·23	0·04	0·10	—	0·11	—	—	0·02	0·10	26
27	Inflammation of the Bronchi	0·01	—	—	—	—	—	—	—	—	0·01	27
28	Other Diseases of the Respiratory System	0·09	0·07	—	0·16	—	0·11	0·03	—	0·05	0·07	28
29	Inflammation of the Tonsils	—	—	—	—	—	—	—	—	—	—	29
30	Other Diseases of the Digestive System	0·18	0·26	0·08	0·16	—	0·33	0·07	0·24	0·17	0·19	30
31	Diseases of the Ear and Nose	0·01	—	—	0·05	—	—	0·03	—	—	0·01	31
32	Diseases of the Eye	0·00	—	—	—	—	—	—	—	—	0·00	32
33	Diseases of the Skin and I.A.T. (excl. Scabies)	0·02	—	0·01	0·05	—	—	—	—	—	0·01	33
34	All Other Diseases	0·23	0·35	0·06	—	0·94	0·55	0·17	0·24	1·36	0·45	34
35	*Total Deaths from Diseases*	1·34	1·75	0·45	0·98	1·11	2·11	0·61	1·18	3·20	1·70	35
36	Injuries—N.E.A.	0·97	1·65	0·45	0·92	0·19	0·67	0·27	0·24	0·22	1·02	36
37	Injuries—E.A.	1·22	0·15	—	—	—	—	0·34	—	0·08	0·60	37
38	*Total Deaths from Injuries*	2·19	1·80	0·45	0·92	0·19	0·67	0·61	0·24	0·30	1·62	38
39	*Total Deaths*	3·54	3·55	0·90	1·90	1·30	2·78	1·22	1·42	3·49	3·31	39

(a) Equivalent annual rates based on deaths for the period June to December.
(b) Equivalent annual rates based on deaths for the period July to December.
(c) Equivalent annual rates based on deaths for the period January to August.

TABLE 80

Middle East Forces. Deaths in Hospital, 1943. By Commands
Annual Rates per 1,000 Strength

Source: Annual Report O.2.E., G.H.Q., M.E.F.

	CAUSES	Egypt, Cyrenaica and Tripolitania	Palestine	Syria	Cyprus	Sudan and Eritrea	Malta	Aden	Total M.E.F.	
1	Diphtheria	0·03	0·01	—	—	—	—	—	0·02	1
2	Dysentery	0·04	—	—	—	—	—	—	0·03	2
3	Enteric Group of Fevers	0·15	0·05	0·08	0·06	0·40	0·07	—	0·13	3
4	Infective Hepatitis	0·06	0·02	0·02	0·06	—	—	—	0·05	4
5	Influenza	—	0·01	—	—	—	—	—	0·00	5
6	Malaria	0·02	0·01	0·03	—	0·20	0·04	—	0·02	6
7	Measles	—	—	—	—	—	—	—	—	7
8	Meningococcal Infection	0·04	0·04	—	—	0·20	—	—	0·03	8
9	Mumps	—	—	—	—	—	—	—	—	9
10	Pneumonia	0·11	0·02	0·06	—	0·20	0·07	0·16	0·09	10
11	P.U.O.	0·01	—	—	—	—	—	—	0·00	11
12	Rheumatic Fever	0·00	—	—	—	—	—	—	0·00	12
13	Sandfly Fever	—	—	—	—	—	—	—	—	13
14	Schistosomiasis	—	—	—	—	—	—	—	—	14
15	Scabies	—	—	—	—	—	—	—	—	15
16	Smallpox	0·04	0·03	0·03	—	—	—	—	0·03	16
17	Tuberculosis	0·20	0·31	0·13	0·50	—	0·04	0·79	0·21	17
18	Typhus Fever	0·09	0·01	0·02	—	—	—	—	0·06	18
19	Venereal Diseases	—	0·01	—	—	—	—	—	0·00	19
20	Effects of Heat	0·01	—	—	—	—	0·04	—	0·01	20
21	Mental Diseases—Psychoses	0·02	—	—	—	—	—	—	0·02	21
22	Mental Diseases—Psychoneuroses	0·01	0·01	—	—	—	—	—	0·01	22
23	Nervous Diseases	0·11	0·07	0·05	0·25	—	0·18	—	0·10	23
24	Valvular Disease of the Heart	0·03	0·10	0·02	0·06	0·40	—	—	0·04	24
25	Other Diseases of the Circulatory System	0·07	0·11	0·08	0·06	—	—	—	0·07	25
26	Inflammation of the Bronchi	0·01	—	—	0·31	—	—	—	0·01	26
27	Other Diseases of the Respiratory System	0·07	0·10	—	—	0·20	0·04	—	0·07	27
28	Inflammation of the Tonsils	0·00	—	—	—	—	—	—	0·00	28
29	Other Diseases of the Digestive System	0·12	0·26	0·10	—	—	0·07	0·16	0·14	29
30	Diseases of the Ear and Nose	0·02	0·01	0·02	—	—	—	—	0·02	30
31	Diseases of the Eye	—	—	—	—	—	—	—	—	31
32	Diseases of the Skin and I.A.T. (excl. Scabies)	0·01	0·01	—	—	—	—	—	0·01	32
33	All Other Diseases	0·31	0·45	0·16	0·12	0·40	0·21	0·32	0·31	33
34	*Total Deaths due to Diseases*	1·58	1·65	0·78	1·44	2·00	0·74	1·42	1·48	34
35	Injuries—N.E.A.	0·65	1·40	0·67	0·56	0·40	0·49	0·32	0·74	35
36	Injuries—E.A.	0·29	0·02	0·02	0·19	—	0·25	—	0·22	36
37	*Total Deaths from Injuries*	0·94	1·42	0·69	0·75	0·40	0·74	0·32	0·96	37
38	*Total Deaths*	2·52	3·07	1·47	2·19	2·41	1·48	1·73	2·44	38

TABLE 81

Middle East Forces. Deaths in Hospitals, 1944. All Troops. By Commands
Annual Rates per 1,000 Strength

Source: Annual Report O.2.E., G.H.Q., M.E.F.

	CAUSES	Egypt	Palestine	Syria	Cyprus	Sudan and Eritrea	Aden	Cyrenaica	Tripolitania	Total M.E.F.	
1	Diphtheria	0·01	0·01	—	—	—	0·19	—	0·07	0·01	1
2	Dysentery	0·03	—	—	—	—	0·19	0·03	—	0·02	2
3	Enteric Group of Fevers	0·07	0·05	0·07	—	—	—	0·03	—	0·06	3
4	Infective Hepatitis	0·08	0·05	0·02	—	—	—	0·07	0·07	0·07	4
5	Influenza	—	—	—	—	—	—	—	—	—	5
6	Malaria	0·03	0·04	0·05	—	—	0·19	0·03	—	0·03	6
7	Measles	0·00	—	—	—	—	—	—	—	0·00	7
8	Meningococcal Infection	0·05	0·04	—	—	—	—	0·17	—	0·05	8
9	Mumps	—	—	—	—	—	—	—	—	—	9
10	Pneumonia	0·10	0·05	—	—	—	0·57	0·35	—	0·10	10
11	P.U.O.	—	—	—	—	—	—	—	—	—	11
12	Rheumatic Fever	—	—	—	—	—	—	—	—	—	12
13	Sandfly Fever	—	—	—	—	—	—	—	—	—	13
14	Schistosomiasis	0·01	—	—	—	—	—	—	—	0·01	14
15	Scabies	—	—	—	—	—	—	—	—	—	15
16	Smallpox	0·05	0·02	—	—	—	—	—	—	0·03	16
17	Tuberculosis	0·58	0·45	0·12	—	—	0·38	0·14	0·27	0·46	17
18	Typhus Fever	0·01	0·01	—	—	—	—	—	—	0·01	18
19	Venereal Diseases	0·00	—	—	—	—	—	—	—	0·00	19
20	Effects of Heat	—	—	—	—	—	—	—	—	—	20
21	Mental Diseases—Psychoses	0·03	—	—	—	—	—	—	—	0·02	21
22	Mental Diseases—Psychoneuroses	0·00	—	—	—	—	—	—	—	0·00	22
23	Nervous Diseases	0·08	0·01	0·05	—	—	0·38	0·07	—	0·06	23
24	Valvular Disease of the Heart	0·11	0·05	0·05	—	—	—	—	0·07	0·08	24
25	Other Diseases of the Circulatory System	0·10	0·10	0·05	0·12	—	0·19	0·14	0·20	0·10	25
26	Inflammation of the Bronchi	0·02	0·04	—	—	—	—	—	—	0·02	26
27	Other Diseases of the Respiratory System	0·07	0·04	0·02	—	—	0·19	—	—	0·05	27
28	Inflammation of the Tonsils	—	—	—	—	—	—	—	—	—	28
29	Other Diseases of the Digestive System	0·12	0·14	0·12	0·12	0·61	0·19	0·14	0·27	0·14	29
30	Diseases of the Ear and Nose	0·01	0·01	—	—	—	—	—	—	0·01	30
31	Diseases of the Eye	—	—	—	—	—	—	—	—	—	31
32	Diseases of the Skin and I.A.T. (excl. Scabies)	0·01	—	—	—	—	—	—	—	0·00	32
33	All Other Diseases	0·40	0·39	0·24	0·36	—	0·19	0·24	0·13	0·35	33
34	*Total Deaths due to Diseases*	2·00	1·48	0·81	0·60	0·61	2·63	1·42	1·07	1·69	34
35	Injuries—N.E.A.	0·64	0·82	0·49	0·72	—	0·38	1·11	0·60	0·69	35
36	Injuries—E.A.	0·02	0·01	—	—	—	—	—	—	0·02	36
37	*Total Deaths from Injuries*	0·67	0·83	0·49	0·72	—	0·38	1·11	0·60	0·70	37
38	*Total Deaths*	2·67	2·31	1·30	1·32	0·61	3·01	2·53	1·67	2·39	38

TABLE 82

Middle East Forces. Deaths in Hospitals, 1945. All Troops. By Commands.
Annual Rates per 1,000 Strength

Source: Annual Report O.2.E., G.H.Q., M.E.F.

	CAUSES	Egypt	Palestine	Syria	Cyprus	Sudan and Eritrea	Aden	Cyren-aica	Tripoli-tania	Persia and Iraq	Total M.E.F.	
1	Diphtheria	—	—	—	—	—	—	—	—	—	—	1
2	Dysentery	0·03	—	—	—	—	—	—	—	—	0·02	2
3	Enteric Group of Fevers	0·05	0·01	—	—	0·22	—	0·05	—	0·04	0·04	3
4	Infective Hepatitis	0·02	0·01	—	—	—	—	0·05	—	0·06	0·02	4
5	Influenza	—	—	—	—	—	—	—	—	—	—	5
6	Malaria	0·00	0·01	0·03	—	0·22	—	—	—	—	0·01	6
7	Measles	—	—	—	—	—	—	—	—	—	—	7
8	Meningococcal Infection	0·03	0·02	—	—	—	—	0·05	—	—	0·02	8
9	Mumps	—	—	—	—	—	—	—	—	—	—	9
10	Pneumonia	0·03	0·05	0·03	—	—	—	0·05	—	0·04	0·04	10
11	P.U.O.	0·00	—	—	—	—	—	—	—	—	0·00	11
12	Rheumatic Fever	—	—	—	—	—	—	—	—	—	—	12
13	Sandfly Fever	—	—	—	—	—	—	—	—	—	—	13
14	Schistosomiasis	—	—	—	—	—	—	—	—	—	—	14
15	Scabies	—	—	—	—	—	—	—	—	—	—	15
16	Smallpox	0·00	—	—	—	—	—	—	—	—	0·00	16
17	Tuberculosis	0·56	0·39	0·06	—	—	—	—	0·40	0·14	0·41	17
18	Typhus Fever	—	—	—	—	—	—	—	—	—	—	18
19	Venereal Diseases	—	—	—	—	—	—	—	—	0·01	0·00	19
20	Effects of Heat	—	—	—	—	—	—	—	—	0·11	0·02	20
21	Mental Diseases—Psychoses	0·03	—	—	—	—	—	—	—	—	0·02	21
22	Mental Diseases—Psychoneuroses	0·01	—	—	—	—	—	—	—	—	0·00	22
23	Nervous Diseases	0·05	0·06	—	—	—	—	0·05	—	0·03	0·05	23
24	Valvular Disease of the Heart	0·06	0·06	—	—	—	—	—	0·10	0·01	0·05	24
25	Other Diseases of the Circulatory System	0·15	0·04	—	—	—	—	0·14	—	0·04	0·10	25
26	Inflammation of the Bronchi	0·01	—	—	—	—	—	—	—	—	0·00	26
27	Other Diseases of the Respiratory System	0·03	0·05	0·03	—	—	0·22	—	—	0·01	0·03	27
28	Inflammation of the Tonsils	0·00	—	—	—	—	—	—	—	—	0·00	28
29	Other Diseases of the Digestive System	0·04	0·14	—	—	—	—	0·05	0·10	0·09	0·11	29
30	Diseases of the Ear and Nose	—	—	0·06	—	—	—	—	—	0·01	0·00	30
31	Diseases of the Eye	0·00	—	—	—	—	—	—	—	—	0·00	31
32	Diseases of the Skin and I.A.T. (excl. Scabies)	0·03	—	—	—	—	—	—	—	0·01	0·02	32
33	All Other Diseases	0·39	0·20	0·09	0·20	—	—	0·15	0·10	0·19	0·28	33
34	*Total Deaths due to Diseases*	1·52	1·04	0·30	0·20	0·44	0·22	0·59	0·70	0·79	1·28	34
35	Injuries—N.E.A.	0·38	0·50	0·40	0·20	0·67	0·45	0·90	0·40	0·90	0·48	35
36	Injuries—E.A.	0·01	0·02	—	—	—	—	—	—	—	0·01	36
37	*Total Deaths from Injuries*	0·39	0·52	0·40	0·20	0·67	0·45	0·90	0·40	0·90	0·49	37
38	*Total Deaths*	1·91	1·56	0·70	0·40	1·11	0·67	1·49	1·10	1·69	1·77	38

CHAPTER VI

WEST AFRICA COMMAND

As in all other Commands, there is no complete morbidity and traumatic data available for West Africa Command for the war years. In so far as the Medical Index maintained by the Hollerith Section of the War Office is concerned, 100 per cent. of Army Forms I.1220 received from the Command for the years 1941 to 1945 were coded. These forms, however, pertained to British Troops only. The preponderance of troops in the theatre was of West African stock. It is therefore necessary, in order to evaluate the relative importance of the incidence of disease among the British and African troops stationed there, to rely upon another source for data. The statistical reports for the period 1941–44 and for 1945 prepared by the local Army Health Authorities are available and this chapter summarises the information contained in these reports.

Both reports are concerned with hospitalisation only (except with regard to Venereal Diseases) and do not include any data relating to low grade morbidity. They are not comprehensive in that only certain diseases and injuries are included. They do not, as do those of some other commands, give the incidence, for instance, of I.A.T., Psychiatric Disorders, Scabies, etc. They do, however, draw an illuminating picture of those diseases which have a greater incidence among personnel of one or other of the two groups concerned.

Apart from the incidence of the Dysenteries occurring among European Troops in 1944 (Table 85), there is no reason to doubt the accuracy of the figures shown in the tables which follow.

Table 83 shows the rates of hospital admissions for both classes of personnel. The Command rate for Europeans was consistently higher than that for Africans, being in 1941 more than twice as high and in 1945 just under 20 per cent. higher. Throughout the period, the Command rate for Europeans steadily declined, whereas that for Africans fluctuated without any characteristic trend. The reason for this was the successful control of Malaria. This is exemplified by the fact that if the Malaria rates are excluded, the figures for Europeans show no steady decline and differ little from those for Africans.

Table 84 shows the comparative importance of different diseases. Africans are relatively immune to Malaria, Bacillary and Amoebic Dysentery. They are, however, relatively prone to V.D., Pneumonia, Chickenpox and Tropical Ulcer. The high rate for Schistosomiasis in 1944 was largely due to a local outbreak in Nigeria.

TABLE 83

West Africa Command, 1941–45
Admissions to Hospitals, All Causes
Annual Rates per 1,000 Strngth

Source: West Africa Annual Statistical Reports, 1944, 1945

Year	Gold Coast	Nigeria	Sierra Leone	Gambia	Whole Command	
					All Causes	Excluding Malaria
Europeans						
1941	1,737	968	1,804	942	1,620	698
1942	1,585	907	1,583	1,852	1,436	680
1943	1,432	1,186	1,017	1,161	1,157	726
1944	1,029	1,332	677	826	1,105	827
1945	812	794	644	686	760	668
Africans						
1941	877	372	1,400	500	632	561
1942	811	409	897	881	721	648
1943	733	654	656	803	663	621
1944	950	1,032	421	852	851	806
1945	764	647	423	866	649	616

TABLE 84

West Africa Command, 1944, 1945
Admissions to Hospitals for Certain Infectious Diseases
Annual Rates per 1,000 Strength

Source: West Africa Annual Statistical Reports, 1944, 1945

	1944			1945		
	(a) Europeans	(b) Africans	Ratio (a)÷(b)	(c) Europeans	(d) Africans	Ratio (c)÷(d)
Malaria . .	278·0	45·0	6·2	91·9	32·8	2·8
Venereal Diseases .	81·2*	386·0*	0·2	82·0	482·4	0·2
Bacillary Dysentery.	65·2	4·6	14·2	24·4	8·9	2·8
Amoebic Dysentery.	26·0	4·9	5·3	4·3	2·3	1·9
Schistosomiasis .	24·3	19·4	1·3	0·2	6·9	—
'Jaundice' . .	7·2	3·5	2·1	6·4	3·4	1·9
Tuberculosis . .	2·7	2·6	1·0	2·9	1·7	1·7
Pneumonia . .	1·9	21·4	0·1	1·2	15·7	0·1
Chickenpox . .	—	17·8	—	—	9·2	—
Tropical Ulcer .	—	8·7	—	—	4·8	—
Trypanosomiasis .	—	1·6	—	—	1·2	—
Cerebro-Spinal Fever	—	1·4	—	—	1·3	—
Smallpox . .	—	0·2	—	—	0·2	—
Enteric Fevers .	—	0·2	—	—	—	—

* This figure includes cases treated in units.

Table 85 summarises available information regarding DYSENTERY among Europeans, the incidence of which fell, being initially (1941) 51

TABLE 85

West Africa Command, 1941–45
Admissions to Hospitals for Dysentery (all types), Europeans only
Annual Rates per 1,000 Strength
Ratios of Bacillary to Amoebic Dysentery, 1941, 1944

Source: West Africa Annual Statistical Reports, 1944, 1945

Year	Gold Coast	Nigeria	Sierra Leone	Gambia	Whole Command
1941	28	25	46	117	51
1942	21	45	85	53	71
1943	28	42	49	51	42
1944	36	13	24	56	27
1945	51	11	23	33	29
Ratio of Bacillary to Amoebic, 1941, 1944	1 : 1	4 : 1	6 : 1	1 : 1	2 : 1

and finally (1945) 29. The ratio of Bacillary to Amoebic Dysentery was much higher in Sierra Leone being 6 to 1 as against a Command ratio of 2 to 1.

The successful control of MALARIA among both classes of troops is shown by the rates in Table 86. Among Europeans, the 1945 rate was

TABLE 86

West Africa Command, 1941–45
Admissions to Hospitals for Malaria
Comparative Rates (1941 = 100)

Source: West Africa Annual Statistical Reports, 1944, 1945

Year	Europeans					Africans
	Gold Coast	Nigeria	Sierra Leone	Gambia	Whole Command	Whole Command
1941	100·0	100·0	100·0	100·0	100·0	100·0
1942	86·9	93·1	76·6	161·2	85·1	102·8
1943	46·0	81·9	37·6	73·0	49·4	59·2
1944	24·3	70·7	6·9	26·4	31·1	63·4
1945	7·4	24·6	6·2	4·4	10·3	46·4

one tenth that of 1941, while the African rate declined by more than half during the period. The reduction was not so remarkable in Nigeria until 1945 when the incidence fell to just over one third the previous year's rate.

The number of cases of BLACKWATER FEVER among Europeans per 1,000 cases of Malaria is given in Table 87 and shows a remarkable

TABLE 87

West Africa Command, 1941–45
Admissions to Hospitals
Number of cases of Blackwater Fever per 1,000 cases of Malaria
Europeans only

Source: West Africa Annual Statistical Reports, 1944, 1945

Year	Gold Coast	Nigeria	Sierra Leone	Gambia	Whole Command
1941	8·4	11·5	3·5	16·0	6·0
1942	13·0	23·0	5·0	8·0	13·0
1943	11·0	10·0	6·0	8·0	9·0
1944	1·5	0·5	—	—	1·0
1945	—	—	—	—	—

decline throughout the Command. After a rise of over 100 per cent. in 1942 there was a rapid fall, and in 1945 there were no recorded cases. Comparable figures for Africans are not available, but it is known that the hospital admission rates for this disease among Africans was 0·4 per 1,000 troops for each of the years 1944 and 1945.

The figures for VENEREAL DISEASES (Tables 88 and 89), include

TABLE 88

West Africa Command, 1941–45
Incidence of Venereal Diseases (all types)
Annual Rates per 1,000 Strength

Source: West Africa Annual Statistical Reports, 1944, 1945

Year	Gold Coast	Nigeria	Sierra Leone	Gambia	Whole Command
Europeans					
1941	71·4	37·2	52·2	23·5	51·6
1942	62·3	47·8	41·8	16·2	45·3
1943	64·8	105·9	39·1	20·7	69·4
1944	68·6	110·2	46·4	21·9	81·2
1945	82·6	85·2	88·6	40·9	82·0
Africans					
1942	319	475	172	86	314
1943	300	359	196	102	296
1944	419	477	280	120	386
1945	491	537	325	614	482

cases treated in all medical units. Apart from a fall in 1942 for Europeans and 1943 for Africans, the incidence rose each year, notably among Africans in Gambia where the 1945 rate was seven times that of 1942. Striking features in Table 89 (1945 compared with 1944)

TABLE 89

West Africa Command, 1944–45
Incidence of Venereal Diseases
Relative Rates

Source: West Africa Annual Statistical Reports, 1944, 1945

	Gold Coast		Nigeria		Sierra Leone		Gambia		Whole Command	
	1944	1945	1944	1945	1944	1945	1944	1945	1944	1945
Europeans										
Syphilis .	8·4	6·4	4·1	2·7	18·0	21·1	23·0	6·3	6·3	8·3
Gonorrhoea and Urethritis .	72·8	71·4	59·2	94·2	70·0	62·4	61·5	74·9	64·4	78·3
Lympho-granuloma .	7·0	4·7	8·8	1·0	3·6	2·7	—	—	9·3	2·7
Chancroid .	11·8	17·5	27·9	2·1	8·4	13·8	15·5	18·8	20·0	10·7
Totals .	100·0	100·0	100·0	100·0	100·0	100·0	100·0	100·0	100·0	100·0
Africans										
Syphilis .	2·3	1·9	2·1	5·8	1·3	3·0	8·5	8·1	1·7	4·1
Gonorrhoea and Urethritis .	76·6	81·5	92·0	79·6	94·0	82·7	65·0	73·4	88·2	80·8
Lympho-granuloma .	11·3	8·8	3·5	8·3	3·5	8·1	—	8·0	5·6	8·2
Chancroid .	9·8	7·8	2·4	6·3	1·2	6·2	26·5	10·5	4·5	6·9
Totals .	100·0	100·0	100·0	100·0	100·0	100·0	100·0	100·0	100·0	100·0

are the rise in Syphilis and Chancroid among Africans and the rise and fall in Gonorrhoea and Chancroid respectively among Europeans.

Table 90 exhibits the relative causes of Evacuation to the United Kingdom of Europeans and that of Invaliding from the Army of

TABLE 90

West Africa Command, 1942–45
Medical Evacuations to the United Kingdom (Europeans)
and Invalidings (Africans)
Relative Rates

Source: West Africa Annual Statistical Reports, 1944, 1945

CAUSES	Europeans (Evacuation to the U.K.)			Africans (Invaliding)			
	1943	1944	1945	1942	1943	1944	1945
Chronic Malaria and Blackwater Fever . .	22·4	11·1	5·8	‡	‡	‡	§
Nervous and Psychiatric Disorders (a) . . .	18·5	17·6	19·2	—	—	11·5	6·4
E.N.T. Diseases . . .	6·8	7·6	5·5	‡	‡	‡	4·0
Accidents	5·3	5·9	6·3	‡	‡	‡	5·4
Tuberculosis . . .	4·8	3·8	4·9	6·8	6·8	10·4	§
Amoebic Dysentery. . .	1·5	7·6	2·0	‡	‡	‡	§
Venereal Diseases . . .	0·8	0·3	0·6	5·7	5·7	4·3	19·7
Yaws	†	*	—	25·2	25·1	4·3	7·2
Guinea Worm . . .	†	*	—	5·9	5·9	1·1	6·1
Leprosy. . . .	†	*	—	2·3	2·4	4·8	§
Other Causes . . .	39·9	46·1	55·7	54·1	54·0	61·5	51·2
Totals	100·0	100·0	100·0	100·0	100·0	100·0	100·0

(a) There are no satisfactory records of African psychiatric cases invalided during 1942 and 1943.
* Less than 0·2 per cent.
† Less than 0·5 per cent.
‡ Less than 1·0 per cent.
§ Not recorded.

Africans. Evacuation to the United Kingdom does not necessarily imply invaliding from the Army, as individuals may be medically unfit for service in West Africa but fit for service in temperate climates. It does, however, represent wastage to the Army in West Africa as does the invaliding of local troops. Invaliding among Africans for Tuberculosis was twice that of evacuation of Europeans, as may be expected from the admission rates (Table 84). Nervous and Psychiatric Disorders, the largest figure among Europeans, accounted for nearly 20 per cent. of the evacuations.

Deaths due to disease (Table 92) among Europeans in 1945 were 20 per cent. of the annual average for the period 1941–44. None were attributable to the diseases shown in the table. One half of the deaths among Europeans in 1941–44 were caused by Malaria and Blackwater Fever as compared with just over 1 per cent. for Africans. The main causes of deaths among Africans were Pneumococcal Infection and Tuberculosis.

TABLE 91

West Africa Command, 1941–45
Medical Evacuations to the United Kingdom (Europeans) and Invalidings (Africans)
Annual Rates per 1,000 Strength

Source: West Africa Annual Statistical Reports, 1944, 1945

Year	Gold Coast	Nigeria	Sierra Leone	Gambia	Whole Command
Europeans (Evacuations to the United Kingdom)					
1941	53	131	91	76	96
1942	44	95	69	54	70
1943	36	62	55	55	59
1944	44	116	67	75	85
1945	55	58	64	62	59
Africans (Invalidings)					
1942	59	51	25	25	44
1943	51	43	23	21	37
1944	52	62	18	34	46
1945	95	140	27	38	100

TABLE 92

West Africa Command, 1942–45
Relative Mortality Rates, 1941–44 and 1945

Source: West Africa Annual Statistical Reports, 1944, 1945

CAUSES	1941–44		1945	
	Europeans	Africans	Europeans	Africans
Blackwater Fever	36·20	0·45	—	1·45
Malaria	13·49	0·83	—	1·12
Pneumonia	4·91	—	—	—
Pneumococcal Infections	—	17·07	—	10·62
Staphylococcal Infections	4·29	7·70	—	*
Neoplasms	3·68	4·46	—	4·92
Infective Hepatitis	3·07	6·42	—	*
Heat Exhaustion	2·46	0·98	—	*
Nephritis	2·45	3·85	—	*
Encephalitis	2·45	1·21	—	0·56
Smallpox	1·84	1·66	—	*
Tuberculosis	1·23	13·22	—	16·20
Bacillary Dysentery	1·23	3·25	—	4·02
Streptococcal Infections	1·23	2·11	—	6·59
Meningococcal Infections	—	10·80	—	5·47
Vitamin Deficiencies	—	0·83	—	*
Others	21·48	25·16	100·00	49·05
Totals	100·00	100·00	100·00	100·00

* Figures not available—included in 'Others'.

CHAPTER VII

EAST AFRICA COMMAND

THE dearth of morbidity statistics from the East Africa Command must result in a somewhat sketchy and incomplete chapter. The tabulations which follow, therefore, can be of only limited value.

Very little data are available prior to 1944. The statistics for that year have been obtained from the 'East Africa Command Health Report, 1944'. The troops in the Command during that year were composed of British, East Africans, Mauritians, Seychellois and others of Colonial stock, with the local East Africans predominating. As the only reliable statistics in the report were for 'All Troops' only, it is impossible to evaluate the incidence of disease among, or make a comparison between, the various classes of troops located in the Command.

East Africa Command was non-operational in 1944. Its chief rôle was the training of reinforcements for East African Units in the Middle East and South East Asia Commands. The Command included Kenya, Tanganyika, Nyasaland, British Somaliland, Northern Rhodesia, Madagascar, Mauritius and the Seychelles, a vast area ranging from the malarious coastal regions to sub-tropical highlands. It would have been both interesting and instructive to have been able to compare the incidence of diseases in the Mombassa area with that in the Nairobi district, or Mauritius with Madagascar. Unfortunately, this is not possible.

The information derived from the report mentioned above is presented in Tables 93 and 94. There is no reason to doubt the accuracy of the data included therein.

Apart from the 1944 Report, the only statistics available are contained in Table 95. These figures relate to British Troops only for 1945 and were obtained from the Hollerith Section of the War Office. All statistics relating to admissions to Hospitals received from the Hollerith Section are based on Army Forms I.1220 received in the War Office. The accuracy of these figures is subject to the limitations mentioned in the introduction to the Army section of this Volume.

As Army Forms I.1220 for British Troops only were sent to the War Office for coding and translation to punched cards, it is not possible to obtain from the Hollerith Section any information regarding the other classes of troops in the Command. A comparison of morbidity rates for all troops for the years 1944 and 1945 cannot, therefore, be made.

The tabulations presented refer to Hospitalisation only and do not include any data relating to low grade morbidity.

Table 93 shows the Annual Rates per 1,000 strength of admissions to

TABLE 93

East Africa Command, 1944
Causes of Admissions to and Deaths in Hospital
All Troops
Annual Rates per 1,000 Strength

Source: East Africa Command Annual Health Report, 1944

CAUSES	Annual Rates	
	Admissions	Deaths
Dysentery	29·16	0·21
Enteric Group of Fevers	0·18	0·08
Influenza	4·39	—
Infective Hepatitis	7·18	0·23
Kala Azar	0·07	0·01
Malaria	100·60	0·24
Cerebro-Spinal Meningitis	1·58	0·29
Pneumonia	14·06	0·66
Relapsing Fever	5·02	0·02
Schistosomiasis	4·81	0·02
Smallpox	1·67	0·01
Tuberculosis	2·00	0·51
Undulant Fever	0·04	—
Venereal Diseases	160·18	0·13
Yaws	0·68	—
Deficiency Diseases	0·16	0·01
Effects of Heat	0·20	—
Nervous Diseases	7·99	0·12
Diseases of the Heart	0·83	0·17
Other Diseases of the Circulatory System	9·50	0·07
Inflammation of the Bronchi	29·34	0·01
Other Diseases of the Respiratory System	4·45	0·14
Pharyngitis and Tonsillitis	13·14	0·02
Enteritis and Diarrhoea	13·36	0·04
Other Diseases of the Digestive System	16·35	0·55
Skin and I.A.T. (including Scabies)	31·67	0·01
Rheumatic Fever and Other Rheumatic Diseases	4·46	—
Other Diseases of the bones and organs of movement	10·82	0·01
Diseases of the Eye	8·35	—
Diseases of the Ear	4·61	0·02
All Other Diseases	84·57	0·86
Total Diseases	571·42	4·44
Injuries—E.A.	0·01	0·01
Injuries—N.E.A.	29·38	1·15
Total Injuries	29·39	1·16
Total Admissions/Deaths	600·81	5·60

TABLE 94

East Africa Command, 1944
Admissions to and Deaths in Hospitals
Breakdown of Certain Diseases Shown in Table 93
All Troops
Annual Rates per 1,000 Strength

Source: East Africa Command Health Report, 1944

DISEASES	Admissions A.R.	Deaths A.R.
Dysentery		
Bacillary	11·03	0·09
Amoebic	3·36	0·04
Other Forms	14·77	0·08
Totals	29·16	0·21
Malaria		
B.T.	4·39	—
Q.	0·33	—
M.T.	52·71	0·04
Blackwater Fever	0·05	0·03
Other Forms	43·12	0·17
Totals	100·60	0·24
Venereal Diseases		
Gonorrhoea	78·65	0·10
Syphilis	28·21	0·01
Other Forms	53·32	0·02
Totals	160·18	0·13

hospitals of ALL TROOPS, while Table 94 analyses certain disease groups.

Due to the absence of major epidemics, the admission rates fell from 681 in 1943 to 601 in 1944. The average admission rate per day was 1·65 per 1,000 troops. The death rate during the year was 5·6 per 1,000 compared with 6·9 in 1943.

Admissions for VENEREAL DISEASES accounted for over one quarter of the total admissions for diseases, the rate being 160 per 1,000 compared with 164 in 1943. The 1944 Report stated 'The V.D. rate is approximately three times as great in Africans as in Europeans . . . nearly 50 per cent. of all V.D. infections in Africans were contracted on leave'.

The admission rate for MALARIA was just over one sixth of the total for diseases. It increased from 91 per 1,000 in 1943 to 101 in 1944. This increase was due to an unusually high number of admissions in the coastal region. Elsewhere in the Command there was a reduction in admissions compared with the previous year.

A decrease in the rate for DYSENTERY was reported for the years 1941 to 1944. Rates per 1,000 were 93 in 1941, 57 in 1942, 59 in 1943 and 29 in 1944. This decline was attributed to the improvement of sanitary conditions in camps and more rigorous sanitary discipline.

Admissions for PNEUMONIA were 29 per 1,000 in 1943 and 14 in 1944. The drop is attributable to there being no marked seasonal increase in 1944 as was experienced in 1943 when pneumonia reached epidemic proportions during the cold season.

TABLE 95

East Africa Command, 1945
British Troops
Causes of Admission to Hospital
Annual Rates per 1,000 Strength

Source: Hollerith Tabulations

CAUSES	Annual Rates	
Common Cold		3·56
Dysentery		17·93
Enteric Fever Group		0·36
Infective Hepatitis		3·56
Malaria		53·44
Pneumonia		2·49
Tuberculosis—Pulmonary		0·36
Tuberculosis—Other Types		0·24
P.U.O.		11·99
Amoebiasis		4·16
Venereal Diseases:		
Gonorrhoea	9·14	
Syphilis	4·99	
Soft Chancre	2·38	
Other Types	3·33	
Total V.D.		19·83
Other Infectious Diseases		3·33
Scabies		0·83
Other Infestations		1·54
Diseases of the Nervous System		2·02
Mental Diseases:		
Psychoses	0·48	
Psychoneuroses	4·51	
Other Types	0·24	
Total Mental Diseases		5·23
Diseases of the Eye		2·26
Diseases of the Ear, Nose, and Throat:		
Otitis Media	1·90	
Otitis Externa	1·66	
Pharyngitis	4·04	
Tonsillitis	16·39	
Other Diseases	3·68	
Total E.N.T. Diseases		27·67

TABLE 95 (*contd.*)

East Africa Command, 1945
British Troops
Causes of Admission to Hospital
Annual Rates per 1,000 Strength

Source: Hollerith Tabulations

CAUSES	Annual Rates	
Diseases of the Cardio-Vascular System		3·68
Diseases of the Blood and Blood-forming Organs		2·85
Diseases of the Respiratory System		4·87
Diseases of the Mouth, Teeth, and Gums		4·63
Diseases of the Digestive System:		
Appendicitis	4·28	
Diarrhoea	1·90	
Enteritis	16·51	
Gastritis and Dyspepsia	6·41	
Hernia	2·26	
Peptic Ulcers	1·07	
Other Diseases	10·09	
Total Diseases of the Digestive System		42.52
Diseases of the Genito-Urinary System		16·74
Diseases of the Musculo-Skeletal System		15·44
I.A.T.		8·91
Diseases of the Skin (excluding Scabies and I.A.T.)		17·58
Effects of Heat		0·71
All Other Diseases		11·40
Total Diseases		290·12
Injuries		24·94
Burns		0·48
Total Admissions		315·54

In 1943, there was an epidemic of CEREBRO-SPINAL MENINGITIS. The peak was reached in July 1943, declined throughout 1944 and by the end of the year, very few cases were reported. This epidemic affected both the civil and military populations in the East African Territories and the decline corresponded in both the populations. The 1944 rate was 1·6 per 1,000 as compared with 6·5 in 1943.

RELAPSING FEVER showed a steady increase throughout the year from 2 per 1,000 in 1943 to 5 in 1944.

An epidemic of INFECTIVE HEPATITIS commenced early in 1944, reached its peak during the middle of the year and then subsided. The rate per 1,000 for the year was 7·18–7·07 in Africans and 8·64 in Europeans.

Table 95 records the hospital admission rates for BRITISH TROOPS only in 1945. No figures prior to 1945 for this class of personnel are available, except that the rate for INFECTIVE HEPATITIS was

TABLE 96

East Africa Command, 1916–18 and 1944
Admissions to Hospital for Certain Diseases
All Troops
Rates per 1,000 Strength

Sources: 1916–18—History of the Great War—Medical Services, Statistical Volume.
1944—East Africa Command Health Report for 1944.

	1916	1917	1918	1944
Dysentery	182·21	277·01	80·28	29·16
Enteric Group	2·91	2·45	1·68	0·18
Malaria	1,039·11	1,422·84	559·09	100·60
Pneumonia	9·48	32·60	49·30	14·06
Cerebro-Spinal Fever	N.A.	5·82	1·83	1·58
Smallpox	N.A.	N.A.	7·34	1·67

8·64 per 1,000. This was revealed in the Annual Report for 1944. The 1945 rate for this disease was 3·56.

During the War of 1914–18, a campaign was conducted in East Africa. In the last war, the rôle of the troops stationed there was mainly that of training. Figures for both wars, therefore, are not comparable, but from the point of view of interest, Table 96 is included. This gives figures for All Troops for certain diseases during the years 1916 to 1918 and 1944. The data for the War of 1914–18 are taken from the Volume of the *History of the Great War, Medical Services, Casualties and Medical Statistics.*

CHAPTER VIII

INDIA COMMAND

INDIA Command consisted, at the outbreak of war, of the Indian Army and that portion of the British Army stationed in India. Both comprised only Regular Soldiers; personnel of the British Army were posted to India for a tour of five years, while personnel of the Indian Army seldom, if ever, left India. Officers of the Indian Army were predominantly of British origin, but this was gradually receding with the Indianisation of the Indian Army.

Shortly after the outbreak of war, both British and Indian Units were sent overseas on active service. Recruiting on a volunteer basis of Indians commenced and eventually India produced the largest volunteer Army known in history. As the war progressed, so the proportion of Indian to British Officers in the Indian Army increased considerably.

India became a vast training ground and it was not until after the entry of Japan into the war in December 1941 that the position of both British and Indian Troops in the Eastern Command rapidly became operational. In April 1942, Eastern Command was renamed Eastern Army. On November 1, 1943 it was partitioned into the Fourteenth Army and Eastern Command, the former passing to the control of South East Asia Command and the latter remaining within the Indian Command. In the figures which follow, those relating to Eastern Army for the whole of the years 1942 and 1943 have been excluded from those of India Command.

Figures for personnel serving in India with units based on S.E.A.C. are not included in this section, neither are those for Indian personnel serving in Middle East, Persia and Iraq, North Africa, Central Mediterranean, etc.—these are presented with statistics relating to the Command concerned. They do, however, include personnel serving in these areas who might have been admitted to hospital while on leave in India.

The statistics set forth in this section are derived from the Annual Reports on the Health of the Army in India for the years 1939 to 1945. These reports are based on monthly statistical returns rendered by hospitals and can be accepted as substantially accurate. If the reports suffer from deficiencies they are, (*a*) seasonal fluctuations except in a few diseases are not given, (*b*) morbidity among Officers is not dealt with in such detail as that among Other Ranks.

The morbidity rates for both British and Indian Armies in India, in general, show an upward trend throughout the war years. Factors which may have affected this are:

(i) The alteration in the composition of the Army due to the great influx of recruits and the recall of reservists. Young soldiers are much more susceptible than seasoned troops to many diseases, especially under war conditions when overcrowding in barracks and tented camps tends to become rife. A large proportion of the British Army, consisting mainly of young soldiers, were serving in India for the first time. DIARRHOEA and mild DYSENTERY is common in new arrivals in India. MALARIA and SANDFLY FEVER might be more likely to affect newcomers to endemic areas.

(ii) The decline in physical fitness due to a relaxation of the peace-time standards of entry, and the tendency to retain in the Army, as long as they could usefully perform duties of any kind, individuals who, before the war, would have been invalided.

(iii) It seems probable that there had been a general lowering of resistance to disease as a result of harder work, longer hours on duty, less leave and more time spent on the plains in the hot weather.

(iv) During the war, the Army was composed mainly of men who were unaccustomed to improvised systems of sanitation and unaware of the necessity for the strict observance of the rules for personal and environmental hygiene, which are so important under semi-active conditions for the prevention of disease. The majority of Officers were new to the Army and much less skilled than the pre-war Regular Officers in the art of maintaining the health of their men.

(v) There was a large increase in the movements of units, often through malarious areas. This led to large numbers of men being exposed to infection in transit.

(vi) Due to the rapid expansion of the Army, camps were often sited outside cantonments in endemic areas. To these were added camps for training in jungle warfare, often in intensely malarious areas.

Table 97 shows the principal causes of admission to Hospitals of Officers and Other Ranks of the British Army. The total rate per 1,000 for Officers rose from 436 in 1939 to a peak of 1,099 in 1942 and fell to 767 in 1945. That for Other Ranks showed a similar rise and fall, 664 in 1939 to 863 in 1945, except that the peak (1,014) was in 1944, two years later than that for Officers. In comparison, the rates during the First World War were (Table 108) Officers 694 in 1915, rising to 1,344 in 1918 and Other Ranks 825 in 1915, rising to 1,030 in 1918. (The high rates for 1918 were due largely to the INFLUENZA Epidemic.)

The admission rate for DENGUE FEVER in respect of Officers is approximately twice that of B.O.Rs. and that of CATARRHAL JAUNDICE from twice to nearly five times. Officers appear to be more prone to DIARRHOEA and DYSENTERY than are Other Ranks. In comparing rates, however, it must be remembered that the age constitution of the Officer group is higher than the Other Rank group. It is possible that some of the higher rate of admissions is accounted for by this greater age. Conversely, the ratios for MALARIA as between Officers and Other Ranks were approximately:

1939 1 : 1·5 *1940* 1 : 1·7 *1941* 1 : 2 *1942* 1 : 1·3
1943 1 : 1·4 *1944* 1 : 1·7 *1945* 1 : 2

The figures for MALARIA show a steady increase from 1939 to 1944 with a dramatic fall in 1945 to roughly half the 1944 rates. Even so, the 1945 rate is twice that of 1939. This trend is also observed in the MALARIA rates for the Indian Army.

The admission rates for SANDFLY FEVER, over the years, show a decrease on the whole, the 1943 rate (the latest available) for Officers being one-half that for 1939, with the 1945 rate for Other Ranks slightly over one sixth that of 1939.

The incidence of VENEREAL DISEASES increased steadily from 51·2 per 1,000 in 1939 to 79·8 per 1,000 in 1945. The figures for 1917 and 1918 were 52 and 62 respectively. Although the rate for Indian Other Ranks increased by 500 per cent. (Table 111) their 1945 rate was just over 50 per cent., the B.O.R. rate.

The rates for HEAT EXHAUSTION (B.O.Rs. only) show a rapid increase from 1939 to 1942 (1·9 to 17·5 per 1,000), a fall to 4·6 in 1943 and a rise in the subsequent two years to 10·5 in 1945. The reason is not difficult to find. The great majority of those attacked were young, unacclimatised soldiers who had been in India only a short time. Accommodation was much below pre-war standards and the hot weather of 1942 was exceptionally severe. The rate for 1942 was the highest ever recorded for British troops in India. That for 1943, although the best of the war years was about double the average for pre-war years. Table 112 shows the incidence of admissions for and deaths from HEAT STROKE and HEAT EXHAUSTION year by year from 1936 to 1945 while Table 113 compares the admissions for B.O.Rs. with that for I.O.Rs. The latter table indicates the comparative racial immunity of the Indians.

Table 98 exhibits the principal causes of DEATHS among B.O.Rs. Total deaths rise from 2·58 per 1,000 in 1939 to a peak of 5·39 in 1942, falling to 2·29 in 1945. Deaths from DYSENTERY in 1942 were thirteen times those in 1939, MALARIA, five times and EFFECTS OF HEAT, seven times.

Table 99 shows the principal causes of INVALIDING to the United Kingdom of British Other Ranks. It must be understood that not all those invalided from India would be invalided from the Army; some would be medically downgraded for service in temperate climates. The main causes for invaliding were PULMONARY TUBERCULOSIS and MENTAL and NERVOUS DISEASES. The total figures for invaliding fell from 1939 to 1941, and rose from 1942 to 1945 when the rate was 16 per 1,000 against 7 for 1939. The low rates in 1940 and 1941 were partly due to the policy of retaining those whose recovery could be completed in India and partly to the shipping situation.

Admissions, deaths and invalidings of Officers and Other Ranks for quinquennial periods from 1910 to 1939 and year by year from 1939 to 1945 are given in Table 100. It is interesting to note that the peak year of deaths for both Officers and Other Ranks was 1942 which was also the peak year for Officer admissions, but the peak of admissions for Other Ranks occurred two years later, in 1944.

The principal causes for ADMISSIONS to hospital of Officers and Other Ranks of the Indian Army are given in Table 102. The peak year for both Officers and Other Ranks was 1942, although the rates for the latter in 1943 and 1944 were only slightly lower. Rates rose, in the case of Officers, from 462 in 1939 to 709 in 1942 and fell to 487 in 1945 and, in the case of Indian Other Ranks from 454 to 747, to 584. DIPHTHERIA was practically non-existent among Other Ranks. The incidence of DIARRHOEA increased yearly to 1942 and fell subsequently. This was paralleled by DYSENTERY, as could be expected. The rates for MALARIA rose considerably (118 in 1939 to 206 in 1942). In 1945 there was a dramatic fall in the incidence, the figure being 76 as against 160 in 1944. This decrease was similar to that experienced with British Other Ranks. Table 114, which exhibits the MALARIA rates for B.O.Rs. and I.O.Rs. for the years 1938 to 1945 shows that in 1938 the Indian rate was twice that of the British. In 1941 and 1943 the rates were almost identical, but in 1945 the Indian rate was less than 60 per cent. that of the British. (In 1946 there was a further fall in the rates, the figures then being B.O.Rs. 34·1 per 1,000 and I.O.Rs. 43·7 per 1,000.)

The great majority of admissions for MUMPS occurred among Gurkha recruits. The incidence of SANDFLY FEVER among officers was from three to five times that among I.O.Rs., whereas the rates between Officers and Other Ranks of the British Army differed only slightly. Admissions for SCABIES increased from 11·9 in 1939 to a peak of 33·2 in 1944. Comparable B.O.R. figures are 2·2 in 1939 to 15·5 in 1942.

In spite of the lowering of standards for enlistment and the environmental hazards resulting from war-time conditions in the Indian Army, the rates for TUBERCULOSIS among Indian Other Ranks remained surprisingly constant (from 2·2 in 1939 to 2·9 in 1942, 1944 and 1945).

As with British Other Ranks, admissions for VENEREAL DISEASES rose considerably, from a peace-time rate of 8·1 in 1938 to 49·8 in 1943.

By 1945 the rate had decreased by 6 per 1,000 to 43·4. Table 111 compares the rates for B.O.Rs. and I.O.Rs.

Indians appear to be more prone to COMMON COLD than do Europeans, admissions being approximately three times for I.O.Rs. than B.O.Rs.

Table 103 shows the principal causes of DEATHS among I.O.Rs. Until 1944, the chief cause of death by disease was PNEUMONIA. In 1944 and 1945, PULMONARY TUBERCULOSIS took pride of place. As might be expected the peak year for deaths was the same as that for admissions, 1942, when the rate was 4·99 per thousand. By 1945 the rate was down to nearly that for 1938, although the rate for admissions had increased by fifty per cent. The total death rates for B.O.Rs. and I.O.Rs. throughout the war years were very similar (Table 107).

The chief cause for Invaliding among I.O.Rs. (Table 104) was PULMONARY TUBERCULOSIS in the initial war years, to be superseded in 1943 by MENTAL DISEASES. The rate for the latter rose from 0·48 in 1939 to 4·13 in 1945 while that for PULMONARY TUBERCULOSIS increased from 1·7 to 2·4 in 1943 decreasing to 1·8 in 1945. The peak years for Invaliding were 1944 and 1945 when the rates were nearly 30 per 1,000. The rates for B.O.Rs. compared favourably with those for I.O.Rs. being approximately one half from 1940 onwards (Table 107).

Table 105 exhibits comparisons between Officers and Other Ranks of the Indian Army in respect of Admissions, Invalidings and Deaths for Quinquennial periods from 1925 to 1939 and annually from 1939 to 1945. A striking aspect of this table is the extremely low rate of invaliding for officers during the period 1940 to 1944, being approximately one fifth of the rate for 1939 and one quarter of the rate for the period 1935–39.

Table 115 compares the incidence of DYSENTERY and DIARRHOEA between (a) Officers of the British Army and Officers of the Indian Army and (b) Other Ranks of the British Army and Other Ranks of the Indian Army for the years 1939 to 1945. This table suggests that personnel of the British Army are more prone to these diseases than personnel of the Indian Army.

Tables 116 to 119 relate to the WOMEN'S SERVICES in India, i.e. members of the Queen Alexandra's Imperial Military Nursing Service and the Womens Auxiliary Corps (India). The table relating to ADMISSIONS shows a steady increase from 1939 to 1945 in respect of members of the Nursing Service (440 in 1939 to 1,233 in 1945) whereas the peak year for admissions of W.A.C.(I.) members was 1942. In 1945 the rate for W.A.C.(I.) was half that for 1942. The DEATH rates do not show any appreciable trend. In 1941 the number of Q.A.I.M.N.S. in India was comparatively small and a slight increase in the actual number of deaths would tend to show a higher proportionate rate per 1,000. This probably occurred in 1941 when the rate for deaths was 10·13. INVALIDS sent Home (Table 118) in respect of Q.A.I.M.N.S. shows a trend similar to that of Officers of the British Army (Table 106) when the peak was in 1943. Here again, invalids sent to the United Kingdom would not necessarily be invalided from the Army on arrival, as opposed to members of the W.A.C.(I.) which was composed of British and Indian Women domiciled in India, the figures for whom are those actually invalided from the Service.

Summary

Broadly speaking the major diseases in India during the war years were:

(a) Among Europeans—Malaria, Venereal Diseases, Dysentery and Diarrhoea.

(b) Among Indians —Malaria, Venereal Diseases, Respiratory Diseases.

Perhaps the most outstanding feature revealed by the tables here presented is that the striking reduction in 1945 of the number of MALARIA cases. That this success in the prevention of this disease was not transitory is emphasised by the figures for 1946 which show a decline on the 1945 rates. The rate for B.O.Rs. in 1946 was 34·1 per 1,000 and that for I.O.Rs. 43·7. These rates were the lowest ever recorded.

TABLE 97

India, 1939–45

British Officers and Other Ranks. British Army in India. Principal Causes of Admission to Hospital

Annual Rates per 1,000 Strength

Source: Annual Reports on the Health of the Army in India

	CAUSES	1939		1940		1941		1942		1943		1944		1945		
		Officers	Other Ranks	Officers	Other Ranks	Officers	Other Ranks	Officers	Other Ranks	Officers	Other Ranks	Officers	Other Ranks	Officers	Other Ranks	
1	Cholera	—	—	—	0·00	—	0·8	—	0·0	—	0·03	—	0·06	—	0·1	1
2	Common Cold	8·5	11·2	8·9	9·3	31·8	19·4	—	13·4	—	14·7	27·9	13·9	21·8	8·8	2
3	Dengue Fever	—	9·6	—	6·7	—	11·1	28·9	11·6	20·7	8·4	33·8	18·7	17·0	9·6	3
4	Diarrhoea	19·8	18·2	—	25·0	121·5	55·4	103·7	72·7	62·1	43·6	68·2	53·2	52·0	45·6	4
5	Dysentery	35·2	28·9	47·6	33·0	70·0	36·9	92·6	50·2	75·8	48·8	104·8	72·5	89·1	72·1	5
6	Enteric Fever	2·1	1·1	—	1·2	—	0·9	—	1·6	—	0·7	—	1·2	—	0·7	6
7	Jaundice, Catarrhal	29·9	6·3	—	9·0	53·4	14·4	44·6	13·4	16·6	8·3	—	4·8	—	2·0	7
8	Influenza	8·0	9·4	9·9	12·1	28·7	11·7	—	11·0	—	4·2	—	2·0	—	0·4	8
9	Malaria	36·3	55·1	44·6	73·4	77·4	144·4	126·7	164·1	144·4	198·4	144·6	248·4	63·1	130·7	9
10	Measles	0·5	0·7	1·5	1·7	—	—	—	—	—	—	—	—	—	—	10
11	Meningococcal Infection	—	0·1	—	0·2	—	—	—	—	—	—	—	—	—	—	11
12	Pneumonia	2·7	4·6	—	6·0	—	6·5	—	4·5	—	3·2	—	4·0	—	3·3	12
13	Pyrexia of Unknown Origin	0·5	0·2	0·5	0·4	—	—	—	—	—	—	—	6·8	—	6·6	13
14	Sandfly Fever	26·7	30·7	21·8	25·7	38·6	38·1	28·1	25·2	13·2	12·1	—	7·5	—	5·3	14
15	Smallpox	—	0·1	—	0·4	—	0·2	—	0·9	—	0·8	—	1·2	—	0·6	15
16	Tuberculosis	3·7	1·3	1·9	2·3	—	2·2	—	1·5	—	1·1	—	1·2	—	1·1	16
17	Typhus Fever	—	0·8	—	0·9	—	0·6	—	0·4	—	0·5	—	2·3	—	10·7	17
18	Venereal Diseases—Syphilis	—	8·5	—	12·7	—	12·6	—	9·5	—	8·2	—	9·4	11·8 (rows 18–20)	11·7	18
19	Venereal Diseases—Gonorrhoea	—	32·4	—	30·9	—	33·8	—	27·1	—	26·3	—	31·6		25·6	19
20	Venereal Diseases—Other	—	10·3	—	14·5	—	18·1	—	33·0	—	29·4	—	31·0		42·5	20
21	Scabies	—	2·2	—	2·7	—	5·0	—	15·5	—	13·6	—	13·2	—	9·8	21
22	Effects of Heat Stroke	—	0·4	—	1·2	—	1·0	—	2·2	—	0·7	—	0·7	—	1·5	22
23	Effects of Heat Exhaustion	—	1·9	—	4·6	—	6·8	—	17·5	—	4·6	—	6·7	8·1	10·5	23
24	Mental Diseases	4·8	2·8	3·9	3·2	—	4·6	—	5·3	—	4·7	—	12·7	—	13·2	24
25	Nervous Diseases	8·5	10·0	14·4	10·8	—	—	—	—	—	—	—	10·6	—	7·9	25
26	Valvular Disease of the Heart	0·5	0·4	—	0·5	—	—	—	—	—	—	—	—	—	—	26
27	Other Diseases of the Circulatory System	2·6	4·4	5·6	5·1	—	—	—	—	—	—	—	—	—	—	27
28	Inflammation of the Bronchi	5·9	19·4	12·4	21·0	—	27·7	—	19·2	—	13·6	15·4	17·3	9·1	14·8	28
29	Other Diseases of the Respiratory System	3·8	4·5	4·2	4·5	—	—	—	—	—	—	—	—	—	—	29
30	Inflammation of the Pharynx	10·7	14·7	17·8	15·3	—	16·7	—	14·9	—	8·9	—	7·7	11·4	8·7	30
31	Inflammation of the Tonsils	21·4	34·6	26·8	43·2	74·3	35·9	62·4	45·0	43·1	27·0	33·3	26·2	29·2	26·3	31
32	Other Diseases of the Digestive System	80·5	77·7	117·5	90·5	—	—	—	—	—	—	—	—	—	—	32
33	Diseases of the Ear and Nose	17·6	28·4	24·7	33·3	—	—	—	—	—	—	—	—	—	—	33
34	Diseases of the Eye	1·1	4·6	5·4	4·0	—	—	—	—	—	—	—	—	—	—	34
35	Skin and I.A.T. (excl. Scabies)	36·3	101·9	42·5	107·8	—	—	—	—	—	—	—	—	—	—	35
36	All Other Diseases	21·6	59·4	64·5	49·97	—	—	—	—	—	—	—	—	—	—	36
37	*Total Diseases*	389·2	596·8	476·4	662·47	—	—	—	—	—	—	—	—	—	—	37
38	Injuries—N.E.A.	46·5	65·8	55·6	59·7	—	—	—	—	—	—	—	—	—	—	38
39	Injuries—E.A.	—	1·3	1·5	1·2	—	—	—	—	—	—	—	—	—	—	39
40	*Total Injuries*	46·5	67·1	57·1	60·9	—	—	—	—	—	—	—	—	—	—	40
41	*Total Admissions*	435·7	663·9	533·5	723·3	975·6	876·1	1,098·9	979·1	930·4	847·2	993·8	1,014·4	767·3	863·3	41

Note: Where a dash is shown the information is not available.

TABLE 98

India, 1939–45. British Army in India. Principal Causes of Death. British Other Ranks
Rates per 1,000 Strength

Source: Annual Reports on the Health of the Army in India

	CAUSES	1939	1940	1941	1942	1943	1944	1945	
1	Cholera	—	0·03	0·01	0·02	—	0·02	0·02	1
2	Dysentery	0·03	0·06	0·11	0·39	0·18	0·02	0·06	2
3	Enteric Fever	0·08	—	0·09	0·23	0·11	0·17	0·07	3
4	Malaria	0·11	—	0·11	0·59	0·24	0·21	0·10	4
5	Meningococcal Infection	0·03	—	—	—	—	0·01	0·01	5
6	Pneumonia	0·11	0·36	0·17	0·23	0·13	0·13	0·08	6
7	Smallpox	—	0·03	—	0·16	0·18	0·17	0·07	7
8	Tuberculosis, Pulmonary	0·11	0·06	0·11	0·33	0·12	0·13	0·07	8
9	Typhus	0·03	0·03	N.A.	N.A.	N.A.	N.A.	N.A.	9
10	Venereal Diseases	0·03	—	—	—	0·01	0·02	—	10
11	Effects of Heat—Heat Stroke	0·06	0·06	0·09	0·44	0·09	0·17	0·16	11
12	Effects of Heat—Heat Exhaustion	0·06	0·15	0·06	0·44	0·06	0·05	0·02	12
13	Nervous Diseases	0·08	0·15	0·29	0·19	0·08	0·08	0·10	13
14	Diseases of the Circulatory System	0·17	0·12	0·38	0·17	0·12	0·11	0·09	14
15	Diseases of the Digestive System	0·37	0·15	0·55	0·48	0·28	0·38	0·24	15
16	Injuries—N.E.A.	0·33	0·66	1·33	1·00	0·79	0·81	0·74	16
	Total Deaths	2·58	2·77	4·19	5·39	3·02	3·38	2·29	

N.A.—No figures available.

TABLE 99

India, 1939–45. British Army in India. Principal Causes of Invaliding to United Kingdom from India of British Other Ranks Rates per 1,000 Strength

Source: Annual Reports on the Health of the Army in India

	CAUSES	1939	1940	1941	1942	1943	1944	1945	
1	Bronchitis	0·22	0·15	N.A.	0·64	0·66	0·50	0·47	1
2	Dysentery	0·06	0·06	N.A.	N.A.	N.A.	N.A.	0·84	2
3	Malaria	—	—	N.A.	N.A.	N.A.	N.A.	3·35	3
4	Pulmonary Tuberculosis	1·03	1·77	1·45	1·63	3·06	1·16	0·08	4
5	Mental Diseases	1·56	1·40	1·25	0·89	2·25	2·68	4·24	5
6	Nervous Diseases	0·81	0·47	0·30	0·45	0·48	0·31	0·33	6
7	Diseases of the Bones and Muscles	0·58	0·34	0·31	0·48	0·20	0·58	0·43	7
8	Diseases of the Circulatory System	0·28	0·42	N.A.	N.A.	N.A.	N.A.	N.A.	8
9	Diseases of the Digestive System	0·45	0·24	N.A.	0·69	0·62	2·10	1·25	9
10	Diseases of the Ear and Nose	0·06	0·09	N.A.	0·25	0·52	0·81	0·98	10
11	Diseases of the Urinary System	0·25	0·34	0·09	0·17	0·25	0·60	0·46	11
12	Injuries—N.E.A.	0·53	0·22	0·09	0·56	0·67	1·08	0·68	12
13	Injuries—E.A.	0·03	0·44	0·06	0·08	N.A.	N.A.	N.A.	13
	Total Invalids	7·06	6·81	5·47	7·80	11·07	15·64	16·10	

N.A.—No Figures available.

TABLE 100

India 1910–45
British Army in India
Comparative Table
Admissions, Deaths and Invalidings
British Officers and British Other Ranks for Quinquennia
Periods from 1910 to 1939 and Year by Year from 1940 to 1945
Annual Rates per 1,000 Strength

Source: Annual Reports on the Health of the Army in India

	Admissions		Deaths		Invalidings	
	Officers	Other Ranks	Officers	Other Ranks	Officers	Other Ranks
1910–1914	567·5	567·2	5·14	4·36	16·30	7·03
1920–1924	676·7	791·9	6·71	5·24	20·99	18·91
1925–1929	589·9	619·4	5·25	2·90	17·44	13·50
1930–1934	428·6	604·7	6·69	2·64	20·09	8·88
1935–1939	436·9	597·4	4·82	2·54	21·24	9·47
1940	533·5	723·3	4·95	2·77	9·91	6·81
1941	975·6	876·1	6·48	4·19	5·24	5·47
1942	1,098·9	979·1	7·43	5·39	14·40	7·80
1943	930·4	847·2	6·16	3·02	26·41	11·07
1944	993·8	1,014·4	5·36	3·33	22·11	15·64
1945	767·3	863·3	4·48	2·29	15·36	16·10

TABLE 101

India, 1935–45
British Army in India
British Officers and British Other Ranks
Average Constantly Sick in Hospital and Barracks
Annual Rates per 1,000 Strength

Sources: Annual Reports on the Health of the Army in India

Year	In Hospital		In Barracks
	Officers	Other Ranks	Other Ranks
1935	18·36	28·36	20·68
1936	15·23	28·59	23·22
1937	N.A.	27·02	N.A.
1938	N.A.	27·61	N.A.
1939	14·88	27·96	25·10
1940	20·34	30·97	23·59
1941	27·83	34·62	22·52
1942	38·41	42·51	17·54
1943	42·30	41·87	13·23
1944	49·01	60·45	15·23
1945	34·18	43·11	7·76

Note: Figures for Officers treated as Out-Patients are not available.

TABLE 102

India, 1938–45. Indian Army in India
Principal Causes of Admissions to Hospital—Officers and Indian Other Ranks
Annual Rates per 1,000 Strength

Source: Annual Reports on the Health of the Army in India

	CAUSES	1938		1939		1940		1941		1942		1943		1944		1945		
		Officers	Other Ranks	Officers	Other Ranks	Officers	Other Ranks	Officers	Other Ranks	Officers	Other Ranks	Officers	Other Ranks	Officers	Other Ranks	Officers	Other Ranks	
1	Bronchitis	—	12·4	9·0	13·2	6·5	15·2	N.A.	27·9	N.A.	31·4	N.A.	33·8	N.A.	27·9	N.A.	23·4	1
2	Common Cold	8·0	13·0	8·1	15·7	9·8	24·7	11·7	39·5	11·9	45·1	11·6	40·5	8·4	39·3	5·1	32·5	2
3	Dengue Fever	N.A.	1·1	3·4	1·1	5·2	1·1	N.A.	0·8	N.A.	2·1	N.A.	1·4	N.A.	1·3	N.A.	0·5	3
4	Diphtheria	N.A.	N.A.	1·3	0·0	0·5	0·0	N.A.	0·0	N.A.	0·0	N.A.	0·0	N.A.	0·0	N.A.	0·1	4
5	Diarrhoea	15·6	5·1	20·9	6·3	24·6	10·9	41·8	23·6	52·9	32·7	41·5	25·7	21·8	20·9	23·3	17·0	5
6	Diseases of the Ear and Nose	12·3	8·4	20·5	9·3	18·8	11·1	23·5	N.A	29·2	N.A	34·0	N.A.	26·8	N.A.	32·2	N.A.	6
7	Dysentery	29·1	17·2	15·8	17·1	28·0	21·8	34·5	21·0	40·6	20·0	35·0	16·0	37·5	16·2	33·3	14·2	7
8	Effects of Heat:																	
	Heat Stroke	N.A.	N.A.	—	—	0·3	0·0	N.A.	0·2	N.A.	0·3	N.A.	0·2	N.A.	0·2	N.A.	} 0·7	8
9	Heat Exhaustion	N.A.	0·2	1·3	0·2	2·3	0·3	N.A.	0·5	N.A.	0·5	N.A.	0·3	N.A.	0·3	4·4		9
10	Enteric Group of Fevers	N.A.	0·8	1·7	0·5	1·6	1·0	N.A.	0·6	N.A.	0·4	N.A.	0·5	N.A.	0·5	N.A.	0·3	10
11	Influenza	7·6	4·2	11·9	3·7	13·5	5·1	16·1	5·1	13·3	4·6	9·2	3·2	2·2	1·6	N.A.	N.A.	11
12	Malaria	40·7	109·7	37·9	118·3	47·9	173·2	54·9	144·6	91·3	206·0	99·8	192·5	73·3	159·5	42·1	76·1	12
13	Meningococcal Infection	N.A.	N.A.	0·4	0·2	0·5	0·5	N.A.	2·4	N.A.	2·7	N.A.	1·6	N.A.	0·6	N.A.	0·3	13
14	Mental Diseases	N.A.	0·9	4·7	1·3	3·7	1·9	N.A.	2·2	N.A.	3·0	N.A.	4·4	N.A.	5·9	12·6	6·8	14
15	Mumps	N.A.	N.A.	5·5	7·0	0·3	9·3	N.A.	20·6	N.A.	15·5	N.A.	14·6	N.A.	12·6	N.A.	11·7	15
16	Pharyngitis	N.A.	19·3	17·5	24·1	13·5	17·5	N.A.	22·2	N.A.	23·1	N.A.	16·2	N.A.	20·0	8·4	20·1	16
17	Pneumonia	N.A.	5·0	3·8	5·4	6·0	8·2	N.A.	11·9	N.A.	11·8	N.A.	11·9	N.A.	8·6	N.A.	8·2	17
18	Sandfly Fever	19·4	4·6	22·6	6·0	16·0	5·9	29·8	10·0	32·0	6·2	15·1	2·4	6·2	2·3	3·8	0·7	18
19	Scabies	N.A.	11·2	—	11·9	—	16·8	N.A.	17·5	N.A.	21·3	N.A.	27·2	N.A.	33·2	N.A.	26·2	19
20	Smallpox	N.A.	N.A.	—	0·2	—	0·1	N.A.	0·1	N.A.	0·3	N.A.	0·5	N.A.	0·9	N.A.	0·5	20
21	Tonsillitis	15·1	6·1	20·5	5·5	22·8	5·0	25·3	4·0	34·8	4·4	26·3	4·0	18·2	5·2	18·6	6·0	21
22	Trachoma	N.A.	1·8	N.A.	2·1	N.A.	1·5	N.A.	1·2	N.A.	1·4	N.A.	2·2	N.A.	2·0	N.A.	2·1	22
23	Tuberculosis	N.A.	1·9	3·8	2·2	1·8	2·6	N.A.	2·4	N.A.	2·9	N.A.	2·8	N.A.	2·9	N.A.	2·9	23
24	Typhus	N.A.	N.A.	0·4	0·6	1·0	0·1	N.A.	0·1	N.A.	0·1	N.A.	0·2	N.A.	0·3	N.A.	0·4	24
	Venereal Diseases:																	
25	Gonorrhoea	N.A.	2·9	—	3·4	0·3	7·5	N.A.	9·4	N.A.	11·0	N.A.	11·4	N.A.	11·5	N.A.	8·2	25
26	Syphilis	N.A.	3·1	0·9	3·4	0·5	6·1	N.A.	8·1	N.A.	10·3	N.A.	9·5	N.A.	12·6	N.A.	11·7	26
27	Chancroid	N.A.	1·5	—	1·2	—	1·4	N.A.	4·1	N.A.	11·6	N.A.	17·5	N.A.	2·1	N.A.	1·4	27
28	Other Forms	N.A.	0·6	—	0·6	—	3·9	N.A.	6·3	N.A.	9·6	N.A.	11·4	N.A.	22·5	N.A.	22·1	28
29	Totals		8·1	0·9	8·6	0·8	18·9		27·9		42·5		49·8	5·0	48·7	10·3	43·4	29
30	All Other Diseases	190·8	131·0	191·7	136·4	193·6	150·3	311·0	191·7	352·0	230·3	332·0	253·4	250·7	278·8	249·0	230·1	30
31	*Total Diseases*	338·6	362·0	403·6	396·9	419·0	503·0	548·6	578·0	658·0	708·6	604·5	705·3	450·1	689·7	443·0	524·2	31
32	Injuries	48·2	59·8	58·5	57·1	49·4	46·0	45·9	37·6	50·9	37·9	50·5	37·4	40·2	43·2	43·8	59·7	32
33	*Total Admissions*	386·8	421·8	462·1	454·0	468·4	549·0	594·5	615·6	708·9	746·5	655·0	742·7	490·3	732·9	486·8	583·9	33

N.A.—Figures not available. Any admissions are included in 'All Other Diseases'.
Note: The term 'Officers' relates to King's Commissioned Officers. Viceroy's Commissioned Officers are included in 'Other Ranks'.

TABLE 103

India, 1938–45
Indian Army in India
Principal Causes of Deaths
*Indian Other Ranks**
Annual Rates per 1,000 Strength

Source: Annual Reports on the Health of the Army in India

CAUSES	1938	1939	1940	1941	1942	1943	1944	1945
Diseases of the Circulatory System	0·15	0·15	0·09	0·16	0·13	0·12	0·12	0·13
Diseases of the Digestive System	0·19	0·13	0·13	0·22	0·37	0·35	0·33	0·26
Diseases of the Nervous System	0·06	0·10	0·03	0·10	0·13	0·16	0·16	0·09
Diseases of the Urinary System	0·04	0·03	0·02	0·05	0·07	0·06	0·05	0·04
Dysentery	0·03	0·04	0·02	0·06	0·36	0·14	0·09	0·02
Enteric Group of Fevers	0·07	0·06	0·05	0·07	0·10	0·09	0·09	0·04
Malaria	0·05	0·04	0·09	0·12	0·45	0·41	0·28	0·11
Meningococcal Infection	0·07	0·04	0·10	0·31	0·38	0·20	0·07	0·04
Pneumonia	0·43	0·29	0·29	0·78	1·05	0·84	0·37	0·23
Tuberculosis—Pulmonary	0·12	0·06	0·11	0·17	0·43	0·46	0·38	0·54
Tuberculosis—Other Forms	0·04	0·04	0·01	0·03	0·09	0·10	0·08	0·07
Injuries	0·62	0·79	0·86	0·72	0·77	0·52	0·60	0·51
All Other Causes	0·34	0·35	0·31	0·69	0·66	0·67	0·68	0·54
Totals	2·21	2·12	2·11	3·48	4·99	4·12	3·30	2·62

* The term 'Indian Other Ranks' includes Viceroy's Commissioned Officers.

TABLE 104

India, 1938–45
Indian Army in India
Principal Causes of Invaliding
*Indian Other Ranks**
Annual Rates per 1,000 Strength

Source: Annual Reports on the Health of the Army in India

CAUSES	1938	1939	1940	1941	1942	1943	1944	1945
Blood and Blood-forming Organs	0·07	0·07	0·21	0·19	0·37	1·09	1·28	0·78
Bones, Joints, Muscles, Fasciae and Bursae	0·34	0·53	1·04	0·75	0·82	1·57	2·10	2·15
Diseases of the Circulatory System	0·14	0·16	0·56	0·43	0·56	0·84	0·95	0·99
Diseases of the Digestive System	0·07	0·27	0·67	0·54	0·59	0·88	1·43	1·20
Diseases of the Nervous System	0·37	0·38	0·96	1·08	1·31	1·91	1·41	0·93
Diseases of the Ear and Nose	0·09	0·09	0·35	0·28	0·31	0·93	1·66	2·03
Diseases of the Eye	0·38	0·36	0·97	0·69	0·82	2·06	1·95	2·03
Diseases of the Urinary System	0·10	0·07	0·18	0·09	0·13	0·14	0·16	0·18
Malaria	0·04	0·02	0·08	0·07	0·12	0·35	0·27	0·22
Mental Diseases	0·37	0·48	0·81	0·77	1·15	2·67	4·41	4·13
Teeth and Gums	0·01	0·11	0·33	0·09	0·10	0·31	0·48	0·54
Tuberculosis—Pulmonary	1·43	1·70	2·02	1·71	1·84	2·41	2·25	1·80
Tuberculosis—Other Forms	0·18	0·21	0·28	0·12	0·25	0·37	0·28	0·27
Other Diseases of the Respiratory System	0·18	0·34	0·80	0·81	1·42	2·78	3·70	3·29
Venereal Diseases	0·05	0·04	0·12	0·03	0·06	0·24	0·20	0·07
Injuries	1·51	1·08	1·58	0·96	1·10	1·92	2·86	4·11
All Other Causes	0·50	0·52	0·91	1·18	1·33	3·30	4·54	5·13
Totals	5·83	6·43	11·86	9·79	12·28	23·87	29·93	29·85

* The term 'Indian Other Ranks' includes Viceroy's Commissioned Officers.

TABLE 105

India, 1925–45
Indian Army in India
Admissions to Hospital, Invalidings and Deaths
*Officers and Indian Other Ranks**
Quinquennial Comparative Table for the period 1925–39 and
Annual Comparative Table Year by Year from 1939 to 1945
Annual Rates per 1,000 Strength

Source: Annual Reports on the Health of the Army in India

Period	Admissions		Invalidings		Deaths	
	Officers	I.O.Rs.	Officers	I.O.Rs.	Officers	I.O.Rs.
1925–29	498·0	385·0	5·22	10·80	4·74	3·48
1930–34	336·7	453·3	12·47	6·55	5·37	2·63
1935–39	383·8	423·3	10·72	5·76	6·05	2·68
1939	462·1	454·0	12·36	6·43	3·85	2·12
1940	466·4	549·0	2·33	11·86	5·17	2·11
1941	594·5	616·6	2·15	9·79	3·48	3·48
1942	708·9	746·5	2·99	12·28	3·49	4·99
1943	655·0	742·7	2·50	23·87	2·65	4·12
1944	490·3	732·9	1·38	29·93	2·15	3·30
1945	486·8	383·9	6·26	29·85	2·57	2·62

* The term 'Indian Other Ranks' includes Viceroy's Commissioned Officers.

TABLE 106

India, 1925–45
Army in India
Admissions to Hospital, Invalidings and Deaths
*Officers, British Army and Officers, Indian Army**
Quinquennial Comparative Table for the period 1925–39 and
Annual Comparative Table Year by Year from 1939 to 1945
Annual Rates per 1,000 Strength

Sources: Annual Reports on the Health of the Army in India

Period	Officers*					
	Admissions		Invalidings		Deaths	
	British Army	Indian Army	British Army	Indian Army	British Army	Indian Army
1925–29	589·9	498·0	17·44	5·22	5·25	4·74
1930–34	428·6	336·7	20·09	12·47	6·69	5·37
1935–39	436·9	383·8	21·24	10·72	4·82	6·05
1939	435·3	462·1	25·09	12·36	2·14	3·85
1940	533·5	466·4	9·91	2·33	4·95	5·17
1941	975·6	594·5	5·24	2·15	6·48	3·48
1942	1,098·9	708·9	14·40	2·99	7·43	3·49
1943	930·4	655·0	26·41	2·50	6·16	2·65
1944	993·8	490·3	22·11	1·38	5·36	2·15
1945	767·3	486·8	15·36	6·26	4·48	2·57

* The term 'Officers' does not include Viceroy's Commissioned Officers.

TABLE 107

India, 1925–45
Army in India
Admissions to Hospital, Invalidings and Deaths
*British Other Ranks and Indian Other Ranks**
Quinquennial Comparative Table for the Period 1925–39 and
Annual Comparative Table Year by Year from 1939 to 1945
Annual Rates per 1,000 Strength

Source: Annual reports on the Health of the Army in India

Period	Admissions		Invalidings		Deaths	
	B.O.Rs.	I.O.Rs.	B.O.Rs.	I.O.Rs.	B.O.Rs.	I.O.Rs.
1925–29	619·4	385·6	13·50	10·80	2·90	3·48
1930–34	604·7	453·3	8·88	6·55	2·64	2·63
1935–39	597·4	423·3	9·47	5·76	2·54	2·68
1939	663·9	454·0	7·06	6·43	2·75	2·12
1940	723·3	549·0	6·81	11·86	2·58	2·11
1941	876·1	615·6	5·47	9·79	4·19	3·48
1942	979·1	746·5	7·80	12·28	5·39	4·99
1943	847·2	742·7	11·07	23·87	3·02	4·12
1944	1,014·4	732·9	15·64	29·93	3·33	3·30
1945	863·3	583·9	16·10	29·85	2·29	2·62

* Includes Viceroy's Commissioned Officers.

TABLE 108

India, 1940–45
British Army in India
Admissions to Hospitals
Comparison between Annual Rates per 1,000 Strength in the Years
1915 to 1918 with those in the Years 1940 to 1945

Source: Annual Reports on the Health of the Army in India

	1915	1916	1917	1918	1940	1941	1942	1943	1944	1945
British Army Officers	694	921	965	1,344	533	976	1,099	930	994	767
British Army Other Ranks	825	772	771	1,030	723	876	979	874	1,014	863
Indian Army Officers	599	626	729	1,050	468	594	708	655	490	487
Indian Army Other Ranks	744	757	741	856	549	616	746	742	733	584

TABLE 109

India, 1939–45. Army in India. Comparison of Principal Causes of Deaths. B.O.Rs. and I.O.Rs.
Annual Rates per 1,000 Strength

Source: Annual Reports on the Health of the Army in India

CAUSES	1939		1940		1941		1942		1943		1944		1945	
	B.O.Rs.	I.O.Rs.	B.O.Rs.	I.O.Rs.	B.O.Rs.	I.O.Rs.	B.O.Rs.	I.O.Rs.	B.O.Rs.	I.O.Rs.	B.O.Rs.	I.O.Rs.	B.O.Rs.	I.O.Rs.
Diseases of the Circulatory System .	0·17	0·15	0·12	0·09	0·38	0·16	0·17	0·13	0·12	0·12	0·11	0·12	0·09	0·13
Diseases of the Digestive System .	0·37	0·12	0·15	0·13	0·55	0·22	0·48	0·37	0·28	0·35	0·38	0·33	0·24	0·26
Diseases of the Nervous System .	0·08	0·10	0·15	0·03	0·29	0·10	0·19	0·13	0·08	0·16	0·08	0·16	0·10	0·09
Dysentery	0·03	0·04	0·06	0·02	0·11	0·06	0·39	0·36	0·18	0·14	0·02	0·09	0·06	0·02
Enteric Group of Fevers . .	0·08	0·06	—	0·05	0·09	0·07	0·23	0·10	0·11	0·09	0·17	0·09	0·07	0·04
Malaria	0·11	0·01	—	0·09	0·11	0·12	0·59	0·45	0·24	0·41	0·21	0·28	0·10	0·11
Meningococcal Infection . .	0·03	0·04	—	0·10	—	0·31	—	0·38	—	0·20	0·01	0·07	0·01	0·04
Pneumonia	0·11	0·29	0·36	0·29	0·17	0·78	0·23	1·05	0·13	0·84	0·13	0·37	0·08	0·23
Tuberculosis—Pulmonary . .	0·11	0·06	0·06	0·11	0·11	0·17	0·33	0·43	0·12	0·46	0·13	0·38	0·07	0·54
Injuries	0·33	0·79	0·66	0·86	1·33	0·72	1·00	0·77	0·79	0·52	0·81	0·60	0·74	0·51
Total Deaths	2·58	2·12	2·77	2·11	4·19	3·48	5·39	4·99	3·02	4·12	3·38	3·30	2·29	2·62

TABLE 110

India, 1939–45

Comparison of Some Causes of Invalidings. B.O.Rs. and I.O.Rs.

Annual Rates per 1,000 Strength

Source: Annual Reports on the Health of the Army in India

CAUSES	1939		1940		1941		1942		1943		1944		1945	
	B.O.Rs.	I.O.Rs.	B.O.Rs.	I.O.Rs.	B.O.Rs.	I.O.Rs.	B.O.Rs.	I.O.Rs.	B.O.Rs.	I.O.Rs.	B.O.Rs.	I.O.Rs.	B.O.Rs.	I.O.Rs.
Diseases of the Bones, Joints, Muscles, etc.	0·58	0·53	0·34	1·04	0·31	0·75	0·48	0·82	0·20	1·57	0·58	2·10	0·43	2·15
Circulatory System	0·28	0·16	0·42	0·56	0·16	0·43	N.A.	0·56	N.A.	0·84	N.A.	0·95	N.A.	0·99
Digestive System	0·45	0·27	0·24	0·67	N.A.	0·54	0·69	0·59	0·62	0·88	2·10	1·43	1·25	1·20
Ear and Nose	0·06	0·09	0·09	0·35	N.A.	0·28	0·25	0·31	0·52	0·93	0·81	1·66	0·98	2·03
Nervous System	0·81	0·38	0·47	0·96	0·30	1·08	0·45	1·31	0·48	1·91	0·31	1·41	0·33	0·93
Mental Diseases	1·56	0·48	1·40	0·81	1·25	0·77	0·89	1·15	2·25	2·67	2·68	4·41	4·24	4·13
Tuberculosis—Pulmonary	1·03	1·70	1·77	2·02	1·45	1·71	1·63	1·84	3·06	2·41	1·16	2·25	0·08	1·80
Injuries	0·56	1·08	0·66	1·58	0·15	0·96	0·64	1·10	0·67	1·92	1·08	2·86	0·68	4·11
Total Invalids	7·06	6·43	6·81	11·86	5·47	9·79	7·80	12·28	11·07	23·87	15·64	29·93	16·10	29·85

TABLE 111

India, 1938–45. Venereal Diseases

Comparison of British Other Ranks with Indian Other Ranks

Annual Rates per 1,000 Strength

Source: Annual Reports on the Health of the Army in India

	1938		1939		1940		1941		1942		1943		1944		1945	
	B.O.Rs.	I.O.Rs.	B.O.Rs.	I.O.Rs.	B.O.Rs.	I.O.Rs.	B.O.Rs.	I.O.Rs.	B.O.Rs.	I.O.Rs.	B.O.Rs.	I.O.Rs.	B.O.Rs.	I.O.Rs.	B.O.Rs.	I.O.Rs.
Gonorrhoea	28·0	2·9	32·4	3·4	30·9	7·5	33·8	9·4	27·1	11·0	26·3	11·4	31·6	11·5	25·6	8·2
Syphilis	7·6	3·1	8·5	3·4	12·7	6·1	12·6	8·1	9·5	10·3	8·2	9·5	9·4	12·6	11·7	11·7
Other Forms	7·9	2·1	10·3	1·8	14·5	5·3	18·6	10·4	33·0	21·2	29·4	28·9	31·0	24·6	42·5	23·5
Total V.D.	43·5	8·1	51·2	8·6	58·1	18·9	65·0	27·9	69·6	42·5	63·9	49·8	72·0	48·7	79·8	43·4

Total V.D. Rates for 1917 and 1918 were:

	B.O.Rs.	I.O.Rs.
1917	52	45
1918	62	

TABLE 112

India, 1936–45
British Army in India
Effects of Heat
British Other Ranks
Annual Rates per 1,000 Strength

Source: Annual Reports on the Health of the Army in India

Year	Heat Stroke		Heat Exhaustion		Total Effects of Heat	
	Cases	Deaths	Cases	Deaths	Cases	Deaths
1936	0·2	0·06	0·7	0·02	0·9	0·08
1937	0·3	0·13	0·8	0·04	1·1	0·17
1938	0·5	0·14	1·5	0·12	2·0	0·25
1939	0·4	0·06	1·9	0·06	2·3	0·12
1940	1·2	0·06	4·9	0·15	6·1	0·21
1941	1·0	0·09	6·8	0·06	7·8	0·15
1942	2·2	0·44	17·5	0·44	19·7	0·88
1943	0·7	0·09	4·6	0·06	5·3	0·15
1944	0·7	0·17	6·7	0·07	7·4	0·24
1945	1·5	0·16	10·5	0·02	12·0	0·18

TABLE 113

India 1936–45. Army in India. Effects of Heat
Comparison between British and Indian Other Ranks. Annual Rates per 1,000 Strength

Source: Annual Reports on the Health of the Army in India

CONDITIONS	1936	1937	1938	1939	1940	1941	1942	1943	1944	1945
Heat Stroke—British Other Ranks	0·2	0·3	0·5	0·4	1·2	1·0	2·2	0·7	0·7	1·5
Heat Exhaustion—British Other Ranks	0·7	0·8	1·5	1·9	4·9	6·8	17·5	4·6	6·7	10·5
Total Effects of Heat—British Other Ranks	0·9	1·1	2·0	2·3	6·1	7·8	19·7	5·3	7·4	12·0
Total Effects of Heat—Indian Other Ranks	0·1	0·3	0·2	0·2	0·3	0·7	0·8	0·5	0·4	0·7

TABLE 114

India, 1938–45
Malaria
Comparison of British Other Ranks with Indian Other Ranks, 1938–45
Annual Rates per 1,000 Strength

Source: Annual Reports on the Health of the Army in India

	1938	1939	1940	1941	1942	1943	1944	1945
B.O.Rs. .	50·4	55·1	73·4	144·4	164·1	198·4	248·4	130·7
I.O.Rs. . .	109·7	118·3	173·4	144·6	206·0	192·5	159·5	76·1

TABLE 115

India 1939–45. Dysentery and Diarrhoea

Comparison of (a) Officers, British Army with Officers, Indian Army (b) Other Ranks, British Army with Other Ranks, Indian Army

Annual Rates per 1,000 Strength

Source: Annual Reports on the Health of the Army in India

	1939		1940		1941		1942		1943		1944		1945	
(a) Officers	B.A.	I.A.	B.A.	I.A.	B.A.	I.A.	B.A.	I.A.	B.A.	I.A.	B.A.	I.A.	B.A.	I.A.
Diarrhoea . .	19·8	20·9	N.A.	24·6	121·5	41·8	103·7	52·9	62·1	41·5	68·2	21·8	52·0	23·2
Dysentery . .	35·2	15·8	47·6	28·0	70·0	34·5	92·6	40·6	75·8	35·5	104·8	37·5	89·1	33·3
Totals . .	55·0	36·7	N.A.	52·6	191·5	76·3	196·3	93·5	137·9	77·0	173·0	59·3	141·1	56·5
(b) Other Ranks														
Diarrhoea . .	18·2	6·3	25·0	10·9	55·4	23·6	72·7	32·7	43·6	25·7	53·2	20·9	45·6	17·0
Dysentery . .	28·9	17·1	33·0	21·8	36·9	21·0	50·2	20·0	48·8	16·0	72·5	16·2	72·1	14·2
Totals . .	47·1	23·4	58·0	32·7	92·3	44·6	122·9	52·7	92·4	41·7	125·7	37·1	117·7	31·2

N.A.—Figures not available.

TABLE 116

India, 1939–45
Army in India
Women's Services
Admissions to Hospital
Annual Rates per 1,000 Strength

Source: Annual Reports on the Health of the Army in India

	1939	1940	1941	1942	1943	1944	1945
Members of Q.A.I.M. Nursing Service . . .	439·6	547·7	638·5	824·8	1,051·3	1,009·9	1,233·3
Women's Auxiliary Corps (India)				1,184·3	510·4	649·8	524·3

TABLE 117

India, 1939–45
Army in India
Women's Services
Deaths in Hospitals
Annual Rates per 1,000 Strength

Source: Annual Reports on the Health of the Army in India

	1939	1940	1941	1942	1943	1944	1945
Members of Q.A.I.M. Nursing Service . . .	—	0·50	10·13	1·39	1·28	2·78	1·64
Women's Auxiliary Corps (India)				2·38	1·64	2·34	2·23

TABLE 118

India, 1939–45
Army in India
Women's Services
Invalids sent Home
Annual Rates per 1,000 Strength

Source: Annual Reports on the Health of the Army in India

	1939	1940	1941	1942	1943	1944	1945
Members of Q.A.I.M. Nursing Service . . .	43·90	1·00	—	12·52	21·82	17·40	31·15
Women's Auxiliary Corps (India)				2·38	7·94	21·45	7·81

TABLE 119

India, 1939–45
Army in India
Women's Services
Average Constantly Sick
Annual Rates per 1,000 Strength

Source: Annual Reports on the Health of the Army in India

	1939	1940	1941	1942	1943	1944	1945
Members of Q.A.I.M. Nursing Service . . .	18·57	22·26	20·24	32·64	35·30	44·04	59·58
Women's Auxiliary Corps (India)				8·56	16·15	22·56	18·92

CHAPTER IX

SOUTH EAST ASIA COMMAND

MEDICAL Statistics for South East Asia Command (S.E.A.C.), presented in this chapter, have been grouped according to the two areas for which data are available, i.e. the Indo-Burma Front and Ceylon. That this is possible is due to administrative considerations and because of it, comparison can be made of the incidence rates among troops of the same stock stationed in areas which differed markedly, not only in geographical conditions, but also in the intensity of operational activity.

The area in which troops on the Indo-Burma Front operated contains some of the worst malaria spots in the world. Climatic conditions ranged from the excessive heat of the plains and the humid coastal and jungle areas, to the colder mountainous regions of the north. It was an area which experienced intense, bitter fighting. In contrast, Ceylon enjoys a more equable climate and enemy action consisted of occasional bombing.

Although this section is designated 'South East Asia Command', statistics herein include casualties sustained before the formation of the Command. Tabulations for both areas have been compiled for the years 1942 to 1945. In 1942 units in the Eastern Command of India became fully operational and were divorced from the Army in India. They became known as the Fourteenth Army, which was later incorporated into S.E.A.C. on the formation of that Command in 1943. The tabulations of the Indo-Burma Front, therefore, contain statistics of the Eastern Command, the Fourteenth Army and the Indo-Burma Front of S.E.A.C. It is possible, too, that they contain some admissions resulting from the Japanese invasion of Burma; they certainly do include all known admissions to hospitals during the operations which resulted in the re-occupation of that country.

The information contained in this section was obtained, originally, from Army Form A.31-B. This was a monthly return devised to show, *inter alia*, the numbers admitted to hospitals, by diseases and deaths in hospitals. It was similar in form, though less detailed, to Army Form A.31 used by hospitals in areas other than operational in India. Transmission of this statistical information followed conventional lines, from hospitals to A.Ds.M.S., to D.Ds.M.S., to D.M.S., S.E.A.C., and thence to D.M.S., G.H.Q.(India). An interesting point in the transmission of these medical statistics was that the D.M.S., S.E.A.C., was not empowered, originally, to send such information direct to the War Office and it was only towards the end of the campaign in this area that the

War Office obtained satisfactory detailed information direct from S.E.A.C.

The statistics which follow relate to admissions direct to hospitals from Units and transfers thereto from other medical units. They take no account of those admissions to such other medical units as Field Ambulances, Casualty Clearing Stations, Malaria Forward Treatment Units, etc., which did not eventually result in transfers to hospitals. Indeed, such information is not available.

A few words must be said with reference to Malaria Forward Treatment Units, and the impact of admissions thereto on the statistics which follow, particularly in relation to Malaria.

In 1942 and 1943, admissions to hospitals on account of Malaria were nearly one half the total patients admitted for disease. Cases were evacuated to hospitals sometimes well to the rear of active operations and many were sent to convalescent camps still further away. For various reasons, it was often a long, difficult, and tedious process to effect a return to units after convalescence. There was thus a colossal wastage of man-hours between discharge from hospital and return to unit and a consequent diminution in fighting strength.

With the object of reducing this wastage and lightening the burden admissions for Malaria had placed on General Hospitals, Malaria Forward Treatment Units were formed. These were mobile units, each of two hundred and fifty beds, which functioned in close proximity to forward troops. They operated in 1944 and 1945. As, finally, there were sixteen of these units functioning on the Indo-Burma Front, admissions to them for Malaria must have been of a very high magnitude, and the incidence rates for this disease in 1944 and, particularly, 1945, shown in the following tabulations are, therefore, far from complete. These units also treated patients suffering from minor diseases when the bed situation allowed. These cases were comparatively few and would have little effect on the incidence rates of such diseases shown in the tabulations.

Apart from these considerations, there appears to be no reason to doubt the accuracy of the statistics here presented.

Troops engaged on the Indo-Burma Front included those of British, Indian, West African, and East African stock. Similar classes (except West Africans) were stationed in Ceylon, where, in addition, there were Ceylonese units. The statistics which follow have been arranged according to these ethnic groups and, where the information is available, sub-divided into Male Officers, Male Other Ranks, and Women's Services. In addition, and in accordance with long established convention, statistics for Indian Other Ranks have been sub-divided into, firstly, Viceroy's Commissioned Officers and Indian Other Ranks (V.C.Os. and I.O.Rs.) and, secondly, Non-Combatants (Enrolled)

(N.Cs.(E)). Tabulations relating to incidence rates for All Troops are included for each of the geographical areas.

Attached to Indian, African and Ceylonese Units were British Officers and Other Ranks of various Corps and Regiments of the British and Indian Armies. Any admissions to hospitals in respect of these personnel are included in the figures relating to British Officers or British Other Ranks (B.O.Rs.). Similarly, admissions of any Indian, African, or Ceylonese personnel attached to British or other units are included in the statistics of their own ethnic group.

Injuries, as in other sections, have been grouped according to whether they were received through enemy action (E.A.), or otherwise (N.E.A.). For 1942 and 1943, no breakdown of N.E.A. injuries are available. During 1944 and 1945 they were broken down as to 'Burns and Scalds' and 'Other Injuries'. Sub-divisions of E.A. injuries were reported for the four years under review as to Blast, Bomb wounds, Gunshot-wounds, and Shell wounds. A tabulation has been prepared for each area showing the sub-division of injuries, according to ethnic grouping, together with the overall detail for All Troops.

In so far as deaths in hospitals are concerned, very little data are available. The only information that can be presented is the annual rates per 1,000 strength, classified ethnically, under two headings, 'Diseases and N.E.A. Injuries' and E.A. Injuries'. The rates quoted relate to deaths in hospitals only. They do not include deaths on the field of battle or in other types of medical units.

Finally, tabulations have been produced showing comparative rates of diseases for each of the ethnic groups.

As in the majority of sections, the rates cited herein have been calculated per 1,000 strength. It will be noted that in some tables Equivalent Annual Rates (E.A.R.) have been computed. This is due firstly, to East and West African Troops being in the Command for only a portion of 1944 and, secondly, to data being available in some cases for nine months only in 1945. Known admissions have been adjusted to equivalent annual rates in order that valid comparisons may be made with the rates of other years.

In the ensuing examination of the tabulations the procedure followed is to consider by each area, firstly, admissions for diseases only for each class of troops. Following this statistics for injuries and then deaths are considered. Finally, the medical ethnography of the area is examined.

The following tables for S.E.A.C. are presented:

CLASS OF TROOPS	Periods Covered	Indo-Burma Front	Ceylon
		Table No.	
(i) *Admissions for Diseases*			
British Officers	1942–45	120	136
British Other Ranks	1942–45	121	137
Q.A.I.M.N.S.	1942–45	122	—
All British Troops	1942–45	123	138
Indian Officers	1942–44	—	139
V.C.Os. and I.O.Rs.	1942–45	124	140
N.Cs.(E.)	1942–45	125	141
V.C.Os., I.O.Rs. and N.Cs.(E.)	1942–45	126	—
W.A.C. (I) and I.M.N.S.	1942–45	127	142
All Indian Troops	1942–45	128	143
W.A.O.Rs.	1944–45	129	—
E.A.O.Rs.	1944–45	130	144
Ceylonese Officers	1943–45	—	145
Ceylonese Other Ranks	1943–45	—	146
All Ceylonese Troops	1943–45	—	147
All Troops	1942–45	131	148
(ii) *Admissions for Injuries*			
All Troops	1942–45	132	149
(iii) *Deaths in Hospitals*			
All Troops	1942–45	133	150
(iv) *Medical Ethnography*			
British and Indian O.Rs.	1942–45	134	151
British, Indian and Ceylonese O.Rs.	1943–45	—	152
All Other Ranks	1944–45	135	153

(1) Indo-Burma Front

BRITISH TROOPS

OFFICERS

Table 120 shows the causes of admissions to hospitals of British Officers. The highest rate of admission for disease occurred in 1943, when the figure was 726 per 1,000. In 1944 and 1945 admissions declined somewhat spectacularly to 521 and 344 respectively, that is, in 1944 to between one quarter and one third less, and in 1945, to slightly more than half, the 1943 rate. Admissions in 1942 were slightly less than in 1943, at 714 per 1,000.

Injuries accounted for rates of 35 in 1942, 48 in 1943, 87 in 1944 and 73 in 1945.

The highest recorded rate of admissions from all causes was 774 per 1,000 in 1943, followed by 748 in 1942, 608 in 1944 and 417 in 1945.

During the first three years, of individual diseases, MALARIA accounted for the highest rate of admissions. In 1942 admissions for this disease were thirty-seven per cent. of the total for all diseases; in 1943 they were thirty per cent.; in 1944, twenty-four per cent.; and finally, in 1945, fell to only nine per cent. To make a further comparison, in 1942 and 1943, the admission rates for Malaria were approximately three times those for Dysentery, which caused the second highest rate of admissions. In 1944 the rate was a little more than twice that of Dysentery, in spite of a decline in the admission rate of the latter disease. In 1945, admissions for Malaria dropped to second place, being four-fifths the rate for Dysentery. The incidence rates for Malaria during the years under review were: 262 per 1,000 in 1942, 221 in 1943, 124 in 1944 and only 30 in 1945 (*See* p.355).

DYSENTERY followed Malaria as next in importance from the point of view of admissions. This disease recorded a steady decline throughout the years from 82 per 1,000 in 1942 to 73 in 1943, 57 in 1944 and 38 in 1945.

The third highest rate of admissions was recorded by Other Diseases of the DIGESTIVE SYSTEM. Here again a steady decline was experienced, from 53 per 1,000 in 1942 to 48 in 1943, 30 in 1944 and 17 in 1945.

It is of interest to note that if the four annual rates of admission in respect of Dysentery and Other Diseases of the Digestive System are plotted, the resultant courses are almost parallel.

Admissions for DIARRHOEA, however, do not conform to this pattern. The rate increased from 29 in 1942 to 36 in 1943 and again to 42 in 1944. There was a fifty per cent. decline in 1945 when the recorded rate was 20.

P.U.O. and N.Y.D. FEVER followed a similar, though more spectacular trend. The rate increased by fifty per cent. in 1943, and this was followed by a sixty per cent. increase. In 1945, the rate, which declined to forty per cent. of the 1944 rate, was very slightly less than that for 1942. Relevant rates were: 1942, 21 per 1,000, 31 in 1943, 50 in 1944 and 20 in 1945.

SEPTIC CONDITIONS were responsible for admissions at 35 per 1,000 in 1942 and 1943, followed by 20 in 1944 and 23 in 1945.

Admissions for INFECTIVE HEPATITIS were comparatively low in 1942, at 10 per 1,000. In the two years which followed the rate increased two and a half times to 25, and there was a slight fall to 23 in 1945.

Diseases of the SKIN (other than Scabies) were responsible for admissions at fairly stable rates during the first three years, at 15, 17 and 14 per 1,000 respectively. In 1945, however, the rate increased somewhat markedly to 23.

Admissions for diseases of the EAR, NOSE and THROAT fluctuated slightly from 11 per 1,000 in 1942 to 17 in 1943, 15 in 1944 and 12 in 1945.

In 1942 the rate of admissions for DENGUE FEVER was 26 per 1,000; it fell to 20 in 1943, and again, to 4 in 1944. This latter rate was maintained in 1945.

Of the numerically minor causes of admission, those for MENTAL, PSYCHONEUROTIC and PERSONALITY DISORDERS tended, on the whole, to increase throughout the period. Admissions in 1942 were 5 per 1,000; in 1945 they had more than doubled to 13. In the intervening years they were 7 in 1943 and 5 in 1944. This tendency to increase is exhibited in all classes of male troops on this front.

Admissions for TUBERCULOSIS, although comparatively few in number, were fairly stable, apart from 1944 when the rate was remarkably low at 0·12 as against 1·07 in 1942, 0·89 in 1943 and 0·91 in 1945.

The rates for DIPHTHERIA fluctuated from 0·21 in 1942 to a peak of 1·25 in 1943.

Admissions for PNEUMONIA in 1943 are not known. Apart from this and although rates are low, they tended to increase. Relevant rates were 0·64 in 1942, 0·75 in 1944 and 1·28 in 1945.

Of the recorded diseases, those due to disorders of NUTRITION showed the lowest rates of admissions, there being none in the years 1942 to 1944 with 0·08 per 1,000 in 1945.

The next lowest was for MUMPS, which recorded rates of 0·21 in 1942, 0·71 in 1943 and 0·45 in 1945. There were no admissions for this disease in 1944.

OTHER RANKS

Table 121 lists the admission rates to hospitals of BRITISH OTHER RANKS.

As in the case of British Officers, the highest rate of admissions for disease occurred in 1943, but, whereas the increase over 1942 for officers was but slight (726 per 1,000 as against 714), admission of other ranks in 1943 rose by seventy per cent. In the following year they decreased by nearly one quarter, while in 1945 they were less than half the peak year of 1943 and a quarter less than the 1942 rate. In 1942, the disease rate was half as much again as that for officers; in 1943 and 1944 it was approximately two and a half times, and in 1945 two and a quarter times the officer rate. The relevant figures are shown in the table below.

Indo-Burma Front. Admissions for Disease.
Comparison of Rates between
(i) *British Officers and* (ii) *British Other Ranks, 1942–45*

		1942	1943	1944	1945
Rates per 1,000 Strength	Officers	714	726	521	344
	Other Ranks	1,021	1,746	1,334	780
Comparative Rates Officer Base	Officers	100	100	100	100
	Other Ranks	143	240	256	227

Of individual diseases, MALARIA was responsible for the highest rate of admissions, they being, in the first three years, approximately one-third and in 1945, about one-sixth of the total admissions for disease. The rates of admission per 1,000 strength of both Officers and Other Ranks together with comparative rates are given below.

Indo-Burma Front. Admissions for Malaria.
Comparison of Rates between
(i) *British Officers and* (ii) *British Other Ranks, 1942–45*

		1942	1943	1944	1945
Rates per 1,000 Strength	Officers	262	221	124	30
	Other Ranks	335	628	406	128
Comparative Rates 1942 Base	Officers	100	84	48	11
	Other Ranks	100	187	121	38
Comparative Rates Officer Base	Officers	100	100	100	100
	Other Ranks	128	284	327	426

Whereas the rates of admissions on account of Malaria for Officers declined each year, those for Other Ranks show that the highest rate recorded was in 1943, followed by 1944, 1942 and 1945. The lowest rate reported for Officers (in 1945) was approximately one-ninth the peak admission rate (in 1942). For Other Ranks the lowest rate, also in 1945, was one-fifth of the highest recorded rate (in 1943). It would seem that 'Anti-Malaria Discipline', the personal precautionary measures to be taken to avoid this disease, was of a much higher order among Officers than among Other Ranks.

DYSENTERY caused the next highest rate of admissions of Other Ranks as in the case of Officers. The Officer rates declined each year, but those for Other Ranks show the peak year to be 1943, with the lowest rate in 1945 at one-half the 1943 rate. The trends follow the patterns exhibited by both classes of personnel in respect of Malaria. Rates of admission, with comparative rates, are indicated below.

Indo-Burma Front. Admissions for Dysentery.
Comparison of Rates between
(i) *British Officers and* (ii) *British Other Ranks, 1942–45*

		1942	1943	1944	1945
Rates per 1,000 Strength	Officers	82	73	57	38
	Other Ranks	88	132	97	65
Comparative Rates 1942 Base	Officers	100	89	70	46
	Other Ranks	100	150	110	74
Comparative Rates Officer Base	Officers	100	100	100	100
	Other Ranks	107	182	170	171

There was very little difference in the 1942 rates, but in the following years admission rates of Other Ranks were approximately one and three-quarters those of Officers. This, as in the case of Malaria, was probably due to more rigid personal discipline among Officers. It is possible that some of the admissions were due to the normal increase in incidence noticed among new arrivals in India, when rates are higher until they become acclimatised.

Next in numerical importance came VENEREAL DISEASES. The peak admission rate occurred in 1943 when it was 158 per 1,000 strength. For the other years under review, the rates were slightly less than one half the 1943 rate at 72 in both 1942 and 1945 and 69 in 1944.

P.U.O. and N.Y.D. FEVER accounted for a large number of admissions, particularly in 1944. Rates increased from 36 in 1942 to 82 in 1943, reached the peak figure of 169 in 1944 and, in 1945, declined sharply to just above the 1942 rate at 42 per 1,000 strength. This trend is similar to, but more extensive than for Officers.

Admissions for DIARRHOEA showed a similar tendency, in that rates increased from 1942 to a peak in 1944 with a sharp decline in 1945. Relevant figures were 42 in 1942, 77 in 1943, 91 in 1944 and 35 in 1945. This again is similar to the trend demonstrated for Officers.

Other Diseases of the DIGESTIVE system were responsible for a comparatively high rate of admissions as were Other Diseases of the RESPIRATORY System. In both cases rates were higher for Other Ranks than for Officers, particularly so in the case of Respiratory Diseases, for whereas the rates for Digestive Diseases were from fifteen to one hundred and six per cent. more than those for Officers, Respiratory Diseases ranged from nearly three hundred to over five hundred per cent. Relevant figures are given below.

Indo-Burma Front. Admissions for (i) *Other Diseases of the Digestive System and* (ii) *Other Diseases of the Respiratory System.*
Comparison of Rates between British Officers and British Other Ranks, 1942–45

(i) *Other Diseases of the Digestive System*		1942	1943	1944	1945
Rates per 1,000 strength	Officers	53	48	30	17
	Other Ranks	61	87	53	35
Comparative Rates Officer Base	Officers	100	100	100	100
	Other Ranks	115	181	177	206
Comparative Rates 1942 Base	Officers	100	91	57	32
	Other Ranks	100	143	87	57
(ii) *Other Diseases of the Respiratory System*					
Rates per 1,000 strength	Officers	14	18	11	9
	Other Ranks	54	69	50	59
Comparative Rates Officer Base	Officers	100	100	100	100
	Other Ranks	386	382	455	656
Comparative Rates 1942 Base	Officers	100	129	79	64
	Other Ranks	100	128	93	109

Diseases of the SKIN (excluding Scabies) accounted for admissions of the order of 42, 50, 36 and 51 per 1,000 during the four years, while the rates for SCABIES were 8, 17, 13 and 5 respectively. The rates for the former were between two and three times, while those for Scabies were from two to sixteen times, the rates for Officers.

The trend of admissions for diseases of the EAR, NOSE and THROAT among Other Ranks was similar to that of Officers. The rates were approximately twice those of Officers and were 19 in 1942, 36 in 1943, 27 in 1944 and 26 in 1945.

SEPTIC CONDITIONS were responsible for admissions at a range of rates from 21 to 36 per 1,000. Although the range was very similar to that of Officers (20 to 35) rates for the latter were, on the average, slightly higher than those for Other Ranks. These were 25 in 1942, 36 in 1943, 22 in 1944 and 21 in 1945.

The admission rates for INFECTIVE HEPATITIS in 1944 and 1945 were over six times that in 1942. The rates, which were 5 per 1,000 in 1942, 27 in 1943 and 31 in 1944 and 1945 were higher than those for Officers. In 1942 it was one half the rate; in 1943 it was slightly higher; in 1944 it was one quarter higher and in 1945 one third higher. Compared with the 1942 rates, Officer admissions rose to a peak of two hundred and fifty per cent. in 1943 and 1944 and fell slightly to two hundred and thirty per cent. in 1945. Other Rank rates, on the other hand, were over five hundred per cent. in 1943 and over six hundred per cent. in 1944 and 1945.

Admissions on account of DENGUE FEVER fell from 38 per 1,000 in 1942 to 25 in 1943. The following year there was a decline to 4, followed by a further decline to 2 in 1945. This trend duplicated that of Officers.

The rates of admissions for COMMON COLD in respect of Other Ranks were from two to three times those of Officers. Rates were 12 in 1942, 21 in 1943, 19 in 1944 and 17 in 1945. Those of Officers were 5, 8, 7 and 5 respectively.

MENTAL, PSYCHONEUROTIC and PERSONALITY DISORDERS were responsible for an increasing rate of admissions from 2·5 in 1942 to 23 in 1945. The comparison between the rates of Other Ranks and those of Officers is interesting. In 1942 the Officer's rate was twice that of Other Ranks. By 1943 the rates were almost equal and in 1944 the Other Ranks rate was twice that of the Officers. This was maintained in 1945. Taking 1942 as the base year, admissions of Officers had risen by 1945 two and a half times, whereas Other Ranks admissions had risen over nine times. It would appear that the increasing *tempo* of war in this area affected British Other Ranks to a far greater degree than it did Officers. Relevant figures are given below.

Indo-Burma Front. Admission Rates for Mental, Psychoneurotic and Personality Disorders.
Comparison of Rates between (i) *British Officers and* (ii) *British Other Ranks, 1942–45*

		1942	1943	1944	1945
Rates per 1,000 strength	Officers	5·0	6·9	5·4	12·6
	Other Ranks	2·5	6·1	10·9	23·2
Comparative Rates 1942 Base	Officers	100	138	108	252
	Other Ranks	100	244	436	928
Comparative Rates Officer Base	Officers	100	100	100	100
	Other Ranks	50	88	202	184

Diseases of the EYE accounted for admissions of the order of 4·6 per 1,000 by 1942. In the following year, it had almost trebled to 13. In 1944 it fell to 10 but increased again to 13 in 1945. Officers' rates were lower at 6·5, 2·9, 2·6 and 5·4 respectively.

Apart from 1943, when the rate rose to 9 per 1,000, admissions for Diseases of the CIRCULATORY System ranged between 5·4 and 5·8. The rates for Officers were 6·7 in 1942, 5·7 in 1943, 1·9 in 1944 and 3·1 in 1945.

The lowest recorded rate for individual diseases, as in the case of Officers, was for MUMPS. Recorded admissions ranged from 0·1 in 1942 to 0·5 in both 1943 and 1945.

Other diseases for which low rates were registered were those due to Disorders of NUTRITION (ranging from 0·0 to 0·8). SMALLPOX (0·4 to 1·01), TUBERCULOSIS (0·4 to 1·0), PNEUMONIA (0·9 to 1·2), DIPHTHERIA (0·7 to 1·2) and the ENTERIC Group of Fevers (0·4 to 1·9). The majority of these ranges are similar to those for Officers.

QUEEN ALEXANDRA'S IMPERIAL MILITARY NURSING SERVICE

Table 122 records the rates of admissions to hospitals of members of the Q.A.I.M.N.S. In 1942, very few members of the Service were located in the area. Comparisons of rates for that year with those of other years when strengths were greatly increased is not satisfactory and, although the rates for 1942 have been included in the table, they are omitted from the discussion on morbidity. Similarly, because of the low strength *vis-à-vis* British Officers and Other Ranks, a comparison with the latter cannot be made, or conclusions drawn, with any degree of validity.

Total admissions for Disease rose from 719 per 1,000 strength in 1943 to 869 in 1944 and fell to 389 in 1954. Three-quarters of the decline in 1945 is accounted for by the remarkable fall in the rates of Malaria, Dysentery and Diarrhoea. These fell by 226, 96 and 44 respectively, a total of 366 per 1,000.

There were no recorded admissions on account of injuries received through enemy action for the three years under review. Those for injuries not caused by enemy action were almost identical in 1943 and 1944 (43·8 and 43·6). In 1945 they dropped to less than half to 20·6.

The peak year of admissions for MALARIA was 1944. This differs from the experience of male troops on this front, when the peak year was 1943, but agrees with members of the W.A.C.(I) and I.M.N.S. The rate in 1943, 87 per 1,000, increased to nearly three times that figure in 1944, when the rate was 229. In conforming to the trend exhibited by all other classes in the Command, there was a remarkable reduction in admissions during the following year when the rate was 23 per 1,000.

The rates for DYSENTERY and DIARRHOEA were also of a high order. Those for Dysentery were 97 in 1943, 142 in 1944 and 45 in 1945. Admissions for Diarrhoea were somewhat lower at 59 in both 1943 and 1944 and 14 in 1945.

Admission rates for Other Diseases of the DIGESTIVE system declined during 1944 and 1945 from 41 in 1943 to 33 in 1944 and finally to 21 in 1945.

A similar decline was also in evidence for TONSILLITIS and SEPTIC CONDITIONS, the rates being:

Tonsillitis	44 in 1943	26 in 1944	19 in 1945
Septic Conditions	31 in 1943	22 in 1944	10 in 1945

Diseases of the EAR, NOSE and THROAT accounted for admissions of the order of 25 in 1943, 26 in 1944 and 10 in 1945. The rates for Other Diseases of the RESPIRATORY SYSTEM were of a comparatively high order at 44 in 1943 and 37 in 1944 and 1945. Admissions for DENGUE FEVER were also comparatively high in 1943 and 1944 at 25 and 31. There was a marked decline in 1945 when the rate was 8 per 1,000.

The trend of admissions for MENTAL, PSYCHONEUROTIC and PERSONALITY Disorders is interesting in that the rates fell in 1944 and 1945. This is at variance with the male Troops in the Command, but agrees with the experience of members of the W.A.C.(I) and I.M.N.S. Relevant rates of Q.A.I.M.N.S. admissions were 6·3 in 1943, 2·2 in 1944 and 2·1 in 1945.

There were no recorded cases of the ENTERIC Group of Fevers, SANDFLY FEVER, SMALLPOX or VENEREAL DISEASES during the three years under review.

ALL BRITISH TROOPS

In Table 123 are presented the annual admission rates per 1,000 strength of all British Troops. As the strength of Other Ranks was many times the combined strength of Officers and members of the

Q.A.I.M.N.S., the trends of admission tend to follow, on the whole, those of B.O.Rs. (Table 121).

The rates given in this table are in many cases slightly lower than those for B.O.Rs. This is due to the rate of admissions for the two other elements being somewhat less. Admissions for some diseases, however, are higher, where the combined rate of admissions for Officers and Q.A.I.M.N.S. were greatly in excess of those for B.O.Rs. This is exemplified in Hepatitis, the Enteric Group of Fevers, Septic Conditions and, in 1943, Mental, Psychoneurotic and Personality Disorders.

INDIAN TROOPS

Data are available, and tabulations presented, for Indian Troops in respect of the following classes:

(i) Viceroy's Commissioned Officers and Indian Other Ranks (V.C.Os. and I.O.Rs.).

(ii) Non-Combatants (Enrolled)—(N.Cs.(E)).

(iii) Members of the Women's Auxiliary Corps (India) and those of the Indian Military Nursing Service (W.A.C.(I.) and I.M.N.S.).

Satisfactory records are not available to produce a separate tabulation for Indian Officers, but such as are available have been included in the statistics for all Indian Troops. The number of Indians commissioned in the Indian Army was comparatively few, particularly in the first two years reviewed here. Any deficiencies of records would, therefore, detract little from the value of the figures presented.

It may be mentioned, as a matter of interest, that Viceroy's Commissioned Officers were peculiar to the Indian Army and were analogous to Warrant Officers in the British Army. Non-Combatants (Enrolled), also peculiar to the Indian Army, and formerly known as Followers, were recruited to undertake menial tasks in the Indian and British Armies. Morbidity statistics of those N.Cs.(E.) and of any V.C.Os. and I.O.Rs. who were attached to the British Army are included in the tabulations which follow.

The Women's Auxiliary Corps (India) was formed in the early years of the war and was comparable with the A.T.S. in the United Kingdom. Members consisted of women chiefly of European, Indian and Anglo-Indian stock. The Indian Military Nursing Service, formed for service in hospitals catering for Indian Troops consisted of women of similar stock as the W.A.C.(I.).

V.C.OS. AND I.O.RS.

Table 124 shows the rates of admissions for V.C.Os. and I.O.Rs. for the years 1942 to 1945. Admissions for diseases rose only in 1943 from

877 per 1,000 strength in 1942 to 1,073 in 1943. This was followed by a decline to 912 in the following year, and in 1945 the rate was reduced by approximately fifty per cent. to 466. Admissions on account of injuries increased annually from 43 in 1942 to 56, 93 and 102 in the succeeding three years. Total admission rates were 921 in 1942, 1,129 in 1943, 1,004 in 1944 and 568 in 1945.

As with other classes of troops in this Command, MALARIA, among individual diseases, was responsible for the largest number of admissions. In 1942 and 1943 the recorded admissions were approximately one-half of those for all diseases and in 1944 it was roughly one-third. Actual rates in these years were 447, 486 and 319. In 1945 there was a dramatic decline of admissions and the rate fell to 68 per 1,000 or one-seventh the total disease rate for that year.

Next in numerical importance to Malaria was P.U.O. and N.Y.D. FEVER, admissions for which rose from 30 in 1942 to 72 in 1943 and 115 in 1944. The rate declined considerably in 1945 to 28. The importance of the impact on admissions of Malaria and P.U.O. and N.Y.D. Fever may be measured by eliminating the rates of these diseases from the total disease rates as under.

Indo-Burma Front. Admissions for (i) *All Diseases and* (ii) *Malaria and P.U.O. and N.Y.D. Fever, 1942–45.*
V.C.Os. and I.O.Rs.

Admissions for:	1942		1943		1944		1945	
(i) All Diseases		877		1,073		912		466
(ii) Malaria	447		486		319		68	
(iii) P.U.O. and N.Y.D. Fever	30	477	72	558	115	434	28	96
(i) less (ii) and (iii)		400		515		478		370

The range of Malaria and P.U.O. and N.Y.D. was 462 (558 less 96). That for the balance of diseases was 145 (515 less 370). The comparatively low range of the balance of diseases indicates:

(a) a fairly stable rate of admissions or

(b) erratic rates of admissions of individual diseases, high rises in some being compensated by equivalent falls in others.

An examination of Table 124 reveals the latter was not the case.

Admissions for VENEREAL DISEASES were high with rates of 39 in 1942, 66 in 1943, 36 in 1944 and 46 in 1945.

DYSENTERY was responsible for a high rate in 1942 at 53 per 1,000. In the following year the rate declined to 34 but rose again in 1944 to 40. There was a marked fall in 1945 when the rate was only 19 per 1,000. This rate compares satisfactorily with 14 per 1,000 recorded for V.C.Os. and I.O.Rs. in India during 1945 and the pre-war Indian rate of 17 per 1,000 (in 1938 and 1939).

Next in importance were admissions for SEPTIC CONDITIONS which recorded rates of 28 in 1942, 40 in 1943, 30 in 1944 and 29 in 1945.

Admissions for other diseases of the DIGESTIVE SYSTEM increased annually to 1944 and then fell to a rate only slightly above that for 1942. Relevant figures were 22 in 1942, followed by 35, 37, and, finally, 23 in 1945.

DIARRHOEA caused admission rates at 28 in 1942 and 1943. In 1944 they rose to 40 per 1,000 but fell in 1945 to 18. The latter rate is slightly higher (by 1·4 per 1,000) than the Indian rate for this class of troops in 1945. This disease did not parallel the experience of Dysentery which recorded a rate in 1945 lower than the Indian rates for 1938 and 1939. Indeed the rates for Diarrhoea in India for these years were at 5 and 6 respectively, one-third of the Indo-Burma Front rates.

Comparatively high in the order of admissions were those for COMMON COLD. These showed an increase of over one hundred per cent. in 1943, from 15 to 35. This was followed by a slight decline to 33 in 1944 and a steeper one in the following year to 24.

Among the diseases of smaller numerical importance, progressively increasing annual rates were experienced by MENTAL, PSYCHONEUROTIC and PERSONALITY DISORDERS. The low 1942 rate of 1·5 per 1,000 was succeeded by 2·9 in 1943, 4·6 in 1944 and 7·33 in 1945. This trend was not peculiar to V.C.Os. and I.O.Rs. Indeed, it was prevalent among all male troops on the Front.

The rates of admission for TUBERCULOSIS were slightly lower than those in India. This was probably due to a strict medical examination of all personnel before being posted to units on active service, in order to exclude the less fit, who were sent to units on garrison duty in India. Relevant rates were 2·1 in 1942, followed by 1·4 in 1943, 1·3 in 1944 and 1·8 in 1945.

INFECTIVE HEPATITIS showed a startling increase in rates from 0·5 in 1942 to 14·7 in 1945. This indicates that for every person admitted for this disease in 1942, twenty-nine were admitted in 1945. The rates for the intermediate years were 2 in 1943 and 12 in 1944.

The rates for PNEUMONIA varied only slightly from 3·5 in 1942 to 2·3 in 1944 and 3·7 in 1945. The 1943 rate is not ascertainable. Very slight changes were also recorded in the rates for TONSILLITIS, which varied from 3 in 1942 and 1944, to 3·4 in 1945 and 3·5 in 1943.

Admissions for MUMPS were less than those for the same class of troops in India. Whereas the rates recorded on the Indo-Burma Front were 11, 4, 5 and 6 respectively for the years 1942 to 1945, those in India were 16, 15, 13 and 12.

SANDFLY and DENGUE FEVERS caused comparatively few admissions. The rates for the former were 0·1, 0·3, 0·1 and 0·7, while those for the latter were 2·5, 0·4, 0·4 and 1·2.

N.CS.(E.)

Table 125 relates to the admissions to hospitals of Non-Combatants (Enrolled).

The total admissions on account of disease only followed the pattern of B.O.Rs. and V.C.Os. and I.O.Rs., in that there occurred a conspicuous rise in 1943 with successive falls in the two following years. Relevant rates were 776 in 1942, 1,083 in 1943, 743 in 1944 and 279 in 1945.

Admissions for Injuries were fairly constant, being 34 in 1942, followed by 38, 35 and, finally, 29 in 1945.

Total admission rates were 811 in 1942, 1,121 in 1943, 776 in 1944 and 308 in 1945.

In the following discussion on disease admission rates, comparisons are made between those for N.Cs.(E.) and those for V.C.Os. and I.O.Rs. (Table 126), hereinafter called I.O.Rs.

Table 126 shows the average rates of admissions for the four years, 1942 to 1945, in respect of I.O.Rs. on the one hand and N.Cs.(E.) on the other, and the order of numerical precedence from the point of view of admissions.

The average rates for I.O.Rs. were generally higher than those for N.Cs.(E.). In only six diseases did the reverse hold good. These were Venereal Diseases, Other Conditions of the Respiratory System, Mumps, Pneumonia, Smallpox and the Enteric Group of Fevers.

A study of the ranking positions reveals the following:

Diseases with similar ranking positions	Malaria, Common Cold, Diseases of the Skin (other than Scabies), Diseases of the Eye, Tuberculosis, Enteric Group of Fevers and Diphtheria.
Diseases with a divergence of one position	P.U.O. and N.Y.D. Fever, Venereal Diseases, Dysentery, Other Diseases of the Digestive Systems, Scabies, E.N.T., Infective Hepatitis, Mumps, Mental, Psychoneurotic and Personality Disorders, Tonsillitis, Dengue Fever, Smallpox, Sandfly Fever, Disorders of Nutrition, Septic Conditions.
Diseases with a divergence of two positions	Diarrhoea, Diseases of the Circulatory System.
Diseases with a divergence of three positions	Pneumonia.
Diseases with a divergence of more than three positions	Other Diseases of the Respiratory System.

Admissions for Diseases for each year except in 1943 were lower than those for I.O.Rs. by 100 to nearly 200 per 1,000. In 1943 admissions of N.Cs.(E.) exceeded those of I.O.Rs. by only 9 per 1,000.

As with other classes of troops, MALARIA caused the greater number of admissions to hospitals. They followed the general pattern on this front with an increase in 1943, a fall in 1944 and a larger one in 1945. Comparison of rates with those for I.O.Rs. reveals only small differences except in 1942 when the rate for I.O.Rs. was one third higher than that for N.Cs.(E.). Relevant rates, with those of I.O.Rs. in brackets were: in 1942, 335 (447), in 1943, 469 (486), in 1944, 278 (319) and in 1945, 37 (68).

The trend of admissions for P.U.O. and N.Y.D. Fever followed that of B.O.Rs. and I.O.Rs. in that increases were experienced in 1943 and 1944 followed by a fall in the following year. The rates were 22 in 1942, 63 in 1943, 85 in 1944 and 20 in 1945. These were lower than those recorded for I.O.Rs. which were 30, 72, 115 and 28 respectively.

A somewhat different tendency was exhibited in the case of VENEREAL DISEASES. In 1942 and 1943 the rates among N.Cs.(E.) were higher than those recorded for I.O.Rs. by slightly over 20 per 1,000. In 1944, the rate was only 2 per 1,000 higher, but in 1945 admissions of I.O.Rs. exceeded those of N.Cs.(E.) by 14 per 1,000. The recorded rates were:

Indo-Burma Front. Admissions for Venereal Diseases among (i) V.C.Os. and I.O.Rs. and (ii) N.Cs.(E.), 1942–45.

	1942	1943	1944	1945
(i) V.C.Os. and I.O.Rs.	39·2	65·7	36·3	46·0
(ii) N.Cs.(E.)	62·4	86·8	38·1	31·5
Differences	+23·2	+21·1	+ 1·8	−14·5

Other Diseases of the RESPIRATORY SYSTEM also accounted for admissions at higher rates except in 1945. In 1943 and 1944 the rate was one third higher than I.O.Rs., but in 1945 admissions declined by over one-half to a rate which was two-thirds that of I.O.Rs. Rates for the two classes are as follows:

Indo-Burma Front. Admissions for Other Diseases of the Respiratory System among (i) V.C.Os. and I.O.Rs. and (ii) N.Cs.(E.), 1942–45.

	1942	1943	1944	1945
(i) V.C.Os. and I.O.Rs.	33·3	32·2	24·2	21·4
(ii) N.Cs.(E.)	36·9	42·1	32·1	14·8
Differences	+ 3·6	+ 9·9	+ 7·9	− 6·6

Admissions for DYSENTERY showed a downward trend during the four years, the 1945 rate being only one quarter of that for 1942.

Rates were 40 in 1942, 35 in 1943, 28 in 1944, and 10 in 1945. These, generally, were lower than those for I.O.Rs., the rates for whom were 53, 34, 40 and 19 respectively.

In 1943, the admission rate for SEPTIC CONDITIONS was the same (28 per 1,000) as that for I.O.Rs. In the succeeding three years, however, the difference in rates progressively increased in favour of N.Cs.(E.) until the difference in 1945 was 13 per 1,000. Recorded rates were:

Indo-Burma Front. Admissions for Septic Conditions among (i) *V.C.Os. and I.O.Rs. and* (ii) *N.Cs.(E.), 1942–45.*

	1942	1943	1944	1945
(i) V.C.Os. and I.O.Rs. . .	28·0	39·6	30·3	29·5
(ii) N.Cs.(E.) . . .	28·0	36·2	23·2	16·3
Differences	NIL	− 3·4	− 7·1	−13·2

The rates for Other Diseases of the DIGESTIVE SYSTEM were lower than those for I.O.Rs. in 1942, 1944 and 1945, but higher in 1943. They were 18 in 1942, 38 in 1943, 29 in 1944 and 12 in 1945 while I.O.Rs. rates were 22, 35, 37 and 23 respectively.

COMMON COLD caused admissions in 1942 and 1943 at rates equivalent to those for I.O.Rs. at 15 and 34 per 1,000 respectively. In 1944, the rate at 29 was 4 per 1,000 less and in 1945 the rate of 15 was 8·5 less than for I.O.Rs.

As in the case of Dysentery, admissions for DIARRHOEA were lower than those for I.O.Rs. at 18 per 1,000 in 1942 as compared with 28, 29 in 1943 (28), 21 in 1944 (40) and 9 in 1945 (18).

The rates of admissions on account of Diseases of the SKIN and for SCABIES among the two classes of troops are given below. Except for 1942 when the difference in rates was but slight, admissions were higher among I.O.Rs. In both cases the rates for N.Cs.(E.) in 1945 were half those of I.O.Rs. There was very little difference in the rates among I.O.Rs. for diseases of the Skin in the three years 1943–45, but admissions of N.Cs.(E.) in 1945 were slightly over one quarter the rate for 1943 whereas among I.O.Rs. it was just under one half.

Indo-Burma Front. Admissions for (a) *Diseases of the Skin (other than Scabies) and* (b) *Scabies among* (i) *V.C.Os. and I.O.Rs. and* (ii) *N.Cs.(E.), 1942–45.*

	1942	1943	1944	1945
(a) *Diseases of the Skin (other than Scabies)*				
V.C.Os. and I.O.Rs.	12·4	25·4	26·7	23·8
N.Cs.(E.)	13·5	20·9	17·6	11·7
(b) *Scabies*				
V.C.Os. and I.O.Rs.	15·9	27·6	23·4	12·6
N.Cs.(E.)	16·9	24·4	14·4	6·5

Diseases of the EAR, NOSE and THROAT were responsible for a slightly higher admission rate in 1942 as compared with I.O.Rs. In 1943 and 1944 the rates were approximately equal, but in 1945 the N.Cs.(E.) rate was less than one half that of I.O.Rs. The rates were 18 in 1942, 20 in 1943, 18 in 1944 and 6 in 1945 as compared with the I.O.Rs. rates of 15, 19, 18 and 14 respectively.

Similar trends were exhibited by both classes of troops with regard to Diseases of the EYE, in that an increase of admissions in 1943 was followed by a decline. Admissions of N.Cs.(E.) were less than I.O.Rs. by slightly over 1 per 1,000 in 1942 and 1943, followed by 4 in 1944 and 6 in 1945. Rates were 10, 18, 10 and 8 respectively.

Of the few diseases admissions for which increased over the years, INFECTIVE HEPATITIS was, perhaps, the most striking. Although not, numerically, very impressive, extensive increases were experienced by both N.Cs.(E.) and I.O.Rs. In the case of the former rates were 0·1 per 1,000 in 1942 and 1943. This was followed by a dramatic rise to 10·2 in 1944 and 7·9 in 1945. Rates for I.O.Rs. were 0·5, 2·1, 12·3 and 14·7 respectively.

The trend of admission of N.Cs.(E.) for MUMPS differed somewhat from that of I.O.Rs. Whereas with the latter a peak rate in 1942 was followed by two comparatively low rates, with a fifty per cent. increase in 1945, the peak year for N.Cs.(E.) occurred in 1943, followed by two successive falls. Relevant rates were:

Indo-Burma Front. Admissions for Mumps among
(i) *V.C.Os. and I.O.Rs. and* (ii) *N.Cs.(E.), 1942–45.*

	1942	1943	1944	1945
(i) V.C.Os. and I.O.Rs.	10·8	4·4	4·6	6·2
(ii) N.Cs.(E.)	7·4	10·4	7·3	6·6

Admission rates for MENTAL, PSYCHONEUROTIC and PERSONALITY Disorders were generally lower than those of I.O.Rs. but, like the latter, registered progressive increases. In both classes, the 1945 rate was approximately five times that for 1942. Rates are as follows:

Indo-Burma Front. Admissions for Mental, Psychoneurotic and Personality Disorders among (i) *V.C.Os. and I.O.Rs. and* (ii) *N.Cs.(E.), 1942–45.*

	1942	1943	1944	1945
(i) V.C.Os. and I.O.Rs.	1·5	2·9	4·6	7·3
(ii) N.Cs.(E.)	1·2	3·5	3·4	6·4

Diseases of the CIRCULATORY SYSTEM among N.Cs.(E.) showed satisfactory successive annual declines from 5·1 per 1,000 in 1942, to

4·5 in 1943, 3·3 in 1944 and, finally, 1·33 in 1945. Among I.O.Rs. rates were at 5 per 1,000 for the first three years and 3 in 1945.

N.Cs.(E.) suffered slightly more admissions on account of PNEUMONIA than did I.O.Rs. Rates for the former were 4·9 in 1942, 4·3 in 1944 and 4 in 1945. Those for I.O.Rs. were 3·5 in 1942, 2·3 in 1944 and 3·7 in 1945. The rates for 1943 are not available.

There was very little variation in the admission rates for TUBERCULOSIS, which ranged from 2·0 in 1942 to 1·1 in 1944. (The 1943 and 1945 rates were 1·7 and 1·2 respectively.) These rates were very similar to those recorded for I.O.Rs.

Diseases which caused admission rates of less than 1 per 1,000 strength were:

> Diphtheria, the Enteric Group of Fevers,
> Smallpox, Sandfly Fever, and those due to disorders of Nutrition.

In all these cases there was very little difference in rates among N.Cs.(E.) and I.O.Rs.

W.A.C.(I.) and I.M.N.S.

Table 127 relates to admissions to hospitals of members of the Women's Auxiliary Corps (India) and those of the Indian Military Nursing Service.

The number of females attached to units in this area was comparatively few, particularly so in 1942 and 1943. Caution must be exercised, therefore, when considering the rates and comparing them with those of male troops. Because of the very small strength in 1942 and 1943 it would be unwise to compare rates of those years with rates of the following years. In view of this, rates for the years 1944 and 1945 only are here discussed.

The table shows there were no admissions for DIPHTHERIA, SANDFLY FEVER, SCABIES, SMALLPOX or Diseases due to DISORDERS of NUTRITION in 1944 or 1945. In 1944 there were no admissions due to PNEUMONIA and, in 1945, none on account of DIARRHOEA, DENGUE FEVER, the ENTERIC Group of Fevers, MUMPS, TUBERCULOSIS, Diseases of the CIRCULATORY SYSTEM or to those of the EAR, NOSE and THROAT.

Diseases for which the admission rates were lower in 1945 than in the previous year were:

MALARIA	which fell from 135 to 28, a fall of 79 per cent.
Other Diseases of the DIGESTIVE System	which fell from 66 to 28, a fall of 58 per cent.
DYSENTERY	which fell from 49 to 38, a fall of 23 per cent.
Other Diseases of the RESPIRATORY System	which fell from 32 to 23, a fall of 28 per cent.
INFECTIVE HEPATITIS	which fell from 9 to 5, a fall of 44 per cent.

MENTAL PSYCHIATRIC and PERSONALITY DISORDERS which fell from 9 to 5, a fall of 44 per cent.
Diseases of the EYE which fell from 6 to 5, a fall of 17 per cent.
Diseases of the SKIN which fell from 6 to 5, a fall of 17 per cent.

The admission rate for DIARRHOEA in 1944 was 29 per 1,000. Surprisingly, there were no recorded admissions for this disease in 1945.

Admission rates of the diseases which follow increased in 1945:

PNEUMONIA from NIL to 9
P.U.O. and N.Y.D. Fever from 37 to 52, a rise of 40 per cent.
TONSILLITIS from 17 to 28, a rise of 65 per cent.
SEPTIC CONDITIONS from 17 to 42, a rise of 147 per cent.

Although some of these increases appear alarming, it must be remembered that, with such a small population, the admission of an additional few cases can increase the rate per 1,000 to a large extent. The reverse applies in considering the reductions noted above.

ALL INDIAN TROOPS

The rates of admission for all Indian Troops are presented in Table 128 which combines Tables 124 to 127.

The peak admission rate for diseases only occurred in 1943 at 1,072 per 1,000 Troops, followed by 1944 when admissions were 868, then by 1942 at 849. In 1945 there occurred a fifty per cent. reduction in admissions at 421 per 1,000.

Admissions for Injuries, however, showed successive annual rises from a rate of 41 in 1942 to an increase of slightly over one hundred per cent. at 84 in 1945. Intervening rates were 50 in 1943 and 78 in 1944.

Total admissions were 890 in 1942, 1,123 in 1943, 946 in 1944 and 505 in 1945.

The trend of admissions was similar to that experienced for all British Troops, but the rates of increase and decrease differ somewhat as indicated in the table below.

Indo-Burma Front. Admissions for All Diseases
Comparison between All British and All Indian Troops, 1942–45

Year	All British Troops			All Indian Troops		
	Rate per 1,000	Percentage increase or decrease over		Rate per 1,000	Percentage increase or decrease over	
		preceding year	1942		preceding year	1942
1942	990	—	—	849	—	—
1943	1,576	+59	+59	1,072	+26	+26
1944	1,218	−23	+23	868	−19	+ 2
1945	689	−43	−30	421	−51	−51

If, however, certain tropical diseases are eliminated—those diseases which characteristically show higher rates for Europeans—the comparison undergoes a complete change and the percentage increases and decreases are not so pronounced. Those eliminated are Malaria, P.U.O. and N.Y.D. Fever, Dysentery and Diarrhoea.

Indo-Burma Front. Admissions for Certain Diseases
Comparison between All British and All Indian Troops, 1942–45

Year	All British Troops			All Indian Troops		
	Rate per 1,000	Percentage increase or decrease over		Rate per 1,000	Percentage increase or decrease over	
		preceding year	1942		preceding year	1942
1942	501	—	—	329	—	—
1943	750	+49	+49	462	+40	+40
1944	525	−30	+5	374	−19	+14
1945	453	−14	−10	302	−19	−8

The above table shows that in 1943 (the peak year of admissions) the percentage increase for British over 1942 was 49 as against 40 for the Indians. This compares with increases of 59 and 26 per cent. as shown on the table for all diseases. It also shows that if 1942 is taken as the basic year, the 1945 rate for British Troops was ten per cent. less as against the Indian eight per cent. It indicates too, that the percentage decrease in 1944 as compared with the preceding year was half as much again among British Troops, but that in 1945 the percentage decrease among Indians, as compared with 1944, was half as much again as the British.

WEST AFRICAN OTHER RANKS

West African Units joined the Indo-Burma Front early in 1944. Because of this, and as data relating to their admissions to hospitals are available only to September 1945, Equivalent Annual Rates based on the known admissions during these years have been computed and are presented in Table 129. These Equivalent Annual Rates will allow of more valid comparisons. The West African Units were led by British Officers and many British Warrant Officers and N.C.Os. were attached to them. Admissions to hospitals of such personnel have been included in the tables relating to British Officers and British Other Ranks.

Admissions for diseases were less than any other class of combatant troops on this front, at 621 and 402 per 1,000 for the two years. This compares with 1,334 and 780 for British Other Ranks, with 912 and 466 for Indian Other Ranks and 741 and 424 for East African Other Ranks. The rates for N.Cs.(E.) were 743 and 279.

Injury rates, which were also lower than those recorded for other classes of active troops, were 50 and 74 per 1,000 respectively.

Total admission rates were 671 in 1944 and 476 in 1945.

Perhaps the most remarkable fact emerging from the table is the low incidence of MALARIA which in 1944 was 39, and, in 1945, 10 per 1,000 troops! Admissions for P.U.O. and N.Y.D. Fever, which may have included some undiagnosed Malaria cases, also compared very favourably with all other classes of Other Ranks. Relevant rates are as follows:

Indo-Burma Front. Admissions of Other Ranks for (i) Malaria and (ii) P.U.O. and N.Y.D. Fever. Comparison between W.A.O.Rs. and Other Classes of O.Rs., 1942–45

	W.A.O.Rs.		B.O.Rs.		I.O.Rs.		N.Cs.(E.)		E.A.O.Rs.	
	1944	1945	1944	1945	1944	1945	1944	1945	1944	1945
(i) *Crude Rates*										
Malaria	39	10	406	128	319	68	278	37	86	13
P.U.O. and N.Y.D. Fever	45	20	169	42	115	28	85	20	99	17
Totals	84	30	575	170	434	96	363	57	185	30
(ii) *Comparative Rates*										
Malaria	100	100	1,041	1,280	818	680	713	370	221	130
P.U.O. and N.Y.D. Fever	100	100	376	210	255	140	189	100	220	85
Totals	100	100	684	566	516	320	432	190	220	100

Admission rates for Malaria in respect of B.O.Rs. *vis à vis* W.A.O.Rs. were ten and thirteen times as high; for I.O.Rs., eight and seven times, N.Cs.(E.) seven and four times; and E.A.O.Rs. twice and one and a quarter times as high.

For P.U.O. and N.Y.D. Fever, the disparity between admission rates is much lower. Among B.O.Rs. they were four times and twice the W.A.O.R. rates; among I.O.Rs. two and a half and one and a half times; among N.Cs.(E.) twice the rate in 1944 and equal in 1945; while among E.A.O.Rs. the 1944 rate was over twice and, in 1945, less at seven-eighths the W.A.O.R. rate.

It is to be noted that the rates for P.U.O. and N.Y.D. Fever among W.A.O.Rs. and E.A.O.Rs. are higher than those for Malaria.

Another interesting feature of this table is the ratio between the rates in 1944 among E.A.O.Rs. For Malaria it was 221 to 100 and for P.U.O. and N.Y.D. Fever, practically identical at 220 to 100.

In contrast to Malaria, the rates for VENEREAL DISEASES were of a relatively high order, being 90 per 1,000 in 1944 and 69 in the following year. The 1944 admission rate was the highest recorded for this group of diseases in that year, and the second highest in the campaign (the highest rate recorded was by B.O.Rs. at 158 in 1943). The rate for 1945, 69 per 1,000, was lower than that for B.O.Rs. at 72, and for

E.A.O.Rs. at 83, but higher than for I.O.Rs. at 46 and N.Cs.(E.) at 32 per 1,000.

High in the admission rates was DYSENTERY at 52 per 1,000 in 1944, but this was more than halved to 22 in 1945. A similar decline was experienced with DIARRHOEA from 29 in 1944 to 13 in 1945.

Other Diseases for which admissions declined in 1945 were:

SEPTIC CONDITIONS	from 32 to 29 per 1,000
INFECTIVE HEPATITIS	from 21 to 6 per 1,000
Other Diseases of the RESPIRATORY System	from 31 to 26 per 1,000
Other Diseases of the DIGESTIVE System	from 23 to 11 per 1,000
SMALLPOX	from 3·2 to 1·2 per 1,000

Admissions for the following diseases registered increases in 1945:

PNEUMONIA	from 14 to 23 per 1,000
Diseases of the EYE	from 9 to 11 per 1,000
MENTAL PSYCHONEUROTIC and PERSONALITY DISORDERS	from 3·3 to 4·5 per 1,000
MUMPS	from 1·4 to 2·5 per 1,000

Diseases for which similar rates were experienced in both years were:

Diseases of the SKIN	16·0 and 16·7 per 1,000
COMMON COLD	6·8 and 6·7 per 1,000
Diseases of the CIRCULATORY System	2·6 and 2·4 per 1,000
TONSILLITIS	1·9 and 1·9 per 1,000
TUBERCULOSIS	0·52 and 0·65 per 1,000

EAST AFRICAN OTHER RANKS

East African Units were first drafted to the Indo-Burma Front in May 1944. Admissions for that year have been adjusted to Equivalent Annual Rates (Table 130). A similar adjustment has been made in 1945 for which year data are available only to September. As with W.A.O.Rs. admissions of British ranks attached to East African Units have been included in the relevant British tables.

Admissions for diseases only were of the order of 741 per 1,000 in 1944 and 424 in 1945. These rates exceeded those for W.A.O.Rs. but were less than for B.O.Rs. and I.O.Rs. The 1944 rate was almost identical with that for N.Cs.(E.), but in 1945 admissions of E.A.O.Rs. were fifty per cent. higher.

Injuries recorded rates of 85 and 74 per 1,000, while total admissions were 827 and 498 respectively.

A notable feature of admissions was the high rate for DYSENTERY at 146 per 1,000 in 1944. This was the highest recorded rate on this Front and, among male troops, compares with 132 per 1,000 for

B.O.Rs. in 1943, the second highest rate. It was nearly three times the rate for All Troops in 1944. In 1945 it declined to 51, which was almost identical with the All Troops rate.

MALARIA accounted for admissions at rates of 86 in 1944 and 13 in 1945 which exceeded those for W.A.O.Rs. but were less than the rates for the other classes.

Admissions for P.U.O. and N.Y.D. Fever were higher than those for Malaria at 99 in 1944 and 17 in 1945. In both cases the decline was over eighty per cent.

The rate for VENEREAL DISEASES increased by over fifty per cent., from 52 in 1944 to 83 in 1945. The latter rate was the highest recorded for this group of diseases on the front in 1945.

Other diseases, admissions for which registered higher rates in 1945 were:

Diseases of the SKIN	from 17	to 25	per 1,000
MENTAL, PSYCHONEUROTIC and PERSONALITY DISORDERS	from 6	to 9	per 1,000
INFECTIVE HEPATITIS	from 5	to 6	per 1,000
TUBERCULOSIS	from 0·29	to 1·03	per 1,000

Other diseases for which admissions declined were:

SEPTIC CONDITIONS	from 48	to 26	per 1,000
DIARRHOEA	from 38	to 10	per 1,000
Other Diseases of the RESPIRATORY SYSTEM	from 30	to 16	per 1,000
COMMON COLD	from 23	to 5	per 1,000
PNEUMONIA	from 13	to 8	per 1,000
Diseases of the EYE	from 11	to 8	per 1,000
Diseases of the EAR, NOSE and THROAT	from 10	to 7	per 1,000

There were little differences in the admission rates of Mumps, Smallpox, Tonsillitis, Diseases of the Circulatory System and Other Diseases of the Digestive System.

ALL TROOPS

Rates of admissions to hospitals for all troops on the Indo-Burma Front for the years 1942 to 1945 are given in Table 131. Admissions during 1945 are known for the first nine months only, and Equivalent Annual Rates have been computed from this data.

Admissions for diseases, in general, followed the trend indicated by the numerically larger classes of troops, and showed an increase in 1943, followed by declines in both the subsequent years. That the rates are similar to those for V.C.Os. and I.O.Rs., particularly in 1942 and 1945, is shown in the table below:

Indo-Burma Front. Admissions for All Diseases of (i) All Troops and (ii) V.C.Os. and I.O.Rs., 1942–45. Crude and Comparative Rates

	1942	1943	1944	1945
(i) *Crude Rates*				
All Troops	885	1,151	993	462
V.C.Os. and I.O.Rs.	877	1,073	911	466
(ii) *Comparative Rates All Troops = 100*				
All Troops	100	100	100	100
V.C.Os. and I.O.Rs.	99	93	92	101
(iii) *Comparative Rates 1942 = 100*				
All Troops	100	130	112	52
V.C.Os. and I.O.Rs.	100	122	104	53
(iv) *Comparative Rates preceding year base*				
All Troops	—	130	86	47
V.C.Os. and I.O.Rs.	—	122	85	51

In 1942 and 1945 there was a difference of only one per cent. between the rates for All Troops and I.O.Rs.; in 1943 it was seven and in 1944 eight per cent. less. Compared with the 1942 rates, in 1943 and 1944 the I.O.Rs. rates were eight per cent. less and in 1945 one per cent. more. When rates are compared with those of the year immediately preceding, admissions of All Troops in 1943 were 130 per cent. of those in 1942, in 1944 they were 86 per cent. and in 1945, 47 per cent. of the previous year's rates. Rates for I.O.Rs. are very similar at 122, 85 and 51 per cent.

Injuries accounted for admissions at rates of 42 per 1,000 in 1942, 54 in 1943, 95 in 1944 and 89 in 1945. Here again, rates correspond closely with those of I.O.Rs. (except in 1945), for whom the rates were 43, 56, 93 and 102 respectively.

The rates of admissions for disease and injuries ranged from 551 in 1945 to 926 in 1942, 1,088 in 1944 to a peak of 1,205 in 1943. That 1943 was the peak year of admissions was to a large extent due to a great increase in the number of Malaria cases, and the rate of 491 per 1,000 must have contained a considerable number of re-admissions due to relapse. As figures of such relapse cases are not available, it is not possible to judge their impact on admissions.

MALARIA with P.U.O. and N.Y.D. Fever were responsible for approximately one-half the admissions for disease during the first three years under review. In 1945, the combined rates were only one fifth of the total. The effect of these diseases on the total disease rates is shown below.

The range of all diseases was 689 (1,151 less 462), but when Malaria and P.U.O. and N.Y.D. Fever were eliminated it was only 218 (590 less 372). Between 1942 and 1944, Other Diseases rates were just over

Indo-Burma Front. Comparison of Admission Rates
All Diseases with Malaria and P.U.O. and N.Y.D. Fever
All Troops, 1942–45.

	1942		1943		1944		1945	
All Diseases . . .		885		1,151		993		462
Malaria	395		491		329		63	
P.U.O. and N.Y.D. Fever	30	425	70	561	120	449	27	90
Other Diseases .		460		590		544		372
Other Diseases as percentages of All Diseases . . .		52		51		55		81

one half of those for All Diseases, but, in 1945, when Malaria and P.U.O. and N.Y.D. Fever admissions had been reduced considerably, the rate was four-fifths that for All Diseases.

The rates for VENEREAL DISEASES remained remarkably steady, except for 1943 when it rose from 50 to 81 per 1,000. For 1944 and 1945 they were 47 and 48. Although it may have been anticipated that the rate would increase in 1945 after the collapse of the Japanese resistance, that this did not occur was probably due in no small way to the crusading efforts of unit medical officers and the establishment of prophylactic centres as well as to the high morale of the troops and the provision of increased amenities.

Admissions for DIARRHOEA and DYSENTERY were considerably less in 1945 than in 1942, the former declining by forty and the latter by sixty per cent. In the case of Diarrhoea, admissions rose in 1943 and again in 1944 from 29 to 35, followed by 46, but declined in 1945 to 18. Admissions on account of Dysentery fell in 1943 from 59 to 48, increased in 1944 to 54 and declined to 25 in the following year. The decrease in 1945 was probably attributable to the acclimatisation of considerable numbers of unseasoned troops arriving in the area, particularly in 1943 and 1944.

INFECTIVE HEPATITIS accounted for a steady increase in the rate of admissions in 1943 and 1944 from 2 per 1,000 to 6 in 1943 and 17 in 1944. The rate for 1945 was slightly less at 15. Information regarding the causes of this increase is lacking, but it is possible that in these figures are included some admissions for Post-arsphenamine Jaundice.

Admissions for MENTAL, PSYCHONEUROTIC and PERSONALITY Disorders also showed a steady increase throughout the period, commencing with 2 in 1942 and followed by 4 in 1943, 6 in 1944 and 9 in 1945. The cause of this increase was, no doubt, the cumulative effect of the stress and strain of war and to more accurate diagnoses, following an increase in the number of psychiatrists available in the Command.

Diseases of the SKIN accounted for admissions at rates of 20 in 1942, 27 in the two subsequent years, and 25 in 1945. Admissions for SCABIES, which are omitted from the foregoing figures, commenced at 14 per 1,000 in 1942, rose to 25 in the following year, and then fell to 20 in 1944 and to 9 in 1945.

Admissions for COMMON COLD fluctuated between 14 and 32 per 1,000, Diseases of the EAR, NOSE and THROAT between 13 and 21, and Diseases of the EYE between 9 and 18 per 1,000. In each case, the higher rate was recorded in 1943.

TONSILLITIS was responsible for admissions at rates which were remarkably constant during the four years at 6, 6, 5 and 5 per 1,000 respectively.

Admissions for SANDFLY FEVER were low at rates which varied from 0·5 per 1,000 in 1945 to 0·8 in 1942 and 1943. In India, the rates for this disease among B.O.Rs. varied between 5·3 and 38·1 per 1,000, and, among I.O.Rs. between 0·7 and 16 per 1,000. The reason for this large difference in rates between the two areas is that this disease is usually mainly associated with the North-West Area of India. Admissions to hospitals in Bengal for Sandfly Fever were usually only a fraction of those in the Punjab and North-West Frontier.

In 1942, admissions for DENGUE FEVER were 11 per 1,000. They declined in 1943 when the rate was 4. This was followed by a further decrease to 1 per 1,000 in both 1944 and 1945.

The appointment of an A.D.M.S. (Nutrition), and the co-operation of civilian nutrition experts, were probably responsible for the decline in admissions from diseases due to Disorders of NUTRITION. The rates recorded were 0·10 per 1,000 in 1942, 0·36 in 1943, 0·03 in 1944 and 0·07 in 1945. To these rates must be linked the fact that recruits to the Indian Army in particular were of a much lower standard in the latter years of the war, and it is not unreasonable to suggest that had not rigorous steps been taken to build up recruits and to combat the diseases, many more admissions would have occurred in 1944 and 1945.

Admissions for SEPTIC CONDITIONS and Other Diseases of the DIGESTIVE and RESPIRATORY Systems followed the general trend of a rise in 1943, with successive falls in the two subsequent years. Rates varied in the case of Septic Conditions from 35 in 1943 to 20 in 1945, in Other Digestive Diseases from 43 in 1943 to 21 in 1945 and in Other Respiratory Diseases from 42 in 1943 to 30 in 1945.

The rates for MUMPS declined from 7 per 1,000 in 1942 to 5 in 1944 and 1945 while those for DIPHTHERIA remained fairly constant ranging from 0·16 in 1944 to 0·29 in 1943.

Admissions for the ENTERIC Group of Fevers showed a gratifying constant decline during the period from 0·95 in 1942 to 0·27 in 1945.

Conclusions

The most gratifying feature of the tables presented in this chapter undoubtedly is the dramatic reduction in the incidence of Malaria. That a similar reduction was experienced in other tropical and subtropical countries does not detract from the remarkable achievement of the medical authorities in reducing admissions from nearly 500 to 63 per 1,000 troops in three years, in a country which contains what is probably one of the worst malarious areas in the world.

Satisfactory results in the campaign against Diarrhoea and Dysentery are indicated in the decrease in admission rates of these diseases.

Against these achievements are recorded increases in the admission rates of Infective Hepatitis from 2 per 1,000 in 1942 to 15 in 1945, and of Mental, Psychoneurotic and Personality Disorders, admission rates of which rose from 1·8 per 1,000 in 1942 to 9·2 in 1945.

INJURIES

Table 132 shows the admission rates on account of Injuries. As with diseases, figures are given separately for all classes of troops in the area and have been broken up into those caused through Enemy Action (E.A.) and those designated Non-Enemy Action (N.E.A.). In the theatre, the criterion for deciding on the attributability of an injury to Enemy Action appears to have been whether it was caused by blast, bombs, gunshot or shell. If the cause was other than this, the injury was classified as N.E.A. The latter was not split into categories up to and including 1943 and even in the two years which followed N.E.A. injuries were broken down only to 'Burns and Scalds' and 'Other'. 'Other' injuries, naturally more numerous than Burns and Scalds, contain interesting data relating to traffic accidents, training injuries, etc., as well as to those which, on other fronts, would be considered as caused by E.A.

Total admissions for injuries ranged from 42 per 1,000 in 1942 to 95 in 1944. The rates for 1943 and 1945 were 54 and 89. In 1942 and 1943 they accounted for slightly under five per cent. of All Admissions, but, in the two years which followed, rose to nine and sixteen per cent. Although an increase in the number of admissions for injuries accounted to a great extent for the percentage increase in 1944, that for the following year was wholly due to the unprecedented decrease in admissions for disease.

N.E.A. Injuries

These were the more numerous, being from fifty to eighty-five per cent. of all injuries. The rates were 36 in 1942, 45 in 1943, 48 in 1944 and 50 in 1945. A condensed table relating to these injuries is given below for comparison purposes.

Indo-Burma Front. Admissions to Hospitals, N.E.A. Injuries
All classes of Male Troops, 1942–45.
Rates per 1,000 Strength

	1942	1943	1944	1945
British Officers	30	33	31	31
British Other Ranks . . .	33	64	55	61
V.C.Os. and I.O.Rs. . .	38	46	48	57
N.Cs.(E.) . . .	33	37	30	26
W.A.O.Rs.			34	36
E.A.O.Rs.			40	53

B.O.Rs. suffered more injuries than any other class of troops. Apart from 1942 when the rate was comparatively low at 33 per 1,000, admissions ranged from 55 to 64. V.C.Os. and I.O.Rs. next in order of admissions produced rates which increased each year from 38 in 1942 to 57 in 1945. The rates of British Officers were fairly constant throughout the years at from 30 to 33 per 1,000. Those for N.Cs.(E.) were 33 in 1942, 37 in 1943, 30 in 1944 and 26 in 1945. The highest rate for N.Cs.(E.) was slightly lower than the lowest for V.C.Os. and I.O.Rs.

W.A.O.Rs. and E.A.O.Rs. who were in the area during 1944 and 1945 only, produced rates which were less than those of B.O.Rs. or V.C.Os. and I.O.Rs.

It is to be noted that, of the troops who were in the area for the four years, the highest rates of admissions were in 1943, except for V.C.Os. and I.O.Rs. among whom the highest rate occurred in 1945.

E.A. Injuries

These were lowest in 1942 and 1943 at 6 and 8 per 1,000 respectively. Admissions rose to 47 in 1944 and fell to 39 in the following year. 1944 also produced the highest rate of N.E.A. Injuries at only 1 per 1,000 more than E.A. Injuries. The table which follows condenses the information shown in Table 136 as to E.A. Injuries by classes of personnel.

Indo-Burma Front. Admissions to Hospitals, E.A. Injuries
All Classes of Male Troops, 1942–45.
Rates per 1,000 Strength

	1942	1943	1944	1945
British Officers	5	15	56	42
British Other Ranks . . .	5	14	102	73
V.C.Os. and I.O.Rs. . .	6	10	45	44
N.Cs.(E.) . . .	1	1	5	2
W.A.O.Rs.			16	38
E.A.O.Rs.			45	21

As with N.E.A. Injuries, B.O.Rs. suffered higher rates of E.A. Injuries than any other class of troops. Rates for them rose from 5 in 1942 to 14 in 1943, to a peak of 102 in 1944 and then declined to 73 in the following year. Rates for V.C.Os. and I.O.Rs. were much less, ranging from 6 in 1942 to 10 in 1943, to 45 in 1944 and finally to 44 in 1945.

British Officers recorded rates which in general were slightly higher than those for V.C.Os. and I.O.Rs.; commencing at 5 in 1942 they rose to 15 in 1943, followed by 56 in 1944 and 42 in 1945.

As might have been expected, rates for N.Cs.(E.) were very low at 1 per 1,000 in both 1942 and 1943, 5 in 1944 and 2 in 1945.

The peak rates of injuries occurred in 1944, except for W.A.O.Rs. whose rate of 38 in 1945 was slightly more than twice the 1944 rate. E.A.O.Rs. rates were 45 in 1944 and 21 in 1945.

Gunshot wounds were predominant in each year. They ranged from fifty to sixty-five per cent. of the total E.A. wounds. During the two years when fighting was at its heaviest, however, in 1944 and 1945, gunshot wounds recorded lower percentages of injuries than in the two previous years. In 1944 and 1945 injuries due to bombs and shells were almost identical and between them accounted for nearly half the injuries.

Conclusions

B.O.Rs. sustained higher rates of injuries, both N.E.A. and E.A., than any other class of troops. In general, E.A. Injuries were far less numerous than N.E.A., although, in 1944 and 1945, E.A. Injuries increased considerably. The greatest number of N.E.A. Injuries occurred in 1945 while E.A. Injuries were more frequent in 1944.

The largest contribution to E.A. Injuries was Gunshot wounds, with Bomb and Shell wounds together almost equalling Gunshot wounds in the last two years of the campaign.

DEATHS

Data regarding deaths in hospitals are very meagre. All that can be ascertained are the rates of deaths by the various categories of troops in each year divided, from 1943, into those caused by diseases and N.E.A. Injuries, and those caused by E.A. Injuries. The rates relating to these deaths are given in Table 133.

It must be emphasised that the statistics in this table relate to deaths in hospitals only, and do not include those which occurred in other medical establishments, or on the field of battle.

Deaths were more numerous in 1944, during which year also occurred the highest rates of admissions on account of injuries. During 1944 and 1945 when fighting was at its highest, there were, in general, more deaths in hospital on account of Disease and N.E.A. Injuries than there were from E.A. Injuries. The only exception to this was in the case of British Officers who recorded rates of 3·3 in 1944 and 2·9 in 1945 from E.A. Injuries as against 3·2 and 1·6 from other causes.

Rates for B.O.Rs. were higher than for any other class, both from E.A. Injuries and from other causes. Deaths from the latter were one and a half times those of the former.

The second highest rates of deaths from Enemy Action was recorded by British Officers. The rate for other causes was approximately fifty per cent. higher on the average during the four years.

Among V.C.Os. and I.O.Rs. the death rate for other causes was nearly three times that for E.A. Injuries.

The rates for N.Cs.(E.) were approximately 0·2 per 1,000 for E.A. Injuries and 3·4 for others. The low rate for the former was to be expected when the low rates of admissions to hospitals for this class are considered.

W.A.O.Rs. recorded death rates of 0·4 in 1944 and 1·2 in 1945 from E.A. Injuries and 3·8 and 3·5 for all other causes. Rates for E.A.O.Rs. were slightly higher at 0·8 and 1·5 for E.A. Injuries and 5·0 and 3·2 for all other causes.

MEDICAL ETHNOGRAPHY ON THE INDO-BURMA FRONT

In relating the ethnic variations of disease on the Indo-Burma Front, the fact that two of the four classes of troops engaged in this area were there for only two years must be taken into account. This is all the more important since rates, in general, were far less in the two final years, and particularly in 1945, owing, chiefly, to the remarkable decrease in admissions for Malaria.

From the data available, and in order to make more valid comparisons this study is divided into two parts:

(i) A comparison between B.O.Rs. and V.C.Os. and I.O.Rs. and

(ii) A comparison between B.O.Rs., V.C.Os. and I.O.Rs., W.A.O.Rs. and E.A.O.Rs.

The first is based on known admissions for the four years 1942 to 1945 and the second on similar information for the two years 1944 and 1945.

To enable comparisons to be made, average rates of admissions have been computed for:

(i) Four years in respect of B.O.Rs. and V.C.Os., and I.O.Rs. and

(ii) Two years in respect of B.O.Rs., V.C.Os. and I.O.Rs., W.A.O.Rs. and E.A.O.Rs.

and comparative tables prepared based on B.O.Rs. who are shown at 100 for each disease. Because of the differing annual rates and more especially as those for 1944 and 1945 were substantially lower than for the previous years, the average rates shown against V.C.Os. and I.O.Rs. for the years 1942 to 1945 will differ somewhat from those for the years 1944 and 1945. These statistics are presented as Tables 134 and 135.

B.O.RS. AND V.C.OS. AND I.O.RS.

Table 134 shows the comparative rates of admissions on account of diseases only for B.O.Rs. and V.C.Os. and I.O.Rs. As the total disease rate among the latter was some seven-tenths that of B.O.Rs., it is not surprising that with only a few diseases were the Indian rates higher.

Of these diseases, MUMPS recorded a much higher incidence, being slightly under twenty times the British rate. PNEUMONIA was three times, TUBERCULOSIS twice and COMMON COLD and Diseases of the EYE both one and a half times the rate for B.O.Rs. These higher incidences were not unexpected having regard to the experiences of these classes of troops in India and elsewhere.

The Indian rate for SCABIES was nearly twice that of B.O.Rs. This is in accord with war-time experience in India and Ceylon but is at variance with that in B.N.A.F. and C.M.F., where the British rate was approximately twice that of the Indians, or in the Middle East, where the rates were roughly equivalent.

At the other end of the scale, admissions of B.O.Rs. for DENGUE FEVER were sixteen times the Indian rate and, for DIPHTHERIA, eight times. The British rates for SANDFLY FEVER, the ENTERIC Group of Fevers and for INFECTIVE HEPATITIS were six, four and three times, respectively, the Indian rate. Admissions for DIARRHOEA and DYSENTERY among B.O.Rs., as might be expected, were from two to three times those of the Indians. Those for MENTAL, PSYCHONEUROTIC and PERSONALITY Disorders were also approximately three times greater.

Diseases which, among Indians, recorded approximately fifty per cent. of the B.O.R's. rates were VENEREAL DISEASES, Other Diseases of the DIGESTIVE System, Diseases of the SKIN, and Other Diseases of the RESPIRATORY System.

Admission rates for SMALLPOX among the Indians were three-fifths of the British rates, as were Diseases of the EAR, NOSE and THROAT.

Rates of admissions on account of SEPTIC Conditions for both classes were practically identical.

MALARIA accounted for Indian admission rates at approximately nine-tenths those of the British, while those for P.U.O. and N.Y.D.

Fever were three-quarters. Comparison of annual rates, as under, leads to some interesting conclusions.

Indo-Burma Front. Admissions of B.O.Rs. and V.C.Os., and I.O.Rs. for (i) Malaria and (ii) P.U.O. and N.Y.D. Fever. Crude and Comparative Rates, 1942–45

	1942	1943	1944	1945
(i) MALARIA				
(a) *Crude Rates*				
B.O.Rs.	335	628	406	128
V.C.Os. and I.O.Rs.	447	486	319	68
(b) *Comparative Rates (B.O.Rs. = 100)*				
B.O.Rs.	100	100	100	100
V.C.Os. and I.O.Rs.	133	77	78	53
(c) *Comparative Rates (1942 = 100)*				
B.O.Rs.	100	185	121	38
V.C.Os. and I.O.Rs.	100	109	71	15
(d) *Comparative Rates (Preceding year = 100)*				
B.O.Rs.		185	65	29
V.C.Os. and I.O.Rs.		109	66	21
(ii) P.U.O. AND N.Y.D. FEVER				
(a) *Crude Rates*				
B.O.Rs.	36	82	169	42
V.C.Os. and I.O.Rs.	30	72	115	28
(b) *Comparative Rates (B.O.Rs. = 100)*				
B.O.Rs.	100	100	100	100
V.C.Os. and I.O.Rs.	83	88	68	69
(c) *Comparative Rates (1942 = 100)*				
B.O.Rs.	100	228	469	117
V.C.Os. and I.O.Rs.	100	240	383	93
(d) *Comparative Rates (Preceding year = 100)*				
B.O.Rs.		228	206	25
V.C.Os. and I.O.Rs.		240	160	24

In 1942 the Malaria rate for Indians was one-third higher than the British rate. During the two following years it was slightly over three-quarters and in 1945 was one-half the rate for B.O.Rs. Compared with 1942, the Indian rate, in 1945, had fallen by eighty-five per cent., while the British rate fell by only sixty per cent. When the rates are compared with those of the preceding year, the fall in the British rate in 1944 was almost seventy per cent. and that of the Indians nearly eighty per cent.

For P.U.O. and N.Y.D. Fever, admission rates of the Indians were lower than those of the British by from ten to thirty per cent. In 1942 and 1943 the Indian rates were eighty-three and eighty-eight per cent. of the British rates and in 1944 and 1945 they were sixty-eight and sixty-nine per cent. Compared with the previous year, the percentages varied little in 1943, while they were almost identical in 1945. In 1944 the British rate was twice and the Indian one and a half times those of 1943. The 1945 rates in each case were one quarter the 1944 rates.

Summary

Morbidity rates on the Indo-Burma Front for B.O.Rs. as compared with V.C.Os. and I.O.Rs. may be summarised as below:

Diseases with comparatively High rates (in descending order)	Diseases with comparatively Low rates (in descending order)	Diseases with little difference in rates
Dengue Fever		
Diphtheria		
Sandfly Fever		
Enteric Group of Fevers		
Infective Hepatitis		
Mental, Psychoneurotic and Personality Disorders	Mumps	Septic Conditions
Dysentery	Pneumonia	Malaria
Diarrhoea	Tuberculosis	Disorders of Nutrition
Diseases of the Skin	Common Cold	P.U.O. and N.Y.D. Fever
Other Diseases of the Digestive System	Diseases of the Eye	Diseases of the Circulatory System
Venereal Diseases		
Other Diseases of the Respiratory System		
Diseases of the Ear, Nose and Throat		
Smallpox		

OTHER RANKS, ALL GROUPS

Table 135 shows the comparative rates of admissions on account of diseases only for B.O.Rs., V.C.Os. and I.O.Rs., W.A.O.Rs., and E.A.O.Rs. As noted above, average rates for two years only have been used in this table, because W.A.O.Rs. and E.A.O.Rs. were in this area for two years only, and because a valid comparison can be made, in this instance, only with data of the same two years relating to the other groups.

The rates of total admissions for Diseases indicates that for every 100 B.O.Rs. admitted to hospital, there were also admitted 65 V.C.Os. and I.O.Rs., 55 E.A.O.Rs., and 48 W.A.O.Rs.

Perhaps the most striking feature of this table is that there were three causes for which the rates of all other groups were higher than those for B.O.Rs. These were PNEUMONIA, MUMPS and TUBERCULOSIS.

Other outstanding features of this table are:

(i) Indian and West African Troops were more prone to SEPTIC Conditions.

(ii) Indian Troops were more liable to SCABIES, COMMON COLD and Diseases of the EYE.

(iii) West Africans were more susceptible to SANDFLY FEVER.

(iv) British and Indian Troops were more liable to contract MALARIA than were Africans.

(v) British Troops were more prone to P.U.O. and N.Y.D. Fever and Other Diseases of the DIGESTIVE System.

(vi) British Troops were more liable to be admitted to hospital with DIARRHOEA, DENGUE FEVER, INFECTIVE HEPATITIS, the ENTERIC Group of Fevers, Diseases of the EAR, NOSE and THROAT, Diseases of the SKIN, and MENTAL, PSYCHONEUROTIC and PERSONALITY Disorders.

(vii) W.A.O.Rs. were more prone to contract VENEREAL DISEASES than B.O.Rs. and E.A.O.Rs. who were twice as likely to contract them than Indians.

(viii) British and East Africans were more liable to DYSENTERY than were Indians or West Africans.

These indications are tabulated below.

DISEASE	Ethnic group	
	Prone	Less Prone
Malaria	British, Indians	Africans
P.U.O. and N.Y.D. Fever	British	West Africans
Sandfly Fever	West Africans	
Dengue Fever	British	Indians, Africans
Enteric Group of Fevers	British	Indians
Common Cold	Indians	Africans
Mumps	Indians, Africans	British
Pneumonia	Indians, Africans	British
Tuberculosis	Indians, Africans	British
Infective Hepatitis	British	Indians, Africans
Scabies	Indians	Africans
Skin Diseases	British	Indians, Africans
Septic Conditions	Indians, West Africans	British, East Africans
Eye Diseases	Indians	
Venereal Diseases	West Africans, British	Indians
Diarrhoea	British	Indians, Africans
Dysentery	British, East Africans	Indians, West Africans
Other Diseases of the Digestive System	British	Africans
Ear, Nose and Throat Diseases	British	Africans
Mental, Psychoneurotic and Personality Disorders	British	Indians, Africans

TABLE 120

South-East Asia Command (Indo-Burma Front)
Causes of Admissions to Hospitals, 1942–45. British Officers
Annual Rates per 1,000 Strength

Source: A.F. A.31-B

	CAUSES	1942	1943	1944	E.A.R. 1945	
1	Common Cold	5·38	7·49	7·21	5·49	1
2	Diarrhoea	29·03	36·31	42·22	20·16	2
3	Dysentery	82·15	72·97	56·58	37·61	3
4	Dengue Fever	25·59	20·25	4·23	3·97	4
5	Diphtheria	0·21	1·25	0·75	0·83	5
6	Enteric Group of Fevers	2·80	1·69	0·31	0·68	6
7	Infective Hepatitis	10·32	25·34	25·25	23·01	7
8	Malaria	261·72	220·71	123·50	30·25	8
9	Mumps	0·21	0·71	—	0·45	9
10	Pneumonia	0·64	*	0·75	1·28	10
11	P.U.O. and N.Y.D. Fever	20·86	30·96	50·37	20·24	11
12	Sandfly Fever	3·23	0·89	0·50	0·31	12
13	Scabies	0·43	1·69	2·92	2·33	13
14	Smallpox	0·86	0·54	0·37	0·68	14
15	Tonsillitis	10·75	12·58	7·34	7·15	15
16	Tuberculosis	1·07	0·89	0·12	0·91	16
17	Venereal Diseases	7·74	13·47	4·36	8·05	17
18	Diseases of the Circulatory System	6·67	5·71	1·93	3·08	18
19	Diseases due to Disorders of Nutrition	—	—	—	0·08	19
20	Diseases of the Ear, Nose and Throat	10·97	16·95	14·68	12·19	20
21	Diseases of the Eye	6·45	2·85	2·55	5·35	21
22	Diseases of the Skin (other than Scabies)	14·62	16·50	14·49	23·17	22
23	Other Diseases of the Digestive System	52·69	47·55	30·22	16·55	23
24	Septic Conditions	34·84	35·14	19·84	22·95	24
25	Other Diseases of the Respiratory System	13·76	17·84	10·69	8·81	25
26	Mental, Psychoneurotic and Personality Disorders	4·95	6·87	5·41	12·64	26
27	All Other Diseases	105·61	128·78	94·71	75·34	27
28	*Total Admissions for Diseases*	713·55	725·93	521·30	343·56	28
29	Injuries—N.E.A.	30·11	32·56	31·15	31·37	29
30	Injuries—E.A.	4·73	15·34	55·72	41·61	30
31	*Total Admissions for Injuries*	34·84	47·90	86·87	72·98	31
32	*Total Admissions*	748·39	773·84	608·17	416·54	32

* Any cases included in "All Other Diseases'.

Note: 1945 rates are equivalent, being based on the known admissions or the first nine months of the year.

TABLE 121

South-East Asia Command (Indo-Burma Front)
Causes of Admissions to Hospitals, 1942–45. British Other Ranks
Annual Rates per 1,000 Strength

Source: A.F. A.31-B

	CAUSES	1942	1943	1944	E.A.R. 1945	
1	Common Cold	11·7	21·3	18·50	16·61	1
2	Diarrhoea	41·7	77·0	91·21	34·83	2
3	Dysentery	87·8	132·0	97·44	64·83	3
4	Dengue Fever	38·2	24·6	4·43	1·81	4
5	Diphtheria	0·8	1·2	0·65	0·69	5
6	Enteric Group of Fevers	1·9	1·4	0·85	0·41	6
7	Infective Hepatitis	5·0	27·0	31·48	31·27	7
8	Malaria	334·7	628·2	405·58	128·35	8
9	Mumps	0·1	0·5	0·24	0·49	9
10	Pneumonia	1·2	*	0·85	0·93	10
11	P.U.O. and N.Y.D. Fever	36·3	82·3	169·34	42·27	11
12	Sandfly Fever	2·8	3·7	0·70	0·39	12
13	Scabies	7·9	16·8	13·38	5·43	13
14	Smallpox	0·4	0·8	0·48	1·01	14
15	Tonsillitis	*	*	*	*	15
16	Tuberculosis	1·0	0·9	0·42	0·64	16
17	Venereal Diseases	72·2	157·9	69·23	72·19	17
18	Diseases of the Circulatory System	5·4	9·0	5·84	5·60	18
19	Diseases due to Disorders of Nutrition	0·0	0·8	0·09	0·68	19
20	Diseases of the Ear, Nose and Throat	19·4	36·4	26·66	26·20	20
21	Diseases of the Eye	4·6	13·1	10·05	13·04	21
22	Diseases of the Skin (other than Scabies)	42·1	50·0	36·13	51·19	22
23	Other Diseases of the Digestive System	61·0	87·1	52·69	34·60	23
24	Septic Conditions	25·2	35·5	21·92	20·68	24
25	Other Diseases of the Respiratory System	53·6	69·0	50·10	58·66	25
26	Mental, Psychoneurotic and Personality Disorders	2·5	6·1	10·88	23·24	26
27	All Other Diseases	163·1	263·3	214·67	143·57	27
28	*Total Admissions for Diseases*	1,020·6	1,745·9	1,333·81	779·61	28
29	Injuries—N.E.A.	33·2	64·4	54·81	60·77	29
30	Injuries—E.A.	4·5	13·9	101·91	73·25	30
31	*Total Admissions for Injuries*	37·7	78·3	156·72	134·03	31
32	*Total Admissions*	1,058·4	1,824·3	1,490·53	913·65	32

* Any cases included in 'All Other Diseases'.

Note: 1945 rates are equivalent, being based on the know admissions for the first nine months of the year.

TABLE 122

South-East Asia Command (Indo-Burma Front)
Causes of Admissions to Hospitals, 1942–45. Q.A.I.M.N.S.
Annual Rates per 1,000 Strength

Source: A.F. A.31-B

	CAUSES	1942	1943	1944	E.A.R. 1945	
1	Common Cold	5·0	6·3	13·1	12·35	1
2	Diarrhoea	*	59·4	58·8	14·40	2
3	Dysentery	65·0	96·9	141·6	45·27	3
4	Dengue Fever	10·0	25·0	30·5	8·23	4
5	Diphtheria	10·0	*	4·4	2·05	5
6	Enteric Group of Fevers	5·0	—	—	—	6
7	Infective Hepatitis	5·0	—	30·7	14·40	7
8	Malaria	70·0	87·0	228·7	22·63	8
9	Mumps	—	—	—	4·12	9
10	Pneumonia	*	*	*	*	10
11	P.U.O. and N.Y.D. Fevers	*	*	37·1	14·40	11
12	Sandfly Fever	—	—	—	—	12
13	Scabies	—	—	—	2·05	13
14	Smallpox	—	—	—	—	14
15	Tonsillitis	20·0	43·8	26·1	18·52	15
16	Tuberculosis	5·0	—	2·2	2·05	16
17	Venereal Diseases	—	—	—	—	17
18	Diseases of the Circulatory System	10·0	9·4	*	2·05	18
19	Diseases due to Disorders of Nutrition	—	3·1	—	—	19
20	Diseases of the Ear, Nose and Throat	5·0	25·0	26·1	10·29	20
21	Diseases of the Eye	*	12·5	2·2	6·17	21
22	Diseases of the Skin (other than Scabies)	15·0	3·1	10·9	12·34	22
23	Other Diseases of the Digestive System	110·0	40·6	32·7	20·57	23
24	Septic Conditions	5·0	31·3	21·8	10·29	24
25	Other Diseases of the Respiratory System	25·0	43·8	37·0	37·03	25
26	Mental, Psychoneurotic and Personality Disorders	*	6·3	2·2	2·05	26
27	All Other Diseases	70·0	225·2	163·2	127·64	27
28	*Total Admissions for Diseases*	435·0	718·7	869·3	388·90	28
29	Injuries—N.E.A.	10·0	43·8	43·6	20·57	29
30	Injuries—E.A.	5·0	—	—	—	30
31	*Total Admissions for Injuries*	15·0	43·8	43·6	20·57	31
32	*Total Admissions*	450·0	762·5	912·9	409·47	32

* Any cases included in 'All Other Diseases'.

Note: 1945 rates are equivalent, being based on the known admissions for the first nine months of the year.

TABLE 123

South-East Asia Command (Indo-Burma Front)
Causes of Admissions to Hospitals, 1942–45. All British Troops
Annual Rates per 1,000 Strength

Source: A.F. A.31-B

	CAUSES	1942	1943	1944	E.A.R. 1945	
1	Common Cold	11·06	19·01	16·90	14·35	1
2	Diarrhoea	40·31	70·35	84·42	31·72	2
3	Dysentery	87·18	122·24	92·53	59·35	3
4	Dengue Fever	36·87	23·86	4·61	2·28	4
5	Diphtheria	0·74	1·17	0·69	0·72	5
6	Enteric Group of Fevers	2·07	1·43	0·77	0·47	6
7	Infective Hepatitis	5·56	26·58	31·02	29·48	7
8	Malaria	326·89	559·64	364·16	107·84	8
9	Mumps	0·12	0·02	0·02	0·52	9
10	Pneumonia	1·18	*	0·84	1·00	10
11	P.U.O. and N.Y.D. Fever	34·64	73·58	151·56	37·64	11
12	Sandfly Fever	2·85	3·22	0·63	0·36	12
13	Scabies	7·17	14·29	11·78	4·79	13
14	Smallpox	0·46	0·72	0·47	0·93	14
15	Tonsillitis	13·70	22·05	12·55	16·27	15
16	Tuberculosis	1·00	0·87	0·38	0·69	16
17	Venereal Diseases	65·92	133·78	59·04	58·76	17
18	Diseases of the Circulatory System	5·60	8·49	5·25	5·07	18
19	Diseases due to Disorders of Nutrition	0·08	1·44	0·14	0·05	19
20	Diseases of the Ear, Nose and Throat	18·54	33·23	25·12	23·27	20
21	Diseases of the Eye	4·76	11·46	8·92	11·44	21
22	Diseases of the Skin (other than Scabies)	39·48	44·35	32·99	45·26	22
23	Other Diseases of the Digestive System	60·39	80·45	49·76	30·87	23
24	Septic Conditions	24·07	32·61	20·42	18·23	24
25	Other Diseases of the Respiratory System	52·16	63·41	45·82	51·33	25
26	Mental, Psychoneurotic and Personality Disorders	2·77	6·19	10·11	20·96	26
27	All Other Diseases	143·99	220·88	186·87	115·42	27
28	*Total Admissions for Diseases*	989·56	1,575·82	1,217·95	689·07	28
29	Injuries—N.E.A.	32·80	58·95	51·54	54·57	29
30	Injuries—E.A.	4·66	14·13	95·46	66·36	30
31	*Total Admissions for Injuries*	37·46	73·08	147·00	120·93	31
32	*Total Admissions*	1,027·01	1,648·90	1,364·95	810·00	32

* Any cases included in 'All Other Diseases'.

Note: 1945 rates are equivalent, being based on the known admissions for the first nine months of the year.

TABLE 124

South-East Asia Command (Indo-Burma Front)
Causes of Admissions to Hospitals, 1942–45. V.C.Os. and I.O.Rs.
Annual Rates per 1,000 Strength

Source: A.F. A.31-B

	CAUSES	1942	1943	1944	E.A. R. 1945	
1	Common Cold	14·5	34·6	33·0	23·99	1
2	Diarrhoea	27·7	27·9	39·6	18·40	2
3	Dysentery	52·8	33·6	40·0	18·51	3
4	Dengue Fever	2·5	0·4	0·4	1·21	4
5	Diphtheria	*	0·2	0·0	0·09	5
6	Enteric Group of Fevers .	0·4	0·5	0·2	0·23	6
7	Infective Hepatitis . .	0·5	2·1	12·3	14·67	7
8	Malaria	447·4	485·6	319·4	68·44	8
9	Mumps	10·8	4·4	4·6	6·23	9
10	Pneumonia	3·5	*	2·3	3·65	10
11	P.U.O. and N.Y.D. Fever .	30·3	72·3	115·0	28·48	11
12	Sandfly Fever . . .	0·1	0·3	0·1	0·67	12
13	Scabies	15·9	27·6	23·4	12·63	13
14	Smallpox	0·2	0·5	0·6	0·40	14
15	Tonsillitis	3·0	3·5	3·0	3·44	15
16	Tuberculosis	2·1	1·4	1·3	1·79	16
17	Venereal Diseases . .	39·2	65·7	36·3	45·96	17
18	Diseases of the Circulatory System	5·2	5·2	5·0	2·92	18
19	Diseases due to Disorders of Nutrition . . .	0·3	0·6	0·1	0·18	19
20	Diseases of the Ear, Nose and Throat . . .	14·8	19·1	17·7	13·55	20
21	Diseases of the Eye . .	11·3	19·6	14·3	14·32	21
22	Diseases of the Skin (other than Scabies) . . .	12·4	25·4	26·7	23·76	22
23	Other Diseases of the Digestive System . .	22·2	34·8	36·9	22·61	23
24	Other Diseases of the Respiratory System . .	33·3	32·2	24·2	21·41	24
25	Septic Conditions . .	28·0	39·6	30·3	29·47	25
26	Mental, Psychoneurotic and Personality Disorders .	1·5	2·9	4·6	7·33	26
27	All Other Diseases . .	97·5	133·4	120·4	81·99	27
28	*Total Admissions for Diseases* . . .	877·4	1,073·4	911·7	466·33	28
29	Injuries—N.E.A. .	37·8	45·7	47·9	57·73	29
30	Injuries—E.A. . .	5·6	9·9	44·7	44·16	30
31	*Total Admissions for Injuries* . . .	43·4	55·6	92·6	101·89	31
32	*Total Admissions* . .	920·8	1,128·9	1,004·3	568·22	32

* Any cases included in 'All Other Diseases'.

Note: 1945 rates are equivalent, being based on the known admissions for the first nine months of the year.

TABLE 125

South-East Asia Command (Indo-Burma Front)
Causes of Admissions to Hospitals, 1942–45. Non-Combatants (Enrolled)
Annual Rates per 1,000 Strength

Source: A.F. A.31-B

	CAUSES	1942	1943	1944	E.A.R. 1945	
1	Common Cold	14·8	34·3	28·9	15·41	1
2	Diarrhoea	18·1	28·6	20·8	9·44	2
3	Dysentery	39·8	34·8	28·3	10·04	3
4	Dengue Fever	1·2	0·2	0·5	0·29	4
5	Diphtheria	*	0·1	0·0	0·04	5
6	Enteric Group of Fevers	0·9	0·5	0·1	0·14	6
7	Infective Hepatitis	0·1	0·1	10·2	7·85	7
8	Malaria	335·3	468·8	278·1	37·28	8
9	Mumps	7·4	10·4	7·3	6·57	9
10	Pneumonia	4·9	*	4·3	3·99	10
11	P.U.O. and N.Y.D. Fever	22·4	62·9	85·0	20·28	11
12	Sandfly Fever	0·0	0·4	0·1	0·07	12
13	Scabies	16·9	24·4	14·4	6·47	13
14	Smallpox	0·1	0·9	1·9	0·39	14
15	Tonsillitis	2·3	3·0	1·9	1·67	15
16	Tuberculosis	2·0	1·7	1·1	1·24	16
17	Venereal Diseases	62·4	86·8	38·1	31·51	17
18	Diseases of the Circulatory System	5·1	4·5	3·3	1·33	18
19	Diseases due to Disorders of Nutrition	—	0·6	—	0·01	19
20	Diseases of the Ear, Nose and Throat	18·3	19·9	17·8	6·41	20
21	Diseases of the Eye	10·1	18·1	10·4	8·19	21
22	Diseases of the Skin (other than Scabies)	13·5	20·9	17·6	11·74	22
23	Other Diseases of the Digestive System	18·3	37·6	28·6	11·79	23
24	Other Diseases of the Respiratory System	36·9	42·1	32·1	14·83	24
25	Septic Conditions	28·0	36·2	23·2	16·29	25
26	Mental, Psychoneurotic and Personality Disorders	1·2	3·5	3·4	6·39	26
27	All Other Diseases	116·2	141·5	85·4	49·19	27
28	*Total Admissions for Diseases*	776·2	1,082·8	742·9	278·85	28
29	Injuries—N.E.A.	33·4	36·9	30·1	26·32	29
30	Injuries—E.A.	1·0	1·2	4·6	2·40	30
31	*Total Admissions for Injuries*	34·3	38·1	34·7	28·72	31
32	*Total Admissions*	810·5	1,120·9	775·5	307·59	32

* Any cases included in 'All Other Diseases'.

Note: 1945 rates are equivalent, being based on the known admissions for the first nine months of the year.

TABLE 126

South-East Asia Command (Indo-Burma Front)
Admissions for Diseases, 1942–45
Crude Average Rates and Order of Precedence of Individual Disease Among
(i) *V.C.Os. and I.O.Rs. and* (ii) *N.Cs.(E.)*

Source: A.F. A.31-B

DISEASES	Average Rates		Order of Precedence	
	V.C.Os. and I.O.Rs.	N.Cs.(E.)	V.C.Os. and I.O.Rs.	N.Cs.(E.)
Malaria	330·2	279·8	1	1
P.U.O. and N.Y.D. Fever	61·5	47·7	2	3
Venereal Diseases	46·8	54·7	3	2
Dysentery	36·2	28·2	4	5
Septic Conditions	31·8	25·9	5	6
Other Diseases of the Digestive System	29·1	24·1	6	7
Diarrhoea	28·4	19·2	7	9
Common Cold	26·5	23·0	8	8
Other Diseases of the Respiratory System	25·3	31·5	9	4
Diseases of the Skin (other than Scabies)	22·1	15·9	10	10
Scabies	19·9	15·5	11	12
Diseases of the Ear, Nose and Throat	16·3	15·6	12	11
Diseases of the Eye	15·0	11·7	13	13
Infective Hepatitis	7·4	4·6	14	15
Mumps	6·5	7·9	15	14
Diseases of the Circulatory System	4·6	3·6	16	17
Mental, Psychoneurotic and Personality Disorders	4·1	3·6	17	17
Tonsillitis	3·2	2·2	18	19
Pneumonia	3·2*	4·4*	19	16
Tuberculosis	1·6	1·5	20	20
Dengue Fever	1·1	0·6	21	22
Smallpox	0·4	0·8	22	21
Enteric Group of Fevers	0·3	0·4	23	23
Sandfly Fever	0·3	0·1	24	25
Diseases due to Disorders of Nutrition	0·3	0·2	25	24
Diphtheria	0·1*	0·1*	26	26
Other Diseases	108·3	98·1		
Average Total Admissions for Diseases	832·2	720·2		

* Based on admissions for three years only.

TABLE 127

South-East Asia Command (Indo-Burma Front)
Causes of Admissions to Hospitals, 1942–45
W.A.C.(I.) and I.M.N.S.

Source: A.F. A.31-B

	CAUSES	1942	1943	1944	E.A.R. 1945	
1	Common Cold	1·67	1·27	14·41	14·08	1
2	Diarrhoea	—	6·97	28·82	—	2
3	Dysentery	1·67	12·05	48·99	37·54	3
4	Dengue Fever	1·67	1·90	8·64	—	4
5	Diphtheria	—	—	—	—	5
6	Enteric Group of Fevers	—	—	2·88	—	6
7	Infective Hepatitis	1·67	—	8·64	4·69	7
8	Malaria	26·67	35·51	135·45	28·17	8
9	Mumps	—	—	2·88	—	9
10	Pneumonia	3·33	—	—	9·39	10
11	P.U.O. and N.Y.D. Fever	—	0·63	37·46	51·64	11
12	Sandfly Fever	—	—	—	—	12
13	Scabies	1·67	—	—	—	13
14	Smallpox	—	—	—	—	14
15	Tonsillitis	—	10·15	17·29	28·17	15
16	Tuberculosis	—	—	2·88	—	16
17	Venereal Diseases	—	—	2·88	—	17
18	Diseases of the Circulatory System	1·67	1·90	5·76	—	18
19	Diseases due to Disorders of Nutrition	—	—	—	—	19
20	Diseases of the Ear, Nose and Throat	5·00	6·34	25·94	—	20
21	Diseases of the Eye	—	—	5·76	4·69	21
22	Diseases of the Skin (other than Scabies)	1·67	1·27	5·76	4·69	22
23	Other Diseases of the Digestive System	8·33	15·22	66·28	28·17	23
24	Other Diseases of the Respiratory System	8·33	15·22	31·70	23·48	24
25	Septic Conditions	4·20	6·98	17·29	42·25	25
26	Mental, Psychoneurotic and Personality Disorders	—	9·6	8·64	4·69	26
27	All Other Diseases	29·12	45·00	129·72	173·75	27
28	*Total Admissions for Diseases*	96·67	169·94	608·07	455·40	28
29	Injuries—N.E.A.	—	6·34	17·29	32·87	29
30	Injuries—E.A.	—	—	—	4·69	30
31	*Total Admissions for Injuries*	—	6·34	17·29	37·56	31
32	*Total Admissions*	96·67	176·28	625·36	492·96	32

Note: Rates for 1945 are equivalent, being based on the known admissions for the first nine months of the year.

TABLE 128

South-East Asia Command (Indo-Burma Front)
Causes of Admissions to Hospitals, 1942–45
All Indian Troops

Source: A.F. A.31-B. Annual rates per 1,000 Strength

	CAUSES	1942	1943	1944	E.A.R. 1945	
1	Common Cold	14·56	34·37	31·91	21·91	1
2	Diarrhoea	25·27	27·97	34·78	34·78	2
3	Dysentery	49·42	33·91	37·00	16·47	3
4	Dengue Fever	2·20	0·33	0·43	0·99	4
5	Diphtheria	*	0·12	0·04	0·08	5
6	Enteric Group of Fevers	0·56	0·53	0·17	0·20	6
7	Infective Hepatitis	0·57	1·88	11·78	13·01	7
8	Malaria	418·33	478·90	315·68	60·84	8
9	Mumps	9·96	6·14	5·31	6·31	9
10	Pneumonia	3·86	*	2·82	3·51	10
11	P.U.O. and N.Y.D. Fever	28·00	69·34	107·25	26·48	11
12	Sandfly Fever	0·10	0·35	0·08	0·55	12
13	Scabies	16·11	26·61	21·09	11·12	13
14	Smallpox	0·17	0·64	0·72	0·40	14
15	Tonsillitis	2·81	3·37	2·73	3·03	15
16	Tuberculosis	2·11	1·53	1·19	1·65	16
17	Venereal Diseases	44·75	71·47	36·67	42·41	17
18	Diseases of the Circulatory System	5·19	4·97	4·56	2·52	18
19	Diseases due to Disorders of Nutrition	0·24	0·59	0·04	0·13	19
20	Diseases of the Ear, Nose and Throat	15·65	19·25	17·69	11·80	20
21	Diseases of the Eye	10·07	19·09	13·28	12·83	21
22	Diseases of the Skin (other than Scabies)	12·63	24·01	24·35	20·83	22
23	Other Diseases of the Digestive System	21·22	35·57	34·80	19·99	23
24	Septic Conditions	34·10	34·95	26·27	19·83	24
25	Other Diseases of the Respiratory System	28·23	38·51	28·45	26·29	25
26	Mental, Psychoneurotic and Personality Disorders	1·41	3·10	4·28	7·11	26
27	All Other Diseases	101·93	134·79	104·82	74·30	27
28	*Total Admissions for Diseases*	849·45	1,072·29	868·19	420·80	28
29	Injuries—N.E.A.	36·59	42·98	43·35	50·09	29
30	Injuries—E.A.	4·46	7·35	34·35	33·99	30
	Total Admissions for Injuries	41·05	50·33	77·70	84·08	31
32	*Total Admissions*	890·50	1,122·63	945·88	504·88	32

* Any cases included in 'All Other Diseases'.

Note: 1945 rates are equivalent, being based on the known admissions for the first nine months of the year.

TABLE 129

South-East Asia Command (Indo-Burma Front)
Causes of Admissions to Hospitals, 1944 and 1945
West African Other Ranks

Source: A.F. A.31-B

	CAUSES	1944 E.A.R.	1945 E.A.R.	
1	Common Cold	6·83	6·71	1
2	Diarrhoea	28·97	12·96	2
3	Dysentery	52·42	22·40	3
4	Dengue Fever	0·48	0·21	4
5	Diphtheria	*	*	5
6	Enteric Group of Fevers	0·16	0·48	6
7	Infective Hepatitis	20·61	6·47	7
8	Malaria	38·84	10·48	8
9	Mumps	1·38	2·52	9
10	Pneumonia	13·96	23·44	10
11	P.U.O. and N.Y.D. Fever	44·54	20·12	11
12	Sandfly Fever	0·48	0·93	12
13	Scabies	4·24	3·04	13
14	Smallpox	3·20	1·17	14
15	Tonsillitis	1·92	1·91	15
16	Tuberculosis	0·52	0·65	16
17	Venereal Diseases	90·05	68·59	17
18	Diseases of the Circulatory System	2·57	2·41	18
19	Diseases due to Disorders of Nutrition	0·04	0·13	19
20	Diseases of the Ear, Nose and Throat	9·37	7·92	20
21	Diseases of the Eye	9·31	11·35	21
22	Diseases of the Skin (other than Scabies)	16·01	16·69	22
23	Other Diseases of the Digestive System	22·84	11·13	23
24	Septic Conditions	32·21	28·80	24
25	Other Diseases of the Respiratory System	31·46	25·79	25
26	Mental, Psychoneurotic and Personality Disorders	3·34	4·49	26
27	All Other Diseases	185·71	111·41	27
28	*Total Admissions for Diseases*	621·46	402·20	28
29	Injuries—N.E.A.	34·22	36·03	29
30	Injuries—E.A.	15·74	37·90	30
31	*Total Admissions for Injuries*	49·97	73·92	31
32	*Total Admissions*	671·44	476·11	32

* Any cases included in 'All Other Diseases'.

Note: The rates shown are equivalent, being based on the known admissions for the last ten months in 1944 and the first nine months in 1945.

TABLE 130

South-East Asia Command (Indo-Burma Front)
Causes of Admissions to Hospitals, 1944 and 1945
East African Other Ranks
Annual Rates per 1,000 Strength

Source: A.F. A.31-B.

	CAUSES	1944 E.A.R.	1945 E.A.R.	
1	Common Cold	23·09	5·32	1
2	Diarrhoea	37·66	10·05	2
3	Dysentery	146·33	50·52	3
4	Dengue Fever	1·51	0·32	4
5	Diphtheria	*	*	5
6	Enteric Group of Fevers	0·53	0·13	6
7	Infective Hepatitis	5·37	6·15	7
8	Malaria	86·26	13·39	8
9	Mumps	0·53	0·45	9
10	Pneumonia	13·06	8·07	10
11	P.U.O. and N.Y.D. Fever	99·33	16·52	11
12	Sandfly Fever	*	*	12
13	Scabies	1·95	2·81	13
14	Smallpox	0·31	0·19	14
15	Tonsillitis	2·42	2·05	15
16	Tuberculosis	0·29	1·03	16
17	Venereal Diseases	52·29	82·92	17
18	Diseases of the Circulatory System	4·37	4·55	18
19	Diseases due to Disorders of Nutrition	*	*	19
20	Diseases of the Ear, Nose and Throat	10·11	7·11	20
21	Diseases of the Eye	11·02	8·13	21
22	Diseases of the Skin (other than Scabies)	16·68	25·11	22
23	Other Diseases of the Digestive System	15·99	16·91	23
24	Septic Conditions	47·61	25·75	24
25	Other Diseases of the Respiratory System	30·03	16·29	25
26	Mental, Psychoneurotic and Personality Disorders	6·19	8·64	26
27	All Other Diseases	128·55	111·30	27
28	*Total Admissions for Diseases*	741·48	423·71	28
29	Injuries—N.E.A.	40·30	52·96	29
30	Injuries—E.A.	44·98	21·07	30
31	*Total Admissions for Injuries*	85·29	74·03	31
32	*Total Admissions*	826·77	497·75	32

* Any cases included in 'All Other Diseases'.

Note: The rates shown below are equivalent, being based on the known admissions for the last seven months in 1944 and the first nine months in 1945.

TABLE 131

South-East Asia Command (Indo-Burma Front)
Causes of Admissions to Hospitals, 1942–45
All Troops
Annual Rates per 1,000 Strength

Source: A.F. A.31-B

	CAUSES	1942	1943	1944	E.A.R. 1945	
1	Common Cold	13·66	31·98	30·21	19·01	1
2	Diarrhoea	29·14	34·56	46·41	18·21	2
3	Dysentery	59·14	47·65	53·86	24·95	3
4	Dengue Fever	11·13	3·99	1·25	1·11	4
5	Diphtheria	0·19	0·29	0·16	0·17	5
6	Enteric Group of Fevers	0·95	0·44	0·30	0·27	6
7	Infective Hepatitis	1·86	5·72	16·01	14·92	7
8	Malaria	394·79	491·46	328·93	63·01	8
9	Mumps	7·42	5·26	4·49	4·88	9
10	Pneumonia	3·17	*	3·63	4·67	10
11	P.U.O. and N.Y.D. Fevers	29·71	69·99	120·42	27·44	11
12	Sandfly Fever	0·81	0·80	0·21	0·52	12
13	Scabies	13·81	24·69	19·72	9·24	13
14	Smallpox	0·24	0·65	0·88	0·53	14
15	Tonsillitis	5·62	6·28	4·67	5·01	15
16	Tuberculosis	1·82	1·42	1·08	1·41	16
17	Venereal Diseases	50·20	81·17	47·43	48·36	17
18	Diseases of the Circulatory System	5·29	5·52	4·95	3·00	18
19	Diseases due to Disorders of Nutrition	0·10	0·36	0·03	0·07	19
20	Diseases of the Ear, Nose and Throat	16·39	21·43	19·85	13·19	20
21	Diseases of the Eye	8·92	17·90	13·33	12·32	21
22	Diseases of the Skin (other than Scabies)	19·55	27·17	27·29	24·59	22
23	Other Diseases of the Digestive System	31·30	42·55	39·27	20·99	23
24	Septic Conditions	31·52	34·59	28·35	20·41	24
25	Other Diseases of the Respiratory System	34·40	42·39	34·23	29·87	25
26	Mental, Psychoneurotic and Personality Disorders	1·76	3·58	5·69	9·19	26
27	All Other Diseases	111·64	148·79	139·76	84·90	27
28	*Total Admissions for Diseases*	884·53	1,150·63	993·01	462·24	28
29	Injuries—N.E.A.	35·61	45·47	47·90	49·93	29
30	Injuries—E.A.	6·18	8·40	47·43	38·92	30
31	*Total Admissions for Injuries*	41·79	53·87	95·33	88·85	31
32	*Total Admissions*	926·32	1,204·50	1,088·34	551·09	32

* Any cases included in 'All Other Diseases.'

Note: 1945 rates are equivalent, being based on the known admissions for the first nine months of the year.

TABLE 132

South-East Asia Command (Indo-Burma Front)
Admissions to Hospitals for Injuries, 1942–45
Annual Rates per 1,000 Strength

Source: A.F. A.31-B

1. BRITISH TROOPS	British Officers				British Other Ranks				Q.A.I.M.N.S.				All British Troops			
	1942	1943	1944	1945 (E.A.R.)	1942	1943	1944	1945 (E.A.R.)	1942	1943	1944	1945 (E.A.R.)	1942	1943	1944	1945 (E.A.R.)
(a) *Non-Enemy Action*																
Burns and Scalds	N.A.	N.A.	1·74	1·65	N.A.	N.A.	3·81	6·36	N.A.	N.A.	N.A.	2·05	N.A.	N.A.	3·51	5·39
Others	N.A.	N.A.	29·41	29·72	N.A.	N.A.	50·99	54·41	N.A.	N.A.	N.A.	18·52	N.A.	N.A.	48·03	49·19
Totals	30·11	32·56	31·15	31·37	33·2	64·4	54·81	60·77	10·0	43·8	43·67	20·57	32·80	58·95	51·54	54·57
(b) *Enemy Action*																
Injuries caused by Blast	—	—	0·31	0·22	—	—	0·82	0·41	—	—	—	—	—	—	0·75	0·37
Bomb Wounds	0·86	3·30	12·56	8·95	0·5	2·4	21·85	12·61	—	—	—	—	0·58	2·56	20·57	11·79
Gunshot Wounds	3·87	9·99	29·60	23·09	3·9	8·8	54·81	40·61	5·0	—	—	—	3·96	8·98	51·28	36·80
Shell Wounds	—	2·05	13·24	9·33	0·1	2·7	24·43	19·61	—	—	—	—	0·12	2·59	22·87	17·40
Totals	4·73	15·34	55·72	41·61	4·5	13·9	101·91	73·25	5·0	—	—	—	4·66	14·13	95·46	66·36
(c) *Total Injuries*	34·84	47·90	86·87	72·99	37·7	78·3	156·72	134·03	15·0	43·8	43·67	20·57	37·46	73·08	147·00	120·93

2. INDIAN TROOPS	V.C.Os. and I.O.Rs.				N.Cs.(E.)				V.C.Os., I.O.Rs. and N.Cs.(E)				W.A.C.(I.) and I.M.N.S.				All Indian Troops			
	1942	1943	1944	1945 (E.A.R.)	1942	1943	1944	1945 (E.A.R.)	1942	1943	1944	1945 (E.A.R.)	1942	1943	1944	1945 (E.A.R.)	1942	1943	1944	1945 (E.A.R.)
(a) *Non-Enemy Action*																				
Burns and Scalds	N.A.	N.A.	2·3	4·32	N.A.	N.A.	1·9	2·48	N.A.	N.A.	2·24	3·88	—	N.A.	N.A.	N.A.	N.A.	N.A.	2·24	3·88
Others	N.A.	N.A.	45·6	53·41	N.A.	N.A.	28·1	23·83	N.A.	N.A.	41·13	46·23	—	N.A.	N.A.	N.A.	N.A.	N.A.	41·11	46·21
Totals	37·8	45·7	47·9	57·73	33·37	36·92	30·09	26·32	36·74	43·14	43·37	50·11	—	6·34	17·29	32·87	36·59	42·98	43·35	50·09
(b) *Enemy Action*																				
Injuries caused by Blast	—	—	0·4	0·12	—	—	0·01	0·13	—	—	0·31	0·12	—	—	—	—	—	—	0·31	0·12
Bomb Wounds	0·0	3·2	11·4	11·72	0·0	0·4	1·66	0·75	0·05	2·38	8·93	9·05	—	—	—	4·69	0·05	2·37	8·93	9·05
Gunshot Wounds	5·0	5·0	21·1	22·56	0·9	0·7	1·73	0·92	4·02	3·79	16·11	17·31	—	—	—	—	4·00	3·77	16·09	17·20
Shell Wounds	0·5	1·7	11·7	9·75	0·0	0·1	1·16	0·60	0·41	1·21	9·02	7·52	—	—	—	—	0·40	1·20	9·01	7·52
Totals	5·61	9·89	44·65	44·16	0·97	1·18	4·56	2·40	4·47	7·38	34·38	34·00	—	—	—	4·69	4·46	7·35	34·35	33·99
(c) *Total Injuries*	43·41	55·59	92·55	102·16	34·34	38·10	34·65	28·72	41·21	51·52	77·75	84·11	—	6·34	17·29	37·56	41·05	50·33	77·70	84·08

3. WEST AFRICAN OTHER RANKS

	1944 (E.A.R.)	1945 (E.A.R.)
(a) *Non-Enemy Action*		
Burns and Scalds	1·57	1·31
Others	32·64	34·71
Totals	34·22	36·03
(b) *Enemy Action*		
Injuries caused by Blast	0·23	0·21
Bomb Wounds	0·90	5·60
Gunshot Wounds	13·15	18·49
Shell Wounds	1·47	13·59
Totals	15·74	37·89
(c) *Total Injuries*	49·97	73·92

4. EAST AFRICAN OTHER RANKS

	1944 (E.A.R.)	1945 (E.A.R.)
(a) *Non-Enemy Action*		
Burns and Scalds	2·49	2·05
Others	37·82	50·91
Totals	40·30	52·96
(b) *Enemy Action*		
Injuries caused by Blast	0·07	0·07
Bomb Wounds	12·06	3·13
Gunshot Wounds	31·17	14·21
Shell Wounds	1·66	3·65
Totals	44·98	21·07
(c) *Total Injuries*	85·29	74·03

5. ALL TROOPS

	1942	1943	1944	1945 (E.A.R.)
(a) *Non-Enemy Action*				
Burns and Scalds	N.A.	N.A.	2·62	3·87
Others	N.A.	N.A.	45·27	46·05
Totals	35·61	45·47	47·90	49·93
(b) *Enemy Action*				
Injuries caused by Blast	—	—	0·41	0·17
Bomb Wounds	1·86	2·40	11·38	9·03
Gunshot Wounds	3·99	4·58	24·01	20·36
Shell Wounds	0·33	1·42	11·64	9·36
Totals	6·18	8·40	47·43	38·92
(c) *Total Injuries*	41·79	53·87	95·35	88·85

TABLE 133

South-East Asia Command (Indo-Burma Front)
Deaths in Hospitals, 1942–45
By Categories of Troops
Annual Rates per 1,000 Strength

Source: A.F. A.31-B

CAUSES	1942	1943	1944	E.A.R. 1945
British Officers				
Diseases and N.E.A. Injuries	N.A.	4·1	3·2	1·6
E.A. Injuries	N.A.	0·5	3·3	2·9
Totals	8·0	4·6	6·5	4·5
British Other Ranks				
Diseases and N.E.A. Injuries	N.A.	5·0	6·6	2·0
E.A. Injuries	N.A.	0·7	4·3	3·5
Totals	5·3	5·6	10·8	5·5
V.C.Os. and I.O.Rs.				
Diseases and N.E.A. Injuries	N.A.	4·8	4·5	2·3
E.A. Injuries	N.A.	0·5	2·1	1·7
Totals	7·8	5·3	6·6	4·0
N.Cs.(E.)				
Diseases and N.E.A. Injuries	N.A.	5·7	3·3	1·2
E.A. Injuries	N.A.	0·3	0·1	0·2
Totals	9·4	6·0	3·4	1·4
W.A.C.(I.) and I.M.N.S.				
Diseases and N.E.A. Injuries	N.A.	0·6	5·8	—
E.A. Injuries	N.A.	—	—	—
Totals	1·7	0·6	5·8	—
All Indian Troops				
Diseases and N.E.A. Injuries	N.A.	5·7	4·2	2·0
E.A. Injuries	N.A.	0·3	1·6	1·3
Totals	8·13	6·0	5·8	3·4
W.A.O.Rs.				
Diseases and N.E.A. Injuries			3·8	3·5
E.A. Injuries			0·4	1·2
Totals			4·3	4·8
E.A.O.Rs.				
Diseases and N.E.A. Injuries			5·0	3·2
E.A. Injuries			0·8	1·5
Totals			5·8	4·7

TABLE 134

South-East Asia Command (Indo-Burma Front)
Admissions to Hospitals for Diseases, 1942–45
Comparative Rates B.O.Rs. and V.C.Os. and I.O.Rs.

Source: A.F. A.31-B

	DISEASES	B.O.Rs.	V.C.Os. and I.O.Rs.	
1	Common Cold	100	156	1
2	Diarrhoea	100	47	2
3	Dysentery	100	38	3
4	Dengue Fever	100	6	4
5	Diphtheria	100	12	5
6	Enteric Group of Fevers	100	26	6
7	Infective Hepatitis	100	31	7
8	Malaria	100	88	8
9	Mumps	100	1,970	9
10	Pneumonia	100	323	10
11	P.U.O. and N.Y.D. Fever	100	75	11
12	Sandfly Fever	100	16	12
13	Scabies	100	183	13
14	Smallpox	100	60	14
15	Tuberculosis	100	216	15
16	Venereal Diseases	100	50	16
17	Diseases of the Circulatory System	100	71	17
18	Diseases due to Disorders of Nutrition	100	77	18
19	Diseases of the Ear, Nose and Throat	100	60	19
20	Diseases of the Eye	100	146	20
21	Diseases of the Skin (Other than Scabies)	100	49	21
22	Other Diseases of the Digestive System	100	49	22
23	Septic Conditions	100	98	23
24	Other Diseases of the Respiratory System	100	55	24
25	Mental, Psychoneurotic and Personality Disorders	100	38	25
26	All Other Diseases	100	57	26
27	*Total Admissions for Diseases*	100	68	27

TABLE 135
South-East Asia Command (Indo-Burma Front)
Admissions to Hospitals for Diseases, 1944–45
Comparative Rates Other Ranks

Source: A.F. A.31-B

	DISEASES	B.O.Rs.	V.C.Os. and I.O.Rs.	W.A.O.Rs.	E.A.O.Rs.	
1	Common Cold	100	162	39	81	1
2	Diarrhoea	100	46	33	37	2
3	Dysentery	100	36	46	121	3
4	Dengue Fever	100	26	11	29	4
5	Diphtheria	100	6	N.A.	N.A.	5
6	Enteric Group of Fevers .	100	33	51	52	6
7	Infective Hepatitis . .	100	43	43	18	7
8	Malaria	100	73	9	19	8
9	Mumps	100	1,503	542	136	9
10	Pneumonia	100	334	2,101	1,181	10
11	P.U.O. and N.Y.D. Fever .	100	68	31	55	11
12	Sandfly Fever	100	70	130	N.A.	12
13	Scabies	100	192	39	25	13
14	Smallpox	100	68	295	34	14
15	Tuberculosis	100	291	166	125	15
16	Venereal Diseases . .	100	58	112	96	16
17	Diseases of the Circulatory System . . .	100	69	44	78	17
18	Diseases due to Disorders of Nutrition . . .	100	37	21	N.A.	18
19	Diseases of the Ear, Nose and Throat . . .	100	59	33	33	19
20	Diseases of the Eye . .	100	124	90	83	20
21	Diseases of the Skin (Other than Scabies) .	100	58	37	48	21
22	Other Diseases of the Digestive System . .	100	68	39	38	22
23	Septic Conditions . .	100	131	143	97	23
24	Other Diseases of the Respiratory System .	100	55	53	43	24
25	Mental, Psychoneurotic and Personality Disorders .	100	35	23	43	25
26	All Other Diseases . .	100	58	56	68	26
27	*Total Admissions for Diseases*	100	65	48	55	27

(ii) **Ceylon**

BRITISH TROOPS

BRITISH OFFICERS

In Table 136 are presented the admission rates of British Officers for the years 1942 to 1945. They include not only those officers on the strength of British Units, but also those who were attached to Indian, Ceylonese and East African Units.

Admissions for diseases were highest in 1942 and lowest in 1945, the rate for which year was slightly over half that for 1942. In 1943, admissions were three-quarters those of 1942 and were almost equal to those in 1944. Rates were 857 in 1942, 632 in 1943, 623 in 1944 and 443 in 1945. Admissions for injuries were also highest in 1942 at 75 per 1,000. The second highest rate occurred in 1944 at 51, followed by 42 in 1943 and 39 in 1945. The majority of injuries were sustained other than by enemy action.Total admissions were 993 per 1,000 in 1942, 674 in 1943 and 1944, and 482 in 1945.

Of those diseases noted in the table, MALARIA caused most admissions, except in 1945, when Diseases of the SKIN took pride of place. Malaria was responsible for admission rates at 135 in 1942 and 132 in 1943. This was followed by a decline of nearly fifty per cent. to 71 in 1944 and a similar fall to 33 in the ensuing year. Rates for P.U.O. and N.Y.D. FEVER are not known for 1942 and 1943, but in 1944 and 1945 they were 58 and 29.

Figures relating to Diseases of the SKIN (other than Scabies) are also not available for 1942 and 1943. Rates for the succeeding years were 43 and 49. DENGUE FEVER was responsible for the high admission rate of 112 per 1,000 in 1942. This was decreased by one-half in 1943 and 1944 to 60 and 58 respectively and, in 1945, to the low rate of 10. SEPTIC CONDITIONS which registered the high rate of 86 in 1942 fell considerably to 18 in 1945 with 28 and 31 in the intervening years.

A trend similar to that exhibited by Septic Conditions was witnessed in Other Diseases of the DIGESTIVE SYSTEM which recorded rates of 73 in 1942, 42 in 1943, 46 in 1944 and 30 in 1945. The rates for DYSENTERY were fairly constant, ranging from 27 in 1944 and 1945 to 29 in 1943. DIARRHOEA showed a decline of 10 per 1,000 from the highest rate of 27 in 1944 to 17 in 1945. Other rates were 26 in 1942 and 20 in 1943.

Admissions for TONSILLITIS were 23 per 1,000 in 1942. In the following year they declined by fifty per cent. to 12 but rose to 15 in 1944 and again to 19 in 1945. INFECTIVE HEPATITIS caused rates at 24 per 1,000 in 1942 and 5 in 1943. This was followed by an increase to 13 in 1944 with a decline by almost fifty per cent. to 7 in 1945. Admissions for COMMON COLD were relatively high at rates which varied from 20 in 1942 to 12 in 1943. They increased to 14 in 1944 and to 16 in the following year.

Other Diseases of the RESPIRATORY SYSTEM registered 9 admissions per 1,000 officers in 1942. This rate declined to 2, then rose to a peak rate of 19 in 1944 and subsided in 1945 to slightly above the 1942 rate to 10 per 1,000. DIPHTHERIA recorded the comparatively high rate of 7 in 1942. By 1944 it had declined to 3 and in the following year was 0·5 per 1,000.

VENEREAL DISEASES produced rates of 9 in 1942, 7 in 1943, 17 in 1944 and 9 in 1945. Rates for Diseases of the EYE fluctuated from 7 in 1942 to 2 in 1943, rose to 8 in 1944 and fell to 4 in 1945. Admissions for MENTAL, PSYCHONEUROTIC and PERSONALITY Disorders also fluctuated from 6 in 1942 to 3 in the following year, then to 6 in 1944 and finally to 9 in 1945. In 1942 the rate for TUBERCULOSIS was 2 per 1,000. This was reduced to 1·3 in 1943 and again to 0·5 in both 1944 and 1945.

There were no admissions over the period for SMALLPOX, SANDFLY FEVER or for Diseases due to Disorders of NUTRITION.

BRITISH OTHER RANKS

Table 137 records the rates of admissions to hospitals of B.O.Rs. Admissions for diseases only were, in general, somewhat higher than those for British Officers. In 1942, 1943 and 1945, they were some thirty per cent. higher. In 1944, however, the rate was three per cent. lower. Rates, which declined each year, were 1,094 in 1942, 813 in 1943, 602 in 1944 and 584 in 1945. Admission rates for Injuries were also higher than those for Officers, except in 1942, at 72, 51, 55 and 47 per 1,000, respectively. Total admission rates were 1,166 in 1942, 865 in 1943, 658 in 1944 and 631 in 1945.

As with officers, MALARIA, individually, caused more admissions than any other disease. The rate in 1942 was 278; it fell slightly to 254 in the following year. By 1944 it had declined by two-thirds to 82 and in 1945 there was a further fall to 36. The 1945 rate was approximately one-eighth that of 1942 and the decline was much steeper than the one experienced by Officers. Rates for P.U.O. and N.Y.D. FEVER are not available for the first two years but were 44 in 1944 and 24 in 1945.

Second in importance to Malaria, in so far as numbers admitted are concerned, were VENEREAL DISEASES. The high rate of 113 per 1,000 in 1942 was followed by a decline of forty-five per cent. in 1943 to 63. There was a further fall during the following year when the rate was 47 but, in 1945, admissions increased to a rate only slightly lower than that of 1943 at 62 per 1,000. The rate of 113 in 1942 was the highest recorded by any class of personnel in this area during the four years.

DENGUE FEVER was responsible for some high admission rates which, on the whole, were lower than those registered by Officers. It was only in 1945 that the rate for Officers was lower. Rates for B.O.Rs. were 79 (as against 112 for Officers) in 1942, 54 (60) in 1943, 53 (58) in 1944 and 20 (10) in 1945. SEPTIC CONDITIONS also caused some high rates, as with Officers, particularly in 1942, when the rate was 88 per 1,000. This was followed by 32 in 1943, 29 in 1944 and 32 in 1945.

Admissions for Other Diseases of the DIGESTIVE SYSTEM, which followed Septic Conditions in importance, were 42 in 1942, and 40 in 1943 with 33 and 31 in the two ensuing years. Admissions for DYSENTERY and DIARRHOEA were much lower than on the Indo-Burma Front. Rates for the former ranged from between 25 (in 1943) and 29 (1944 and 1945) while those for Diarrhoea were 35 in 1942, 15 in 1943, 17 in 1944 and 21 in 1945.

TONSILLITIS rates registered by British Officers in 1943 were approximately one half the 1942 rate. This was duplicated by B.O.Rs. whose rates for the two years were 33 and 15. A further decline occurred in 1944 to 13, but in 1945 there was a slight rise to 16 per 1,000. COMMON COLD recorded an admission rate of 30 in 1942 as against 20 for Officers. This decreased each year until by 1945 the rate was 8 per 1,000. The trend was rather different to that of Officers which showed successive increases in the last two years following a decline in 1943. Other Diseases of the RESPIRATORY SYSTEM caused admissions at rates of 8 in 1942 and 3 in 1943. In the two following years admissions were much heavier at 16 in 1914 and 14 in 1945.

Admissions for Diseases of the EYE fell from 11 to 7 in 1943 and to 6 in 1944 but increased to 10 in 1945. The rates for INFECTIVE HEPATITIS, contrary to those recorded on the Indo-Burma Front, were fairly stable at between 8 and 10 per 1,000 except in 1943, when the rate was 6. In general they were lower than those for Officers.

The rates for SCABIES varied between 4 and 7. Those for Diseases of the SKIN rose from 48 in 1944 to 69 in 1945. The rates for the first two years are not available. There were no admissions for diseases due to Disorders of NUTRITION during the first three years, none for SMALLPOX in 1942 and 1943 or from MUMPS in 1943.

ALL BRITISH TROOPS

Table 138 gives the Annual rates of admissions to hospitals for All British Troops. As the strength of Other Ranks was greatly in excess of that of Officers, the rates tend to follow those of B.O.Rs. in Table 137.

Compared with the rates for All British Troops on the Indo-Burma Front, admissions for diseases were, in general, not so heavy, in spite of the 1942 rates which, in Ceylon, were greater by 90 per 1,000. On the Indo-Burma Front admissions in 1943 had risen by nearly 600 per 1,000 to a peak rate of 1,576. The same year, in Ceylon, witnessed a decline of admissions by over one quarter those of the previous year. In 1944 the difference in rates was some 600 per 1,000, but in 1945 was only 130. In Ceylon, the 1945 rate was fifty-one per cent. that of 1942, while on the Indo-Burma Front, it was seventy per cent. If, however, the 1945 rates are compared with admissions in peak years, the figures are fifty-one and forty-four per cent. respectively.

It is perhaps worthy of mention that success in the fight against MALARIA, among British Troops at least, appeared one year earlier in Ceylon where the rate in 1943 of 238 was followed by 80 in 1944, a reduction of sixty-six per cent. The decline of admissions in 1944 on the Indo-Burma Front was thirty-five per cent. The overall decline in

Ceylon was nearly ninety per cent., while that on the Indo-Burma Front was under seventy per cent. Annual rates were lower in Ceylon being 267 (as compared with 327 on the Indo-Burma Front) in 1942, 238 (560) in 1943, 80 (364) in 1944 and 36 (108) in 1945.

Admissions on account of DIARRHOEA and DYSENTERY were much less in Ceylon but rates for DENGUE FEVER were considerably in excess. On the Indo-Burma Front, admissions for INFECTIVE HEPATITIS increased year by year from 6 in 1942 to 29 per 1,000 in 1945. In Ceylon, rates varied from 6 to 10 with the second lowest rate in 1945.

Rates for SMALLPOX were less that those recorded on the Indo-Burma Front, there being none in 1942 or 1943, while the rates for the following years at 0.16 and 0·11 per 1,000 compared with 0·47 and 0·93. TONSILLITIS caused higher rates of admission in Ceylon, especially in 1942 as did SEPTIC CONDITIONS with 89 per 1,000 as against 24. During the other years, rates varied much less.

Perhaps the greatest differences in rates were registered by Other Diseases of the RESPIRATORY SYSTEM. In Ceylon, the rates were 8 per 1,000 in 1942, 4 in 1943, 0·16 in 1944 and 13 in 1945, while on the Indo-Burma Front they were 52, 64, 46 and 51 respectively. Although, in 1942, the rate of admissions in Ceylon on account of MENTAL, PSYCHONEUROTIC and PERSONALITY DISORDERS was twice that on the Indo-Burma Front, by 1945 the position was reversed and the rate in Ceylon was 10, as compared with 21 per 1,000.

Summary

Rates of admission to hospitals were, generally, less in Ceylon than on the Indo-Burma Front. Among individual diseases, lower rates were recorded for Diarrhoea, Dysentery, Infective Hepatitis, Smallpox and, particularly, Malaria. Admission rates were higher for Tonsillitis, Septic Conditions and, more especially, for Dengue Fever.

INDIAN TROOPS

INDIAN OFFICERS

Table 139 records the admission rates of Indian Officers to hospitals in Ceylon. As information for 1945 is unobtainable, only those rates for the three years 1942 to 1944 have been recorded.

There were very few Indian Officers stationed in Ceylon. Because of this and for reasons which have already been discussed, a comparison between Indian Officer rates and those of other classes of troops is invalid as is, indeed, a comparison between the annual rates among those Officers. The purpose of including the table is to make the statistical survey of morbidity in this area as complete as possible.

VICEROY'S COMMISSIONED OFFICERS AND INDIAN OTHER RANKS

Admission rates of V.C.Os. and I.O.Rs. are shown in Table 140. As with British Troops, a successive annual decrease was experienced. Rates for disease were 867 in 1942, 703 in 1943, 614 in 1944 and 464 in 1945. The overall decline was forty-six per cent. Injuries accounted for rates at 66, 48, 52 and 43 per 1,000 respectively.

Of individual diseases, MALARIA accounted for the highest rates with 195 in 1942, followed by 189 in 1943 and 156 in 1944. In the following year, the rate declined to one third the 1942 rate at 65. Admission rates for P.U.O. and N.Y.D. FEVER are available only for 1944 and 1945 when they were 67 and 35.

Next to Malaria in order of numerical importance were admissions for VENEREAL DISEASES. There was comparatively little variation in the rates which decreased annually from 47 in 1942 to 37 in 1945. SEPTIC CONDITIONS were also responsible for high rates of admissions at 72 per 1,000 in 1942. Successive declines in the two following years were recorded at rates of 44 and 22 but in 1945 a slight rise brought admissions to 25 per 1,000. Other Diseases of the DIGESTIVE SYSTEM registered rates of 50 in 1942, 28 in both 1943 and 1945, and 32 in 1944. The rates for DYSENTERY were lower at 19, 23, 25 and 19 respectively, while those for DIARRHOEA were, on the average, still lower at 31, 22, 14 and 11 per 1,000.

Admissions for Diseases of the EAR, NOSE and THROAT are known only for 1944 and 1945, and were comparatively high at 25 and 28 per 1,000. Although the rates for Other Diseases of the RESPIRATORY SYSTEM decreased in 1943 from 17 to 7, they rose in 1944 to 27 per 1,000 and, in 1945, to 28. Admissions for Diseases of the EYE were 23 in 1942. They declined in 1943 to 16 and again in the following year to 13, but increased to 19 in 1945.

COMMON COLD recorded comparatively low rates in the second and fourth years of the period with 9 and 8 in 1943 and 1945 against 18 and 26 per 1,000 in 1942 and 1944. Admissions for SCABIES were consistent at 16 per 1,000 except in 1944 when the rate was 10. The rate for Diseases of the SKIN in 1944 and 1945 was 21 while those for the previous years are not available. In spite of a rise from 11 in 1943 to 16 in 1944, a large decrease in admission rates over the four years was recorded by DENGUE FEVER from 17 in 1942 to 4 in 1945. The rates for INFECTIVE HEPATITIS ranged from 4 to 7 and those for TONSILLITIS were even less varied at from 4 to 5.

The high rate of 10 per 1,000 was recorded for TUBERCULOSIS in 1943, following a rate of 4 in the previous year. Those in the ensuing years were 1·70 and 1·19. A similar trend, but of lesser magnitude was experienced among N.Cs.(E.) at 3, 7, 1·16 and 0·60 per 1,000 over the four years.

MENTAL, PSYCHONEUROTIC and PERSONALITY DISORDERS were responsible for rates which increased from 3 per 1,000 in 1942 and 1943, to 5 in 1944 and 6 in 1945. Admissions for MUMPS were comparatively high in 1942 and 1945 at 2·12 and 2·65 with 0·78 and 1·41 in 1943 and 1945.

Of the other diseases noted in the table with low rates, admissions for diseases due to Disorders of NUTRITION were recorded only in 1944 at 1·05 per 1,000; there were no admissions in 1945 for SANDFLY FEVER or for the ENTERIC Group of Fevers and none for DIPHTHERIA in 1943.

NON-COMBATANTS (ENROLLED)

In presenting the rates of admissions to hospitals of N.Cs.(E.) in Table 141 it must be mentioned that the figures include some labourers, civilians from Southern India, mainly Travancore State, employed by the Government of India in clearing and levelling ground for air-strips, etc. The number included is not known, but it is certain that there were not many and insufficient to affect the rates cited to any marked degree. The figures in the table then, to all intents and purposes, reflect the morbidity state among N.Cs.(E.).

Rates for diseases decreased annually from 778 in 1942, to 667 in 1943 and from 361 in 1944 to 209 in 1945. These were lower than the rates for I.O.Rs. by from 100 in 1942 to 250 in 1945. The overall rate of decrease from 1942 to 1945 was seventy-three per cent. as against forty-six per cent. for I.O.Rs. Injury rates which were predominantly N.E.A., varied from 39 in 1942 to 14 in 1945.

As with B.O.Rs. and I.O.Rs., MALARIA was, individually, responsible for more admissions than any other disease and followed the normal trend of successive annual declines. Rates were 210, 156, 97 and 61 per 1,000. The 1942 rate was slightly higher than that for I.O.Rs. but other rates were less, although in 1945 the difference was only 3 per 1,000. The fall in 1944 was thirty-eight per cent., compared with eighteen per cent. among I.O.Rs., but in 1945 the decline among I.O.Rs. was greater by twenty per cent. Admissions for P.U.O. and N.Y.D. FEVER, known only for 1944 and 1945 were 37 and 22 per 1,000.

Following Malaria in numerical importance were admissions for VENEREAL DISEASES. The rates were higher than those for I.O.Rs. in 1942 and 1943, but lower in the two ensuing years. They were 72 (as against 47 for I.O.Rs.) in 1942, 56 (44) in 1943, 21 (40) in 1944 and the extremely low rate of 9 (37) in 1945.

Admissions for Other Diseases of the DIGESTIVE SYSTEM increased by over fifty per cent. in 1943, from 32 to 51. In 1944 they declined to 17 and by 1945 were only 9 per 1,000. The rates for DIARRHOEA followed the general trend, in that they declined annually, and were 21, 11, 8 and 4 respectively. Those for DYSENTERY, however, increased from 10 in

1942 to 13 in 1943 and to 19 in the following year, before falling to 10 in 1945. In all these diseases the rates for I.O.Rs. were somewhat higher.

In 1942 and 1943, admissions for DENGUE FEVER were heavier among N.Cs.(E.) when rates of 25 and 13 were recorded, as against 17 and 11 for I.O.Rs. During 1944 and 1945, however, admissions of the former were 6 and 1 in contrast to 16 and 4 for I.O.Rs. Admissions for COMMON COLD rose in 1943 by nearly fifty per cent., from 13 to 18, declined in 1944 to 11 and, in 1945, to 3 per 1,000. In contrast, admissions among I.O.Rs. fell in 1943 by fifty per cent., rose in 1944 and in 1945 decreased to approximately the 1943 rate.

Diseases of the EYE recorded an admission rate of 17 in 1942, which declined by one third to 11 in the following year and to 5 per 1,000 in 1944 and 1945. The corresponding rates for I.O.Rs. were higher at 23, 16, 13 and 19 respectively.

SCABIES recorded admission rates which were approximately half those for I.O.Rs. and which ranged between 6 and 10 per 1,000, while diseases of the SKIN (during the two years for which figures are available) were 9 and 6.

The rate for TUBERCULOSIS was unusually high in 1943 at 7 per 1,000. Other rates were 3 in 1942, 1·16 in 1944 and 0·60 in 1945. The trend of admissions on account of MENTAL, PSYCHONEUROTIC and PERSONALITY DISORDERS was different from that recorded by I.O.Rs. Whereas rates for the latter increased annually, those for N.Cs.(E.) increased only in 1943 (from 1·5 to 4) and decreased to 3 and 2 in the following years. The rates for INFECTIVE HEPATITIS, which were approximately one-half of those for I.O.Rs., showed no particular trend, and ranged between 2 and 4, while those for TONSILLITIS were lower at between 1 and 3 and were also less than those reported for I.O.Rs.

Of other diseases whose admission rates were relatively low, there were very few cases of SMALLPOX recorded in 1942, 1944 or 1945 and none in 1943; there were no admissions for DIPHTHERIA in 1945, of the ENTERIC Group of FEVERS in 1942, or for Disorders of NUTRITION in 1942 and 1943.

INDIAN MILITARY NURSING SERVICE

Table 142 records the annual rates of known admissions to hospitals in Ceylon of members of the Indian Military Nursing Service.

The strength of the I.M.N.S. in Ceylon during the years 1942 to 1945 was particularly small and care must be taken in endeavouring to compare morbidity rates of this class of personnel with another, all the more so as much information is missing, especially in 1944 and 1945. The missing information, however, does not affect the rates for total admissions for disease.

ALL INDIAN TROOPS

The admission rates for All Indian Troops are recorded in Table 143. Admission rates and trends tend to follow, in general, those of V.C.Os. and I.O.Rs., who were the predominating numerical component of Indian Troops.

Compared with the rates for this class of troops serving on the Indo-Burma Front, admissions for diseases only were slightly higher in 1942 (by 14 per 1,000) and in 1945 (by 43 per 1,000). In 1943 and 1944, however, those in Ceylon were lower by 372 and 258 per 1,000 respectively. Compared with 1942, the decrease in Ceylon by 1945 was forty-six per cent. as against fifty per cent. on the Indo-Burma Front. If, however, the peak year of admissions is taken for comparison, the decline on the Indo-Burma Front is even more striking at sixty-one per cent. as against forty-six per cent. in Ceylon. Admissions for Injuries were less in Ceylon. That this is due to the much lower rate on account of injuries sustained through Enemy Action is offset by the higher rates, in Ceylon, of N.E.A. injuries by, on the average, 8 per 1,000.

Rates for MALARIA were, in general, much higher on the Indo-Burma Front. In 1945, however, the rate in Ceylon was 4 per 1,000 more. The 1945 rate in Ceylon was roughly one-third that in 1942 as against approximately one-seventh on the Indo-Burma Front.

Apart from 1943, when admissions for VENEREAL DISEASES on the Indo-Burma Front increased from 45 to 71, rates differed but little. In Ceylon they ranged from 37 to 46 as against 37 to 45. Admissions on account of SEPTIC CONDITIONS were higher in Ceylon, particularly in 1942, when the rate was 71 as compared with 34. Apart from this admissions in Ceylon varied from 22 to 44 and, on the Indo-Burma Front, from 20 to 35 per 1,000.

Other Diseases of the DIGESTIVE SYSTEM were also higher in 1942 at 50 as compared with 21. In 1943 and 1944 rates were twenty-five and ten per cent. lower but in 1945 were again higher by thirty per cent. Rates for DIARRHOEA and DYSENTERY were lower in Ceylon by twenty-three and thirty-eight per cent. respectively. Admissions on account of Other Diseases of the RESPIRATORY SYSTEM fluctuated between 7 in 1943 and 28 in 1945. Except in 1945 when they were slightly higher, rates were, in general, much lower in Ceylon and differences ranged from 31 in 1943 to 1 in 1944.

Diseases of the EYE produced rates which, in general, were higher in Ceylon. In 1942 the rate was 23 (compared with 10 on the Indo-Burma Front), in 1943 it was 16 (19), in 1944 it was 13 (13) and 19 (13) in 1945. Admissions for COMMON COLD were less in Ceylon by, on the average, 10 per 1,000. The greatest differences in rate occurred in 1943 and 1945 when rates in Ceylon were 9 and 8, while those on the Indo-Burma

Front were 34 and 22 respectively. Rates for SCABIES were also slightly lower.

DENGUE FEVER produced rates which were considerably higher in Ceylon. Whereas rates on the Indo-Burma Front varied from 2·20 in 1942 to 0·99 in 1945, those in Ceylon ranged from 17 to 4 per 1,000. Admissions for TONSILLITIS were also higher in Ceylon, but differences in rates much less. The highest rate of admission was 5·4 as against 3·4 on the Indo-Burma Front. INFECTIVE HEPATITIS was responsible for rates which, on the Indo-Burma Front, rose from 0·57 in 1942 to 13 in 1945. In Ceylon rates were highest at 7 in 1942, lowest at 4 in 1943 while in 1944 and 1945 they were slightly under 6 per 1,000.

Apart from 1944 and 1945 when there was little difference in the rates, admissions for TUBERCULOSIS were higher in Ceylon, particularly in 1943 when the rate was extremely high at 9·92 per 1,000. In that year the rates for both I.O.Rs. and N.Cs.(E.) were unprecedented. MENTAL, PSYCHONEUROTIC and PERSONALITY DISORDERS were responsible for admissions which rose from 2·6 in 1942 to 5·9 in 1944 as compared with those on the Indo-Burma Front which increased from 1·4 to 7·1.

MUMPS caused less admissions in Ceylon with rates recorded at 0·78 to 2·65 as against 5·31 to 9·96. Admissions for diseases of the CIRCULATORY SYSTEM were also considerably less, except in 1944 when the rates were almost identical. Apart from 1944, rates varied from 0·13 to 0·77 as against 2·52 to 5·19 on the Indo-Burma Front.

Summary

Indian Troops were, in general, healthier in Ceylon than on the Indo-Burma Front. Of individual diseases, there were less admissions in Ceylon for Malaria, Diarrhoea, Dysentery, Common Cold, Infective Hepatitis, Diseases of the Circulatory System and Other Diseases of the Respiratory System. Higher admission rates were registered in Ceylon by Diseases of the Eye, Tonsillitis and, in particular, Dengue Fever.

EAST AFRICAN TROOPS

EAST AFRICAN OTHER RANKS

East African Units were stationed in Ceylon from 1944 and rates of admissions in hospitals for 1944 and 1945 are presented in Table 144. As on the Indo-Burma Front, admissions of British Officers, Warrant Officers and N.C.Os. attached to these units have been excluded from this table and incorporated in their own tabulations. Admissions for Diseases were at the rates of 411 in 1944 and 388 per 1,000 in 1945. Those for Injuries were 34 and 46 respectively.

The highest rate of admissions was caused by VENEREAL DISEASES at rates of 79 and 92 per 1,000. This was exceptional in that, for all other classes of male troops, MALARIA took pride of place as causing the greatest number of admissions. Indeed, Malaria, among this class of troops was comparatively low at fifth place in the order of admissions at only 19 in 1944 and 14 in 1945.

After Venereal Diseases in numerical importance, DYSENTERY was responsible for admission rates of 37 and 17 and Other Diseases of the RESPIRATORY SYSTEM at 31 and 19. The rates for P.U.O. and N.Y.D. FEVER varied but little at 19 and 21. Admissions for Diseases of the EAR, NOSE and THROAT increased from 12 to 16 and Diseases of the EYE from 7 to 16, while those for COMMON COLD and SEPTIC CONDITIONS decreased from 16 to 11 and from 17 to 10 respectively.

Other diseases for which admissions increased in 1945 were:

Other Diseases of the DIGESTIVE SYSTEM	from	7	to	13	per 1,000
MENTAL, PSYCHONEUROTIC and PERSONALITY DISORDERS	from	3·2	to	7·1	per 1,000
INFECTIVE HEPATITIS	from	2·1	to	4·3	per 1,000
SANDFLY FEVER	from	0·65	to	2·51	per 1,000

Admissions for the following diseases decreased in 1945:

DIARRHOEA	from	17	to	5	per 1,000
Diseases of the SKIN	from	12	to	8	per 1,000
Diseases of the CIRCULATORY SYSTEM	from	5	to	2	per 1,000
TONSILLITIS	from	4	to	3	per 1,000
DENGUE FEVER	from	3·1	to	0·9	per 1,000
SCABIES	from	1·8	to	0·9	per 1,000

In 1944 there were no admissions for Disorders of NUTRITION and in 1945 none for DIPHTHERIA, MUMPS, SMALLPOX or TUBERCULOSIS.

Compared with the E.A.O.Rs. on the Indo-Burma Front, admissions for diseases were forty-four per cent. lower in 1944 and nine per cent. lower in 1945.

Admissions for Malaria were less in Ceylon in 1944 where the rate was 19 per 1,000 compared with 86 on the Indo-Burma Front, but in the following year there was but little difference in the rates. The rates for Dysentery were also higher on the Indo-Burma Front at four times in 1944 and three times in 1945. P.U.O. and N.Y.D. Fever on the Indo-Burma Front was over five times the Ceylon rate in 1944, but in 1945 was 5 per 1,000 less.

On the other hand, admissions for Venereal Diseases were higher in Ceylon by 27 per 1,000 in 1944 and 10 in 1945.

CEYLONESE TROOPS

CEYLONESE OFFICERS

Table 145 records the annual admission rates for Ceylonese Officers. The strength of these officers was comparatively small and care should be taken in drawing conclusions when comparing these rates with those of other classes of troops. Admissions for diseases only were highest in 1944 at 387 per 1,000, as were those for Injuries at 57.

MALARIA was responsible for more admissions than any other disease at an average rate of 55 per 1,000. This was followed by Other Diseases of the DIGESTIVE SYSTEM at approximately one-half the Malaria rates. COMMON COLD produced rates at 22 in 1944 and 14 in 1945.

Other diseases for which admissions decreased in 1945 were:

P.U.O. and N.Y.D. FEVER	from 35	in 1944 to	14	in 1945
SEPTIC CONDITIONS	from 10	in 1944 to	5	in 1945
INFECTIVE HEPATITIS	from 8	in 1944 to	5	in 1945
TUBERCULOSIS	from 3·38	in 1944 to	1·57	in 1945

Increases in admissions were recorded by:

Diseases of the EAR, NOSE and THROAT	from 14	in 1944 to	17	in 1945
Other Diseases of the RESPIRATORY SYSTEM	from 16	in 1944 to	19	in 1945
DIARRHOEA	from 10	in 1944 to	13	in 1945

CEYLONESE OTHER RANKS

Annual rates of admissions to hospitals in respect of Ceylonese Other Ranks are recorded in Table 146. Admissions on account of diseases declined annuallyfrom 868 in 1943 to 771 in 1944 and to 618 in 1945. The decrease in 1944 was just over ten per cent. of the 1943 rate and that in 1945 one-fifth of the previous year. Admissions for Injuries, mainly N.E.A., varied from 41 to 48 per 1,000.

As with Officers, the largest number of admissions was caused by MALARIA. The high rate of 215 in 1943 was exceeded only by British Other Ranks at 278 with Non-Combatants (Enrolled) a close third with 210. A decline of one-third to 144 was recorded in 1943 and a further fall in 1945 took the rate to 109 per 1,000. Rates for P.U.O. and N.Y.D. FEVER were 71 in 1944 and 33 in 1945.

Admission rates for COMMON COLD were surprisingly high at 82 in 1943, 90 in 1944 and 81 in 1945, as were those of Other Diseases of the RESPIRATORY SYSTEM at 29, 42 and 35 per 1,000 respectively. Other diseases of the DIGESTIVE SYSTEM caused admissions at rates of 40 in 1943, 42 in 1944 and 39 in 1945.

Next in numerical importance were VENEREAL DISEASES, admissions for which rose slightly in 1944 from 24 to 26 per 1,000. In 1945 an increase of one-third was registered and admissions rose to 33. Rates for DIARRHOEA decreased from 31 in 1943 to 25 in 1944 and 19 in 1945, and DYSENTERY from 26 to 19 and 12 respectively. Admissions for SEPTIC CONDITIONS also declined by fifty per cent. from 30 to 15.

Diseases of the EYE were responsible for rates which increased annually from 16 in 1943 to 20 in 1945. A similar trend occurred with SCABIES from 11 to 18, with MUMPS from 8 to 12, TONSILLITIS from 5 to 8 and with INFECTIVE HEPATITIS from 3 to 5 per 1,000.

Admissions for MENTAL, PSYCHONEUROTIC and PERSONALITY DISORDERS increased from 2·60 in 1943 to 4·00 in 1944 and declined to 2·51 in 1945. Rates for Diseases of the CIRCULATORY SYSTEM rose considerably in 1944, from 0·14 to 7·18 and decreased in 1945 to 0·98. DENGUE FEVER rates were comparatively low and varied little at 1·30, 1·76 and 0·81 respectively. Admissions for TUBERCULOSIS were relatively low in 1943 at 0·28 but rose to 0·90 and 0·94 in the two ensuing years.

No admissions were recorded for SANDFLY FEVER or for the ENTERIC Group of FEVERS in 1945 and there were none for SMALLPOX or for Disorders of NUTRITION in 1943 and 1944.

ALL CEYLONESE TROOPS

In Table 147 are presented the admission rates to hospitals for All Ceylonese Troops. As their composition was predominantly Other Ranks, rates and trends tend to follow those of the Other Ranks (*see* Table 146).

Rates of admissions for diseases experienced by these troops were higher than those for any other class of troops. Admission rates of British Troops were from eighty to ninety-three per cent. those of Ceylonese and Indians from seventy-six to eighty-two per cent. A comparative table is given below.

Ceylon
Comparative Table of Admissions
All Ceylonese, British and Indian Troops, 1943–45

	1943	1944	1945
Ceylonese Troops	100	100	100
British Troops	93	80	91
Indian Troops	82	80	76

Except for COMMON COLD, admissions for which were, on the average, over 60 per 1,000 in excess of those of British or Indian Troops, no individual diseases were responsible for excessive admissions among Ceylonese Troops.

ALL TROOPS

Table 148 records the admission rates to hospitals of All Troops in Ceylon. Rates for diseases only decreased annually from 702 to 418, a decline of forty per cent. This compares with rates on the Indo-Burma Front from 1,151 (in 1943) to 462, a decline of sixty per cent.

In each year, MALARIA caused the greatest number of admissions among individual diseases. Rates increased in 1943 from 156 to 166. This was due to the inclusion, in that year, of Ceylonese Troops whose Other Ranks were responsible for the high admission rate of 215 per 1,000. In 1944 there was a decline by slightly over forty per cent. to 96, and in the following year the rate was even lower at 70. A comparison of these rates with those for All Troops on the Indo-Burma Front is interesting.

Admissions for Malaria. All Troops
Comparison of Rates on the Indo-Burma Front with Ceylon, 1942–45

	1942	1943	1944	1945
Crude rates				
Indo-Burma Front	395	491	329	63
Ceylon	156	166	96	70
Comparative Rates (Indo-Burma Front = 100)				
Indo-Burma Front .	100	100	100	100
Ceylon	40	34	29	111
Comparative Rates (1942 = 100)				
Indo-Burma Front	100	124	83	16
Ceylon	100	106	62	45
Comparative Rates (Preceding year = 100)				
Indo-Burma Front	—	124	67	19
Ceylon	—	106	58	73

During the years 1942 to 1944 the Ceylon rate for Malaria was between thirty and forty per cent. of that on the Indo-Burma Front, but in 1945 it was ten per cent. higher. Taking the 1942 rates as a base, the Ceylon rate in 1943 and 1944 was eighteen and twenty-one points lower but in 1945 was twenty-nine points higher. When compared with rates of the preceding year, in 1943 the Ceylon rate was 106 against 124, in 1944, 55 against 67 and in 1945, 73 compared with 19. It would appear that the Anti-Malaria campaign was somewhat more successful in Ceylon in 1944, but this was overshadowed by the overwhelming reduction of admissions on the Indo-Burma Front in 1945.

The decline in admissions in respect of DENGUE FEVER was also impressive. In 1942 there were 37 admissions per 1,000 troops; in 1943 and 1944 rates of 15 and 12 were recorded. In 1945 admissions had fallen to under 4 per 1,000, at ten per cent. the rate for 1942. Admissions for SEPTIC CONDITIONS also declined considerably from 53 to 16 per 1,000, as did DIARRHOEA from 25 to 12, TONSILLITIS from 12 to 6, and Other Diseases of the DIGESTIVE SYSTEM from 33 to 24. Rates for VENEREAL DISEASES were 51 in 1942, 40 in 1943, 42 in 1944 and 30 in 1945.

Among British and Indian Troops, admissions for COMMON COLD declined, in general, over the years. That this is not duplicated in Table 148 is due to the abnormally high rates experienced by Ceylonese Other Ranks at over 80 per 1,000 during the last three years of the period under review. This caused the All Troops rate of 28 in 1942 to increase in 1943 and again in 1944 when it was 33, before declining to 27 in 1945.

Increases in admission rates were recorded by Other Diseases of the RESPIRATORY SYSTEM from 13 to 21, SCABIES from 7 to 12, and MENTAL, PSYCHONEUROTIC and PERSONALITY DISORDERS from 2·7 to 4·0 per 1,000.

INJURIES

Table 149 records the rates of admissions to hospitals on account of injuries. As on the Indo-Burma Front, injuries have been classified according to whether they were caused by enemy action (E.A.) or otherwise (N.E.A.). The former have been sub-divided into Bomb, Gunshot, and Shell wounds, but N.E.A. Injuries were not sub-divided until 1945 and then only as to 'Burns and Scalds' and 'Others'.

Admissions for Injuries ranged from 49 per 1,000 in 1942 to 32 in 1945, with 38 and 41 respectively in the two intervening years. In 1942 they accounted for six per cent. of the total admissions; in 1943 they were less by one per cent., but in 1944 and 1945 they represented seven per cent. of all admissions. This increase in relative rates is, of course, due to the decline in admissions from disease.

N.E.A. Injuries

As Ceylon suffered comparatively little from enemy action, admissions on account of N.E.A. Injuries were much higher than those for E.A. Injuries, being from ninety-six to ninety-nine per cent. of all injuries. The table below relating to N.E.A. Injuries, and condensed from Table 149, compares the admission rates by the various categories of troops.

As on the Indo-Burma Front, British Other Ranks suffered more injuries than any other class of troops. Indeed, only once were they

Admissions to Hospital. N.E.A. Injuries
All categories of Male Troops, 1942–45. Crude and Comparative Rates

	Crude Rates				Comparative Rates (B.O.Rs. = 100)			
	1942	1943	1944	1945	1942	1943	1944	1945
British Other Ranks	66	51	55	47	100	100	100	100
British Officers	66	41	50	38	100	80	93	81
V.C.Os. and I.O.Rs.	65	47	52	43	98	92	96	91
N.Cs.(E.)	38	25	27	14	58	49	50	30
Ceylonese Officers	—	43	57	30	—	84	106	64
Ceylonese Other Ranks	—	41	48	43	—	80	89	91
E.A.O.Rs.	—	—	34	45	—	—	63	96

exceeded, in 1944, by Ceylonese Officers. B.O.Rs. produced rates which varied between 66 per 1,000 in 1942 and 47 in 1945. This compares with 33 to 64 on the Indo-Burma Front. N.E.A. Injury rates for V.C.Os. and I.O.Rs. were over ninety per cent. of those for B.O.Rs., at from 66 to 43 per 1,000. Those for British Officers were also comparatively high from 65 to 38 per 1,000. Admissions for N.Cs.(E.) were lowest with rates which varied from 38 per 1,000 in 1942 to 14 in 1945. This low rate of 14 per 1,000 was the lowest recorded for any class of troops in Ceylon, India, or on the Indo-Burma Front.

E.A. Injuries

Rates of admission on account of Enemy Action Injuries were 1·80 in 1942, 0·44 in 1943, 0·31 in 1944 and 0·07 in 1945. The majority of admissions in 1942 were among British Troops whose rate was 5·66. Very few casualties occurred among Ceylonese Troops or East African Other Ranks and among Non-Combatants (Enrolled) E.A., injuries were recorded only in 1942.

DEATHS

Information regarding deaths in hospitals is even more meagre than is similar data for the Indo-Burma Front. All that is known are the rates per 1.000, by class of personnel, for each year (Table 150).

The highest mortality rates were recorded by E.A.O.Rs. at 3·56 in 1944 and 2·29 in 1945. N.Cs.(E.) provided the next highest rates which varied from 2·13 to 3·22. This is surprising as they registered, on the whole, admission rates which were lower than any other class. Rates recorded by British Officers varied from 1·77 to 3·85 and those for British Other Ranks were 1·66 to 2·72. There was but little difference between the rates for V.C.Os. and I.O.Rs. and those for Ceylonese

Other Ranks at the range from 1·54 to 2·36 per 1,000. No deaths occurred among Indian Officers or members of the I.M.N.S. during the four years or among Ceylonese Officers in 1943.

MEDICAL ETHNOGRAPHY IN CEYLON

Due to the varying periods in which the various classes of troops were stationed in Ceylon, it is not possible to present an ethnographical comparison of admissions for all groups based on a period of longer than two years. Some classes were on the Island for two and others for three and four years and as, naturally, assumptions based on long periods are more valid than others, the following discussion has been divided into three parts:

(i) B.O.Rs. and V.C.Os. and I.O.Rs. for the four years, 1942 to 1945.
(ii) B.O.Rs., V.C.Os. and I.O.Rs., and Ceylonese Other Ranks for the three years, 1943 to 1945, and
(iii) B.O.Rs., V.C.Os. and I.O.Rs., Ceylonese Other Ranks, and East African Other Ranks for the two years 1944 and 1945.

B.O.RS., V.C.OS., AND I.O.RS.

Table 151 records the comparative rates of admissions to hospitals, on account of diseases only, in respect of B.O.Rs., V.C.Os. and I.O.Rs. The rates are based on average admissions of the four years, 1942 to 1945.

The total disease rate of I.O.Rs. was between eighty and ninety per cent. of that for B.O.Rs. Of the twenty-five diseases and disease groups listed in the table, nine recorded rates which, among Indians, were higher than those for B.O.Rs. Experience elsewhere indicated that the incidence of MUMPS among Indians was likely to be very much more than among the British and that the rates of admission for SCABIES, TUBERCULOSIS and DISEASES of the EYE would probably be twice as high. These indications were fully realised. The Indian rate for MUMPS was twelve times that for B.O.Rs., that for SCABIES three times, and TUBERCULOSIS and Diseases of the EYE were twice as high. Also double the B.O.R. rate was that for Diseases of the RESPIRATORY SYSTEM. Other diseases which registered rates above those of B.O.Rs. were P.U.O. and N.Y.D. FEVER, Diseases due to Disorders of NUTRITION, Diseases of the EAR, NOSE and THROAT, and SMALLPOX. Rates for these were between twenty-five and fifty per cent. higher than those for B.O.Rs.

At the other end of the scale, the ENTERIC Group of FEVERS caused admissions among B.O.Rs. at rates which were fourteen times those of I.O.Rs., with DENGUE FEVER and TONSILLITIS at four times, and Other Diseases of the SKIN at three times, the Indian rates. Admissions for VENEREAL DISEASES and DIPHTHERIA among I.O.Rs. were approximately three-fifths those of B.O.Rs.; those for INFECTIVE HEPATITIS and MENTAL, PSYCHONEUROTIC and PERSONALITY DISORDERS were slightly higher, with DYSENTERY and Diseases of the CIRCULATORY SYSTEM at three-quarters of the British rate.

There was but little difference in the rates for other diseases included in the table.

Summary

Morbidity rates in Ceylon for B.O.Rs. as compared with V.C.Os. and I.O.Rs. may be summarised as below.

Diseases with a comparatively high rate (in descending order)	Diseases with a comparatively low rate (in descending order)	Diseases with little differences in rates
Enteric Group of Fevers	P.U.O. and N.Y.D. Fever	Diarrhoea
Dengue Fever	Diseases of the Respiratory System	Sandfly Fever
Tonsillitis	Diseases of the Eye	Other Diseases of the Digestive System
Diseases of the Skin	Tuberculosis	Malaria
Venereal Diseases	Scabies	Septic Conditions
Diphtheria	Mumps	Common Cold

B.O.RS., CEYLONESE O.RS. AND V.C.OS. AND I.O.RS.

In Table 152 are the comparative rates of admission of British, Ceylonese and Indian Other Ranks. As these rates are based on the three years 1943 to 1945 the rates shown for Indian Other Ranks differ somewhat from those given in Table 151, which were based on admissions for four years. This is exemplified in the total admissions for disease for which the comparative Indian rate for 1942–45 was 86 and, for 1943–45 it was 89. Again the comparative Indian rate for Mumps for 1942–45 was 1,243 whereas for the shorter period it increased to 1,936.

Although it produced admission rates of a relatively low order, MUMPS, much more predominant among Ceylonese, was highest on the list of comparative rates for both the non-European classes. COMMON COLD was also prevalent among Ceylonese at between five and seven times the British rates. Other Diseases of the RESPIRATORY SYSTEM, and Diseases due to Disorders of NUTRITION were other diseases, the rates for which were high among the Ceylonese, lower among Indians and still lower for B.O.Rs.

There was little difference between the non-European rates for SCABIES, or for Diseases of the EYE which were nearly three times and double the British rate respectively. Admission rates for P.U.O. and N.Y.D. Fever among the Ceylonese and Indians were one and a half times those for B.O.Rs. while the Ceylonese rate for MALARIA was twenty-five and the Indian ten per cent. higher than the British rate. The SANDFLY FEVER rate among Indians was approximately one and a half times that for the other two groups.

Admissions for DYSENTERY among non-Europeans were in the vicinity of three-quarters of the British rate, but while the Indian rate for DIARRHOEA was ten per cent. lower, that for Ceylonese was fourteen per cent. higher.

TUBERCULOSIS provided the only example of a disease the rate for which was high among one class of non-Europeans and low among the other. Compared with B.O.Rs. the Indian rate was twice as high, whereas that for the Ceylonese was one-third. The high Indian rate was partly due to an unusually large number of admissions in 1942. Had the disease followed the normal trend, the rates of British admissions to Indian and Ceylonese may have been in the region of 3 : 2·5 : 1.

VENEREAL DISEASES and MENTAL, PSYCHONEUROTIC and PERSONALITY DISORDERS produced comparative rates of approximately 70 among Indians and 50 among Ceylonese, while there was little difference in the rates for Diseases of the SKIN at 40, and TONSILLITIS at one-third the British rate. Admissions of Non-Europeans for DIPHTHERIA were one-twentieth of the rate for B.O.Rs. and the comparative rates for DENGUE FEVER were 3 for Ceylonese as against 24 for Indians.

BRITISH, EAST AFRICAN, INDIAN AND CEYLONESE OTHER RANKS

Comparative rates of admissions to hospitals for disease in respect of these classes of troops are contained in Table 153, and are based on the average of known admissions for 1944 and 1945. The order of admissions was Ceylonese at 117, British at 100, Indians at 91 and East Africans at 34.

In only two diseases were the admission rates of each of the non-European groups higher than those for B.O.Rs. These were Mumps and Common Cold. The comparative rates for MUMPS were extremely high at 7,200 for Ceylonese, 1,600 for Indians and 600 for East Africans. For COMMON COLD, the Ceylonese again took pride of place at over eight times, with Indians at approximately one and a half times and East African slightly above, the British rate.

Other features of this table are:

(i) B.O.Rs. were more liable to be admitted for VENEREAL DISEASES, the ENTERIC Group of FEVERS, INFECTIVE HEPATITIS, SEPTIC CONDITIONS, SMALLPOX and TUBERCULOSIS. They were also prone to MENTAL, PSYCHONEUROTIC and PERSONALITY DISORDERS, TONSILLITIS, Diseases of the SKIN, DENGUE FEVER and DIPHTHERIA.

(ii) British and East African troops were more prone to DYSENTERY.

(iii) British and Ceylonese were more liable to contract DIARRHOEA and Diseases of the CIRCULATORY SYSTEM.

(iv) Indians and Ceylonese were more susceptible to Diseases of the EYE, Other Diseases of the RESPIRATORY SYSTEM, MALARIA, P.U.O. and N.Y.D. FEVER, Diseases due to Disorders of NUTRITION, and SCABIES.

(v) Ceylonese Other Ranks were more prone to Other Diseases of the DIGESTIVE SYSTEM.

(vi) East Africans were less likely to contract Diseases of the EAR, NOSE and THROAT.

These indications may be summarised as below:

DISEASE	Prone	Less Prone
Mumps	Ceylonese, Indians, East Africans	British
Common Cold	Ceylonese, Indians	British
Other Diseases of the Respiratory System	Ceylonese, Indians	British, East Africans
Diseases of the Eye	Ceylonese, Indians	British, East Africans
Malaria	Ceylonese, Indians	British, East Africans
P.U.O. and N.Y.D. Fever	Ceylonese, Indians	East Africans
Disorders of Nutrition	Ceylonese, Indians	East Africans
Dysentery	British, East Africans	Ceylonese
Diseases of the Ear, Nose and Throat	Indians, British, Ceylonese	East Africans
Venereal Diseases	British	Ceylonese
Enteric Group of Fevers	British	Indians, Ceylonese, East Africans
Mental, Psychoneurotic and Personality Disorders	British	East Africans, Ceylonese
Infective Hepatitis	British	East Africans
Smallpox	British	East Africans, Ceylonese
Tuberculosis	British	East Africans, Ceylonese
Septic Conditions	British	East Africans, Ceylonese
Tonsillitis	British	East Africans, Indians, Ceylonese
Diseases of the Skin	British	East Africans, Indians, Ceylonese
Diphtheria	British	East Africans, Indians, Ceylonese
Dengue Fever	British	East Africans, Ceylonese, Indians
Diarrhoea	Ceylonese, British	East Africans, Indians
Diseases of the Circulatory System	Ceylonese, British	East Africans
Other Diseases of the Digestive System	Ceylonese	East Africans
Scabies	Ceylonese, Indians	East Africans, British

TABLE 136

South-East Asia Command (Ceylon)
Causes of Admissions to Hospitals, 1942–45
British Officers. Annual Rates per 1,000 Strength

Source: A.F. A.31-B

	CAUSES	1942	1943	1944	1945	
1	Common Cold	19·65	11·50	13·95	15·83	1
2	Diarrhoea	25·96	20·35	26·94	17·27	2
3	Dysentery	27·92	29·20	27·42	26·86	3
4	Dengue Fever	111·69	60·18	57·72	10·07	4
5	Diphtheria	7·24	*	3·37	0·48	5
6	Enteric Group of Fevers	—	0·44	0·96	—	6
7	Infective Hepatitis	23·78	5·31	12·51	7·19	7
8	Malaria	135·47	132·30	70·71	33·09	8
9	Mumps	1·03	0·88	—	0·48	9
10	Pneumonia	*	*	*	0·96	10
11	P.U.O. and N.Y.D. Fever	*	*	58·20	28·78	11
12	Sandfly Fever	—	—	—	—	12
13	Scabies	—	1·33	1·44	0·48	13
14	Smallpox	—	—	—	—	14
15	Tonsillitis	22·75	11·50	14·91	19·18	15
16	Tuberculosis	2·07	1·33	0·48	0·48	16
17	Venereal Diseases	9·31	7·08	17·32	8·63	17
18	Diseases of the Circulatory System	—	0·44	2·89	4·80	18
19	Diseases due to Disorders of Nutrition	—	—	—	—	19
20	Diseases of the Ear, Nose and Throat	*	*	14·91	6·23	20
21	Diseases of the Eye	7·23	1·77	7·69	4·32	21
22	Diseases of the Skin (other than Scabies)	*	*	43·29	49·40	22
23	Other Diseases of the Digestive System	73·42	41·59	45·69	29·74	23
24	Other Diseases of the Respiratory System	9·31	2·21	19·24	9·59	24
25	Septic Conditions	85·83	28·32	30·78	18·22	25
26	Mental, Psychoneurotic and Personality Disorders	6·20	3·10	6·25	8·63	26
27	All Other Diseases	288·43	273·03	146·23	141·98	27
28	*Total Admissions for Diseases*	857·29	631·86	622·90	442·69	28
29	Injuries—N.E.A.	65·15	41·15	50·02	38·37	29
30	Injuries—E.A.	10·34	1·33	1·44	0·48	30
31	*Total Admissions for Injuries*	75·49	42·48	51·46	38·85	31
32	*Total Admissions*	932·78	674·34	674·36	481·53	32

* Any cases included in 'All Other Diseases'.

TABLE 137

South-East Asia Command (Ceylon)
Causes of Admissions to Hospitals, 1942–45
British Other Ranks. Annual Rates per 1,000 Strength

Source: A.F. A.31-B

	CAUSES	1942	1943	1944	1945	
1	Common Cold	29·88	17·44	12·57	7·71	1
2	Diarrhoea	35·20	15·34	16·61	21·03	2
3	Dysentery	27·81	25·23	29·37	29·34	3
4	Dengue Fever	78·83	54·11	53·08	19·81	4
5	Diphtheria	1·58	0·68	3·93	0·15	5
6	Enteric Group of Fevers	2·46	0·31	0·77	0·30	6
7	Infective Hepatitis	8·50	5·87	9·79	9·38	7
8	Malaria	278·13	253·80	81·97	36·00	8
9	Mumps	0·32	—	0·10	0·15	9
10	Pneumonia	*	*	*	—	10
11	P.U.O. and N.Y.D. Fever	*	*	44·06	24·23	11
12	Sandfly Fever	2·15	0·37	1·06	0·45	12
13	Scabies	4·85	4·45	3·84	6·96	13
14	Smallpox	—	—	0·19	0·15	14
15	Tonsillitis	33·38	15·15	12·67	16·49	15
16	Tuberculosis	1·35	1·55	3·36	1·51	16
17	Venereal Diseases	112·68	62·52	46·84	61·56	17
18	Diseases of the Circulatory System	0·08	0·18	3·17	3·93	18
19	Diseases due to Disorders of Nutrition	—	—	—	0·76	19
20	Diseases of the Ear, Nose and Throat	*	*	20·73	19·81	20
21	Diseases of the Eye	11·44	7·30	6·43	9·68	21
22	Diseases of the Skin (other than Scabies)	*	*	47·99	68·82	22
23	Other Diseases of the Digestive System	42·04	40·01	33·02	31·16	23
24	Other Diseases of the Respiratory System	8·18	3·46	16·03	13·76	24
25	Septic Conditions	88·37	31·72	29·28	31·62	25
26	Mental, Psychoneurotic and Personality Disorders	5·48	3·77	4·89	10·29	26
27	All Other Diseases	321·22	269·97	120·48	159·28	27
28	*Total Admissions for Diseases*	1,093·93	813·23	602·23	584·33	28
29	Injuries—N.E.A.	66·43	50·96	54·62	46·89	29
30	Injuries—E.A.	5·32	0·49	0·67	0·15	30
31	*Total Admissions for Injuries*	71·75	51·45	55·29	47·04	31
32	*Total Admissions*	1,165·69	864·69	657·52	631·37	32

* Any cases included in 'All Other Diseases'.

TABLE 138

South-East Asia Command (Ceylon)
Causes of Admissions to Hospitals, 1942–45
All British Troops. Annual Rates per 1,000 Strength

Source: A.F. A.31-B

	CAUSES	1942	1943	1944	1945	
1	Common Cold	29·49	16·99	12·83	9·73	1
2	Diarrhoea	34·93	16·01	18·24	20·81	2
3	Dysentery	28·24	25·81	29·32	29·09	3
4	Dengue Fever	82·28	55·56	54·49	19·69	4
5	Diphtheria	1·98	0·59	3·90	0·22	5
6	Enteric Group of Fevers	2·28	0·32	0·80	0·34	6
7	Infective Hepatitis	9·63	5·79	10·36	8·73	7
8	Malaria	267·22	238·22	79·91	35·91	8
9	Mumps	0·37	0·11	0·08	0·34	9
10	Pneumonia	*	*	*	0·22	10
11	P.U.O. and N.Y.D. Fever	*	*	46·21	28·64	11
12	Sandfly Fever	1·98	0·32	0·88	0·34	12
13	Scabies	4·49	4·06	3·43	5·26	13
14	Smallpox	—	—	0·16	0·11	14
15	Tonsillitis	32·72	15·09	13·07	17·79	15
16	Tuberculosis	1·40	1·51	2·95	1·23	16
17	Venereal Diseases	104·93	55·56	41·75	47·75	17
18	Diseases of the Circulatory System	0·07	0·22	3·11	4·25	18
19	Diseases due to Disorders of Nutrition	—	—	—	—	19
20	Diseases of the Ear, Nose and Throat	*	*	19·84	16·78	20
21	Diseases of the Eye	11·17	6·60	6·62	8·17	21
22	Diseases of the Skin (other than Scabies)	*	*	47·24	63·55	22
23	Other Diseases of the Digestive System	44·34	40·20	34·97	32·33	23
24	Other Diseases of the Respiratory System	8·31	3·52	0·16	12·75	24
25	Septic Conditions	88·61	31·43	28·60	25·17	25
26	Mental, Psychoneurotic and Personality Disorders	5·51	3·79	5·18	9·96	26
27	All Other Diseases	319·47	272·00	142·66	158·68	27
28	*Total Admissions for Diseases*	1,079·42	793·70	606·76	557·84	28
29	Injuries—N.E.A.	66·40	49·94	53·62	43·97	29
30	Injuries—E.A.	5·66	0·59	0·80	0·22	30
31	*Total Admissions for Injuries*	72·06	50·53	54·42	44·19	31
32	*Total Admissions*	1,151·48	844·24	661·17	602·04	32

* Any cases included in 'All Other Diseases'.

TABLE 139

South-East Asia Command (Ceylon)
Causes of Admissions to Hospitals, 1942–44
Indian Officers. Annual Rates per 1,000 Strength

Source: A.F. A.31-B

	CAUSE	1942	1943	1944	
1	Common Cold	—	—	—	1
2	Diarrhoea	*	11·1	*	2
3	Dysentery	41·2	33·3	6·8	3
4	Dengue Fever	51·6	11·1	6·8	4
5	Diphtheria	—	—	—	5
6	Enteric Group of Fevers	—	—	—	6
7	Infective Hepatitis	—	—	—	7
8	Malaria	72·2	66·7	40·5	8
9	Mumps	—	—	—	9
10	Pneumonia	—	—	—	10
11	P.U.O. and N.Y.D. Fever	—	—	6·8	11
12	Sandfly Fever	—	—	—	12
13	Scabies	—	—	—	13
14	Smallpox	—	—	—	14
15	Tonsillitis	20·6	*	*	15
16	Tuberculosis	—	11·1	—	16
17	Venereal Diseases	*	22·2	*	17
18	Diseases of the Circulatory System	*	*	6·8	18
19	Diseases due to Disorders of Nutrition	—	—	—	19
20	Diseases of the Ear, Nose and Throat	*	*	20·3	20
21	Diseases of the Eye	—	—	—	21
22	Diseases of the Skin (other than Scabies)	*	*	13·5	22
23	Other Diseases of the Digestive System	10·3	44·4	27·0	23
24	Other Diseases of the Respiratory System	20·6	*	13·5	24
25	Septic Conditions	20·6	11·1	20·3	25
26	Mental, Psychoneurotic and Personality Disorders	*	22·2	*	26
27	All Other Diseases	154·6	133·3	81·1	27
28	*Total Admissions for Diseases*	391·8	366·7	243·2	28
29	Injuries—N.E.A.	41·2	11·1	33·8	29
30	Injuries—E.A.	—	—	—	30
31	*Total Admissions for Injuries*	41·2	11·1	33·8	31
32	*Total Admissions*	433·0	377·8	277·0	32

* Any cases included in 'All Other Diseases'.

Note: No data are available for 1945

TABLE 140

South-East Asia Command (Ceylon)
Causes of Admissions to Hospitals, 1942–45
V.C.Os. and I.O.Rs. Annual Rates per 1,000 Strength

Source: A.F. A.31-B

	CAUSES	1942	1943	1944	1945	
1	Common Cold	17·78	8·96	25·96	8·38	1
2	Diarrhoea	31·38	22·13	14·01	11·38	2
3	Dysentery	18·97	22·52	24·79	18·78	3
4	Dengue Fever	16·79	10·61	15·82	3·77	4
5	Diphtheria	0·06	—	0·12	0·21	5
6	Enteric Group of Fevers	0·13	0·08	0·06	—	6
7	Infective Hepatitis	6·77	3·61	5·63	5·86	7
8	Malaria	194·66	188·96	155·54	64·56	8
9	Mumps	2·12	0·78	1·41	2·65	9
10	Pneumonia	*	*	*	3·28	10
11	P.U.O. and N.Y.D. Fever	*	*	66·63	34·76	11
12	Sandfly Fever	1·26	1·13	1·58	—	12
13	Scabies	15·86	15·96	10·14	16·47	13
14	Smallpox	0·06	0·13	0·06	0·14	14
15	Tonsillitis	5·31	4·13	4·57	5·02	15
16	Tuberculosis	3·52	9·96	1·70	1·19	16
17	Venereal Diseases	46·64	44·48	39·85	36·85	17
18	Diseases of the Circulatory System	0·13	0·22	4·45	0·77	18
19	Diseases due to Disorders of Nutrition	—	—	1·05	—	19
20	Diseases of the Ear, Nose and Throat	*	*	25·02	28·06	20
21	Diseases of the Eye	22·89	16·17	12·66	18·64	21
22	Diseases of the Skin (other than Scabies)	*	*	20·92	21·64	22
23	Other Diseases of the Digestive System	50·42	28·22	31·53	28·34	23
24	Other Diseases of the Respiratory System	16·52	7·35	27·20	27·99	24
25	Septic Conditions	71·66	44·13	21·80	24·50	25
26	Mental, Psychoneurotic and Personality Disorders	2·65	2·87	4·57	5·86	26
27	All Other Diseases	341·38	270·93	96·77	94·57	27
28	*Total Admissions for Diseases*	867·04	703·33	613·84	463·67	28
29	Injuries—N.E.A.	65·09	47·22	51·63	42·93	29
30	Injuries—E.A.	0·67	0·83	0·35	0·07	30
31	*Total Admissions for Injuries*	65·76	48·05	51·98	43·00	31
32	*Total Admissions*	932·79	751·38	665·82	506·67	32

* Any cases included in 'All Other Cases'.

TABLE 141

South-East Asia Command (Ceylon)
Causes of Admissions to Hospitals, 1942–45
Non-Combatants (Enrolled). Annual Rates per 1,000 Strength

Source: A.F. A.31-B

	CAUSES	1942	1943	1944	1945	
1	Common Cold	12·78	17·60	10·90	2·56	1
2	Diarrhoea	21·00	10·64	8·46	4·09	2
3	Dysentery	10·35	12·77	18·54	9·75	3
4	Dengue Fever	24·95	12·77	5·74	1·20	4
5	Diphtheria	0·30	0·19	0·08	—	5
6	Enteric Group of Fevers	—	0·19	0·16	0·20	6
7	Infective Hepatitis	2·13	2·32	4·29	1·90	7
8	Malaria	210·29	156·32	97·36	61·22	8
9	Mumps	0·91	0·97	0·99	2·03	9
10	Pneumonia	*	*	*	0·63	10
11	P.U.O. and N.Y.D. Fever	*	*	36·99	21·50	11
12	Sandfly Fever	0·91	0·39	0·25	—	12
13	Scabies	7·00	9·87	5·82	7·59	13
14	Smallpox	0·30	—	0·04	0·07	14
15	Tonsillitis	2·43	3·48	3·43	1·16	15
16	Tuberculosis	2·74	6·96	1·16	0·60	16
17	Venereal Diseases	72·43	56·10	21·39	9·48	17
18	Diseases of the Circulatory System	—	0·97	1·94	0·17	18
19	Diseases due to Disorders of Nutrition	—	—	0·74	0·10	19
20	Diseases of the Ear, Nose and Throat	*	*	9·50	10·35	20
21	Diseases of the Eye	17·04	10·64	4·95	4·56	21
22	Diseases of the Skin (other than Scabies)	*	*	8·67	5·62	22
23	Other Diseases of the Digestive System	31·95	50·69	17·34	8·85	23
24	Other Diseases of the Respiratory System	8·52	6·38	22·46	11·21	24
25	Septic Conditions	33·47	27·66	20·07	11·21	25
26	Mental, Psychoneurotic and Personality Disorders	1·52	4·06	3·18	2·23	26
27	All Other Diseases	316·52	276·08	56·41	30·31	27
28	*Total Admissions for Diseases*	777·54	667·05	360·86	208·59	28
29	Injuries—N.E.A.	38·34	24·76	26·80	13·84	29
30	Injuries—E.A.	0·30	—	—	—	30
31	*Total Admissions for Injuries*	38·64	24·76	26·80	13·84	31
32	*Total Admissions*	816·19	691·82	387·65	222·43	32

* Any cases included in 'All Other Diseases'.

TABLE 142

South-East Asia Command (Ceylon)
Causes of Admissions to Hospitals, 1942–45
Indian Military Nursing Services. Annual Rates per 1,000 Strength

Source: A.F. A.31-B

	CAUSES	1942	1943	1944	1945	
1	Common Cold	—	11·9	*	*	1
2	Diarrhoea	—	11·9	*	*	2
3	Dysentery	—	23·8	29·4	*	3
4	Dengue Fever	—	—	29·4	—	4
5	Diphtheria	—	—	—	—	5
6	Enteric Group of Fevers	—	—	—	—	6
7	Infective Hepatitis	—	—	—	—	7
8	Malaria	—	23·8	29·4	*	8
9	Mumps	—	—	—	—	9
10	Pneumonia	—	—	—	—	10
11	P.U.O. and N.Y.D. Fever	—	—	—	—	11
12	Sandfly Fever	—	—	—	—	12
13	Scabies	—	—	—	—	13
14	Smallpox	—	—	—	—	14
15	Tonsillitis	—	—	—	—	15
16	Tuberculosis	—	—	—	—	16
17	Venereal Diseases	—	—	—	—	17
18	Diseases of the Circulatory System	—	—	—	—	18
19	Diseases due to Disorders of Nutrition	—	—	—	—	19
20	Diseases of the Ear, Nose and Throat	—	—	29·4	55·6	20
21	Diseases of the Eye	—	11·9	*	*	21
22	Diseases of the Skin (excluding Scabies)	—	—	—	—	22
23	Other Diseases of the Digestive System	50·0	23·8	29·4	*	23
24	Other Diseases of the Respiratory System	—	—	29·4	*	24
25	Septic Conditions	100·0	71·4	*	*	25
26	Mental, Psychoneurotic and Personality Disorders	—	—	—	—	26
27	All Other Diseases	100·0	119·1	206·0	277·8	27
28	*Total Admissions for Diseases*	250·0	297·6	382·4	333·3	28
29	Injuries—N.E.A.	—	11·9	—	—	29
30	Injuries—E.A.	—	—	—	—	30
31	*Total Admissions for Injuries*	—	11·9	—	—	31
32	*Total Admissions*	250·0	309·5	382·4	333·3	32

* Any cases included in 'All Other Diseases'.

TABLE 143

South-East Asia Command (Ceylon)
Causes of Admissions to Hospitals, 1942–45
All Indian Troops. Annual Rates per 1,000 Strength

Source: A.F. A.31-B

	CAUSES	1942	1943	1944	1945	
1	Common Cold	17·64	8·93	25·69	8·36	1
2	Diarrhoea	31·14	22·05	13·86	11·36	2
3	Dysentery	19·09	22·57	24·64	18·75	3
4	Dengue Fever	16·99	10·97	15·77	3·76	4
5	Diphtheria	0·07	0·00	0·12	0·21	5
6	Enteric Group of Fevers	0·13	0·09	0·06	—	6
7	Infective Hepatitis	6·71	3·58	5·57	5·86	7
8	Malaria	193·63	187·89	154·30	64·48	8
9	Mumps	2·11	0·78	1·39	2·65	9
10	Pneumonia	*	*	*	3·28	10
11	P.U.O. and N.Y.D. Fever	*	*	65·99	34·72	11
12	Sandfly Fever	1·25	1·12	1·57	0·00	12
13	Scabies	15·73	15·84	10·03	16·45	13
14	Smallpox	0·07	0·13	0·06	0·14	14
15	Tonsillitis	5·40	4·10	4·52	5·02	15
16	Tuberculosis	3·49	9·92	1·68	1·18	16
17	Venereal Diseases	46·28	44·23	39·43	36·81	17
18	Diseases of the Circulatory System	0·13	0·22	4·46	0·77	18
19	Diseases due to Disorders of Nutrition	—	—	1·04	0·00	19
20	Diseases of the Ear, Nose and Throat	*	*	24·99	26·09	20
21	Diseases of the Eye	22·72	16·10	12·52	18·62	21
22	Diseases of the Skin (other than Scabies)	*	*	20·99	21·61	22
23	Other Diseases of the Disgestive System	50·17	28·27	31·49	28·30	23
24	Other Diseases of the Respiratory System	16·52	7·29	27·08	27·95	24
25	Septic Conditions	71·37	44·10	22·49	24·54	25
26	Mental, Psychoneurotic and Personality Disorders	2·63	2·93	4·52	5·86	26
27	All Other Diseases	339·92	269·45	95·95	96·74	27
28	*Total Admissions for Diseases*	863·19	700·56	610·21	463·51	28
29	Injuries—N.E.A.	64·85	46·95	51·38	42·87	29
30	Injuries—E.A.	0·66	0·82	0·36	0·07	30
31	*Total Admissions for Injuries*	65·51	47·77	51·74	42·94	31
32	*Total Admissions*	928·70	748·33	661·93	506·45	32

* Any cases included in 'All Other Diseases'.

TABLE 144

South East Asia Command (Ceylon)
Causes of Admissions to Hospitals, 1944–45
East African Other Ranks. Annual Rates per 1,000 Strength

Source: A.F. A.31-B

	CAUSES	1944	1945	
1	Common Cold	16·04	10·97	1
2	Diarrhoea	16·93	5·03	2
3	Dysentery	36·85	17·15	3
4	Dengue Fever	3·12	0·91	4
5	Diphtheria	0·04	—	5
6	Enteric Group of Fevers	4·86	*	6
7	Infective Hepatitis	2·06	4·34	7
8	Malaria	19·27	14·40	8
9	Mumps	1·58	—	9
10	Pneumonia	*	2·29	10
11	P.U.O. and N.Y.D. Fever	18·99	21·03	11
12	Sandfly Fever	0·65	2·51	12
13	Scabies	1·82	0·91	13
14	Smallpox	0·04	—	14
15	Tonsillitis	3·81	2·74	15
16	Tuberculosis	0·57	—	16
17	Venereal Diseases	79·33	92·13	17
18	Diseases of the Circulatory System	5·26	2·06	18
19	Diseases due to Disorders of Nutrition	—	0·23	19
20	Diseases of the Ear, Nose and Throat	11·58	16·46	20
21	Diseases of the Eye	6·59	16·23	21
22	Diseases of the Skin (other than Scabies)	12·39	7·77	22
23	Other Diseases of the Digestive System	7·17	13·26	23
24	Other Diseases of the Respiratory System	30·69	18·52	24
25	Septic Conditions	16·56	10·06	25
26	Mental, Psychoneurotic and Personality Disorders	3·20	7·09	26
27	All Other Diseases	111·69	121·88	27
28	*Total Admissions for Diseases*	411·09	387·97	28
29	Injuries—N.E.A.	33·65	45·04	29
30	Injuries—E.A.	0·53	0·46	30
31	*Total Admissions for Injuries*	34·18	45·50	31
32	*Total Admissions*	445·27	433·47	32

* Any cases included in 'All Other Diseases'.

TABLE 145

South-East Asia Command (Ceylon)
Causes of Admissions to Hospitals, 1943–45
Ceylonese Officers. Annual Rates per 1,000 Strength

Source: A.F. A.31-B

	CAUSES	1943	1944	1945	
1	Common Cold	14·90	21·96	14·13	1
2	Diarrhoea	11·59	10·13	12·96	2
3	Dysentery	4·97	6·76	4·71	3
4	Dengue Fever	3·31	5·07	3·14	4
5	Diphtheria	—	—	—	5
6	Enteric Group of Fevers	—	—	—	6
7	Infective Hepatitis	—	8·45	4·71	7
8	Malaria	62·91	57·43	45·53	8
9	Mumps	—	1·69	1·57	9
10	Pneumonia	—	—	—	10
11	P.U.O. and N.Y.D. Fever	*	35·47	14·13	11
12	Sandfly Fever	—	—	—	12
13	Scabies	—	—	7·85	13
14	Smallpox	—	—	—	14
15	Tonsillitis	9·93	1·69	4·71	15
16	Tuberculosis	—	3·38	1·57	16
17	Venereal Diseases	8·28	—	6·26	17
18	Diseases of the Circulatory System	—	3·38	1·57	18
19	Diseases due to Disorders of Nutrition	—	—	4·71	19
20	Diseases of the Ear, Nose and Throat	*	13·51	17·27	20
21	Diseases of the Eye	6·62	8·45	9·42	21
22	Diseases of the Skin (other than Scabies)	*	18·58	20·41	22
23	Other Diseases of the Digestive System	21·52	38·85	21·98	23
24	Other Diseases of the Respiratory System	4·97	16·27	18·84	24
25	Septic Conditions	—	10·13	4·71	25
26	Mental, Psychoneurotic and Personality Disorders	—	1·69	—	26
27	All Other Diseases	102·66	123·93	86·34	27
28	*Total Admissions for Diseases*	251·66	386·82	306·12	28
29	Injuries—N.E.A.	43·05	57·43	29·83	29
30	Injuries—E.A.	—	—	1·57	30
31	*Total Admissions for Injuries*	43·05	57·43	31·40	31
32	*Total Admissions*	294·70	444·26	337·52	32

* Any cases included in 'All Other Diseases'.

TABLE 146

South-East Asia Command (*Ceylon*)
Causes of Admissions to Hospitals, 1943–45
Ceylonese Other Ranks. Annual Rates per 1,000 Strength

Source: A.F. A.31-B

	CAUSES	1943	1944	1945	
1	Common Cold	81·85	89·51	80·94	1
2	Diarrhoea	30·61	25·41	18·87	2
3	Dysentery	26·11	18·87	11·59	3
4	Dengue Fever	1·30	1·76	0·81	4
5	Diphtheria	0·09	0·04	0·13	5
6	Enteric Group of Fevers .	0·14	0·30	—	6
7	Infective Hepatitis . .	3·25	4·99	5·11	7
8	Malaria	214·90	144·07	109·01	8
9	Mumps	7·61	5·63	12·40	9
10	Pneumonia	*	*	3·07	10
11	P.U.O. and N.Y.D. Fever .	*	70·55	32·80	11
12	Sandfly Fever . . .	0·42	1·33	—	12
13	Scabies	10·57	13·46	18·40	13
14	Smallpox	—	—	0·13	14
15	Tonsillitis	4·59	3·70	7·71	15
16	Tuberculosis	0·28	0·90	0·94	16
17	Venereal Diseases	24·35	26·44	33·48	17
18	Diseases of the Circulatory System .	0·14	7·18	0·98	18
19	Diseases due to Disorders of Nutrition .	—	—	1·66	19
20	Diseases of the Ear, Nose and Throat .	*	17·58	19·72	20
21	Diseases of the Eye	15·68	16·51	19·72	21
22	Diseases of the Skin (other than Scabies)	*	26·78	23·34	22
23	Other Diseases of the Digestive System .	40·49	42·48	38·68	23
24	Other Diseases of the Respiratory System	29·21	42·39	35·39	24
25	Septic Conditions	30·05	15·05	14·61	25
26	Mental, Psychoneurotic and Personality Disorders	2·60	4·00	2·51	26
27	All Other Diseases	344·05	192·22	125·81	27
28	*Total Admissions for Diseases* .	868·29	771·15	617·81	28
29	Injuries—N.E.A.	41·09	47·72	42·55	29
30	Injuries—E.A.	0·05	0·13	—	30
31	*Total Admissions for Injuries* .	41·14	47·85	42·55	31
32	*Total Admissions*	909·43	819·00	660·36	32

* Any cases included in 'All Other Diseases'.

TABLE 147

South-East Asia Command (Ceylon)
Causes of Admissions to Hospitals, 1943–45
All Ceylonese Troops. Annual Rates per 1,000 Strength

Source: A.F. A.31-B

	CAUSES	1943	1944	1945	
1	Common Cold	80·03	87·83	79·17	1
2	Diarrhoea	30·09	25·03	18·70	2
3	Dysentery	25·53	18·57	11·40	3
4	Dengue Fever	1·35	1·84	0·87	4
5	Diphtheria	0·09	0·04	0·12	5
6	Enteric Group of Fevers	0·13	0·29	—	6
7	Infective Hepatitis	3·16	5·07	5·10	7
8	Malaria	210·76	141·92	107·33	8
9	Mumps	7·40	5·53	12·11	9
10	Pneumonia	*	*	2·99	10
11	P.U.O. and N.Y.D. Fever	*	69·68	32·31	11
12	Sandfly Fever	0·41	1·30	—	12
13	Scabies	10·29	13·12	18·12	13
14	Smallpox	—	—	0·12	14
15	Tonsillitis	4·74	3·65	7·63	15
16	Tuberculosis	0·27	0·96	0·95	16
17	Venereal Diseases	23·91	25·78	32·76	17
18	Diseases of the Circulatory System	0·13	7·08	0·99	18
19	Diseases due to Disorders of Nutrition	—	—	1·74	19
20	Diseases of the Ear, Nose and Throat	*	17·48	16·66	20
21	Diseases of the Eye	15·20	17·48	16·83	21
22	Diseases of the Skin (other than Scabies)	*	26·58	23·27	22
23	Other Diseases of the Digestive System	39·97	42·39	38·24	23
24	Other Diseases of the Respiratory System	28·55	41·84	34·97	24
25	Septic Conditions	29·23	14·92	14·35	25
26	Mental, Psychoneurotic and Personality Disorders	2·53	3·94	2·45	26
27	All Other Diseases	337·72	189·29	130·39	27
28	*Total Admissions for Diseases*	851·49	761·61	609·57	28
29	Injuries—N.E.A.	41·14	47·96	42·22	29
30	Injuries—E.A.	0·04	0·13	0·04	30
31	*Total Admissions for Injuries*	41·18	48·09	42·26	31
32	*Total Admissions*	892·68	809·70	651·83	32

* Any cases included in 'All Other Diseases'.

TABLE 148

South-East Asia Command (Ceylon). Causes of Admissions to Hospitals, 1942–45 All Troops. Annual Rates per 1,000 Strength

Source: A.F. A.31-B

	CAUSES	1942	1943	1944	1945	
1	Common Cold	27·61	28·88	32·68	27·33	1
2	Diarrhoea	24·95	20·18	16·42	11·52	2
3	Dysentery	14·90	36·11	25·28	14·28	3
4	Dengue Fever	36·60	15·44	11·85	3·61	4
5	Diphtheria	0·59	0·15	0·53	0·10	5
6	Enteric Group of Fevers	0·86	0·22	1·38	0·11	6
7	Infective Hepatitis	5·46	3·01	4·88	4·40	7
8	Malaria	155·97	166·12	96·14	69·95	8
9	Mumps	3·56	2·35	2·15	4·80	9
10	Pneumonis	—	—	—	1·83	10
11	P.U.O. and N.Y.D. Fever	*	*	46·20	27·68	11
12	Sandfly Fever	1·00	0·48	0·88	0·17	12
13	Scabies	7·39	8·36	6·96	11·60	13
14	Smallpox	0·02	0·03	0·05	0·10	14
15	Tonsillitis	11·87	5·80	4·94	5·64	15
16	Tuberculosis	1·72	3·41	1·27	0·84	16
17	Venereal Diseases	51·06	39·82	41·79	29·63	17
18	Diseases of the Circulatory System	0·06	0·19	4·50	1·08	18
19	Diseases due to Disorders of Nutrition	—	—	0·70	1·10	19
20	Diseases of the Ear, Nose and Throat	*	*	15·80	17·21	20
21	Diseases of the Eye	12·56	10·73	9·45	12·39	21
22	Diseases of the Skin (other than Scabies)	*	*	20·51	20·01	22
23	Other Diseases of the Digestive System	33·48	29·45	25·29	23·71	23
24	Other Diseases of the Respiratory System	13·10	10·13	28·98	21·46	24
25	Septic Conditions	53·19	29·19	19·59	16·27	29
26	Mental, Psychoneurotic and Personality Disorders	2·72	2·65	3·82	4·03	26
27	All Other Diseases	243·78	244·47	115·51	87·63	27
28	*Total Admissions for Diseases*	702·45	657·17	537·55	418·48	28
29	Injuries—N.E.A.	46·93	37·22	40·77	32·16	29
30	Injuries—E.A.	1·80	0·44	0·81	0·07	30
31	*Total Admissions for Injuries*	48·73	37·66	41·58	32·23	31
32	*Total Admissions*	751·18	694·83	579·14	450·71	32

* Any cases included in 'All Other Diseases'.

TABLE 149

South-East Asia Command (Ceylon). Admissions to Hospitals for Injuries, 1942–45. Annual Rates per 1,000 Strength

Source: A.F. A.31-B

1. BRITISH TROOPS	Officers				Other Ranks				All British Troops			
	1942	1943	1944	1945	1942	1943	1944	1945	1942	1943	1944	1945
(a) *Non-Enemy Action*												
Burns and Scalds	N.A.	N.A.	N.A.	0·96	N.A.	N.A.	N.A.	2·57	N.A.	N.A.	N.A.	2·13
Others	N.A.	N.A.	N.A.	37·41	N.A.	N.A.	N.A.	44·32	N.A.	N.A.	N.A.	41·84
Totals	66·15	41·15	50·02	38·37	66·43	50·96	54·62	46·89	66·40	49·94	53·62	43·97
(b) *Enemy Action*												
Bomb Wounds	3·10	—	0·96	—	1·67	—	0·10	—	1·76	—	0·24	—
Gunshot Wounds	3·10	0·88	0·48	0·48	3·26	0·31	0·38	0·15	3·23	0·38	0·40	0·22
Shell Wounds	4·14	0·44	—	—	0·40	0·18	0·19	—	0·66	0·22	0·16	—
Totals	10·34	1·33	1·44	0·48	5·32	0·49	0·67	0·15	5·66	0·59	0·80	0·22
(c) *Total Injuries*	75·49	42·48	51·46	38·85	71·75	51·45	55·29	47·04	72·06	50·53	54·42	44·19

2. INDIAN TROOPS	V.C.Os. and I.O.Rs.				N.Cs.(E.)				I.M.N.S.				All Indian Troops			
	1942	1943	1944	1945	1942	1943	1944	1945	1942	1943	1944	1945	1942	1943	1944	1945
a) *Non-Enemy Action*																
Burns and Scalds	N.A.	N.A.	N.A.	1·19	N.A.	N.A.	N.A.	0·13	—	N.A.	—	—	N.A.	N.A.	N.A.	1 18
Others	N.A.	N.A.	N.A.	41·74	N.A.	N.A.	N.A.	13·71	—	N.A.	—	—	N.A.	N.A.	N.A.	41·69
Totals	65·09	47·22	51·63	42·93	38·34	24·76	26·80	13·84	—	11·9	—	—	64·85	46·95	51·38	42·87
(b) *Enemy Action*																
Bomb Wounds	0·07	—	—	—	0·30	—	—	—	—	—	—	—	0·07	—	—	—
Gunshot Wounds	0·60	0·78	0·35	0·07	—	—	—	—	—	—	—	—	0·59	0·78	0·35	0·07
Shell Wounds	—	0·04	—	—	—	—	—	—	—	—	—	—	—	0·04	—	—
Totals	0·67	0·83	0·35	0·07	0·30	—	—	—	—	—	—	—	0·66	0·82	0·35	0·07
(c) *Total Injuries*	65·76	48·05	51·98	43·00	38·64	24·76	26·80	13·84	—	11·9	—	—	65·51	47·77	51·74	42·94

TABLE 149 (*contd.*)

South-East Asia Command (Ceylon). Admissions to Hospitals for Injuries, 1942–45. Annual Rates per 1,000 Strength

Source: A.F. A.31-B

3. CEYLONESE TROOPS	Officers			Other Ranks			All Ceylonese Troops		
	1943	1944	1945	1943	1944	1945	1943	1944	1945
(a) *Non-Enemy Action*									
Burns and Scalds	N.A.	N.A.	N.A.	N.A.	N.A.	2·00	N.A.	N.A.	1·95
Others	N.A.	N.A.	N.A.	N.A.	N.A.	40·55	N.A.	N.A.	40·27
Totals	43·05	57·43	29·83	41·09	47·72	42·55	41·14	47·96	42·22
(b) *Enemy Action*									
Bomb Wounds	—	—	—	—	—	—	—	—	—
Gunshot Wounds	—	—	1·57	0·05	0·13	—	0·04	0·13	0·04
Shell Wounds	—	—	—	—	—	—	—	—	—
Totals	—	—	1·57	0·05	0·13	—	0·04	0·13	0·04
(c) *Total Injuries*	43·05	57·43	31·40	41·14	47·85	42·55	41·18	48·09	42·26

4. EAST AFRICAN OTHER RANKS	1944	1945
(a) *Non-Enemy Action*		
Burns and Scalds	N.A.	N.A.
Others	N.A.	N.A.
Totals	33·65	45·04
(b) *Enemy Action*		
Bomb Wounds	—	—
Gunshot Wounds	0·36	0·46
Shell Wounds	0·16	—
Totals	0·53	0·46
(c) *Total Injuries*	34·18	45·50

5. ALL TROOPS	1942	1943	1944	1945
(a) *Non-Enemy Action*				
Burns and Scalds	N.A.	N.A.	N.A.	1·06
Others	N.A.	N.A.	N.A.	31·10
Totals	46·93	37·22	40·77	32·16
(b) *Enemy Action*				
Bomb Wounds	0·53	—	0·03	—
Gunshot Wounds	1·08	0·39	0·22	0·07
Shell Wounds	0·18	0·05	0·06	—
Totals	1·80	0·44	0·31	0·07
(c) *Total Injuries*	48·73	37·66	41·08	32·23

TABLE 150

South-East Asia Command (Ceylon)
Deaths in Hospitals, 1942–45. All Causes
Annual Rates per 1,000 Strength

	1942	1943	1944	1945
British				
Officers	2·07	1·77	3·85	1·92
Other Ranks	2·22	2·72	1·82	1·66
Indian				
Officers	—	—	—	—
V.C.Os. and I.O.Rs.	1·86	2·35	1·95	1·54
N.Cs.(E.)	2·13	2·90	3·22	2·16
I.M.N.S.	—	—	—	—
Ceylonese				
Officers		—	1·69	1·57
Other Ranks		2·36	1·55	1·96
East African				
Other Ranks			3·56	2·29

TABLE 151

South-East Asia Command (Ceylon). Admissions to Hospitals for Diseases, 1942–45
Comparative Rates B.O.Rs. and V.C.Os. and I.O.Rs.

Source: A.F. A.31-B

	DISEASES	B.O.Rs.	V.C.Os. and I.O.Rs.	
1	Mumps	100	1,243	1
2	Scabies	100	291	2
3	Tuberculosis	100	211	3
4	Diseases of the Eye	100	202	4
5	Other Diseases of the Respiratory System	100	191	5
6	P.U.O. and N.Y.D. Fever*	100	148	6
7	Diseases due to Disorders of Nutrition	100	137	7
8	Diseases of the Ear, Nose and Throat*	100	131	8
9	Smallpox	100	125	9
10	Diarrhoea	100	98	10
11	Sandfly Fever	100	98	11
12	Other Diseases of the Digestive System	100	95	12
13	Malaria	100	93	13
14	Septic Conditions	100	90	14
15	Common Cold	100	90	15
16	Dysentery	100	76	16
17	Diseases of the Circulatory System	100	76	17
18	Infective Hepatitis	100	65	18
19	Mental, Psychoneurotic and Personality Disorders	100	65	19
20	Diphtheria	100	63	20
21	Venereal Diseases	100	59	21
22	Diseases of the Skin (other than Scabies)*	100	36	22
23	Tonsillitis	100	25	23
24	Dengue Fever	100	23	24
25	Enteric Group of Fevers	100	7	25
26	All Other Diseases	100	92	26
27	*Total Admissions for Diseases*	100	86	27

* Based on admissions for two years only.

TABLE 152

South-East Asia Command (Ceylon). Admissions to Hospitals for Diseases, 1943–45
Comparative Rates British, Ceylonese and Indian Other Ranks

Source: A.F. A.31-B

	DISEASES	British	Ceylonese	Indian	
1	Mumps	100	10,256	1,936	1
2	Common Cold	100	669	115	2
3	Other Diseases of the Respiratory System	100	322	188	3
4	Scabies	100	278	279	4
5	Diseases of the Eye	100	222	203	5
	Diseases due to Disorders of Nutrition	100	218	138	6
7	P.U.O. and N.Y.D. Fever*	100	151	148	7
8	Malaria	100	126	110	8
9	Other Diseases of the Digestive System	100	117	85	9
10	Diarrhoea	100	114	90	10
11	Diseases of the Circulatory System	100	114	75	11
12	Sandfly Fever	100	93	144	12
13	Diseases of the Ear, Nose and Throat*	100	92	131	13
14	Dysentery	100	67	79	14
15	Septic Conditions	100	64	98	15
16	Infective Hepatitis	100	53	60	16
17	Venereal Diseases	100	49	71	17
18	Mental, Psychoneurotic and Personality Disorders	100	48	70	18
19	Diseases of the Skin (other than Scabies)*	100	43	36	19
20	Smallpox	100	38	97	20
21	Tonsillitis	100	36	31	21
22	Tuberculosis	100	33	200	22
23	Enteric Group of Fevers	100	32	10	23
24	Diphtheria	100	5	7	24
25	Dengue Fever	100	3	24	25
26	All other Diseases	100	120	84	26
27	*Total Admissions for Diseases*	100	113	89	27

* Based on admissions for two years only.

TABLE 153

South-East Asia Command (Ceylon). Admissions to Hospitals for Diseases, 1944–45 Comparative Rates of British, East African, Indian and Ceylonese Other Ranks

Source: A.F. A.31-B

	DISEASES	British	East African	Indian	Ceylonese	
1	Mumps	100	632	1,624	7,212	1
2	Common Cold	100	113	169	860	2
3	Sandfly Fever	100	105	105	88	3
4	Dysentery	100	92	74	52	4
5	Other Diseases of the Respiratory System	100	83	185	261	5
6	Venereal Diseases	100	79	71	55	6
7	Diseases of the Eye	100	71	194	225	7
8	Diarrhoea	100	58	67	118	8
9	Diseases of the Circulatory System	100	52	74	115	9
10	Enteric Group of Fevers	100	45*	6	28	10
11	Diseases of the Ear, Nose and Throat	100	35	131	92	11
12	Mental, Psychoneurotic and Personality Disorders	100	34	69	43	12
13	Infective Hepatitis	100	33	60	53	13
14	Malaria	100	29	187	215	14
15	P.U.O. and N.Y.D. Fever	100	29	148	151	15
16	Septic Conditions	100	22	76	49	16
17	Other Diseases of the Digestive System	100	16	93	126	17
18	Diseases due to Disorders of Nutrition	100	14	138	218	18
19	Scabies	100	13	246	295	19
20	Tonsillitis	100	11	33	39	20
21	Diseases of the Skin (other than Scabies)	qoo	9	36	43	21
22	Dengue Fever	100	6	27	4	22
23	Smallpox	100	6	59	38	23
24	Tuberculosis	100	6	59	38	24
25	Diphtheria	100	1	8	4	25
26	All Other Diseases	100	24	68	114	26
27	*Total Admissions for Diseases*	100	34	91	117	27

* Admissions for one year only.

CHAPTER X

Discharges from the Army on Medical Grounds

THE statistics which follow were prepared from Hollerith tabulations, the basic data for which were contained on Army Forms B.3978. Presidents of Medical Boards were required, as from September 1, 1942, to complete these forms for all cases approved for invaliding from the Army, that is, those placed in Medical Category E.

As discharges on medical grounds could be effected only in the United Kingdom, medical boards convened overseas could only recommend for transfer home as invalids those cases they considered should be invalided out of the Army. On arrival in the United Kingdom, the patients continued to receive medical treatment in hospitals, appeared before medical boards and were either:

(a) placed in Medical Category E,

(b) medically up- or down-graded and returned to duty, or,

(c) graded temporarily unfit as requiring further hospital in-patient treatment.

Patients admitted to medical units in the United Kingdom considered by their medical officers as suitable for invaliding received similar administrative treatment.

Presidents of medical boards were empowered only to recommend discharge from the Army; approval was vested in the local medical administrative officers, while discharges were carried out by the medical units in which the patients were being treated.

Data from all Army Forms B.3978 received in the War Office were transferred to Hollerith punched cards. In view of the known limitations of war-time medical statistics produced by the Hollerith machines, and in common with other Hollerith tabulations, overall figures have been checked against another source of information. The result showed a high degree of similarity, albeit there was evidence of a slight leakage of the forms in transit.

Comparison is also possible with statistics on this subject published in the *Statistical Report on the Health of the Army*, 1943–45. The differences existing between the two sets of figures are reasonably small, so that it may be said that the tabulations which follow are substantially correct. Data are grouped as to males (Officers and Other Ranks combined) and females (A.T.S. Officers and Other Ranks combined). No rates can be quoted for the discharge of nurses and V.A.D. members due to the lack of accurate strength figures.

MALES

Discharge rates of males are cited in Tables 154 to 158. It must be emphasised that these rates are for the whole army and not that part stationed in the United Kingdom only.

A summary of discharge rates is given in Table 154. Invalidings on account of diseases only increased by 3 per 1,000 each year, from 18 in 1943 to 24 in 1945. Injuries produced rates of 3, 5 and 9 per 1,000 respectively and accounted for some fourteen, twenty and twenty-seven per cent. of discharges for all medical reasons. Total discharges rose in 1944 by 5 per 1,000 to 26 and to 33 in the following year.

By far the largest number of discharges in each year was on account of MENTAL DISORDERS (Table 155). In 1943, thirty-five per cent. of all discharges through disease were attributable to this cause. During the following year, the proportion rose to forty-one per cent. and in 1945 it declined very slightly to forty per cent. Expressed as rates per 1,000 strength, discharges rose from 6 in 1943 to 8·6 in 1944 and finally to 9·4 in 1945. Discharges due to this group are analysed below.

Discharges from the Army on Medical Grounds, 1943–45
Mental Disorders. Relative Rates

Source: Hollerith Tabulations

	1943	1944	1945
Psychoses:			
Manic Depressive	6·39	3·83	2·89
Schizophrenia	6·24	6·67	5·69
Paranoid State	0·49	0·32	0·47
Others	0·16	0·02	0·07
Psychoneuroses:			
Anxiety State	39·98	46·21	53·30
Hysteria	20·05	19·56	16·34
Others	2·12	1·33	1·56
Psychopathic Personality	17·18	15·79	13·79
Mental Deficiency	6·64	6·19	5·72
Other Mental Disorders	0·75	0·09	0·17
	100	100	100

ANXIETY STATE contributed to between forty and fifty per cent. of discharges due to mental disorders, and HYSTERIA to between sixteen and twenty per cent. PSYCHOPATHIC PERSONALITY accounted for approximately fifteen per cent. and SCHIZOPHRENIA and MENTAL DEFICIENCY for six per cent. each. There was a marked decline over the three years in discharges due to MANIC DEPRESSIVE Psychosis, the number in 1945 being slightly over one-half those in 1943 (the mean strength in 1945 was some five per cent. less than that in 1943). This was reflected in a decline in the relative rates from six to less than three per cent.

Next in numerical importance came Diseases of the DIGESTIVE SYSTEM, discharges for which, producing rates at around 3 per 1,000 strength were almost one-third those for mental disorders. An analysis of these discharges follows.

Discharges from the Army on Medical Grounds, 1943–45
Diseases of the Digestive System. Relative Rates

Source: Hollerith Tabulations

	1943	1944	1945
Gastric Ulcer	12·64	12·75	12·72
Duodenal Ulcer	62·64	60·83	57·42
Peptic Ulcer—unspecified	2·40	3·63	3·84
Perforated Ulcer	3·68	4·59	5·77
Dyspepsia and Gastritis	6·73	5·69	4·87
Hernia	2·73	2·47	2·85
Appendicitis	0·23	0·23	0·50
Haemorrhoids	0·19	0·14	0·10
Other Diseases of the Digestive System	8·76	9·67	11·93
	100	100	100

Four-fifths of these discharges were due to Ulcers, sixty per cent. to DUODENAL Ulcers, twelve per cent. to GASTRIC and eight per cent. to PERFORATED and UNSPECIFIED Ulcers. Six per cent. were due to DYSPEPSIA and GASTRITIS and nearly three per cent. to HERNIAS. It is worthy of notice that in a group of diseases which caused such a large number of discharges, relative rates of individual diseases within the group varied but little. Indeed, in the largest component of the group, the variation is only five per cent.; among the next largest component, the variation is as low as 0·11 per cent.

Discharges due to Diseases of the RESPIRATORY SYSTEM were between seven and eight per cent. of all those due to disease, at rates which varied little from 1·4 per 1,000 in 1943 to 1·6 in 1945. The following analysis show that from fifty to sixty per cent. of these discharges were due to BRONCHITIS, at least three quarters of which were chronic. ASTHMA provided between fifteen and twenty per cent. of the total and PLEURISY an average of three per cent. over the period.

Discharges from the Army on Medical Grounds, 1943–45
Diseases of the Respiratory System. Males. Relative Rates

Source: Hollerith Tabulations

	1943	1944	1945
Bronchitis	61·63	60·32	50·29
Asthma	15·27	14·56	21·52
Pleurisy	2·37	2·55	4·39
Other Diseases of the Respiratory System	20·72	22·57	23·80
	100	100	100

Diseases of the MUSCULO-SKELETAL SYSTEM were responsible for discharges at rates within the range 1·4 to 1·6 per 1,000 strength and representing approximately seven per cent. of all discharges for disease. They are analysed below.

Discharges from the Army on Medical Grounds, 1943–45
Diseases of the Musculo-Skeletal System. Males. Relative Rates

Source: Hollerith Tabulations

	1943	1944	1945
Diseases of the Joints:			
Synovitis	1·50	1·48	1·78
Arthritis	11·81	11·87	12·21
I.D.K.	5·67	5·86	6·96
Others	4·60	4·24	3·24
Diseases of the Bone	9·51	9·58	9·60
Diseases of the Spine	11·46	12·42	11·31
Diseases of the Muscles	0·69	0·76	0·68
Diseases of Fasciae, Tendons, Tendon Sheaths and Bursae	0·94	1·12	0·90
Diseases and Deformities of the Limbs:			
Infected Fingers	0·11	0·21	0·25
Hallus Valgus, etc.	4·30	2·99	2·91
Hammer Toe	0·19	0·03	0·08
Pes Cavus	5·96	4·24	3·94
Pes Planus	6·12	4·92	6·48
Others	0·27	0·42	2·11
Rheumatic Conditions:			
Non-Articular	8·42	8·12	9·05
Articular	28·73	31·74	28·49
	100	100	100

Nearly forty per cent. of these discharges were due to RHEUMATIC CONDITIONS, other than Rheumatic fever. Of these, between one-quarter and one-third were of the articular type. Both ARTHRITIS and Diseases of the SPINE were responsible for twelve per cent., while Diseases of the BONE accounted for nearly ten per cent. each year. Discharges for INTERNAL DERANGEMENT of the KNEE were some six per cent. of the group total with PES PLANUS slightly less.

Discharges on account of TUBERCULOSIS increased annually from 1·2 to 1·5 per 1,000 and were between six and seven per cent. of the group total. Rates for PULMONARY Tuberculosis were 1·02 per 1,000 in 1943, 1·23 in 1944 and 1·31 in 1945. Those for other forms of tuberculosis remained stationary at 0·19 per 1,000.

Diseases of the NERVOUS SYSTEM accounted for approximately six per cent. of all discharges for disease, with rates increasing slightly from 1·13 in 1943 to 1·29 in 1945. The table which follows analyses this group to component diseases or sub-groups.

Discharges from the Army on Medical Grounds, 1943–45
Diseases of the Nervous System. Males. Relative Rates

Source: Hollerith Tabulations

	1943	1944	1945
Sciatica	14·27	19·56	23·36
Other forms of Neuritis	1·04	2·87	2·04
Migraine	2·75	3·92	4·88
Epilepsy	38·58	34·06	28·34
Other Diseases of Uncertain Pathology	4·25	1·50	1·73
Effect Syndrome	1·81	1·26	2·01
Diseases of Cerebral Meninges	2·11	1·88	2·53
Diseases of the Brain	5·93	6·58	5·38
Disorders of Cranial Nerves	19·96	16·33	16·10
Other Causes	9·30	12·04	13·63
	100	100	100

Between thirty and forty per cent. of discharges in this group were due to EPILEPSY. Next in numerical importance were disorders of the CRANIAL NERVES at from sixteen to twenty per cent. and SCIATICA increasing from fourteen per cent. in 1943 to twenty-three in 1945. Disorders of the BRAIN were comparatively low at 6 per cent.

Slightly over four per cent. of discharges for disease were attributable to Diseases of the CARDIO-VASCULAR System, and produced rates at 0·9 per 1,000 strength in 1943 and 1944 and 0·96 in 1945. VALVULAR DISEASE of the HEART was responsible for one third of the group total in 1943, one quarter in 1944, and one-fifth in 1945 and VARICOSE VEINS for seven, eight and twelve per cent. respectively.

Next in numerical order of discharges were Diseases of the SKIN, discharges for which increased from 0·57 per 1,000 in 1943 to more than double in 1945. An analysis appears in the tabulation below.

Discharges from the Army on Medical Grounds, 1943–45
Diseases of the Skin. Males. Relative Rates

Source: Hollerith Tabulations

	1943	1944	1945
Impetigo	1·39	0·73	0·75
Dermatitis	36·90	44·96	48·97
Boils	0·79	0·77	0·29
Eczema	24·62	24·32	18·24
Psoriasis	7·39	4·57	6·82
Tinea	1·65	1·15	1·01
Diseases of the Sebaceous Glands	3·70	4·36	4·32
Diseases of the Sweat Glands and Ducts	1·25	1·32	1·95
Diseases of the Hair and Follicles	5·68	5·43	3·86
Other Diseases of the Skin	16·63	12·39	13·79
	100	100	100

The increase in discharges during 1945 as compared with 1943 was due almost entirely to DERMATITIS which rose from a little over one-third of the total in 1943 to nearly one-half in 1945. Comparatively high rates were also attributable to ECZEMA which, with Dermatitis, accounted for between sixty and seventy per cent. of the group total.

Diseases of the EAR, NOSE and THROAT provided discharges at rates which increased from 0·72 per 1,000 in 1943 to 0·80 in 1945, and were between three and four per cent. of discharges for disease. The following table analyses the statistics of this group.

Discharges from the Army on Medical Grounds, 1943–45
Diseases of the Ear, Nose and Throat. Males. Relative Rates

Source: Hollerith Tabulations

	1943	1944	1945
Otitis Media	69·36	66·08	65·27
Otosclerosis	10·67	9·20	6·84
Middle Ear Deafness	5·02	7·29	6·24
Diseases of the Mastoid Process	3·80	3·32	4·14
Other Diseases of the Ear	1·74	2·46	2·59
Diseases of the Accessory Sinuses	6·71	8·09	9·88
Other Diseases of the Nose	1·27	1·80	3·14
Diseases of the Throat	1·43	1·76	1·90
	100	100	100

Between eight-five and ninety per cent. of discharges within the group were due to Diseases of the Ear. As could be expected, OTITIS MEDIA was responsible for the greater portion of these discharges at from sixty-five to seventy per cent. OTOSCLEROSIS accounted for about nine per cent., MIDDLE EAR DEAFNESS for six per cent. and Diseases of the MASTOID PROCESS under four per cent. Diseases of the NOSE contributed one-tenth of the group total and Diseases of the THROAT under two per cent.

Diseases of the EYE were responsible for approximately two per cent. of discharges due to diseases with rates per 1,000 strength which decreased from 0·45 in 1943 to 0·33 in 1945.

Nearly one half each year were placed under SYMPTOMATIC DISTURBANCES of VISION. Among other causes for discharge within this group were Diseases of the CORNEA, some fourteen per cent., Diseases of the RETINA about nine per cent. and Diseases of the CHOROID slightly lower.

Table 157 records the annual rates per 1,000 strength of discharges of Male Troops through INJURIES, while Table 158 cites relative rates. Discharges increased from 3 per 1,000 in 1943, to 9 in 1945. This increase is not unremarkable in view of the opening of the Second Front in Europe in 1944, and the offensive campaign against the Japanese, culminating in the liberation of Burma and Malaya.

Discharges due to injuries caused through enemy action (E.A.) in 1945 were five times those in 1943 (1·33 per 1,000 against 6·75) while those not caused through enemy action (N.E.A.) increased only slightly over the period (1·6 to 2·2 per 1,000). In 1943, the former was forty-six per cent. of all discharges on account of injury; by 1945 it had risen to seventy-five per cent.

FRACTURES other than to the head, both E.A. and N.E.A., were responsible for the majority of discharges and, while rates per 1,000 strength increased in 1944 and 1945, the proportion of E.A. injuries to the total declined from fifty-one to thirty-two per cent. In contrast, the proportion of N.E.A. fractures to the whole rose from twenty-four to fifty-two per cent. A similar situation is witnessed among Head Injuries, Burns and Scalds, and Old Injuries and is caused by the very large increase in discharges due to 'Other Injuries (E.A.)'. These rose from 0·44 per 1,000 in 1943 to 4·04 in 1945 while 'Other Injuries (N.E.A.)' decreased from 1·11 to 0·59 in the same period.

The statistics cited above and in the tabulations do not tell the full story of medical discharges. They do not, for instance, record the varying DEGREES of DISABLEMENT as shown on discharge documents or, which is closely related, figures regarding FITNESS for CIVIL EMPLOYMENT. Neither are any RECOVERY RATES quoted. What follows is an attempt, in some small way, to furnish this information, in so far as E.A. Injuries are concerned.

For this purpose an investigation was pursued among data of all British Other Ranks wounded in North-West Europe during 1944 and 1945, i.e., from the landings in Normandy to the cessation of hostilities. It was necessary to isolate two classes of personnel, those who died of their wounds and those who were invalided from the Army because of their wounds. It was not possible to trace deaths through the medium of Hollerith tabulations because 'result on discharge' (from hospital) had ceased to be coded. This information was obtainable from another source and figures relating to degrees of disablement and fitness for civil employment were obtainable from the Hollerith tabulations.

From the Adjutant General's Statistical Branch at the War Office (A.G. Stats.) casualty figures revealed that seven per cent. of all B.O.Rs. wounded in North-West Europe subsequently died of their wounds. Thus the chances of SURVIVAL were ninety-three per cent., i.e., ninety-three per cent. of wounded were either returned to duty or invalided from the Army with a disability which might, to some extent, affect their earning power.

From the point of view of army wastage, to this seven per cent. must be added the invaliding rate. For North-West Europe, the proportion invalided was fourteen per cent. That this is somewhat higher than in previous campaigns (the figure for the First World War was eight per cent.) may partly be explained by:

(i) the end of hostilities is likely to have brought with it a relaxation in the criteria for invaliding,

(ii) the advance of medical science (in e.g. penicillin) in saving the lives of many who, in other campaigns, would have died, would increase the proportion of seriously wounded among the survivors and thus raise the invaliding rate.

Thus, the wastage from the army point of view was:

Deaths . . 7 per cent.
Invalidings 14 per cent.
Total . 21 per cent.

and the recovery rate was therefore seventy-nine per cent.

The question must also be considered from a national point of view. To do this, allowance must be made for those who, as invalids from the Army point of view, are still capable of useful employment in civil life. An analysis of the degree of disablement recorded on discharge documents is of material assistance in this respect. Of those discharged as invalids

Analyses of Invalidings due to Wounds—North-West Europe—Other Ranks
Degree of Disablement, June 1944–July 1947

1. *Degree of Disablement*	Medical Boards in				Averages	Cumulative
	1944	1945	1946	1947		
0	0·1	0·0	—	—	0·0	0·0
10	0·4	0·4	0·4	0·5	0·4	0·4
20	2·3	4·2	3·7	4·3	3·9	4·3
30	8·2	13·6	15·3	13·3	12·9	17·2
40	17·9	18·3	18·4	21·9	18·3	35·5
50	13·9	13·4	9·3	11·9	13·0	48·5
60	9·7	10·3	7·8	12·4	10·0	58·5
70	9·9	7·4	6·4	7·1	7·7	66·2
80	5·4	4·4	4·4	4·3	4·5	70·7
90	1·2	0·8	1·2	1·4	0·9	71·6
100	31·0	27·2	33·1	22·9	28·4	100
Totals	100	100	100	100	100	100

2. *Fitness for Civil Employment*

	1944	1945	1946	1947	Total
(*a*) Yes	24·7	19·6	13·3	9·5	19·6
(*b*) No	42·4	41·1	34·8	22·4	40·4
(*c*) Yes, qualified . . .	32·9	39·3	51·9	68·1	40·0
Totals . . .	100	100	100	100	100

from the Army on account of wounds received in North-West Europe, the tabulation shows the relative rates of degrees of disablement.

The higher the degree of disablement, the more restricted is the occupational scope. If a disability of forty per cent. or less is taken as a standard for a reasonably wide range of employment, a little more than one-third of all the invalids fall into this category. As the overall invaliding figure was fourteen per cent. it may be assumed that approximately five per cent. made a good recovery. This figure, no doubt, increased as some of those with an initial high degree of disability were rehabilitated with the passage of time.

In the final analysis, therefore, on the assumptions stated, wastage in North-West Europe from wounds was approximately:

Deaths	7 per cent.
Invalids fit for no, or restricted, civil employment	9 per cent.
Totals	16 per cent.

The recovery rate was thus of the order of eighty-four per cent.

AUXILIARY TERRITORIAL SERVICE

Tables 159 to 161 relate to discharges from the Army on Medical grounds of all ranks of the A.T.S. Discharges on account of disease were 20 per 1,000 in 1943, and 21 in 1944 and 1945. They were slightly higher, by 2 per 1,000, than males in 1943, but lower by 2·5 in 1945. Apart from a few instances rates varied but little during the three years, even less than did those for males. Injuries accounted for approximately two per cent. of all discharges.

The main cause of discharges, as with males, were MENTAL DISORDERS, rates increasing by 1 per 1,000 to 10·5 in 1945. This compares with an increase among males by fifty per cent. from 6·2 to 9·4. Discharges for this group accounted for one half the total for disease. TUBERCULOSIS which, at 2 per 1,000 accounted for nine per cent. of discharges, was at a slightly higher rate than for men at 1·4. Diseases of the GENITO-URINARY System provided rates of discharges which, though not of a high order, were three times those for males (an average of 1·06 against 0·36).

In contrast, the female rate of 0·7 per 1,000 for discharges due to the DIGESTIVE System was one-quarter that for males.

SUMMARY

1. MENTAL DISORDERS were responsible for nearly forty per cent. of discharges for disease among males and one half among A.T.S.

2. Discharges due to Diseases of the DIGESTIVE System was of a much higher order among males.

3. TUBERCULOSIS accounted for a higher percentage of female discharges.

4. INJURIES negligible among women were responsible for fourteen per cent. of all discharges among males in 1943 and twenty-eight per cent. in 1945.

5. The recovery rate from wounds incurred in North-West Europe was approximately eighty-four per cent.

TABLE 154

Discharges from the Army on Medical Grounds—Males. 1943–45
Annual Rates per 1,000 Strength and Relative Rates

Source: Hollerith Tabulations

1. *Rates per 1,000 Strength*	1943		1944		1945	
Diseases		17·78		20·76		23·63
Injuries:						
E.A.	1·35		3·38		6·75	
N.E.A.	1·60		1·74		2·21	
Total Injuries		2·95		5·12		8·96
Total Discharges		20·73		25·88		32·59
2. *Relative Rates*						
Diseases		85·77		80·22		72·51
Injuries:						
E.A.	6·51		13·06		20·71	
N.E.A.	7·72		6·72		6·78	
Total Injuries		14·23		19·78		27·49
Total Discharges		100		100		100

TABLE 155

Discharges from the Army on Medical Grounds—Males. 1943–45, Diseases.
Annual Rates per 1,000 Strength

Source: Hollerith Tabulations

CAUSES	1943	1944	1945
Mental Disorders	6·24	8·55	9·42
Diseases of the Digestive System	2·76	2·56	3·05
Diseases of the Respiratory System	1·39	1·57	1·58
Diseases of the Musculo-Skeletal System	1·42	1·40	1·59
Tuberculosis	1·21	1·41	1·50
Diseases of the Nervous System	1·13	1·22	1·29
Diseases of the Cardio-Vascular System	0·91	0·90	0·96
Diseases of the Skin	0·57	0·85	1·23
Diseases of the Ear, Nose and Throat	0·72	0·73	0·80
Diseases of the Eye	0·45	0·38	0·33
Diseases of the Genito-Urinary System	0·31	0·34	0·44
Rheumatic Fever	0·05	0·06	0·07
All Other Diseases	0·62	0·79	1·37
Total Discharges for Diseases	17·78	20·76	23·63

TABLE 156

Discharges from the Army on Medical Grounds, 1943–45. Diseases, Males. Relative Rates

Source: Hollerith Tabulations

	CAUSES	1943	1944	1945	
1	Diphtheria	0·02	0·07	0·08	1
2	Dysentery	0·07	0·05	0·13	2
3	Jaundice, Catarrhal	0·01	0·03	0·05	3
4	Malaria	0·03	0·08	0·98	4
5	Meningococcal Infection	0·06	0·04	0·04	5
6	Pneumonia	0·08	0·09	0·17	6
7	Rheumatic Fever	0·30	0·31	0·29	7
8	Tuberculosis—Pulmonary	5·76	5·93	5·56	8
9	Tuberculosis—Other	1·09	0·85	0·79	9
10	Venereal Diseases	0·54	0·34	0·28	10
11	Other Diseases due to Infection	0·42	0·87	1·32	11
12	Diseases due to Infestation	0·09	0·05	0·08	12
13	Diseases of the Nervous System	6·36	5·88	5·46	13
14	Mental Conditions	35·08	41·17	39·84	14
15	Diseases of the Eye	2·52	1·83	1·40	15
16	Diseases of the Ear, Nose, and Throat	4·03	3·50	3·38	16
17	Diseases of the Cardio-Vascular System	5·12	4·33	4·06	17
18	Diseases of the Blood and Blood-forming Organs	0·39	0·38	0·44	18
19	Diseases of the Endocrine System	0·53	0·40	0·42	19
20	Diseases of the Respiratory System	7·81	7·58	6·69	20
21	Diseases of the Digestive System	15·50	12·35	12·91	21
22	Disorders of Nutrition and Metabolism	0·69	0·67	0·87	22
23	Diseases of the Genito-Urinary Tract	1·77	1·62	1·88	23
24	Diseases of the Musculo-Skeletal System	7·97	6·76	6·72	24
25	Diseases of the Areolar Tissue	0·12	0·11	0·08	25
26	Diseases of the Skin	3·23	4·11	5·20	26
27	All Other Diseases	0·40	0·60	0·87	27
28	*Total Discharges for Diseases*	100	100	100	28

TABLE 157

Discharges from the Army on Medical Grounds, 1943–45. Injuries, Males. Annual Rates per 1,000 Strength

Source: Hollerith Tabulations

1. *Injuries caused through Enemy Action*

CAUSES	1943	1944	1945
Head Injuries	0·16	0·36	0·45
Fractures (other than to the head)	0·69	0·89	2·17
Burns and Scalds	0·02	0·03	0·07
Old Injuries	0·04	0·01	0·04
Other Injuries	0·44	2·09	4·04
Totals	1·35	3·38	6·75

2. *Injuries not caused through Enemy Action*

CAUSES	1943	1944	1945
Head Injuries	0·09	0·27	0·26
Fractures (other than to the head)	0·38	0·87	1·16
Burns and Scalds	0·01	0·06	0·08
Old Injuries	0·01	0·07	0·12
Other Injuries	1·11	0·47	0·59
Totals	1·60	1·74	2·21

3. *All Injuries*

CAUSES	1943	1944	1945
Head Injuries	0·24	0·63	0·69
Fractures (other than to the head)	1·07	1·76	3·34
Burns and Scalds	0·04	0·09	0·14
Old Injuries	0·05	0·08	0·15
Other Injuries	1·55	2·56	4·64
Totals	2·95	5·12	8·96

TABLE 158

Discharges from the Army on Medical Grounds, 1943–45. Injuries, Males. Relative Rates

Source: Hollerith Tabulations

1. *Injuries caused through Enemy Action*

CAUSES	1943	1944	1945
Head Injuries	11·63	10·55	6·33
Fractures (other than to the head)	51·09	26·28	32·21
Burns and Scalds	1·77	0·88	0·99
Old Injuries	3·00	0·25	0·58
Other Injuries	32·51	62·04	59·89
Totals	100	100	100

2. *Injuries not caused through Enemy Action*

CAUSES	1943	1944	1945
Head Injuries	5·49	15·41	11·99
Fractures (other than to the head)	23·92	50·23	52·32
Burns and Scalds	0·66	3·55	3·52
Old Injuries	0·47	3·72	5·22
Other Injuries	69·46	27·09	26·95
Totals	100	100	100

3. *All Injuries*

CAUSES	1943	1944	1945
Head Injuries	8·29	12·20	7·72
Fractures (other than to the head)	36·34	34·42	37·17
Burns and Scalds	1·17	1·78	1·62
Old Injuries	1·63	1·43	1·72
Other Injuries	52·57	50·17	51·77
Totals	100	100	100

TABLE 159

Discharges from the Army on Medical Grounds, 1943–45. A.T.S. All Ranks. Annual Rates per 1,000 Strength and Relative Rates

Source: Hollerith Tabulations

1. *Rates per 1,000 Strength*	1943		1944		1945	
Diseases		19·61		21·13		21·03
Injuries:						
E.A.	0·35		0·32		0·55	
N.E.A.	0·01		0·03		0·04	
Total Injuries		0·36		0·35		0·59
Total Discharges		19·97		21·48		21·62
2. *Relative Rates*						
Diseases		98·20		98·37		97·27
Injuries:						
E.A.	1·75		1·49		2·54	
N.E.A.	0·05		0·14		0·19	
Total Injuries		1·80		1·63		2·73
Total Discharges		100		100		100

TABLE 160

Discharges from the Army on Medical Grounds—Diseases, 1943–45. A.T.S. All Ranks. Rates per 1,000 Strength

Source: Hollerith Tabulations

CAUSES	1943	1944	1945
Mental Disorders	9·71	10·76	10·52
Tuberculosis	2·15	2·10	2·07
Diseases of the Nervous System	1·20	1·29	1·24
Diseases of the Respiratory System	0·99	1·22	1·27
Diseases of the Musculo-Skeletal System	0·97	1·19	1·21
Diseases of the Genito-Urinary System	1·08	1·12	0·99
Diseases of the Digestive System	0·59	0·70	0·86
Diseases of the Cardio-Vascular System	0·82	0·56	0·63
Diseases of the Skin	0·44	0·45	0·51
Diseases of the Endocrine System	0·40	0·40	0·44
Diseases of the Ear, Nose and Throat	0·33	0·41	0·43
Diseases of the Eye	0·25	0·18	0·11
Rheumatic Fever	0·14	0·11	0·07
All Other Diseases	0·54	0·64	0·68
Total Discharges for Disease	19·61	21·13	21·03

TABLE 161

Discharges from the Army on Medical Grounds—Diseases, 1943–45. A.T.S. All Ranks. Relative Rates

Source: Hollerith Tabulations

	CAUSES	1943	1944	1945	
1	Malaria	—	0·02	0·08	1
2	Meningococcal Infection	0·03	0·07	0·05	2
3	Pneumonia	0·10	0·09	0·11	3
4	Rheumatic Fever	0·73	0·53	0·33	4
5	Tuberculosis—Pulmonary	8·78	7·97	7·96	5
6	Tuberculosis—Other	2·20	1·98	1·87	6
7	Venereal Diseases	0·25	0·26	0·05	7
8	P.U.O.	0·10	—	0·03	8
9	Other diseases due to Infection	0·53	0·44	0·62	9
10	Diseases of the Nervous System	6·10	6·09	5·89	10
11	Mental Disorders	49·52	50·93	50·03	11
12	Diseases of the Eye	1·26	0·86	0·54	12
13	Diseases of the Ear, Nose and Throat	1·69	1·93	2·04	13
14	Diseases of the Cardio-Vascular System	4·20	2·67	2·99	14
15	Diseases of the Blood and Blood-forming Organs	0·53	0·77	0·82	15
16	Diseases of the Endocrine System	2·02	1·88	2·09	16
17	Diseases of the Breast	0·18	0·21	0·16	17
18	Diseases of the Respiratory System	5·03	5·76	6·05	18
19	Diseases of the Digestive System	3·01	3·33	4·10	19
20	Disorders of Nutrition and Metabolism	0·43	0·60	0·43	20
21	Diseases of the Genito-Urinary Tract	5·49	5·30	4·70	21
22	Diseases of the Musculo-Skeletal System	4·93	5·63	5·75	22
23	Diseases of the Areolar Tissue	0·13	0·07	0·11	23
24	Diseases of the Skin	2·25	2·14	2·44	24
25	All Other Diseases	0·51	0·47	0·76	25
		100	100	100	

The Royal Air Force Medical Services

MEDICAL STATISTICS

by Group Captain S. C. Rexford Welch,
M.A., M.Sc., M.R.C.S., L.R.C.P.

CONTENTS

I. ROYAL AIR FORCE

CHARTS

I. Royal Air Force

INTRODUCTION

THE collection of Royal Air Force medical statistics at the outbreak of war in 1939 was undertaken by Branch M.A.7 of Air Ministry. In 1941 this function was taken over by the Central Statistical Branch but this was a change in name only as the methods employed did not alter.

The system of medical documentation employed in the R.A.F. in 1939 proved as useful under conditions of war as it had been in peace and few modifications had to be made. These modifications were aimed at easing the burden on staff and transport, for example, stations and commands were required to submit monthly summaries of sickness instead of the weekly returns of peace-time.

It is interesting to note that the Inter-Services Committee on Medical Documentation which was formed after the war based its recommendations largely on the existing R.A.F. system.*

The medical documents of each officer and airman were contained in a Medical History Envelope (Form 48) at the man's unit. During the relatively static conditions of peace-time there was rarely a delay of more than twenty-four hours between the arrival of a man at a new unit and the receipt of his Medical History Envelope. During war-time, with a vastly increased force and an overloaded communications system, there was often a considerable delay between the man's arrival and the receipt of his medical documents. Medical officers, however, usually had a complete record of a man's medical history available eventually. One fault of the system was that the Medical History Envelope carried no record of minor but often significant illnesses not requiring admission to sick quarters or hospital; all such ailments were recorded in the station sick book at Sick Parade. (Since the war the sick book has been superseded by Treatment Cards for the recording of minor illnesses and these cards accompany the rest of a man's documents.)

Many Service patients admitted to station sick quarters or hospitals were suffering from minor illnesses for which civilian patients would be treated at home, but with which the airman could rarely remain sick in quarters. These cases of forty-eight hours' duration or less were not fully documented but brief notes on diagnosis and treatment were made in the sick book. Exceptions to this rule were made in certain diseases, such as gonorrhoea, which, though requiring only a very brief in-patient treatment, were nevertheless of special interest. Patients were classified

* The system of documentation for W.A.A.F. personnel was identical with that described here for the R.A.F.

as (1) 'admitted'—i.e. in hospital or sick quarters or sick at home for more than forty-eight hours; (2) 'detained'—i.e. in sick quarters for forty-eight hours or less; and (3) 'excused duty'—i.e. merely off duty and not necessarily in sick quarters.

For cases which were admitted all records were prepared in triplicate. A manuscript copy (Form 41) was prepared in the first instance by the medical officer and from this were typed a card copy and a flimsy copy (Forms 39). The original manuscript copy was retained at the unit, the flimsy copy was inserted in the Medical History Envelope (Form 48) and the card copy forwarded to Air Ministry.

The cards on arrival at Air Ministry were analysed on to coding slips from which Hollerith machine cards were punched. Numerical codes were used for everything—trades, age groups, Commands, disposal, disease, etc.

A source of error in the collection of R.A.F. medical records resulted from the admission of R.A.F. patients to Emergency Medical Services (E.M.S.) hospitals. Many outlying units relied almost entirely on E.M.S. hospitals for the treatment of patients and, of course, survivors of air crashes were taken to the nearest hospital, civilian or Service. Men taken ill when on leave and requiring hospital treatment were usually admitted to civilian hospitals. Many of the latter were over-burdened and under-staffed and it was obviously asking too much to expect them to conform to the varied and complicated systems of medical documentation required by the Services.

It is also obvious that human error or enemy action prevented some medical cards from reaching Air Ministry.

Before and during the war period the R.A.F. used its own Disease and Injury classification (which is therefore used in this publication); the International Statistical Classification of Diseases, Injuries and Causes of Death (W.H.O.) was adopted in 1948 and came into use in 1950.

Statistical classification has always been a difficult problem and attempts at improvement have been continuous since the first International Congress in Brussels in 1856. Criticism may therefore be levelled at the war-time system of coding. For instance, only the principal disease leading to admission was coded and no allowance was made for complications of the disease or for secondary disease or injury. Difficulties and inaccuracies in such a method spring to mind. A man admitted with lacerations develops tetanus; is he classified as an injury or as a case of tetanus? A man under treatment for a depressive psychosis takes an overdose of phenobarbitone; is he classified as a psychosis or as an attempted suicide? Again, no differentiation was made between admissions for fresh diseases and recurrent admissions for the same disease. Thus it is right that a man admitted several times during the year for the common cold should represent so many fresh cases of the common cold, but if a man were admitted several times during the year for recurrent episodes of peptic ulcer pain then his classification each time as a fresh case gives a false impression of the incidence of peptic ulcer. This is a common statistical problem and although the R.A.F. has made attempts to remedy it by secondary tabulations, auxiliary codes, etc., no satisfactory solution has as yet been found.

Parallel with the collection of cards and flimsies was the system of summaries of sickness submitted by all stations to their Commands, weekly at first, but later monthly (Form 38); the Commands consolidated these and forwarded them to Air Ministry. These records showed the number of admissions for each particular disease, the number of days spent in hospital or sick quarters and the final disposal of the patient. From these unit records the Principal Medical Officer at Command Headquarters was able to form an up-to-date picture of the health of the Command as a whole. Any undue incidence of a particular disease could be noted and possible preventive measures taken. There was but slight delay in the receipt of these Command records by Air Ministry and a fairly accurate summary of the health of the Royal Air Force was available at any time.

From the medical cards Air Ministry prepared annual reports on the health of the R.A.F. and the W.A.A.F. It is from the tables in these annual reports and from the general library of medical record cards that the present statistical survey has been prepared. For the years 1944 and 1945, when the strength of the R.A.F. was over one million and when staffing problems at Air Ministry were acute, it was found impossible to prepare statistics for the whole force and a 10 per cent. sample was taken, except for figures relating to deaths and medical boards, all of which were examined. The sampling was done by analysing the medical records of every officer and airman who had 0 as the last figure in his Service number; the sample, of course, was large enough to make error insignificant.

These statistics provide the basis for medical planning. They show the trend of diseases, major sources of wastage, the efficacy of different types of treatment and the need for special prophylactic measures. They give now an accurate picture of the health of a known population in defined age groups under known conditions. It is admitted that we are ignorant of morbidity rates in large populations and that our social medicine is founded on mortality statistics. For the country as a whole an attempt has been made to remedy this by analysing certificates of incapacity for work. This covers the whole of the working population, both employed and self-employed. There are, however, inherent inaccuracies in this scheme of collecting statistical data which do not apply to the R.A.F. system. The figures are based on claims for benefit supported by a doctor's certificate. This cannot be a confidential document and is not designed to be an accurate diagnostic record. In many instances doctors are reluctant to disclose a grave diagnosis to a patient. Illness causing absence from work of less than four days does not make the patient eligible for benefit. Ministry of Health surveys have shown that 94 per cent. of illness is of less than four days' duration and that more than three-quarters of those with such illness do not consult their doctors.

But, above all, the following tables show how important a part was played by the medical services in maintaining the R.A.F. as a fully effective fighting force throughout the war and in all parts of the world. Throughout history battles have been won and lost and armies decimated through disease and epidemics. In the South African War typhoid affected more than a quarter of the British Army and over eight thousand men died as a result; dysentery may fairly be said to have been one of the most important causes of failure of the Gallipoli campaign in the War of 1914–18. In the Second World War, however, medicine at last was in the ascendant over disease.

Sickness in the R.A.F., 1939–45

Sickness in the Royal Air Force for the war period 1939–45 is analysed by geographical areas in Tables 1 and 2.

The word sickness used in this report includes disease, accidents and wounds.

The geographical areas included under the heading 'Mediterranean Littoral' in Table 2 are Aden, Egypt and North Africa, Kenya, Malta, Palestine and Trans-Jordan and the Sudan; Italy was included in this group from 1943. Units based in France and Germany in 1944 and 1945 are included under the 'Force at Home'.

The first section of each table is an analysis of all cases of sickness where treatment meant absence from duty, i.e. excused duty, detained in sick quarters for forty-eight hours or less, or admitted to hospital or sick quarters for over forty-eight hours. It does not, of course, refer to all those who were seen and treated on the daily sick parades but who were able to carry on with their duties. The second section of the tables analyses cases of over forty-eight hours' duration.

Final invalidings and deaths are also recorded in these tables.

A comparison of sickness rates in pre-war days with those during war-time is interesting and Chart 1 shows sickness in the total force during the ten years 1936–45. Before the war the R.A.F. was a small, compact and reasonably static force living under relatively good conditions. Every man was a volunteer and morale and discipline were of a high order. The peace-time expansion to meet the German threat was more than adequately catered for in the construction of suitable permanent accommodation at the new stations. It is not surprising, therefore, that sickness rates for the years 1936–39 show a steady and progressive decrease, and it would have been reasonable to expect a considerable increase in sickness rates under war conditions. There was a rapid increase in strength with men drawn from all walks of life. Peace-time standards of accommodation went by the board.* There was often serious overcrowding and the floor space allowed per man in a barrack room or hut had to be reduced from the peace-time standard of 60 sq. ft. to 32 sq. ft. Many men had to live in tents and the temporary huts, erected by a building industry whose resources were strained to the utmost, were often inadequate, draughty and ill-ventilated. Black-out restrictions added severely to the problems of ventilation.† The policy of dispersal of buildings used as a counter-measure to the threat of bombing resulted in men having long walks through the open to reach working areas, dining halls and washhouses. The need for fuel economy meant that only rarely were there adequate facilities for drying damp

* *See R.A.F. Medical Services* Vol. I. Accommodation, pp. 356–358, 362.

† *See R.A.F. Medical Services* Vol. II, No. 60 Group, pp. 665–667.

CHART I

R.A.F. SICKNESS IN THE TOTAL FORCE DURING THE TEN YEARS, 1936–45

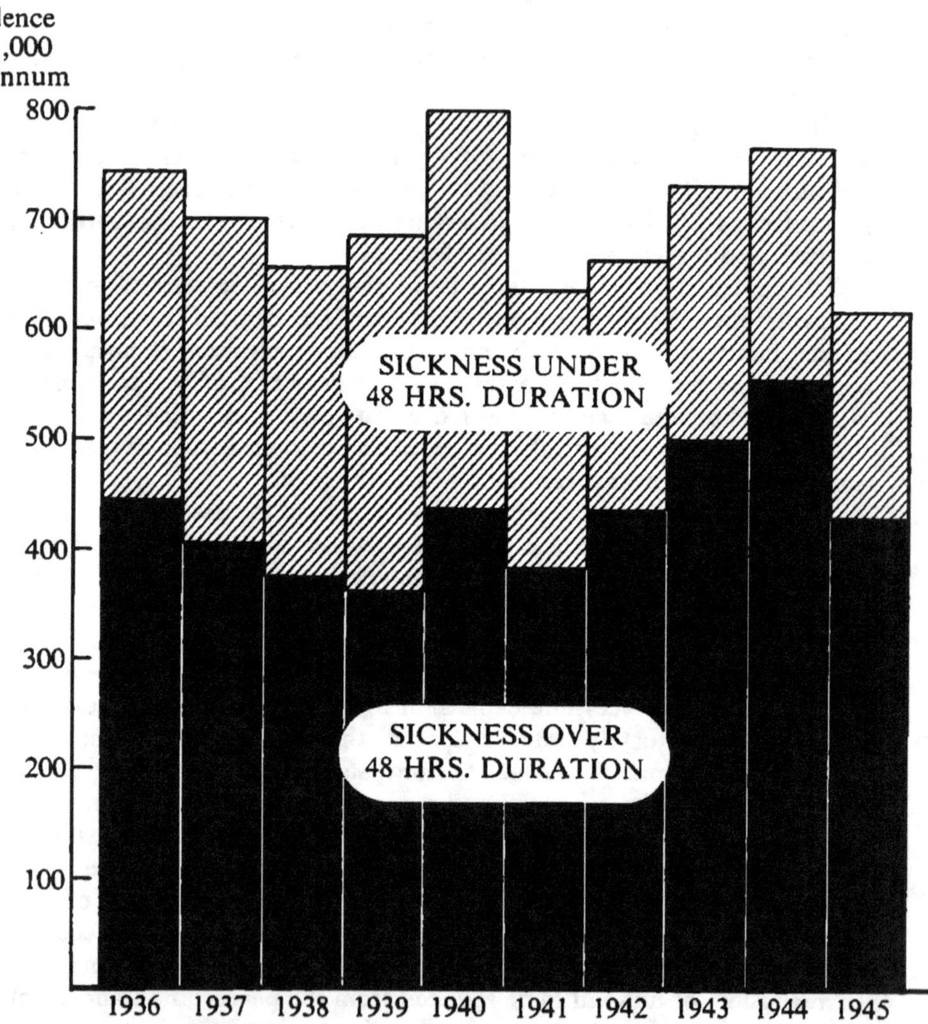

clothing. The problems of feeding large numbers with existing facilities and of providing an adequate diet were considerable. Sewage disposal, particularly on new sites far from existing civil sewerage services, was another big problem and many instances are recorded of sewerage plants being dangerously overloaded. Increased hours of work and the added strain and fatigue of war-time duties were further hazards to health. Added to this, the first winter of the war in 1940 was very severe.

Sickness rates did rise in 1940 but in view of the circumstances the rise was surprisingly small. The total sickness incidence reached a peak for the ten year period at 798 cases per 1,000 of strength which compares favourably with the 1936 figure of 750 cases per 1,000 of strength. Sickness of over 48 hours' duration in 1940 was at the rate of 435 cases per 1,000 of strength which was, in fact, slightly lower than the 1936 rate. In 1941 sickness rates fell considerably and the figure for all sickness of 636 cases per 1,000 of strength was lower than for any of the pre-war years mentioned. Sickness of over 48 hours' duration at 382 cases per 1,000 of strength was lower than the rates for 1936 and 1937. Thereafter, there was a steady rise in sickness rates to 1944 when the total figure was 764 cases per 1,000 of strength and the figure for cases of over 48 hours' duration 551 cases per 1,000 of strength. This can be correlated with the larger percentage of men serving overseas; the sickness rates for the force at home do not show the same trend. In 1945

CHART 2

R.A.F. NUMBER OF SICK DAILY PER 1,000 OF STRENGTH AT HOME AND ABROAD, 1938–45

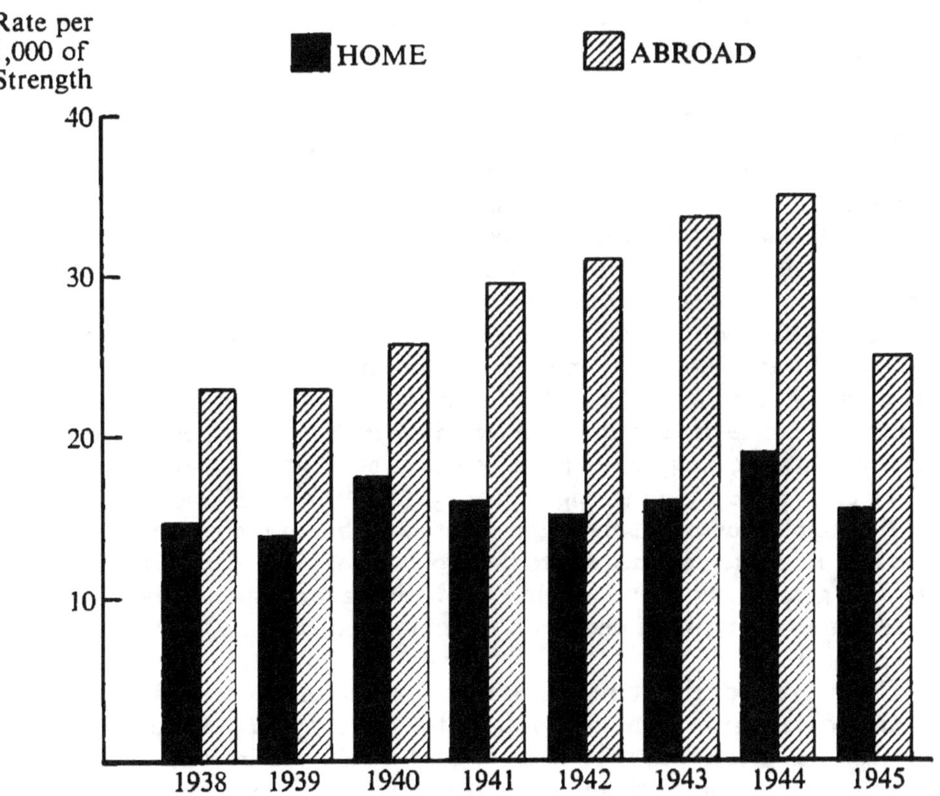

TABLE I

	TOTAL FORCE						
	1939†	1940	1941	1942	1943	1944	1945†
Average Strength	140,862	324,398	662,772	860,747	971,439	1,002,593	933,922
TOTAL SICKNESS							
Number of Cases	96,649	259,015	421,576	568,130	708,494	766,079	572,212
Incidence per 1,000 of strength	686	798	636	660	729	764	613
Average duration in days of each case returned to duty	8.2	9·5	9·5	9·5	9·5	10·8	10·0
Average number of days sickness per head	5·6	6·8	6·5	6·9	7·9	8·8	6·8
Number of sick daily per 1,000 of strength	15·4	18·7	17·8	19·0	21·5	24·2	18·7
*SICKNESS (excluding cases of 48 hours and under)							
Number of Cases	50,276	141,170	253,225	370,388	483,813	552,303	397,644
Incidence per 1,000 of strength	357	435	382	430	498	551	426
Average duration in days of each case returned to duty	14·4	14·5	15·1	14	14	15	14
Average number of days sickness per head	5·1	6·3	6·1	6·6	7·5	8·6	6·6
Number sick daily per 1,000 of strength	14·1	17·3	16·8	18·1	20·7	23·5	18·1
Cases of sickness of 48 hours and under	46,373	117,845	168,351	197,742	224,681	213,776	174,568
FINAL INVALIDINGS							
Numbers	1,173	3,497	10,017	12,875	13,181	15,177	17,946
Incidence per 1,000 of strength	8·3	10·8	15·1	15·0	13·6	15·1	19·2
INVALIDINGS TO THE UNITED KINGDOM							
Numbers	—	—	—	—	—	—	—
Incidence per 1,000 of strength	—	—	—	—	—	—	—
DEATHS							
Numbers	950	6,343	9,892	12,973	18,625	19,665	7,758
Incidence per 1,000 of strength	6·7	19·6	14·9	15·1	19·2	19·6	8·3

* Includes cases resulting in death or invaliding irrespective of duration.
† The whole year.

there was a considerable fall to 613 cases per 1,000 of strength for all sickness and to 426 cases per 1,000 of strength in sickness of over 48 hours' duration. The tonic effect of winning the war must have contributed largely to this, accompanied, as it was, by a general improvement in living conditions and the lessening of operational demands.

Chart 2 records the number of sick daily as rates per 1,000 of strength at home and abroad during the years 1938–45. In other words it represents the average daily wastage of man-power from disease and injury. In the force at home there is surprisingly little difference between the rate for 1938 and that for the war years. Abroad, there was a steady increase in the number of sick daily from 23 cases per 1,000 of strength in 1939 to 35 cases per 1,000 of strength in 1944, with a fall to 25 cases per 1,000 of strength in 1945. (*See* Table 1.) This increase in the number of sick daily is largely attributable to the expansion of the R.A.F. in the Far East where the problems of tropical medicine are at their greatest. For the force in the Mediterranean Littoral the peak year was in 1941 with a decline in the number of sick daily after that. (*See* Table 2.)

Chart 3 records the average number of days sickness per head before return to duty, at home and abroad, for the years 1938–45. At home the average was greatest in 1940 when it was 6·0 days and in 1944 when it was 6·9 days. Abroad there was a steady increase from an average of

R.A.F. Total Sickness at Home and Abroad

FORCE AT HOME							FORCE ABROAD						
1939†	1940	1941	1942	1943	1944	1945†	1939†	1940	1941	1942	1943	1944	1945†
123,430	292,668	584,924	658,334	662,600	683,816	639,269	17,432	31,730	77,848	202,413	308,839	318,777	294,653
80,866	227,871	327,174	322,584	345,699	386,660	293,770	15,783	31,144	94,402	245,546	362,795	379,419	278,442
655	779	559	490	522	565	460	905	982	1,213	1,213	1,175	1,190	945
8·0	8·4	9·6	10·3	10·6	11·9	11·5	9·4	9·6	8·8	8·3	8·8	9·1	8·1
5·2	6·5	5·9	5·6	5·9	7·0	5·8	8·5	9·4	10·9	11·3	12·3	12·8	9·2
14·3	17·9	16·2	15·3	16·3	19·1	15·8	23·2	25·7	29·8	31·0	33·6	35·1	25·1
41,385	123,160	202,520	228,350	267,632	311,927	232,518	8,891	18,010	50,705	142,038	216,181	240,376	165,126
335	421	346	347	404	456	364	510	568	651	702	700	754	560
14·2	14·3	15·2	15	14	15	15	15·5	15·5	14·5	14	14	14	13
4·7	6·0	5·6	5·4	5·8	6·9	5·6	7·9	8·8	10·2	10·6	11·6	12·2	8·6
13·0	16·5	15·4	14·7	15·8	18·8	15·5	21·7	24·1	27·9	29·0	31·8	33·5	23·7
39,481	104,711	124,654	94,234	78,067	74,733	61,252	6,892	13,134	43,697	103,508	146,614	139,043	113,316
1,089	3,398	9,908	12,477	12,286	13,489	16,267	84	99	109	398	895	1,689	1,679
8·8	11·6	16·9	19·0	18·5	19·7	25·4	4·8	3·1	1·4	2·0	2·9	5·2	5·7
—	—	—	—	—	—	—	322	648	600	1,220	3,410	7,146	5,545
—	—	—	—	—	—	—	18·5	20·4	7·7	6·0	11·0	22·4	18·8
828	5,229	8,113	9,896	15,030	16,278	5,641	122	1,114	1,779	3,077	3,595	3,387	2,117
6·7	17·9	13·9	15·0	22·7	23·8	8·8	7·0	35·1	22·9	15·2	11·6	10·6	7·2

7·9 days in 1939 to 12·2 days in 1944 with a fall to 8·6 days in 1945. (*See* also Table 1.) Again this is correlated with the increasing size of the R.A.F. in the Far East.

During the war when the number of civilian hospital beds often proved inadequate to deal with the demand, criticism was occasionally levelled at the R.A.F. policy of maintaining a large number of beds and retaining patients for long periods. The explanation, of course, is that all R.A.F. patients had to be kept in hospital or sick quarters until they were completely fit for duty and life under rigorous conditions. The development of medical rehabilitation units and convalescent units did much to ease the demand on hospital beds, but Service medical officers were very rightly reluctant to return men to duty when they were still semi-convalescent.

The various causes of invaliding are analysed in Table 16 and discussed in the section relating thereto (page 595). The considerably higher incidence of invaliding from the force at home is a result of the system of retaining all men with limited medical categories in the United Kingdom; obviously, men with past histories of medical complaints tended to make up the majority of invalidings.

The high incidence of invaliding in 1945 was a natural concomitant of victory. Men who were content to suffer their disabilities in the national interest during the war years realised in 1945 that herein lay

TABLE 2

R.A.F. Sickness by Geographical Areas

	MEDITERRANEAN LITTORAL							IRAQ						
	1939	1940	1941	1942	1943	1944	1945	1939	1940	1941	1942	1943	1944	1945
Average Strength	7,305	12,471	39,731	90,351	140,714	154,845	130,932	2,053	1,999	3,324	9,935	8,313	3,610	3,254
TOTAL SICKNESS														
Number of cases	6,662	14,105	62,744	120,826	152,467	158,276	98,538	1,923	1,546	4,594	12,464	10,326	5,825	5,255
Incidence per 1,000 of strength	912	1,131	1,579	1,337	1,084	1,022	753	937	773	1,382	1,255	1,242	1,614	1,615
Average duration in days of each case returned to duty	8·9	9·4	8·0	7·2	9·4	9·1	8·3	10·1	11·2	7·5	9·7	11·1	10·3	8·7
Average number of days sickness per head	8·2	10·6	13·9	11·4	11·4	10·4	7·2	9·5	8·7	12·0	13·8	16·0	18·8	16·2
Number of sick daily per 1,000 of strength	22·3	29·2	38·1	31·3	31·1	28·6	19·6	25·9	23·7	33·0	37·9	43·8	51·4	44·3
*SICKNESS (excluding cases of 48 hours and under)														
Number of cases	3,851	8,337	29,574	58,629	92,379	101,734	61,643	1,398	1,094	2,875	8,744	6,528	4,122	3,495
Incidence per 1,000 of strength	527	669	744	649	657	657	471	681	547	865	880	785	1,142	1,074
Average duration in days of each case returned to duty	14·4	14·9	16·1	14·5	15·1	13·7	12·7	13·3	15·1	11·3	13·4	17·0	14·2	12·6
Average number of days sickness per head	7·6	10·0	12·8	10·4	10·8	10·0	6·8	9·1	8·3	11·3	13·2	14·5	18·1	15·5
Number of sick daily per 1,000 of strength	20·8	27·3	35·0	28·6	29·6	27·3	18·6	24·9	22·5	31·0	36·4	42·1	49·7	42·1
Cases of sickness of 48 hours and under	2,811	5,768	33,170	62,197	60,088	56,542	36,895	525	452	1,719	3,720	3,798	1,703	1,760
FINAL INVALIDINGS														
Numbers	21	16	64	178	439	734	685	3	—	6	12	41	16	11
Incidence per 1,000 of strength	2·9	1·3	1·6	2·0	3·1	4·7	5·2	1·5	—	1·8	1·2	4·9	4·4	3·4
INVALIDINGS TO THE UNITED KINGDOM														
Numbers	71	61	431	492	1,603	2,573	1,612	24	8	21	56	134	111	20
Incidence per 1,000 of strength	9·7	4·9	10·8	5·4	11·4	16·6	12·3	11·7	4·0	6·3	5·6	16·1	30·7	6·1
DEATHS														
Numbers	41	308	1,236	1,742	2,233	2,027	797	8	4	56	48	45	36	14
Incidence per 1,000 of strength	5·6	24·7	31·1	19·3	15·9	13·1	6·1	3·9	2·0	16·8	4·8	5·4	10·0	4·3

* Includes cases resulting in death or invaliding irrespective of duration.

	A.C.S.E.A.		INDIA					SOUTH AFRICA AND SOUTHERN RHODESIA				WEST AFRICA			CANADA	
	1944	1945	1939	1940	1941	1942	1943	1942	1943	1944	1945	1943	1944	1945	1944	1945
Average Strength	93,219	126,846	1,983	1,891	2,952	30,317	82,643	22,575	27,435	28,239	16,759	9,451	8,245	5,141	24,387	5,714
TOTAL SICKNESS																
Number of cases	152,860	146,633	1,541	1,570	2,523	43,293	98,834	22,941	23,661	21,328	6,538	15,774	10,349	3,935	12,311	11,659
Incidence per 1,000 of strength	1,640	1,156	777	830	855	1,428	1,196	1,016	862	755	390	1,669	1,255	765	505	290
Average duration in days of each case returned to duty	9·5	7·9	9·6	9·5	9·7	9·7	11·1	8·3	8·0	9·6	10·2	8·2	7·7	8·2	13·4	12·9
Average number of days sickness per head	18·6	11·3	7·5	7·9	8·5	15·3	14·9	7·9	9·3	10·1	6·0	14·2	11·8	7·9	6·9	4·9
Number of sick daily per 1,000 of strength	50·9	31·1	20·5	21·2	23·4	41·8	40·9	21·5	22·9	27·9	16·4	38·9	32·4	21·4	19·0	13·3
*SICKNESS (excluding cases of 48 hours and under)																
Number of cases	93,227	84,142	936	1,044	1,688	27,524	64,531	12,439	13,247	14,350	4,386	9,091	6,645	2,589	12,311	11,659
Incidence per 1,000 of strength	1,000	663	472	552	572	908	781	551	483	508	262	962	806	504	505	290
Average duration in days of each case returned to duty	15·1	13·3	14·9	13·5	13·8	14·8	16·7	11·9	13·5	14·0	15·0	13·3	11·5	12·1	13·4	12·9
Average number of days sickness per head	17·7	10·7	7·0	7·4	8·1	14·5	14·4	7·5	7·8	9·8	5·8	13·2	11·2	7·5	6·9	4·9
Number of sick daily per 1,000 of strength	48·5	29·3	19·3	20·1	22·2	39·8	39·4	20·5	21·5	27·0	15·9	36·3	30·7	20·4	19·0	13·3
Cases of sickness of 48 hours and under	59,633	62,491	605	526	835	15,769	34,303	10,502	10,414	6,978	2,152	6,683	3,704	1,346	—	—
FINAL INVALIDINGS																
Numbers	535	718	3	1	1	18	121	32	76	161	101	24	42	57	141	77
Incidence per 1,000 of strength	5·7	5·7	1·5	0·5	0·3	0·6	1·5	1·4	2·8	5·7	6·0	2·5	5·1	11·1	5·8	13·5
INVALIDINGS TO THE UNITED KINGDOM																
Numbers	3,211	3,276	11	3	5	141	772	108	247	495	208	198	276	104	288	127
Incidence per 1,000 of strength	34·4	25·8	5·5	1·6	1·7	4·7	9·3	4·8	9·0	17·5	12·4	21·0	33·5	20·2	11·8	22·2
DEATHS																
Numbers	982	1,124	10	18	14	277	559	166	192	139	65	82	43	12	110	22
Incidence per 1,000 of strength	10·5	8·9	5·0	9·5	4·7	9·1	6·8	7·4	7·0	4·9	3·9	8·7	5·2	2·3	4·5	3·9

* Includes cases resulting in death or invaliding irrespective of duration.

CHART 3
R.A.F. AVERAGE NUMBER OF DAYS SICKNESS PER HEAD AT HOME AND ABROAD, 1938–45

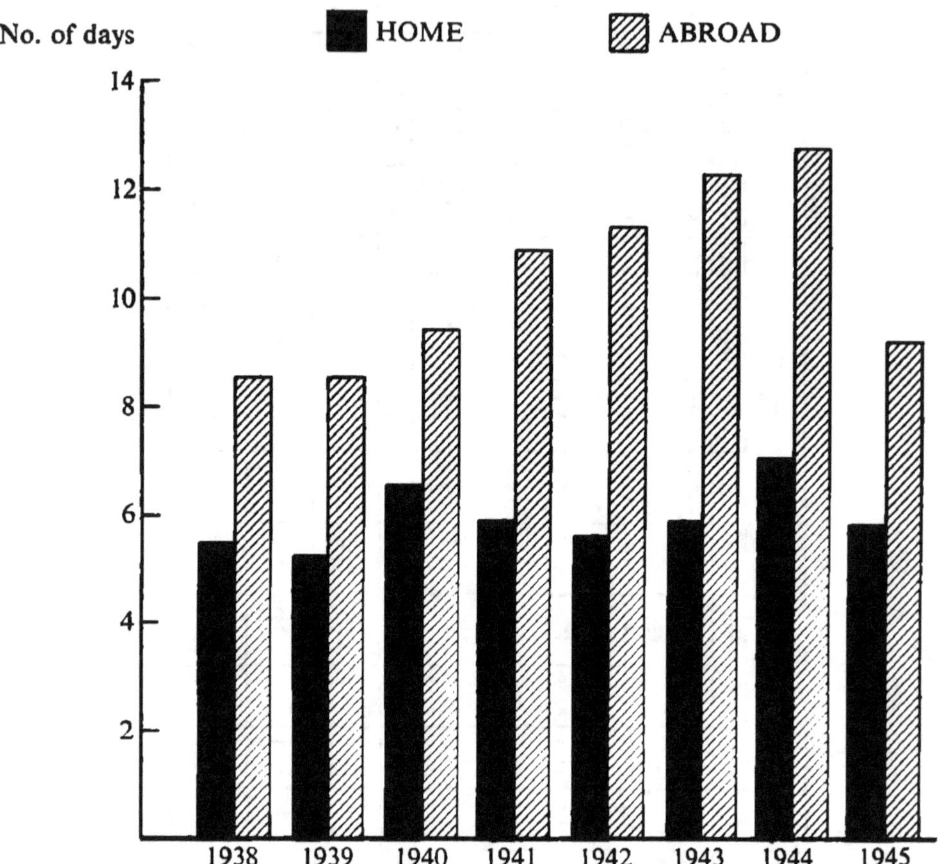

the opportunity of quick release to civilian life and the avoiding of the tedious process of group demobilisation. It is also probably true to say that the invaliding medical boards tended to take a more lenient view of borderline cases when the end of the war was in sight. (*See R.A.F. Medical Services* Vol. III, India and Far East, pp. 629–633, 694.)

SICKNESS AS A WHOLE

Tables 3a, 3b and 3c are the main nosological tables analysing the incidence of diseases and injuries for the Royal Air Force as a whole and for the Commands at home and abroad. The tables show diseases in groups according to the system of the body in which the main lesion is present and the groups are further divided on an anatomical or pathological basis; in some instances individual diseases have been specified. The group of infectious diseases shows the more important tropical diseases separately and the remainder, with the exception of infections of the nervous system, are recorded under the type of organism causing the infection.

TABLE 3(a)
R.A.F. Nosological Table for Total Force
Period of Second World War, September 3, 1939 to August 15, 1945
Fresh Cases

	1939*		1940		1941		1942		1943		1944		1945*		Totals	
	Number of Cases	Incidence per 1,000 per annum	Number of Cases	Incidence per 1,000 per annum	Number of Cases	Incidence per 1,000 per annum	Number of Cases	Incidence per 1,000 per annum	Number of Cases	Incidence per 1,000 per annum	Number of Cases	Incidence per 1,000 per annum	Number of Cases	Incidence per 1,000 per annum	Number of Cases	Incidence per 1,000 per annum
INFECTIOUS DISEASES																
Amoebic Dysentery	2	0·03	30	0·09	120	0·18	1,027	1·19	2,745	2·83	4,363	4·35	2,088	3·46	10,375	2·31
Bacillary Dysentery	27	0·42	279	0·86	1,975	2·98	6,171	7·17	8,469	8·72	8,897	8·87	6,044	10·00	31,862	7·09
Enteric Group	6	0·09	16	0·05	150	0·23	388	0·45	419	0·43	562	0·56	304	0·50	1,845	0·41
Enteritis	420	6·57	2,661	8·20	7,495	11·31	6,550	7·61	1,299	1·34	1,730	1·73	1,290	2·14	21,445	4·78
Malaria	158	2·47	945	2·91	3,637	5·49	12,489	14·51	24,126	24·84	26,220	26·15	7,142	11·82	74,717	16·64
Other Tropical Infections	254	3·98	677	2·09	3,680	5·55	8,786	10·21	9,464	9·74	8,919	8·90	3,938	6·52	35,718	7·95
Bacillary Infections (other than Typhoid and Dysentery)	25	0·39	169	0·52	450	0·68	656	0·76	716	0·74	1,189	1·19	332	0·55	3,537	0·79
Staphylococcal and Streptococcal Infections	114	1·79	832	2·57	891	1·34	1,185	1·38	2,024	2·09	2,024	2·02	399	0·66	7,469	1·66
Virus Infections	462	7·23	7,782	23·99	4,230	6·38	6,600	7·67	4,275	4·40	6,460	6·44	3,362	5·57	33,171	7·39
Metazoan Parasite Infections	10	1·16	64	0·20	97	0·15	263	0·30	473	0·49	623	0·62	430	0·71	1,960	0·44
Infections of Unknown or Doubtful Origin	219	3·43	1,125	3·47	2,825	4·26	5,737	6·67	11,936	12·27	13,276	13·24	3,992	6·61	39,110	8·71
Central Nervous System Infections	120	1·88	922	2·84	1,633	2·46	1,882	2·19	2,165	2·23	3,118	3·11	1,554	2·57	11,394	2·54
Totals	1,817	29·44	15,502	47·79	27,183	41·01	51,734	60·11	68,111	70·12	77,381	77·18	30,875	51·11	272,603	60·71

INFECTIONS OF RESPIRATORY TRACT																
Common Cold, Naso-Pharyngitis and Sore Throat	2,154	33·71	18,899	58·26	27,140	40·95	32,970	38·30	51,287	52·80	44,635	44·52	20,800	34·43	197,885	44·07
Influenza	1,473	23·05	17,693	54·54	20,117	30·35	16,454	19·12	29,857	30·73	17,535	17·49	5,020	8·31	108,149	24·09
Tonsillitis	2,015	31·54	10,476	32·29	17,976	27·12	26,502	30·79	33,303	34·28	38,472	38·37	18,470	30·57	147,214	32·79
Vincent's Angina	40	0·63	395	1·22	1,802	2·72	3,177	3·69	2,750	2·83	2,531	2·53	1,120	1·85	11,815	2·63
Upper Respiratory Tract Infections Totals	5,682	88·93	47,463	146·31	67,035	101·14	79,103	91·90	117,197	120·64	103,173	102·91	45,410	75·16	465,063	103·58
PNEUMONIA	136	2·13	1,183	3·65	2,859	4·31	3,093	3·59	3,557	3·66	6,542	6·53	2,183	3·61	19,553	4·35
PULMONARY TUBERCULOSIS	97	1·52	416	1·28	967	1·46	1,624	1·89	2,030	2·09	1,417	1·41	1,101	1·82	7,652	1·70
TUBERCULOSIS OTHER THAN PULMONARY	16	0·25	103	0·32	294	0·44	366	0·43	400	0·41	574	0·57	210	0·35	1,963	0·44
VACCINIA AND POST INOCULATION EFFECTS	461	7·22	2,409	7·43	2,433	3·67	1,231	1·43	2,947	3·03	2,958	2·95	820	1·36	13,259	2·95
CARRIERS	3	0·05	18	0·06	31	0·05	45	0·05	95	0·10	145	0·14	200	0·33	537	0·12
CONTACTS	11	0·17	153	0·47	216	0·33	240	0·28	346	0·36	391	0·39	120	0·20	1,477	0·33
VENEREAL DISEASES																
Gonorrhoea	584	9·14	2,273	7·01	4,617	6·96	7,066	8·21	8,678	8·93	13,311	13·28	9,658	15·99	46,187	10·29
Syphilis	46	0·72	250	0·77	647	0·98	1,195	1·39	1,397	1·44	2,404	2·40	1,736	2·87	7,675	1·71
Syphilis with Gonorrhoea	—	—	—	—	—	—	3	0·003	68	0·07	144	0·14	20	0·03	235	0·05
Others	42	0·66	110	0·34	292	0·44	497	0·58	727	0·75	2,321	2·31	1,310	2·17	5,299	1·18
Totals	672	10·52	2,633	8·12	5,556	8·38	8,761	10·18	10,870	11·19	18,180	18·13	12,724	21·06	59,396	13·25
SEPTIC CONDITIONS (Areolar Tissues, Lymphatic Channels and Breasts)																
Conditions due to Pyogenic Organisms	1,178	18·44	6,435	19·83	12,326	18·60	19,812	23·02	23,857	24·56	29,989	29·91	13,780	22·81	107,377	23·91
Other Conditions	15	0·23	145	0·45	385	0·58	834	0·97	1,165	1·20	1,573	1·57	845	1·40	4,962	1·11
Breasts	4	0·06	13	0·04	41	0·06	83	0·09	88	0·09	119	0·12	50	0·08	398	0·09
Totals	1,197	18·73	6,593	20·32	12,752	19·24	20,729	24·08	25,110	25·85	31,681	31·60	14,675	24·29	112,737	25·11

* Figures for 1939 and 1945 are for the war periods of the years only, *viz.* 1939—from September 3 to December 31; 1945—from January 1 to August 15.

TABLE 3(a)—(*contd.*)

R.A.F. Nosological Table for Total Force
Period of Second World War, September 3, 1939 to August 15, 1945
Fresh Cases

	1939*		1940		1941		1942		1943		1944		1945*		Totals	
	Number of Cases	Incidence per 1,000 per annum	Number of Cases	Incidence per 1,000 per annum	Number of Cases	Incidence per 1,000 per annum	Number of Cases	Incidence per 1,000 per annum	Number of Cases	Incidence per 1,000 per annum	Number of Cases	Incidence per 1,000 per annum	Number of Cases	Incidence per 1,000 per annum	Number of Cases	Incidence per 1,000 per annum
ALIMENTARY SYSTEM DISEASES																
Dental Conditions	119	1·86	672	2·07	1,463	2·21	1,885	2·19	2,155	2·22	2,222	2·22	1,090	1·80	9,606	2·14
Mouth, Pharynx and Oesophagus	45	0·71	261	0·80	745	1·13	1,165	1·35	1,305	1·34	1,652	1·65	1,118	1·85	6,291	1·40
Gastric Ulcer and its Complications	101	1·58	443	1·37	849	1·28	563	0·65	477	0·49	643	0·64	304	0·50	3,380	0·75
Other Gastric Conditions	379	5·93	2,271	7·00	4,588	6·92	6,629	7·70	7,238	7·45	9,206	9·18	4,711	7·80	35,022	7·80
Duodenal Ulcer and its Complications	191	2·99	694	2·14	2,014	3·04	2,612	3·03	2,885	2·97	3,716	3·71	2,283	3·78	14,395	3·21
Duodenitis	18	0·28	104	0·32	161	0·24	300	0·35	280	0·29	204	0·20	191	0·32	1,258	0·28
Appendicitis, All Types	421	6·59	2,105	6·49	3,671	5·54	4,569	5·31	4,910	5·06	6,257	6·24	2,474	4·09	24,407	5·43
Other Intestinal Conditions	185	2·90	799	2·46	1,518	2·29	12,141	14·11	21,598	22·23	22,347	22·29	15,668	25·93	74,256	16·54
Rectum and Anus	199	3·11	1,183	3·65	2,685	4·05	4,268	4·96	4,890	5·03	6,500	6·48	3,203	5·30	22,928	5·11
Hernia, All Types	222	3·47	1,632	5·03	4,264	6·43	5,877	6·83	4,982	5·13	6,190	6·17	2,814	4·66	25,981	5·79
Liver and Gall Bladder	26	0·41	122	0·38	327	0·49	722	0·84	1,322	1·36	1,616	1·61	480	0·80	4,615	1·03
Pancreas	—	—	2	0·01	8	0·01	6	0·01	7	0·01	43	0·04	13	0·02	79	0·02
Peritoneum	4	0·06	23	0·07	32	0·05	98	0·11	86	0·09	146	0·15	36	0·06	425	0·09
Totals	1,910	29·89	10,311	31·79	22,325	33·68	40,835	47·44	52,135	53·67	60,742	60·58	34,385	56·91	222,643	49·59

CIRCULATORY SYSTEM DISEASES																
Pericardium	—	—	17	0·05	15	0·02	25	0·03	40	0·04	23	0·02	24	0·04	144	0·03
Endocarditis and Valvular Disease of the Heart	54	0·85	180	0·56	279	0·42	406	0·47	405	0·42	395	0·40	166	0·27	1,885	0·42
Myocardium	38	0·59	162	0·50	208	0·31	231	0·27	277	0·29	295	0·30	131	0·22	1,342	0·30
Cardiac Arrhythmias	28	0·44	160	0·49	243	0·37	263	0·31	246	0·25	374	0·37	126	0·21	1,440	0·32
Disordered Action of the Heart	37	0·58	199	0·61	460	0·70	657	0·76	674	0·69	765	0·76	341	0·56	3,133	0·70
Totals	157	2·46	718	2·21	1,205	1·82	1,582	1·84	1,642	1·69	1,852	1·85	788	1·30	7,944	1·77
Blood Vessels	174	2·72	934	2·88	2,487	3·75	4,014	4·66	4,336	4·46	4,850	4·84	3,182	5·27	19,977	4·45
Circulatory System Totals	331	5·18	1,652	5·09	3,692	5·57	5,596	6·50	5,978	6·15	6,702	6·69	3,970	6·57	27,921	6·22
BLOOD, BLOOD-FORMING ORGANS, SPLEEN AND RETICULO-ENDOTHELIAL SYSTEM																
Anaemias	8	0·12	44	0·13	117	0·18	179	0·21	246	0·25	190	0·19	145	0·24	929	0·20
Leukaemias	2	0·03	10	0·03	15	0·02	21	0·02	20	0·02	45	0·05	7	0·01	120	0·03
Purpuras	3	0·05	9	0·03	21	0·03	37	0·04	48	0·05	61	0·06	33	0·06	212	0·05
Other Diseases of the Blood	3	0·05	12	0·04	25	0·04	30	0·03	72	0·08	86	0·09	56	0·09	284	0·06
Lymphatic Glands	1	0·02	15	0·05	37	0·06	110	0·13	37	0·04	85	0·08	62	0·10	347	0·08
Spleen and Reticulo-Endothelial System	3	0·05	8	0·02	23	0·03	57	0·07	82	0·08	133	0·13	10	0·02	316	0·07
Totals	20	0·31	98	0·30	238	0·36	434	0·50	505	0·52	600	0·60	313	0·52	2,208	0·49
RESPIRATORY SYSTEM DISEASES																
Larynx and Trachea	3	0·05	9	0·03	24	0·04	647	0·75	1,147	1·18	1,334	1·33	703	1·17	3,867	0·86
Bronchi	708	11·08	3,676	11·33	5,637	8·50	10,001	11·62	13,713	14·12	17,135	17·09	8,188	13·55	59,058	13·15
Lungs	51	0·80	195	0·60	396	0·60	1,290	1·50	1,335	1·37	1,644	1·64	580	0·96	5,491	1·22
Pleura	139	2·17	817	2·52	1,698	2·56	2,087	2·42	1,899	1·95	3,145	3·14	1,010	1·67	10,795	2·41
Mediastinum	—	—	—	—	—	—	8	0·01	6	0·01	1	0·001	2	0·003	17	0·003
Totals	901	14·10	4,697	14·48	7,755	11·70	14,033	16·30	18,100	18·63	23,259	23·20	10,483	17·35	79,228	17·64

* Figures for 1939 and 1945 are for the war periods of the years only, *viz.* 1939—from September 3 to December 31; 1945—from January 1 to August 15.

TABLE 3(a)—(*contd.*)

R.A.F. Nosological Table for Total Force
Period of Second World War, September 3, 1939 to August 15, 1945
Fresh Cases

	1939*		1940		1941		1942		1943		1944		1945*		Totals	
	Number of Cases	Incidence per 1,000 per annum	Number of Cases	Incidence per 1,000 per annum	Number of Cases	Incidence per 1,000 per annum	Number of Cases	Incidence per 1,000 per annum	Number of Cases	Incidence per 1,000 per annum	Number of Cases	Incidence per 1,000 per annum	Number of Cases	Incidence per 1,000 per annum	Number of Cases	Incidence per 1,000 per annum
ALLERGY, DISEASES OF																
Asthma	119	1·86	525	1·62	1,205	1·82	1,301	1·51	1,197	1·23	1,777	1·77	834	1·38	6,958	1·55
Hay Fever	—	—	13	0·04	49	0·07	32	0·04	46	0·05	48	0·05	52	0·09	240	0·05
Urticaria	29	0·45	222	0·68	395	0·60	639	0·74	756	0·78	935	0·93	565	0·93	3,541	0·79
Others	1	0·02	14	0·04	25	0·04	99	0·12	121	0·12	101	0·10	36	0·06	397	0·09
Totals	149	2·33	774	2·38	1,674	2·53	2,071	2·41	2,120	2·18	2,861	2·85	1,487	2·46	11,136	2·48
URINARY SYSTEM DISEASES																
Anomalies of Urinary Secretion	75	1·17	358	1·10	767	1·16	1,348	1·57	1,461	1·50	1,652	1·65	859	1·42	6,520	1·45
Nephritis, All Forms	33	0·52	151	0·47	249	0·37	331	0·38	333	0·34	420	0·42	173	0·29	1,690	0·38
Kidney	55	0·86	308	0·95	600	0·90	801	0·93	1,019	1·05	1,073	1·07	661	1·09	4,517	1·01
Urinary Calculi and Urinary Colic	68	1·06	303	0·93	648	0·98	861	1·00	1,116	1·15	1,430	1·43	841	1·39	5,267	1·17
Bladder	49	0·77	227	0·70	640	0·97	839	0·97	1,149	1·18	1,365	1·36	649	1·08	4,918	1·09
Others	2	0·03	10	0·03	25	0·04	22	0·03	35	0·04	55	0·05	39	0·06	188	0·04
Totals	282	4·41	1,357	4·18	2,929	4·42	4,202	4·88	5,113	5·26	5,995	5·98	3,222	5·33	23,100	5·14
GENERATIVE SYSTEM DISEASES																
Prostate	8	0·12	30	0·09	74	0·11	201	0·23	272	0·28	439	0·44	264	0·44	1,288	0·29
Urethra	136	2·13	783	2·42	1,587	2·39	2,045	2·38	2,602	2·68	2,268	2·26	540	0·89	9,961	2·22
Penis	136	2·13	641	1·98	1,371	2·07	2,135	2·48	2,338	2·40	2,665	2·66	1,680	2·78	10,966	2·44
Spermatic Cord, Testis and Epididymis	88	1·38	478	1·47	1,297	1·96	1,953	2·27	2,281	2·35	2,808	2·80	1,582	2·62	10,487	2·33
Totals	368	5·76	1,932	5·96	4,329	6·53	6,334	7·36	7,493	7·71	8,180	8·16	4,066	6·73	32,702	7·28

LOCOMOTOR SYSTEM DISEASES																
Muscles	26	0·41	131	0·41	227	0·34	284	0·33	287	0·29	286	0·29	183	0·30	1,424	0·32
Rheumatic Group	255	3·99	1,610	4·96	3,087	4·66	4,084	4·75	4,795	4·94	7,014	6·99	3,690	6·11	24,535	5·47
Deformities	92	1·44	620	1·91	1,627	2·46	1,363	1·58	1,126	1·16	1,826	1·82	664	1·0	7,318	1·63
Joints	218	3·41	1,289	3·97	2,901	4·38	5,009	5·82	6,389	6·58	5,301	5·29	3,211	5·32	24,318	5·42
Internal Derangement of Knee Joint	24	0·37	154	0·48	463	0·70	1,080	1·25	1,466	1·51	1,545	1·54	713	1·18	5,445	1·21
Bones and Cartilages	25	0·39	227	0·70	473	0·71	570	0·66	594	0·61	680	0·68	367	0·61	2,936	0·65
Ligaments and Tendons	47	0·74	315	0·97	717	1·08	739	0·86	461	0·47	576	0·57	444	0·73	3,299	0·73
Effects of Old Injuries	—	—	—	—	—	—	—	—	—	—	2,604	2·60	1,519	2·51	4,123	0·92
Totals	687	10·75	4,346	13·40	9,495	14·33	13,129	15·25	15,118	15·56	19,832	19·78	10,791	17·76	73,398	16·35
NERVOUS SYSTEM AND MENTAL DISEASES																
Psychoneuroses	267	4·18	1,680	5·18	4,230	6·38	6,047	7·02	6,893	7·10	8,851	8·83	5,233	8·66	33,201	7·39
Psychoses	96	1·50	255	0·79	488	0·74	516	0·60	645	0·66	831	0·83	315	0·52	3,146	0·70
Psychopathic Personality	49	0·77	266	0·82	508	0·77	711	0·83	1,039	1·07	1,841	1·83	1,142	1·89	5,556	1·24
Mental Defect	1	0·02	23	0·07	180	0·27	190	0·22	185	0·19	169	0·17	112	0·19	860	0·19
Epilepsies	84	1·31	323	0·99	689	1·04	661	0·77	645	0·66	578	0·58	324	0·54	3,304	0·74
Indefinite Aetiology	87	1·36	487	1·50	1,120	1·69	1,485	1·73	1,669	1·72	1,704	1·70	969	1·60	7,521	1·68
Totals	584	9·14	3,034	9·35	7,215	10·89	9,610	11·17	11,076	11·40	13,974	13·94	8,095	13·40	53,588	11·94
ORGANIC NERVOUS DISEASES																
Brain, Diseases of	30	0·47	89	0·27	207	0·31	239	0·28	310	0·32	403	0·40	173	0·29	1,451	0·32
Organic Diseases Indefinite	11	0·17	53	0·16	169	0·25	132	0·15	142	0·15	188	0·19	91	0·15	786	0·17
Cranial Nerves	15	0·24	100	0·31	222	0·34	284	0·33	310	0·32	360	0·36	325	0·54	1,616	0·36
Spinal Cord	16	0·25	38	0·12	102	0·15	76	0·09	103	0·10	56	0·06	39	0·06	430	0·10
Spinal and Peripheral Nerves	103	1·61	567	1·75	1,048	1·58	1,520	1·76	1,902	1·96	2,791	2·78	1,257	2·08	9,188	2·05
Others	—	—	23	0·07	17	0·03	58	0·07	—	—	—	—	—	—	98	0·02
Totals	175	2·74	870	2·68	1,765	2·66	2,309	2·68	2,767	2·85	3,798	3·79	1,885	3·12	13,569	3·02
Nervous System and Mental Diseases Totals	759	11·88	3,904	12·03	8,980	13·55	11,919	13·85	13,843	14·25	17,772	17·73	9,980	16·52	67,157	14·96

* Figures for 1939 and 1945 are for the war periods of the years only *viz.* 1939—from September 3 to December 31; 1945—from January 1 to August 15.

TABLE 3(a)—(*contd.*)

R.A.F. Nosological Table for Total Force
Period of Second World War, September 3, 1939 to August 15, 1945
Fresh Cases

	1939*		1940		1941		1942		1943		1944		1945*		Totals	
	Number of Cases	Incidence per 1,000 per annum	Number of Cases	Incidence per 1,000 per annum	Number of Cases	Incidence per 1,000 per annum	Number of Cases	Incidence per 1,000 per annum	Number of Cases	Incidence per 1,000 per annum	Number of Cases	Incidence per 1,000 per annum	Number of Cases	Incidence per 1,000 per annum	Number of Cases	Incidence per 1,000 per annum
EYE DISEASES																
Defects of Vision	9	0·14	125	0·39	401	0·60	600	0·70	734	0·76	673	0·67	506	0·84	3,048	0·68
Inflammatory Conditions	115	1·80	578	1·78	1,157	1·75	1,599	1·86	2,110	2·17	3,077	3·07	1,637	2·71	10,273	2·29
Others	89	1·39	472	1·45	959	1·45	1,294	1·50	1,518	1·56	1,888	1·88	968	1·60	7,188	1·60
Totals	213	3·33	1,175	3·62	2,517	3·80	3,493	4·06	4,362	4·49	5,638	5·62	3,111	5·15	20,509	4·57
EAR DISEASES																
Deafness	—	—	—	—	—	—	340	0·40	361	0·37	379	0·38	328	0·54	1,408	0·31
Otitis Media, Acute	126	1·98	1,125	3·47	2,020	3·05	3,041	3·53	3,063	3·15	3,570	3·56	1,455	2·41	14,400	3·21
Otitis Media, Chronic	64	1·00	448	1·38	1,311	1·98	1,592	1·85	2,161	2·23	2,961	2·95	1,660	2·75	10,197	2·27
Otitis Externa	86	1·35	303	0·93	661	1·00	1,263	1·47	2,180	2·24	2,879	2·87	1,865	3·09	9,237	2·06
Perforated Tympanic Membrane	4	0·06	75	0·23	216	0·33	95	0·11	31	0·03	48	0·05	31	0·05	500	0·11
Mastoiditis, Acute	6	0·09	72	0·22	194	0·29	173	0·20	203	0·21	377	0·38	116	0·19	1,141	0·25
Mastoiditis, Chronic	4	0·06	15	0·05	39	0·06	77	0·09	60	0·06	93	0·09	49	0·08	337	0·08
Others	32	0·50	44	0·14	162	0·24	142	0·16	172	0·18	226	0·23	164	0·27	942	0·21
Totals	322	5·04	2,082	6·42	4,603	6·95	6,723	7·81	8,231	8·47	10,533	10·51	5,668	9·38	38,162	8·5
NOSE AND THROAT DISEASES																
Nasal Passages }									2,673	2·75	3,028	3·02	1,694	2·80	7,395	1·65
Sinuses }	161	2·52	1,539	4·74	3,321	5·01	4,913	5·71	3,442	3·54	4,415	4·40	1,948	3·22	19,739	4·39
Naso-Pharynx }									3,472	3·58	3,513	3·51	1,540	2·55	8,525	1·90
Throat }	78	1·22	603	1·86	1,638	2·47	2,971	3·45	15	0·02	29	0·03	10	0·02	5,344	1·19
Totals	239	3·74	2,142	6·60	4,959	7·48	7,884	9·16	9,602	9·89	10,985	10·96	5,192	8·59	41,003	9·13

SKIN DISEASES																
Scabies	295	4·62	2,126	6·55	7,346	11·08	8,973	10·42	4,862	5·01	3,186	3·18	1,330	2·20	28,118	6·26
Impetigo	281	4·40	1,313	4·05	3,220	4·86	5,612	6·52	6,180	6·36	7,154	7·13	3,563	5·90	27,323	6·09
Pediculosis and Pediculitis	30	0·47	209	0·64	352	0·53	323	0·38	157	0·16	180	0·18	70	0·12	1,321	0·29
Tinea Cruris	82	1·29	324	1·00	675	1·02	670	0·78	577	0·60	960	0·96	533	0·88	3,821	0·85
Tinea, Others	57	0·89	248	0·76	655	0·99	1,450	1·68	2,257	2·32	2,545	2·54	1,840	3·05	9,052	2·02
Dermatitis and Eczema	130	2·03	962	2·97	2,167	3·27	4,283	4·98	5,461	5·62	7,048	7·03	3,453	5·71	23,504	5·23
Pityriasis and Erythemata	73	1·14	485	1·50	1,057	1·60	1,068	1·24	701	0·72	876	0·87	579	0·96	4,839	1·08
Psoriasis	18	0·28	85	0·26	248	0·37	349	0·41	392	0·40	527	0·52	271	0·45	1,890	0·42
Ingrowing Toenail	59	0·92	253	0·78	557	0·84	968	1·12	1,163	1·20	1,109	1·11	570	0·94	4,679	1·04
Other Conditions	162	2·54	581	1·79	1,432	2·16	2,321	2·70	3,293	3·39	5,111	5·10	3,091	5·12	15,991	3·56
Totals	1,187	18·58	6,586	20·30	17,709	26·72	26,017	30·23	25,043	25·78	28,696	28·62	15,300	25·33	120,538	26·84
ENDOCRINE DISEASES																
General Endocrine Disturbances	—	—	5	0·02	6	0·01	27	0·03	32	0·03	31	0·03	29	0·05	130	0·03
Male Gonads	3	0·05	23	0·07	166	0·25	202	0·23	165	0·17	261	0·26	181	0·30	1,001	0·22
Parathyroid	—	—	—	—	—	—	4	0·004	5	0·01	11	0·01	11	0·02	31	0·01
Pituitary	1	0·02	4	0·01	22	0·03	15	0·02	27	0·03	40	0·04	24	0·04	133	0·03
Suprarenal	—	—	5	0·02	4	0·01	6	0·01	8	0·01	11	0·01	6	0·01	40	0·01
Thymus	1	0·02	—	—	—	—	1	0·001	2	0·002	10	0·01	2	0·003	16	0·004
Thyroid	15	0·23	70	0·21	165	0·25	204	0·24	191	0·19	287	0·29	124	0·21	1,056	0·24
Totals	20	0·31	107	0·33	363	0·55	459	0·53	430	0·44	651	0·65	377	0·63	2,407	0·54
DISEASES OF METABOLISM	34	0·53	89	0·27	167	0·25	230	0·27	280	0·29	303	0·30	222	0·37	1,325	0·30
DEFICIENCY DISEASES	—	—	10	0·03	5	0·01	47	0·05	224	0·23	571	0·57	270	0·45	1,127	0·25
EFFECTS OF TOXIC SUBSTANCES†	10	0·16	—	—	—	—	130	0·15	144	0·15	138	0·14	200	0·33	622	0·14
PHYSICAL AGENTS, EFFECTS OF†	—	—	—	—	—	—	6	0·01	27	0·03	—	—	—	—	33	0·01
CYSTS AND TUMOURS																
Cysts	33	0·51	226	0·70	441	0·67	766	0·89	1,112	1·14	1,382	1·38	773	1·28	4,733	1·06
Tumours, Benign	28	0·44	123	0·38	300	0·45	499	0·58	573	0·59	590	0·59	420	0·69	2,533	0·56
Tumours, Malignant	12	0·19	78	0·24	161	0·24	211	0·24	281	0·29	401	0·40	234	0·39	1,378	0·31
Tumours, Unspecified	3	0·05	13	0·04	20	0·03	109	0·13	222	0·23	312	0·31	132	0·22	811	0·18
Totals	76	1·19	440	1·36	922	1·39	1,585	1·84	2,188	2·25	2,685	2·68	1,559	2·58	9,455	2·11

* Figures for 1939 and 1945 are for the war periods of the years only *viz.* 1939—from September 3 to December 31; 1945—from January 1 to August 15.

† *See* R.A.F. Vol. II, Chap. 7, *Maintenance Command*, pp. 513–26.

TABLE 3(a)—(*contd.*)

R.A.F. Nosological Table for Total Force
Period of Second World War, September 3, 1939 to August 15, 1945
Fresh Cases

	1939*		1940		1941		1942		1943		1944		1945*		Totals	
	Number of Cases	Incidence per 1,000 per annum	Number of Cases	Incidence per 1,000 per annum	Number of Cases	Incidence per 1,000 per annum	Number of Cases	Incidence per 1,000 per annum	Number of Cases	Incidence per 1,000 per annum	Number of Cases	Incidence per 1,000 per annum	Number of Cases	Incidence per 1,000 per annum	Number of Cases	Incidence per 1,000 per annum
INDEFINITE AND GENERAL CONDITIONS																
Observation and No Apparent Disease	254	3·97	1,677	5·17	5,384	8·12	7,770	9·03	7,598	7·82	8,644	8·62	4,890	8·09	36,217	8·06
Debility	46	0·72	414	1·28	723	1·09	944	1·10	1,050	1·08	1,151	1·15	1,050	1·74	5,378	1·20
Pyrexia of Uncertain Origin	79	1·24	375	1·15	823	1·24	1,185	1·37	3,301	3·40	3,859	3·85	3,072	5·08	12,694	2·83
Accidental Contamination from Noxious Gases**	—	—	3	0·01	8	0·01	35	0·04	54	0·06	37	0·03	30	0·05	167	0·04
Others	26	0·41	234	0·72	367	0·56	860	1·00	1,905	1·96	2,976	2·97	2,462	4·08	8,830	1·96
Totals	405	6·34	2,703	8·33	7,305	11·02	10,794	12·54	13,908	14·32	16,667	16·62	11,504	19·04	63,286	14·09
Total, All Diseases	18,005	282·79	120,878	372·62	219,293	330·87	322,847	375·08	415,507	427·72	465,252	464·05	230,418	381·29	1,792,200	399·15

GENERAL INJURIES																
Multiple Injuries with Fractures	211	3·30	1,754	5·41	2,629	3·97	3,260	3·79	3,567	3·67	4,826	4·81	2,304	3·81	18,551	4·13
Multiple Injuries with Burns	82	1·28	526	1·62	996	1·50	1,412	1·64	1,754	1·81	1,467	1·46	647	1·07	6,884	1·53
Multiple Wounds	6	0·09	58	0·18	99	0·15	183	0·21	175	0·18	209	0·21	92	0·15	822	0·18
Fractured Skull with Other Injuries	75	1·18	382	1·18	637	0·96	446	0·52	224	0·23	97	0·10	68	0·11	1,929	0·43
Missile Wounds, Multiple	6	0·09	200	0·62	239	0·36	222	0·26	178	0·18	97	0·10	32	0·05	974	0·23
Minor Injuries	102	1·60	624	1·92	1,263	1·90	1,131	1·31	851	0·88	1,006	1·00	570	0·94	5,547	1·23
Burns Generalised	34	0·53	264	0·81	287	0·43	368	0·43	587	0·60	693	0·69	293	0·49	2,526	0·56
Burns of Face and Hands	4	0·06	73	0·22	187	0·28	262	0·30	235	0·24	246	0·25	163	0·27	1,170	0·26
Scalds	3	0·05	17	0·05	28	0·04	17	0·02	15	0·02	—	—	—	—	80	0·02
Frostbite in Aircrew during Flight**	4	0·06	22	0·07	38	0·06	42	0·05	84	0·09	28	0·03	37	0·06	255	0·06
Exposure to Natural Elements	2	0·03	1	0·003	10	0·02	75	0·09	120	0·12	114	0·11	40	0·07	362	0·08
Drowning, including Effects of Immersion	31	0·49	136	0·42	257	0·39	243	0·28	252	0·26	186	0·19	103	0·17	1,208	0·27
Injuries to Tissues and Specialised Structures†	—	—	—	—	—	—	1,138	1·32	3,599	3·70	4,773	4·76	2,148	3·56	11,658	2·60
Chemical Agents, Effects of Contact with††	—	—	—	—	—	—	86	0·10	106	0·11	113	0·11	54	0·09	359	0·08
Other Injuries	3	0·05	187	0·58	225	0·34	1,016	1·18	2,729	2·81	3,730	3·72	1,380	2·29	9,270	2·06
Missing, Presumed Dead	255	3·99	3,182	9·81	4,936	7·45	6,925	8·05	12,111	12·47	13,015	12·98	3,112	5·15	43,536	9·70
Totals	818	12·80	7,426	22·89	11,831	17·85	16,826	19·55	26,587	27·37	30,600	30·52	11,043	18·28	105,131	23·42
LOCALISED INJURIES: CRANIUM																
Contusions and Wounds	83	1·30	373	1·15	721	1·09	1,063	1·23	1,237	1·28	1,575	1·57	577	0·96	5,629	1·25
Fractures of Skull, Vault / Fractures of Skull, Base	54	0·85	296	0·91	413	0·62	957	1·11	429	0·44	599	0·60	212	0·35	2,960	0·66
Concussion	340	5·32	1,278	3·94	1,831	2·76	1,583	1·84	2,169	2·23	2,432	2·42	1,070	1·77	10,703	2·38
Missile Wounds	4	0·06	89	0·28	103	0·15	60	0·07	108	0·11	116	0·12	75	0·12	555	0·13
Burns and Scalds	2	0·03	6	0·02	4	0·01	23	0·03	7	0·01	—	—	10	0·02	52	0·01
Others	11	0·17	79	0·24	104	0·16	76	0·09	—	—	—	—	—	—	270	0·06
Totals	494	7·73	2,121	6·54	3,176	4·79	3,762	4·37	3,950	4·07	4,722	4·71	1,944	3·22	20,169	4·49
FACE AND MOUTH																
Contusions and Wounds	73	1·14	302	0·93	582	0·88	796	0·93	822	0·84	1,226	1·22	590	0·98	4,391	0·98
Fractures, Fracture-Dislocations and Dislocations	35	0·55	230	0·71	476	0·72	600	0·70	701	0·72	1,056	1·06	431	0·72	3,529	0·79
Missile Wounds	1	0·02	8	0·02	20	0·03	27	0·03	20	0·02	10	0·01	21	0·03	107	0·02
Tooth Injuries	2	0·03	7	0·02	9	0·01	12	0·01	1	0·001	20	0·02	20	0·03	71	0·01
Burns and Scalds	9	0·14	92	0·29	136	0·21	159	0·18	181	0·19	313	0·31	260	0·43	1,150	0·26
Totals	120	1·88	639	1·97	1,223	1·85	1,594	1·85	1,725	1·77	2,625	2·62	1,322	2·19	9,248	2·06

* Figures for 1939 and 1945 are for the war periods of the years only, *viz.* 1939—from September 3 to December 31; 1945—from January 1 to August 15.
** *See* R.A.F. Vol. II, Chap. 1, *Bomber Command*, pp. 109–120.
† Includes injuries to nerves, muscles, ligaments and tendons.
†† *See* R.A.F. Vol. II, Chap. 7, *Maintenance Command*, pp. 513–526 (Industrial Medical Problems).

TABLE 3(a)—(*contd.*)

R.A.F. Nosological Table for Total Force
Period of Second World War, September 3, 1939 to August 15, 1945
Fresh Cases

	1939*		1940		1941		1942		1943		1944		1945*		Totals	
	Number of Cases	Incidence per 1,000 per annum	Number of Cases	Incidence per 1,000 per annum	Number of Cases	Incidence per 1,000 per annum	Number of Cases	Incidence per 1,000 per annum	Number of Cases	Incidence per 1,000 per annum	Number of Cases	Incidence per 1,000 per annum	Number of Cases	Incidence per 1,000 per annum	Number of Cases	Incidence per 1,000 per annum
EYES																
Eyelids, Injuries of	13	0·20	96	0·30	109	0·16	159	0·18	131	0·14	134	0·13	110	0·19	752	0·17
Eye, Substance, Superficial Wounds of	16	0·25	125	0·38	265	0·40	398	0·46	341	0·35	566	0·57	181	0·30	1,892	0·42
Eye, Substance, Injury to Eyeball	17	0·27	63	0·19	103	0·16	184	0·21	356	0·37	427	0·43	303	0·50	1,453	0·32
Eye, Substance, Injuries Resulting in Removal of Eye	2	0·03	15	0·05	23	0·04	14	0·02	29	0·03	51	0·05	29	0·05	163	0·04
Missile Wounds	—	—	7	0·02	14	0·02	16	0·02	26	0·03	19	0·02	24	0·04	106	0·02
Burns and Scalds of Eyelids and Eyes	4	0·06	18	0·06	47	0·07	75	0·09	43	0·04	69	0·07	50	0·08	306	0·07
Chemical Injuries of Eyelids and Eyes	—	—	—	—	—	—	6	0·01	33	0·03	75	0·07	20	0·03	134	0·03
Totals	52	0·81	324	1·00	561	0·85	852	0·99	959	0·99	1,341	1·34	717	1·19	4,806	1·07
EARS																
Pinna, Injuries to	3	0·05	7	0·02	24	0·04	19	0·02	11	0·01	10	0·01	—	—	74	0·02
Rupture of Tympanic Membranes	5	0·08	18	0·06	22	0·03	37	0·05	37	0·04	79	0·08	41	0·07	239	0·05
Burns and Scalds	—	—	—	—	1	0·001	1	0·001	—	—	—	—	10	0·02	12	0·003
Totals	8	0·13	25	0·08	47	0·07	57	0·07	48	0·05	89	0·09	51	0·09	325	0·07

NECK																
Contusions and Wounds	4	0·06	23	0·07	25	0·04	39	0·05	40	0·04	131	0·13	30	0·05	292	0·07
Cut Throat	1	0·02	2	0·01	3	0·004	9	0·01	6	0·01	3	0·002	3	0·004	27	0·01
Missile Wounds	—	—	12	0·04	18	0·03	21	0·02	16	0·02	6	0·01	11	0·02	84	0·01
Burns and Scalds, Internal and External	1	0·02	2	0·01	3	0·004	7	0·01	7	0·01	20	0·02	—	—	40	0·01
Others	4	0·06	21	0·05	32	0·05	43	0·05	3	0·003	10	0·01	—	—	113	0·02
Totals	10	0·16	60	0·18	81	0·12	119	0·14	72	0·07	170	0·17	44	0·07	556	0·12
CHEST																
Contusion and Superficial Wounds	33	0·52	166	0·51	243	0·37	298	0·35	298	0·31	364	0·36	140	0·23	1,542	0·34
Compression and Blast Injury	2	0·03	13	0·04	15	0·02	17	0·02	22	0·02	26	0·03	1	0·001	96	0·02
Penetrating Wounds	—	—	13	0·04	18	0·03	18	0·02	13	0·01	28	0·03	21	0·03	111	0·02
Fractures, Fracture-Dislocations and Dislocations	33	0·52	121	0·38	191	0·29	205	0·24	224	0·23	208	0·21	164	0·28	1,146	0·26
Missile Wounds	2	0·03	69	0·21	88	0·13	81	0·09	84	0·09	71	0·07	54	0·09	449	0·10
Burns and Scalds	—	—	4	0·01	7	0·01	19	0·02	13	0·01	20	0·02	20	0·03	83	0·02
Totals	70	1·10	386	1·19	562	0·85	638	0·74	654	0·67	717	0·72	400	0·66	3,427	0·76
BACK AND VERTEBRAL COLUMN																
Contusions and Superficial Wounds	61	0·95	317	0·97	537	0·81	596	0·69	440	0·44	613	0·61	200	0·33	2,764	0·61
Contusions and Wounds involving Viscera	—	—	19	0·06	18	0·03	8	0·01	56	0·06	10	0·01	10	0·02	121	0·03
Wounds involving Spinal Cord	—	—	1	0·003	2	0·003	—	—	2	0·002	—	—	—	—	5	0·001
Spinal Concussion	1	0·02	9	0·03	2	0·003	10	0·01	17	0·02	20	0·02	136	0·22	195	0·04
Fractures, Fracture-Dislocations and Dislocations, Body of Vertebrae	23	0·36	142	0·44	239	0·36	305	0·36	359	0·37	427	0·43	112	0·19	1,607	0·36
Fractures of Process and Coccyx	—	—	—	—	—	—	11	0·01	8	0·01	22	0·02	20	0·03	61	0·01
Missile Wounds involving Vertebral Column	—	—	32	0·10	12	0·02	22	0·03	8	0·01	3	0·002	—	—	77	0·02
Burns and Scalds	2	0·03	2	0·01	8	0·01	19	0·02	15	0·02	10	0·01	20	0·03	76	0·02
Totals	87	1·36	522	1·61	818	1·23	971	1·13	905	0·93	1,105	1·10	498	0·82	4,906	1·09

* Figures for 1939 and 1945 are for the war periods of the years only *viz.* 1939—from September 3 to December 31; 1945—from January 1 to August 15.

TABLE 3(a)—(*contd.*)

R.A.F. Nosological Table for Total Force
Period of Second World War, September 3, 1939 to August 15, 1945
Fresh Cases

	1939*		1940		1941		1942		1943		1944		1945*		Totals	
	Number of Cases	Incidence per 1,000 per annum	Number of Cases	Incidence per 1,000 per annum	Number of Cases	Incidence per 1,000 per annum	Number of Cases	Incidence per 1,000 per annum	Number of Cases	Incidence per 1,000 per annum	Number of Cases	Incidence per 1,000 per annum	Number of Cases	Incidence per 1,000 per annum	Number of Cases	Incidence per 1,000 per annum
ABDOMEN																
Contusion and Superficial Wounds	16	0·25	73	0·22	85	0·13	112	0·12	94	0·09	80	0·08	112	0·19	572	0·13
Contusion and Wounds involving Viscera	6	0·09	22	0·07	43	0·06	32	0·04	66	0·07	69	0·07	14	0·02	252	0·06
Wounds	3	0·05	7	0·02	6	0·01	—	—	—	—	—	—	—	—	16	0·004
Missile Wounds	—	—	39	0·12	40	0·06	54	0·06	38	0·04	54	0·05	14	0·02	239	0·05
Burns and Scalds	—	—	3	0·01	6	0·01	5	0·01	9	0·01	30	0·03	40	0·07	93	0·02
Totals	25	0·39	144	0·44	180	0·27	203	0·23	207	0·21	233	0·23	180	0·30	1,172	0·26
BUTTOCKS AND PELVIS																
Contusions and Wounds	6	0·09	39	0·12	52	0·08	89	0·10	87	0·09	121	0·12	40	0·06	434	0·10
Contusions and Wounds of Generative Organs	12	0·19	77	0·24	103	0·15	132	0·15	143	0·15	177	0·17	30	0·05	674	0·15
Contusions and Wounds of Other Organs	2	0·03	4	0·01	7	0·01	13	0·02	18	0·02	1	0·001	31	0·05	76	0·02
Fracture, Fracture-Dislocations and Dislocations	10	0·16	40	0·12	73	0·11	82	0·10	81	0·08	211	0·21	63	0·10	560	0·12
Missile Wounds	—	—	18	0·06	13	0·02	38	0·04	44	0·04	29	0·03	22	0·04	164	0·04
Burns and Scalds	—	—	3	0·01	4	0·01	13	0·02	16	0·02	29	0·03	10	0·02	75	0·02
Totals	30	0·47	181	0·56	252	0·38	367	0·43	389	0·40	568	0·56	196	0·32	1,983	0·45

UPPER LIMB, HAND AND WRIST																
Contusions and Wounds	76	1·19	291	0·90	567	0·86	975	1·13	1,223	1·26	1,537	1·53	751	1·24	5,420	1·21
Sprains	14	0·22	46	0·14	65	0·10	87	0·10	89	0·09	119	0·12	30	0·05	450	0·10
Fractures, Fracture-Dislocations and Dislocations	54	0·84	264	0·81	546	0·82	814	0·95	1,042	1·07	1,494	1·49	642	1·06	4,856	1·08
Amputations	10	0·16	61	0·19	153	0·23	108	0·13	50	0·05	—	—	—	—	382	0·08
Missile Wounds	4	0·06	80	0·25	90	0·14	92	0·11	285	0·30	107	0·11	55	0·09	713	0·16
Burns and Scalds	11	0·17	120	0·37	200	0·30	331	0·38	263	0·27	693	0·69	300	0·50	1,918	0·43
Totals	169	2·64	862	2·66	1,621	2·45	2,407	2·80	2,952	3·04	3,950	3·94	1,778	2·94	13,739	3·06
UPPER LIMB, REST OF LIMB																
Contusions and Wounds	35	0·55	177	0·55	335	0·51	501	0·58	461	0·48	495	0·49	263	0·43	2,267	0·51
Sprains and Strains, Traumatic Synovitis, Muscle Fibre Tears	22	0·34	115	0·35	154	0·23	122	0·14	37	0·04	60	0·06	40	0·07	550	0·12
Fracture, Fracture-Dislocations and Dislocations	177	2·77	881	2·71	1,584	2·39	2,117	2·46	2,427	2·50	3,250	3·24	1,745	2·89	12,181	2·71
Amputations	—	—	3	0·01	5	0·01	—	—	—	—	—	—	—	—	8	0·002
Missile Wounds	7	0·11	116	0·36	113	0·17	149	0·17	158	0·16	169	0·17	92	0·15	804	0·18
Burns and Scalds	3	0·05	28	0·09	93	0·14	143	0·17	209	0·22	306	0·31	140	0·23	922	0·21
Multiple Fractures of Whole Upper Limb	—	—	4	0·01	27	0·04	3	0·003	6	0·001	10	0·01	—	—	50	0·01
Multiple Missile Wounds of Whole Upper Limb	—	—	25	0·08	31	0·05	—	—	6	0·001	—	—	—	—	62	0·01
Totals	244	3·82	1,349	4·16	2,342	3·54	3,035	3·52	3,304	3·40	4,290	4·28	2,280	3·77	16,844	3·75
LOWER LIMB, FOOT AND ANKLE																
Contusions and Wounds	72	1·13	314	0·97	693	1·04	1,068	1·24	1,369	1·41	1,376	1·37	921	1·53	5,813	1·29
Sprains and Strains	213	3·33	1,004	3·09	1,712	2·58	2,565	2·98	2,885	2·97	3,703	3·69	1,730	2·86	13,812	3·08
Fractures, Fracture-Dislocations and Dislocations	69	1·08	362	1·12	688	1·04	1,037	1·21	1,445	1·49	2,069	2·06	741	1·23	6,411	1·43
Amputations	—	—	6	0·02	10	0·02	2	0·002	—	—	—	—	—	—	18	0·004
Missile Wounds	1	0·02	92	0·28	95	0·14	115	0·13	105	0·11	77	0·08	23	0·04	508	0·11
Burns and Scalds	15	0·23	108	0·33	257	0·39	392	0·46	402	0·41	477	0·48	220	0·36	1,871	0·42
Totals	370	5·79	1,886	5·81	3,455	5·21	5,179	6·02	6,206	6·39	7,702	7·68	3,635	6·02	28,433	6·33

* Figures for 1939 and 1945 are for the war periods of the years only *viz.* 1939—from September 3 to December 31; 1945—from January 1 to August 15.

TABLE 3(a)—(contd.)

R.A.F. Nosological Table for Total Force
Period of Second World War, September 3, 1939 to August 15, 1945
Fresh Cases

	1939*		1940		1941		1942		1943		1944		1945*		Totals	
	Number of Cases	Incidence per 1,000 per annum	Number of Cases	Incidence per 1,000 per annum	Number of Cases	Incidence per 1,000 per annum	Number of Cases	Incidence per 1,000 per annum	Number of Cases	Incidence per 1,000 per annum	Number of Cases	Incidence per 1,000 per annum	Number of Cases	Incidence per 1,000 per annum	Number of Cases	Incidence per 1,000 per annum
LOWER LIMB, REST OF LIMB																
Contusions and Wounds	139	2·17	657	2·03	1,293	1·95	1,832	2·13	1,661	1·71	2,347	2·34	1,092	1·81	9,021	2·01
Sprains and Strains	121	1·89	433	1·33	666	1·00	613	0·71	383	0·40	645	0·64	260	0·43	3,121	0·69
Internal Derangement of Knee Joint	276	4·32	1,283	3·96	2,019	3·05	2,359	2·74	1,672	1·72	2,710	2·70	1,232	2·04	11,551	2·57
Fracture, Fracture-Dislocations and Dislocations	237	3·71	1,062	3·27	1,917	2·89	2,315	2·69	2,305	2·37	3,601	2·59	1,384	2·29	12,821	2·86
Amputations	3	0·05	17	0·05	32	0·05	—	—	—	—	—	—	—	—	52	0·01
Missile Wounds	9	0·14	284	0·88	290	0·44	291	0·34	238	0·25	280	0·28	158	0·26	1,550	0·35
Burns and Scalds	5	0·08	68	0·21	153	0·23	333	0·39	447	0·46	646	0·65	200	0·33	1,852	0·41
Multiple Fractures of Whole Lower Limb	1	0·02	29	0·09	79	0·12	4	0·004	4	0·004	10	0·01	1	0·001	128	0·03
Missile Wounds of Whole Lower Limb	1	0·02	33	0·10	40	0·06	—	—	28	0·03	9	0·01	10	0·02	121	0·03
Totals	792	12·40	3,866	11·92	6,489	9·79	7,747	9·00	6,738	6·94	10,248	9·22	4,337	7·18	40,217	8·96
Total of All Injuries	3,289	51·48	19,791	61·01	32,638	49·25	43,757	50·31	54,696	56·30	68,360	67·18	28,425	47·05	250,956	55·89

UNCLASSIFIED CONDITIONS																
Heat Exhaustion and Heat Hyperpyrexia	2	0·03	104	0·32	387	0·58	1,602	1·86	1,172	1·21	909	0·90	1,285	2·13	5,461	1·22
Surgical Amputations and Fitting of Artificial Appliances	—	—	—	—	—	—	133	0·15	180	0·19	218	0·22	167	0·28	698	0·15
Late Complications of Trauma	—	—	—	—	—	—	22	0·03	30	0·03	47	0·05	21	0·03	120	0·03
Prolonged Loss of Senses immediately following Injury	—	—	—	—	—	—	4	0·004	3	0·003	1	0·001	32	0·05	40	0·01
Totals	2	0·03	104	0·32	387	0·58	1,761	2·04	1,385	1·43	1,175	1·17	1,505	2·49	6,319	1·41
Grand Total of all Disabilities	21,296	334·30	140,773	433·95	252,318	380·70	368,365	427·43	471,588	485·45	534,787	532·40	260,348	430·83	2,049,475	456·45

* Figures for 1939 and 1945 are for the war periods of the years only *viz.* 1939—from September 3 to December 31; 1945—from January 1 to August 15.

TABLE 3(b)

R.A.F. Nosological Table for Home Force
Period of Second World War, September 3, 1939 to August 15, 1945

	1939*		1940		1941		1942		1943		1944		1945*		Totals	
	Number of Cases	Incidence per 1,000 per annum	Number of Cases	Incidence per 1,000 per annum	Number of Cases	Incidence per 1,000 per annum	Number of Cases	Incidence per 1,000 per annum	Number of Cases	Incidence per 1,000 per annum	Number of Cases	Incidence per 1,000 per annum	Number of Cases	Incidence per 1,000 per annum	Number of Cases	Incidence per 1,000 per annum
INFECTIOUS DISEASES																
Amoebic Dysentery	1	0·02	5	0·02	15	0·03	33	0·05	82	0·12	234	0·34	500	1·20	870	0·26
Bacillary Dysentery	1	0·02	21	0·07	95	0·16	224	0·34	479	0·72	543	0·79	401	0·97	1,764	0·53
Enteric Group	2	0·03	6	0·02	46	0·08	34	0·05	19	0·03	19	0·03	10	0·02	136	0·04
Enteritis	217	3·69	1,617	5·52	3,280	5·61	1,631	2·48	228	0·34	257	0·38	270	0·65	7,500	2·24
Malaria	18	0·31	62	0·21	393	0·67	341	0·52	546	0·83	2,476	3·62	1,241	2·99	5,077	1·51
Other Tropical Infections	5	0·08	22	0·07	50	0·09	86	0·13	68	0·10	98	0·14	115	0·28	444	0·13
Bacillary Infections (other than Typhoid and Dysentery)	23	0·39	142	0·49	350	0·60	277	0·42	226	0·34	378	0·55	81	0·19	1,477	0·44
Staphylococcal and Streptococcal Infections	109	1·85	787	2·69	791	1·35	650	0·99	1,026	1·55	1,369	2·00	343	0·83	5,075	1·51
Virus Infections	459	7·80	7,377	25·21	3,995	6·83	5,513	8·37	3,177	4·80	5,351	7·83	2,830	6·82	28,702	8·55
Metazoan Parasite Infections	2	0·03	43	0·15	61	0·10	117	0·18	106	0·16	190	0·28	90	0·22	609	0·18
Infections of Unknown or Doubtful Origin	139	2·36	913	3·12	1,869	3·19	2,255	3·43	2,625	3·96	2,918	4·27	1,351	3·25	12,070	3·60
Central Nervous System Infections	108	1·84	846	2·89	1,498	2·56	1,504	2·28	1,429	2·16	1,997	2·92	1,173	2·83	8,555	2·55
Totals	1,084	18·42	11,841	40·46	12,443	21·27	12,665	19·24	10,011	15·11	15,830	23·15	8,405	20·25	72,279	21·54

INFECTIONS OF RESPIRATORY TRACT																
Common Cold, Nasopharyngitis and Sore Throat	1,864	31·68	17,351	59·29	23,851	40·78	22,852	34·71	35,373	53·39	28,100	41·09	13,740	33·11	143,131	42·65
Influenza	1,364	23·18	16,519	56·44	18,502	31·63	12,437	18·89	25,147	37·95	14,390	21·04	4,480	10·80	92,839	27·66
Tonsillitis	1,783	30·31	9,396	32·11	14,048	24·02	15,751	23·92	19,224	29·01	24,752	36·20	12,280	29·59	97,234	28·97
Vincent's Angina	31	0·53	364	1·24	1,634	2·79	2,683	4·08	2,238	3·38	2,069	3·03	910	2·19	9,929	2·96
Upper Respiratory Tract Infections—Totals	5,042	85·70	43,630	149·08	58,035	99·22	53,723	81·60	81,982	123·73	69,311	101·36	31,410	75·69	343,133	102·24
PNEUMONIA	114	1·94	1,087	3·71	2,540	4·34	2,207	3·35	2,498	3·76	5,023	7·35	1,264	3·05	14,733	4·39
PULMONARY TUBERCULOSIS	83	1·41	386	1·32	855	1·46	1,260	1·91	1,549	2·34	1,192	1·75	849	2·05	6,174	1·84
TUBERCULOSIS (OTHER THAN PULMONARY)	16	0·27	95	0·32	270	0·46	298	0·45	305	0·46	456	0·67	184	0·44	1,624	0·48
VACCINIA AND POST-INOCULATION EFFECTS	453	7·70	2,363	8·07	2,317	3·96	944	1·43	2,151	3·24	2,070	3·03	460	1·11	10,758	3·21
CARRIERS	2	0·03	11	0·04	26	0·05	23	0·04	45	0·07	30	0·04	10	0·02	147	0·04
CONTACTS	9	0·15	137	0·47	177	0·30	169	0·26	178	0·27	199	0·29	100	0·24	969	0·29
VENEREAL DISEASES																
Gonorrhoea	290	4·93	1,611	5·51	3,484	5·95	3,917	5·95	3,899	5·89	5,870	8·58	5,815	14·01	24,886	7·41
Syphilis	20	0·34	158	0·54	478	0·82	644	0·98	575	0·87	938	1·37	983	2·37	3,796	1·13
Syphilis with Gonorrhoea	—	—	—	—	—	—	—	—	27	0·04	40	0·06	—	—	67	0·02
Others	7	0·12	13	0·04	76	0·13	64	0·10	48	0·07	148	0·22	150	0·36	506	0·15
Totals	317	5·39	1,782	6·09	4,038	6·90	4,625	7·03	4,549	6·87	6,996	10·23	6,948	16·74	29,255	8·71
SEPTIC CONDITIONS (Areolar Tissues, Lymphatic Channels and Breasts)																
Conditions due to Pyogenic Organisms	871	14·81	5,487	18·75	9,214	15·75	11,510	17·48	12,351	18·64	15,979	23·37	7,389	17·80	62,801	18·71
Other Conditions	9	0·15	115	0·39	239	0·41	372	0·57	450	0·68	621	0·91	374	0·90	2,180	0·65
Breasts	4	0·07	11	0·04	28	0·05	51	0·08	40	0·06	60	0·09	40	0·10	234	0·07
Totals	884	15·03	5,613	19·18	9,481	16·21	11,933	18·13	12,841	19·38	16,660	24·37	7,803	18·80	65,215	19·43

*Figures for 1939 and 1945 are for the war periods of the years only *viz.* 1939—from September 3 to December 31; 1945—from January 1 to August 15.

TABLE 3(b)—(*contd.*)

R.A.F. Nosological Table for Home Force
Period of Second World War, September 3, 1939 to August 15, 1945

	1939*		1940		1941		1942		1943		1944		1945*		Totals	
	Number of Cases	Incidence per 1,000 per annum	Number of Cases	Incidence per 1,000 per annum	Number of Cases	Incidence per 1,000 per annum	Number of Cases	Incidence per 1,000 per annum	Number of Cases	Incidence per 1,000 per annum	Number of Cases	Incidence per 1,000 per annum	Number of Cases	Incidence per 1,000 per annum	Number of Cases	Incidence per 1,000 per annum
ALIMENTARY SYSTEM DISEASES																
Dental Conditions	86	1·45	597	2·04	1,177	2·01	1,261	1·91	1,337	2·02	1,365	1·99	700	1·69	6,523	1·94
Mouth, Pharynx and Oesophagus	37	0·63	220	0·75	623	1·06	868	1·32	1,002	1·51	1,120	1·64	816	1·97	4,686	1·40
Gastric Ulcer and its Complications	79	1·34	406	1·39	805	1·38	502	0·76	411	0·62	555	0·81	286	0·69	3,044	0·91
Other Gastric Conditions	284	4·83	2,019	6·90	3,905	6·68	4,860	7·38	4,631	6·99	5,764	8·43	3,127	7·53	24,590	7·33
Duodenal Ulcer and its Complications	160	2·72	656	2·24	1,926	3·29	2,364	3·59	2,479	3·74	3,274	4·79	2,082	5·02	12,941	3·86
Duodenitis	14	0·24	101	0·35	146	0·25	268	0·41	220	0·33	164	0·24	181	0·44	1,094	0·33
Appendicitis, All Types	360	6·12	1,889	6·45	3,007	5·14	3,039	4·62	2,909	4·39	4,130	6·04	1,659	4·00	16,993	5·06
Other Intestinal Conditions	136	2·31	624	2·13	1,089	1·86	5,728	8·70	6,816	10·29	8,889	13·0	6,675	16·08	29,957	8·93
Rectum and Anus	157	2·67	1,018	3·48	2,276	3·89	3,018	4·58	2,978	4·49	4,204	6·15	1,953	4·70	15,604	4·64
Hernia, All Types	184	3·13	1,542	5·27	4,046	6·92	5,277	8·01	4,046	6·11	4,900	7·16	2,353	5·67	22,348	6·65
Liver and Gall Bladder	18	0·31	97	0·33	221	0·38	426	0·65	594	0·89	733	1·07	263	0·63	2,352	0·70
Pancreas	—	—	1	0·003	6	0·01	5	0·01	4	0·01	32	0·05	3	0·01	51	0·02
Peritoneum	3	0·05	19	0·07	25	0·04	63	0·10	54	0·08	67	0·10	8	0·02	239	0·07
Totals	1,518	25·80	9,189	31·40	19,252	32·91	27,679	42·04	27,481	41·47	35,197	51·47	20,106	48.45	140,422	41·84

CIRCULATORY SYSTEM DISEASES																
Pericardium	—	—	16	0·05	12	0·02	15	0·02	30	0·05	12	0·02	24	0·06	109	0·03
Endocarditis and Valvular Diseases of the Heart	46	0·77	176	0·60	255	0·44	296	0·45	286	0·43	255	0·37	144	0·34	1,458	0·43
Myocardium	29	0·49	150	0·51	187	0·32	188	0·29	204	0·31	209	0·31	121	0·29	1,088	0·32
Cardiac Arrhythmias	23	0·39	130	0·45	210	0·36	191	0·29	168	0·25	276	0·40	62	0·15	1,060	0·32
Disordered Action of the Heart	29	0·49	174	0·60	400	0·68	493	0·75	458	0·69	458	0·67	190	0·46	2,202	0·66
Totals	127	2·16	646	2·21	1,064	1·82	1,183	1·80	1,146	1·73	1,210	1·77	541	1·30	5,917	1·76
Blood Vessels	140	2·38	864	2·95	2,265	3·87	3,321	5·04	3,157	4·76	3,492	5·11	2,424	5·84	15,663	4·67
Circulatory System Totals	267	4·54	1,510	5·16	3,329	5·69	4,504	6·84	4,303	6·49	4,702	6·88	2,965	7·14	21,580	6·43
BLOOD, BLOOD-FORMING ORGANS, SPLEEN AND RETICULO-ENDOTHELIAL SYSTEM																
Anaemias	6	0·10	32	0·11	84	0·15	96	0·15	117	0·17	75	0·11	118	0·28	528	0·16
Leukaemias	2	0·03	6	0·02	14	0·02	19	0·03	17	0·03	40	0·06	7	0·02	105	0·03
Purpuras	1	0·02	8	0·03	20	0·03	25	0·04	31	0·05	20	0·03	23	0·06	128	0·04
Other Diseases of the Blood	1	0·02	9	0·03	22	0·04	22	0·03	50	0·07	61	0·09	42	0·10	207	0·06
Lymphatic Glands	1	0·02	15	0·05	30	0·05	83	0·13	27	0·04	41	0·06	52	0·12	249	0·08
Spleen and Reticulo-Endothelial System	2	0·03	6	0·02	16	0·03	36	0·05	37	0·06	75	0·11	7	0·02	179	0·05
Totals	13	0·22	76	0·26	186	0·32	281	0·43	279	0·42	312	0·46	249	0·60	1,396	0·42
RESPIRATORY SYSTEM DISEASES																
Larynx and Trachea	3	0·05	8	0·03	20	0·03	573	0·87	891	1·34	1,150	1·68	563	1·36	3,208	0·96
Bronchi	612	10·40	3,366	11·50	5,022	8·59	7,920	12·03	9,653	14·57	12,738	18·63	5,852	14·10	45,163	13·46
Lungs	41	0·70	182	0·62	352	0·60	1,107	1·68	1,012	1·53	1,180	1·72	506	1·22	4,380	1·30
Pleura	128	2·18	755	2·58	1,501	2·57	1,484	2·25	1,184	1·79	2,241	3·28	639	1·54	7,932	2·36
Mediastinum	—	—	—	—	—	—	6	0·01	3	0·004	1	0·001	2	0·004	12	0·004
Totals	784	13·33	4,311	14·73	6,895	11·79	11,090	16·84	12,743	19·23	17,310	25·31	7,562	18·22	60,695	18·08

* Figures for 1939 and 1945 are for the war periods of the years only *viz.* 1939—from September 3 to December 31; 1945—from January 1 to August 15.

TABLE 3(b)—(*contd.*)

R.A.F. Nosological Table for Home Force
Period of Second World War, September 3, 1939 to August 15, 1945

	1939*		1940		1941		1942		1943		1944		1945*		Totals	
	Number of Cases	Incidence per 1,000 per annum	Number of Cases	Incidence per 1,000 per annum	Number of Cases	Incidence per 1,000 per annum	Number of Cases	Incidence per 1,000 per annum	Number of Cases	Incidence per 1,000 per annum	Number of Cases	Incidence per 1,000 per annum	Number of Cases	Incidence per 1,000 per annum	Number of Cases	Incidence per 1,000 per annum
ALLERGY, DISEASES OF																
Asthma	105	1·79	494	1·69	1,085	1·86	1,050	1·59	940	1·42	1,457	2·13	700	1·69	5,831	1·74
Hay Fever	—	—	13	0·04	45	0·08	19	0·03	34	0·05	20	0·03	42	0·10	173	0·05
Urticaria	22	0·37	183	0·63	288	0·49	372	0·57	381	0·57	521	0·76	355	0·86	2,122	0·63
Others	—	—	12	0·04	14	0·02	53	0·08	64	0·10	23	0·03	26	0·06	192	0·06
Totals	127	2·16	702	2·40	1,432	2·45	1,494	2·27	1,419	2·14	2,021	2·95	1,123	2·71	8,318	2·48
URINARY SYSTEM DISEASES																
Anomalies of Urinary Secretion	60	1·02	314	1·07	652	1·12	948	1·44	841	1·27	932	1·36	528	1·27	4,275	1·27
Nephritis, All Forms	29	0·49	138	0·47	219	0·38	243	0·37	236	0·36	319	0·47	127	0·31	1,311	0·39
Kidney	41	0·70	267	0·92	504	0·86	567	0·86	629	0·95	650	0·95	376	0·91	3,034	0·90
Urinary Calculi and Urinary Colic	58	0·99	243	0·83	473	0·81	427	0·65	404	0·61	530	0·78	369	0·89	2,504	0·75
Bladder	39	0·66	194	0·66	540	0·92	573	0·87	744	1·12	891	1·30	407	0·98	3,388	1·01
Others	—	—	9	0·03	20	0·03	13	0·02	24	0·04	15	0·02	38	0·09	119	0·04
Totals	227	3·86	1,165	3·98	2,408	4·12	2,771	4·21	2,878	4·34	3,337	4·88	1,845	4·45	14,631	4·36

GENERATIVE SYSTEM DISEASES																
Prostate	6	0·10	24	0·08	58	0·10	101	0·16	138	0·21	283	0·42	194	0·47	804	0·24
Urethra	83	1·41	537	1·84	1,120	1·91	1,160	1·76	1,596	2·41	1,287	1·88	260	0·63	6,043	1·80
Penis	76	1·29	458	1·56	939	1·61	1,062	1·61	904	1·36	1,206	1·76	780	1·88	5,425	1·62
Spermatic Cord, Testis and Epididymis	72	1·23	416	1·42	1,172	2·00	1,515	2·30	1,464	2·21	1,869	2·73	1,022	2·46	7,530	2·24
Totals	237	4·03	1,435	4·90	3,289	5·62	3,838	5·83	4,102	6·19	4,645	6·79	2,256	5·44	19,802	5·90
LOCOMOTOR SYSTEM DISEASES																
Muscles	23	0·39	121	0·41	189	0·32	212	0·32	161	0·24	158	0·23	103	0·25	967	0·29
Rheumatic Group	187	3·18	1,427	4·88	2,760	4·72	3,112	4·73	3,229	4·87	4,871	7·12	2,704	6·52	18,290	5·45
Deformities	73	1·24	574	1·96	1,507	2·58	1,078	1·64	806	1·22	1,378	2·02	467	1·12	5,883	1·75
Joints	181	3·08	1,183	4·04	2,560	4·38	3,844	5·84	4,323	6·53	3,706	5·42	2,473	5·96	18,270	5·44
Internal Derangement of Knee Joint	19	0·32	137	0·47	405	0·69	880	1·33	1,066	1·61	1,008	1·47	551	1·33	4,066	1·21
Bones and Cartilages	15	0·25	219	0·75	418	0·72	428	0·65	399	0·60	504	0·74	249	0·60	2,232	0·67
Ligaments and Tendons	40	0·68	283	0·97	592	1·01	528	0·80	350	0·53	461	0·67	343	0·83	2,597	0·77
Effects of Old Injuries	—	—	—	—	—	—	—	—	—	—	1,784	2·61	1,184	2·85	2,968	0·89
Totals	538	9·14	3,944	13·48	8,431	14·42	10,082	15·31	10,334	15·60	13,870	20·28	8,074	19·46	55,273	16·47
NERVOUS SYSTEM AND MENTAL DISEASES																
Psychoneuroses	204	3·47	1,497	5·11	3,759	6·43	4,964	7·54	5,246	7·92	6,424	9·39	4,003	9·65	26,097	7·77
Psychoses	76	1·29	213	0·73	430	0·73	342	0·52	395	0·60	439	0·64	245	2·59	2,140	0·64
Psychopathic Personality	43	0·73	255	0·87	479	0·82	591	0·90	862	1·30	1,628	2·38	970	2·34	4,828	1·44
Mental Defect	1	0·02	23	0·08	172	0·29	177	0·27	158	0·24	161	0·24	77	0·19	769	0·23
Epilepsies	72	1·22	302	1·03	641	1·10	548	0·83	508	0·76	426	0·62	251	0·60	2,748	0·82
Indefinite Aetiology	65	1·11	416	1·42	960	1·64	1,095	1·66	973	1·47	1,026	1·50	793	1·91	5,328	1·59
Totals	461	7·84	2,706	9·24	6,441	11·01	7,717	11·72	8,142	12·29	10,104	14·77	6,339	17·28	41,910	12·49

* Figures for 1939 and 1945 are for the war periods of the years only *viz.* 1939—from September 3 to December 31; 1945—from January 1 to August 15.

TABLE 3(b)—(*contd.*)

R.A.F. Nosological Table for Home Force
Period of Second World War, September 3, 1939 to August 15, 1945

	1939*		1940		1941		1942		1943		1944		1945*		Totals	
	Number of Cases	Incidence per 1,000 per annum	Number of Cases	Incidence per 1,000 per annum	Number of Cases	Incidence per 1,000 per annum	Number of Cases	Incidence per 1,000 per annum	Number of Cases	Incidence per 1,000 per annum	Number of Cases	Incidence per 1,000 per annum	Number of Cases	Incidence per 1,000 per annum	Number of Cases	Incidence per 1,000 per annum
ORGANIC NERVOUS DISEASES																
Brain, Diseases of	29	0·49	81	0·28	182	0·31	174	0·26	208	0·31	247	0·36	127	0·30	1,048	0·31
Organic Diseases Indefinite	8	0·14	49	0·17	151	0·26	94	0·14	104	0·16	111	0·16	82	0·20	599	0·18
Cranial Nerves	10	0·17	89	0·30	196	0·33	210	0·32	214	0·32	210	0·31	252	0·61	1,181	0·35
Spinal Cord	13	0·22	36	0·12	92	0·16	64	0·10	72	0·11	52	0·08	33	0·08	362	0·11
Spinal and Peripheral Nerves	82	1·39	514	1·76	913	1·56	1,190	1·81	1,315	1·99	1,956	2·86	902	2·17	6,872	2·05
Others	—	—	23	0·08	16	0·03	58	0·09	—	—	—	—	—	—	97	0·03
Totals	142	2·41	792	2·71	1,550	2·65	1,790	2·72	1,913	2·89	2,576	3·77	1,396	3·36	10,159	3·03
Nervous System and Mental Diseases—Totals	603	10·25	3,498	11·95	7,991	13·66	9,507	14·44	10,055	15·18	12,680	18·54	7,735	20·64	52,069	15·51
EYE DISEASES																
Defects of Vision	7	0·12	110	0·38	346	0·59	469	0·71	477	0·72	428	0·62	227	0·55	2,064	0·61
Inflammatory Conditions	88	1·50	500	1·71	945	1·62	1,038	1·58	1,283	1·94	1,885	2·76	957	2·30	6,696	2·00
Others	79	1·34	428	1·46	858	1·47	929	1·41	934	1·41	1,168	1·71	676	1·63	5,072	1·51
Totals	174	2·96	1,038	3·55	2,149	3·68	2,436	3·70	2,694	4·07	3,481	5·09	1,860	4·48	13,832	4·12

EAR DISEASES																
Deafness	—	—	—	—	—	—	309	0·47	281	0·42	258	0·38	265	0·65	1,117	0·33
Otitis Media, Acute	108	1·84	987	3·37	1,527	2·61	1,706	2·59	1,618	2·44	2,294	3·35	875	2·11	9,115	2·72
Otitis Media, Chronic	52	0·89	407	1·39	1,225	2·09	1,272	1·93	1,358	2·05	1,951	2·85	1,239	2·98	7,504	2·23
Otitis Externa	34	0·58	167	0·57	391	0·67	518	0·79	721	1·09	1,097	1·60	734	1·77	3,662	1·09
Perforated Tympanic Membrane	2	0·03	66	0·22	197	0·34	66	0·10	17	0·03	38	0·06	11	0·03	397	0·12
Mastoiditis, Acute	6	0·10	61	0·21	110	0·19	108	0·17	124	0·19	226	0·19	86	0·21	721	0·21
Mastoiditis, Chronic	2	0·03	14	0·05	33	0·06	55	0·08	42	0·06	72	0·11	35	0·08	253	0·08
Others	25	0·42	40	0·14	143	0·24	101	0·15	106	0·16	187	0·27	104	0·25	706	0·21
Totals	229	3·89	1,742	5·95	3,626	6·20	4,135	6·28	4,267	6·44	6,123	8·95	3,353	8·08	23,475	6·99
NOSE AND THROAT DISEASES																
Nasal Passages } Sinuses	127	2·16	1,339	4·58	2,796	4·78	3,343	5·08	1,780	2·68	2,049	3·00	1,174	2·83	5,003	1·49
Sinuses									1,986	3·00	2,673	3·91	1,121	2·70	13,385	3·99
Naso-Pharynx } Throat	69	1·17	542	1·85	1,358	2·32	2,128	3·23	2,384	3·60	2,405	3·52	1,210	2·92	5,999	1·79
Throat									12	0·02	29	0·04	10	0·02	4,148	1·23
Totals	196	3·33	1,881	6·43	4,154	7·10	5,471	8·31	6,162	9·30	7,156	10·47	3,515	8·47	28,535	8·50
SKIN DISEASES																
Scabies	270	4·59	1,962	6·70	6,335	10·83	6,139	9·33	2,862	4·32	1,710	2·50	580	1·40	19,858	5·92
Impetigo	231	3·93	1,115	3·81	2,526	4·32	3,565	5·42	3,544	5·35	3,920	5·73	1,523	3·67	16,424	4·89
Pediculosis and Pediculitis	17	0·29	187	0·64	279	0·48	159	0·24	74	0·11	100	0·15	10	0·02	826	0·25
Tinea Cruris	64	1·09	259	0·88	436	0·74	316	0·48	165	0·25	278	0·41	120	0·29	1,638	0·49
Tinea, Others	25	0·42	154	0·53	304	0·52	420	0·64	638	0·96	706	1·03	509	1·23	2,756	0·82
Dermatitis and Eczema	84	1·43	805	2·75	1,694	2·90	2,541	3·86	2,799	4·23	3,908	5·71	1,901	4·58	13,732	4·09
Pityriasis and Erythemata	63	1·07	435	1·49	887	1·51	704	1·07	456	0·69	560	0·82	379	0·91	3,484	1·04
Psoriasis	15	0·25	73	0·25	212	0·36	254	0·39	240	0·36	341	0·50	219	0·53	1,354	0·40
Ingrowing Toenail	49	0·83	221	0·76	405	0·69	514	0·78	450	0·68	496	0·72	230	0·55	2,365	0·71
Other Conditions	138	2·35	490	1·67	1,160	1·98	1,299	1·97	1,474	2·22	2,378	3·48	1,326	3·20	8,265	2·46
Totals	956	16·25	5,701	19·48	14,238	24·34	15,911	24·18	12,702	19·17	14,397	21·05	6,797	16·38	70,702	21·07

* Figures for 1939 and 1945 are for the war periods of the years only *viz.* 1939—from September 3 to December 31; 1945—from January 1 to August 15.

TABLE 3(b)—(*contd.*)

R.A.F. Nosological Table for Home Force
Period of Second World War, September 3, 1939 to August 15, 1945

	1939*		1940		1941		1942		1943		1944		1945*		Totals	
	Number of Cases	Incidence per 1,000 per annum	Number of Cases	Incidence per 1,000 per annum	Number of Cases	Incidence per 1,000 per annum	Number of Cases	Incidence per 1,000 per annum	Number of Cases	Incidence per 1,000 per annum	Number of Cases	Incidence per 1,000 per annum	Number of Cases	Incidence per 1,000 per annum	Number of Cases	Incidence per 1,000 per annum
ENDOCRINE DISEASES																
General Endocrine Disturbances	—	—	4	0·01	4	0·01	26	0·04	26	0·04	31	0·05	19	0·04	110	0·03
Male Gonads	3	0·05	23	0·08	155	0·26	185	0·28	138	0·21	198	0·29	143	0·34	845	0·25
Parathyroid	—	—	—	—	—	—	3	0·004	4	0·01	1	0·001	11	0·03	19	0·01
Pituitary	—	—	3	0·01	21	0·04	14	0·02	19	0·03	31	0·05	23	0·06	111	0·03
Suprarenal	—	—	4	0·01	4	0·01	6	0·01	2	0·003	1	0·001	3	0·01	20	0·01
Thymus	1	0·02	—	—	—	—	1	0·001	1	0·002	10	0·01	2	0·004	15	0·004
Thyroid	14	0·24	63	0·22	149	0·25	152	0·23	138	0·21	260	0·38	82	0·20	858	0·26
Totals	18	0·31	97	0·33	333	0·57	387	0·59	328	0·50	532	0·78	283	0·68	1,978	0·59
DISEASES OF METABOLISM	29	0·49	81	0·27	151	0·26	181	0·28	222	0·33	266	0·39	186	0·45	1,116	0·33
DEFICIENCY DISEASES	—	—	5	0·02	2	0·003	19	0·03	35	0·05	135	0·20	71	0·17	267	0·08
EFFECTS OF TOXIC SUBSTANCES†	10	0·17	—	—	—	—	42	0·06	52	0·08	50	0·07	30	0·07	184	0·05
PHYSICAL AGENTS, EFFECTS OF†	—	—	—	—	—	—	2	0·003	15	0·02	—	—	—	—	17	0·01
CYSTS AND TUMOURS																
Cysts	27	0·46	205	0·70	382	0·65	521	0·79	663	1·00	783	1·15	333	0·80	2,914	0·87
Tumours, Benign	25	0·42	114	0·39	250	0·43	352	0·53	394	0·60	406	0·59	250	0·60	1,791	0·53
Tumours, Malignant	8	0·14	68	0·23	147	0·25	172	0·26	218	0·33	340	0·50	218	0·53	1,171	0·35
Tumours, Unspecified	3	0·05	12	0·04	17	0·03	90	0·14	159	0·24	225	0·33	116	0·28	622	0·19
Totals	63	1·07	399	1·36	796	1·36	1,135	1·72	1,434	2·17	1,754	2·57	917	2·21	6,498	1·94

INDEFINITE AND GENERAL CONDITIONS																
Observation and No Apparent Disease	193	3·28	1,353	4·62	4,354	7·44	5,004	7·60	3,683	5·56	4,987	7·29	2,960	7·14	22,534	6·71
Debility	34	0·58	378	1·29	602	1·03	659	1·00	678	1·03	870	1·27	660	1·59	3,881	1·16
Pyrexia of Uncertain Origin	61	1·04	248	0·85	440	0·75	376	0·57	446	0·67	717	1·05	602	1·45	2,890	0·86
Accidental Contamination from Noxious Gases**	—	—	3	0·01	4	0·01	30	0·05	41	0·06	28	0·04	30	0·07	136	0·04
Others	25	0·42	186	0·64	321	0·55	665	1·01	1,305	1·97	2,161	3·16	2,047	4·93	6,710	2·00
Totals	313	5·32	2,168	7·41	5,721	9·78	6,734	10·23	6,153	9·29	8,763	12·81	6,299	15·18	36,151	10·77
Total All Diseases	14,306	243·16	105,887	361·80	174,565	298·44	195,546	297·03	223,767	337·71	254,498	372·18	132,659	321·67	1,101,228	328·12
GENERAL INJURIES																
Multiple Injuries with Fractures	184	3·13	1,534	5·24	2,107	3·60	2,006	3·05	2,421	3·65	3,663	5·36	1,714	4·13	13,629	4·06
Multiple Injuries with Burns	78	1·33	483	1·65	887	1·52	1,195	1·82	1,425	2·15	1,163	1·70	461	1·11	5,692	1·70
Multiple Wounds	6	0·10	48	0·17	77	0·13	95	0·14	66	0·10	154	0·23	36	0·09	482	0·14
Fractured Skull with Other Injuries	73	1·24	355	1·21	576	0·98	376	0·57	122	0·18	72	0·11	49	0·12	1,623	0·48
Missile Wounds, multiple	4	0·07	167	0·57	145	0·25	121	0·18	97	0·15	68	0·10	25	0·06	627	0·19
Minor Injuries	88	1·50	560	1·91	1,066	1·82	816	1·24	530	0·80	707	1·03	400	0·96	4,167	1·24
Burns Generalised	21	0·36	203	0·69	174	0·30	148	0·23	197	0·30	287	0·42	124	0·30	1,154	0·34
Burns of Face and Hands	—	—	52	0·18	156	0·27	199	0·30	164	0·25	174	0·25	122	0·29	867	0·26
Scalds	3	0·05	13	0·05	18	0·03	5	0·01	2	0·003	—	—	—	—	41	0·01
Frostbite in Aircrew during Flight**	2	0·03	18	0·06	29	0·05	24	0·04	60	0·09	28	0·04	27	0·07	188	0·06
Exposure to Natural Elements	—	—	1	0·003	7	0·01	34	0·05	62	0·09	93	0·14	20	0·05	217	0·06
Drowning, including Effects of Immersion	25	0·42	119	0·41	221	0·38	171	0·26	156	0·24	109	0·16	49	0·12	850	0·25
Injuries to Tissues and Specialised Structures‡	—	—	—	—	—	—	764	1·16	2,311	3·49	2,978	4·35	1,317	3·17	7,370	2·20
Chemical Agents, Effects of contact with††	—	—	—	—	—	—	68	0·10	51	0·08	56	0·08	34	0·08	209	0·06
Other Injuries	—	—	158	0·54	174	0·30	539	0·82	1,427	2·15	2,013	2·94	694	1·67	5,005	1·49
Missing, Presumed Dead	238	4·04	2,429	8·30	4,028	6·88	5,801	8·81	10,568	15·95	11,275	16·49	2,429	5·85	36,768	10·96
Totals	722	12·27	6,140	20·98	9,665	16·52	12,362	18·78	19,659	29·67	22,840	33·40	7,501	18·07	78,889	23·50

* Figures for 1939 and 1945 are for the war periods of the years only *viz.* 1939—from September 3 to December 31; 1945—from January 1 to August 15.
** *See* p. 483.
†*See* p. 481.
†† *See* p. 483.
‡ *See* p. 483.

TABLE 3(b)—(*contd.*)

R.A.F. Nosological Table for Home Force
Period of Second World War, September 3, 1939 to August 15, 1945

	1939*		1940		1941		1942		1943		1944		1945*		Totals	
	Number of Cases	Incidence per 1,000 per annum	Number of Cases	Incidence per 1,000 per annum	Number of Cases	Incidence per 1,000 per annum	Number of Cases	Incidence per 1,000 per annum	Number of Cases	Incidence per 1,000 per annum	Number of Cases	Incidence per 1,000 per annum	Number of Cases	Incidence per 1,000 per annum	Number of Cases	Incidence per 1,000 per annum
LOCALISED INJURIES																
CRANIUM																
Contusions and Wounds	68	1·16	336	1·15	615	1·05	757	1·15	827	1·25	1,075	1·57	287	0·69	3,965	1·18
Fractures of Skull, Vault }							347	0·53	261	0·39	399	0·58	} 61	0·15	} 1,068	} 0·32
Fractures of Skull, Base }	50	0·85	279	0·95	362	0·62							109	0·26	800	0·24
Concussion	292	4·96	1,159	3·96	1,599	2·73	1,547	2·35	1,474	2·22	1,864	2·73	770	1·86	8,705	2·59
Missile Wounds	1	0·02	70	0·24	81	0·14	59	0·09	67	0·10	76	0·11	56	0·14	410	0·12
Burns and Scalds	2	0·03	5	0·02	3	0·01	7	0·01	4	0·01	—	—	10	0·02	31	0·01
Others	8	0·14	77	0·26	91	0·15	76	0·11	—	—	—	—	—	—	252	0·08
Totals	421	7·16	1,926	6·58	2,751	4·70	2,793	4·24	2,633	3·97	3,414	4·99	1,293	3·12	15,231	4·54
FACE AND MOUTH																
Contusions and Wounds	64	1·09	265	0·91	507	0·87	579	0·88	543	0·82	935	1·37	420	1·01	3,313	0·99
Fractures, Fracture-Dislocations and Dislocations	27	0·46	201	0·69	407	0·70	406	0·62	429	0·65	607	0·89	221	0·54	2,298	0·68
Missile Wounds	1	0·02	7	0·02	15	0·02	24	0·03	13	0·02	10	0·01	10	0·02	80	0·02
Tooth Injuries	2	0·03	5	0·02	7	0·01	8	0·01	—	—	—	—	10	0·02	32	0·01
Burns and Scalds	7	0·12	77	0·26	123	0·21	130	0·20	113	0·17	205	0·30	170	0·41	825	0·25
Totals	101	1·72	555	1·90	1,059	1·81	1,147	1·74	1,098	1·66	1,757	2·57	831	2·00	6,548	1·95

EYES																
Eyelids, Injuries of	10	0·17	87	0·30	92	0·16	107	0·16	89	0·13	77	0·11	100	0·24	562	0·17
Eye Substance, Superficial Wounds of	12	0·20	111	0·38	225	0·39	298	0·45	226	0·34	391	0·57	101	0·24	1,364	0·41
Eye Substance, Injury to Eyeball	17	0·29	47	0·16	89	0·15	124	0·19	213	0·32	291	0·43	191	0·46	972	0·29
Eye Substance, Injuries Resulting in Removal of Eye	2	0·03	12	0·04	16	0·03	10	0·02	20	0·03	42	0·06	25	0·06	127	0·04
Missile Wounds	—	—	4	0·01	12	0·02	7	0·01	21	0·03	19	0·03	24	0·06	87	0·02
Burns and Scalds of Eyelids and Eyes	4	0·07	14	0·05	36	0·06	55	0·09	23	0·04	50	0·07	40	0·10	222	0·07
Chemical Injuries of Eyelids and Eyes	—	—	—	—	—	—	3	0·004	16	0·02	58	0·09	—	—	77	0·02
Totals	45	0·76	275	0·94	470	0·81	604	0·92	608	0·92	928	1·36	481	1·16	3,411	1·02
EARS																
Pinna, Injuries to	3	0·05	6	0·02	19	0·03	11	0·02	6	0·01	—	—	—	—	45	0·01
Rupture of Tympanic Membranes	4	0·07	14	0·05	15	0·03	17	0·02	24	0·04	39	0·06	11	0·03	124	0·04
Burns and Scalds	—	—	—	—	1	0·001	—	—	—	—	—	—	10	0·02	11	0 003
Totals	7	0·12	20	0·07	35	0·06	28	0·04	30	0·05	39	0·06	21	0·05	180	0·05
NECK																
Contusions and Wounds	1	0·02	18	0·06	21	0·04	23	0·04	22	0·03	81	0·12	10	0·02	176	0·05
Cut Throat	1	0·02	2	0·01	2	0·003	9	0·01	4	0·01	1	0·001	2	0·004	21	0·01
Missile Wounds	—	—	9	0·03	10	0·02	14	0·02	12	0·02	4	0·01	11	0·03	60	0·02
Burns and Scalds, Internal and External	1	0·02	2	0·01	2	0·003	3	0·004	6	0·01	20	0·03	—	—	34	0·01
Others	2	0·03	18	0·06	29	0·05	29	0·05	1	0·001	—	—	—	—	79	0·02
Totals	5	0·09	49	0·17	64	0·11	78	0·12	45	0·07	106	0·16	23	0·06	370	0·11

*Figures for 1939 and 1945 are for the war periods of the years only *viz.* 1939—from September 3 to December 31; 1945—from January 1 to August 15

TABLE 3(b)—(*contd.*)

R.A.F. Nosological Table for Home Force
Period of Second World War, September 3, 1939 to August 15, 1945

	1939*		1940		1941		1942		1943		1944		1945*		Totals	
	Number of Cases	Incidence per 1,000 per annum	Number of Cases	Incidence per 1,000 per annum	Number of Cases	Incidence per 1,000 per annum	Number of Cases	Incidence per 1,000 per annum	Number of Cases	Incidence per 1,000 per annum	Number of Cases	Incidence per 1,000 per annum	Number of Cases	Incidence per 1,000 per annum	Number of Cases	Incidence per 1,000 per annum
CHEST																
Contusion and Superficial Wounds	28	0·48	142	0·49	207	0·36	199	0·30	185	0·28	258	0·37	110	0·27	1,129	0·34
Compression and Blast Injury	2	0·03	13	0·04	12	0·02	9	0·01	9	0·01	12	0·02	—	—	57	0·02
Penetrating Wounds	—	—	12	0·04	18	0·03	7	0·01	7	0·01	5	0·01	—	—	49	0·01
Fractures, Fracture-Dislocations and Dislocations	23	0·39	104	0·36	159	0·27	135	0·21	144	0·22	142	0·21	113	0·27	820	0·24
Missile Wounds	2	0·03	59	0·20	66	0·11	49	0·07	39	0·06	65	0·09	39	0·10	319	0·10
Burns and Scalds	—	—	3	0·01	2	0·003	12	0·02	2	0·003	—	—	10	0·02	29	0·01
Totals	55	0·93	333	1·14	464	0·79	411	0·62	386	0·58	482	0·70	272	0·66	2,403	0·72
BACK AND VERTEBRAL COLUMN																
Contusions and Superficial Wounds	44	0·75	279	0·95	448	0·77	431	0·65	286	0·43	398	0·58	160	0·39	2,046	0·61
Contusions and Wounds involving Viscera	—	—	10	0·03	7	0·01	5	0·01	27	0·04	10	0·01	10	0·02	69	0·02
Wounds involving Spinal Cord	—	—	1	0·003	2	0·003	—	—	2	0·003	—	—	—	—	5	0·001
Spinal Concussion	1	0·02	9	0·03	2	0·003	9	0·01	9	0·01	10	0·01	126	0·30	166	0·05
Fractures, Fracture-Dislocations and Dislocations Body of Vertebrae	20	0·34	130	0·45	202	0·35	209	0·32	209	0·32	291	0·43	20	0·05	1,081	0·32
Fractures of Process and Coccyx	—	—	—	—	—	—	11	0·02	8	0·01	22	0·04	—	—	41	0·01
Missile Wounds	—	—	32	0·11	12	0·02	2	0·003	—	—	—	—	—	—	46	0·01
Burns and Scalds	2	0·03	2	0·01	5	0·01	10	0·02	5	0·01	—	—	—	—	24	0·01
Totals	67	1·14	463	1·58	678	1·16	677	1·03	546	0·82	731	1·07	316	0·76	3,478	1·04

ABDOMEN																
Contusion and Superficial Wounds	15	0·25	64	0·22	74	0·13	71	0·11	67	0·10	49	0·07	52	0·13	392	0·11
Contusions and Wounds involving Viscera	5	0·09	22	0·07	38	0·06	24	0·04	44	0·07	48	0·07	13	0·03	194	0·06
Wounds	3	0·05	7	0·02	6	0·01	—	—	—	—	—	—	—	—	16	0·004
Missile Wounds	—	—	34	0·12	30	0·05	32	0·05	15	0·02	38	0·06	9	0·02	158	0·05
Burns and Scalds	—	—	2	0·01	6	0·01	2	0·003	3	0·004	—	—	10	0·02	23	0·01
Totals	23	0·39	129	0·44	154	0·26	129	0·20	129	0·19	135	0·20	84	0·20	783	0·23
BUTTOCKS AND PELVIS																
Contusions and Wounds	5	0·09	29	0·10	46	0·07	61	0·09	53	0·08	82	0·12	30	0·07	306	0·09
Contusions and Wounds of Generative Organs	11	0·19	68	0·23	86	0·15	101	0·15	80	0·12	139	0·20	20	0·05	505	0·15
Contusions and Wounds of Other Organs	—	—	4	0·01	5	0·01	10	0·02	7	0·01	1	0·001	11	0·03	38	0·01
Fractures, Fracture-Dislocations and Dislocations	9	0·14	38	0·13	56	0·09	57	0·09	47	0·07	109	0·16	53	0·12	369	0·11
Missile Wounds	—	—	16	0·05	9	0·02	17	0·02	23	0·04	29	0·04	12	0·03	106	0·03
Burns and Scalds	—	—	2	0·01	4	0·01	5	0·01	8	0·01	19	0·03	—	—	38	0·01
Totals	25	0·42	157	0·53	206	0·35	251	0·38	218	0·33	379	0·55	126	0·30	1,362	0·40
UPPER LIMB, HAND AND WRIST																
Contusions and Wounds	54	0·92	245	0·84	464	0·79	650	0·98	766	1·15	977	1·43	471	1·14	3,627	1·08
Sprains	7	0·12	27	0·09	52	0·09	45	0·07	32	0·05	50	0·07	20	0·05	233	0·07
Fractures, Fracture-Dislocations and Dislocations	45	0·76	232	0·79	478	0·82	545	0·83	614	0·93	953	1·39	321	0·77	3,188	0·95
Amputations	8	0·14	57	0·20	131	0·22	85	0·13	—	—	—	—	—	—	281	0·08
Missile Wounds	3	0·05	61	0·21	66	0·11	58	0·09	63	0·09	93	0·14	55	0·13	399	0·12
Burns and Scalds	6	0·10	97	0·33	167	0·29	204	0·31	263	0·40	478	0·70	210	0·51	1,425	0·43
Totals	123	2·09	719	2·46	1,358	2·32	1,587	2·41	1,738	2·62	2,551	3·73	1,077	2·60	9,153	2·73

* Figures for 1939 and 1945 are for the war periods of the years only *viz.* 1939—from September 3 to December 31; 1945—from January 1 to August 15.

TABLE 3(b)—(*contd.*)

R.A.F. Nosological Table for Home Force
Period of Second World War, September 3, 1939 to August 15, 1945

	1939*		1940		1941		1942		1943		1944		1945*		Totals	
	Number of Cases	Incidence per 1,000 per annum	Number of Cases	Incidence per 1,000 per annum	Number of Cases	Incidence per 1,000 per annum	Number of Cases	Incidence per 1,000 per annum	Number of Cases	Incidence per 1,000 per annum	Number of Cases	Incidence per 1,000 per annum	Number of Cases	Incidence per 1,000 per annum	Number of Cases	Incidence per 1,000 per annum
UPPER LIMB, REST OF LIMB																
Contusions and Wounds	29	0·49	157	0·54	252	0·43	305	0·46	254	0·38	366	0·54	141	0·34	1,504	0·45
Sprains and Strains, Traumatic Synovitis, Muscle Fibre Tears	21	0·36	103	0·35	141	0·24	88	0·14	23	0·04	30	0·04	40	0·10	446	0·13
Fractures, Fracture-Dislocations and Dislocations	132	2·24	775	2·65	1,338	2·29	1,510	2·29	1,528	2·30	2,054	3·00	1,169	2·82	8,506	2·54
Amputations	—	—	2	0·01	4	0·01	—	—	—	—	—	—	—	—	6	0·002
Missile Wounds	4	0·07	88	0·30	69	0·12	86	0·13	77	0·12	121	0·18	72	0·17	517	0·15
Burns and Scalds	1	0·02	23	0·08	69	0·12	82	0·13	86	0·13	178	0·26	80	0·19	519	0·16
Multiple Fractures of Whole Upper Limb	—	—	4	0·01	26	0·04	2	0·003	3	0·003	10	0·01	—	—	45	0·01
Multiple Missile Wounds of Whole Upper Limb	—	—	19	0·06	20	0·03	—	—	4	0·01	—	—	—	—	43	0·01
Totals	187	3·18	1,171	4·00	1,919	3·28	2,073	3·15	1,975	2·98	2,759	4·03	1,502	3·62	11,586	3·45
LOWER LIMB, FOOT AND ANKLE																
Contusions and Wounds	55	0·93	255	0·87	557	0·96	701	1·07	854	1·29	808	1·18	611	1·47	3,841	1·15
Sprains and Strains	156	2·65	857	2·93	1,416	2·42	1,773	2·69	1,885	2·84	2,634	3·85	1,000	2·41	9,721	2·90
Fractures, Fracture-Dislocations and Dislocations	61	1·04	310	1·06	578	0·99	760	1·15	967	1·46	1,506	2·20	487	1·18	4,669	1·39
Amputations	—	—	5	0·02	7	0·01	2	0·003	—	—	—	—	—	—	14	0·004
Missile Wounds	1	0·02	79	0·27	71	0·12	56	0·09	57	0·09	62	0·09	13	0·03	339	0·10
Burns and Scalds	12	0·20	91	0·31	169	0·29	195	0·30	181	0·27	292	0·43	150	0·36	1,090	0·32
Totals	285	4·84	1,597	5·46	2,798	4·79	3,487	5·30	3,944	5·95	5,302	7·75	2,261	5·45	19,674	5·86

LOWER LIMB, REST OF LIMB																
Contusions and Wounds	111	1·89	578	1·97	1,010	1·73	1,102	1·67	969	1·46	1,497	2·19	769	1·85	6,036	1·80
Sprains and Strains	91	1·55	374	1·28	543	0·93	445	0·68	223	0·34	426	0·62	160	0·39	2,262	0·68
Internal Derangement of Knee Joint	202	3·43	1,123	3·84	1,761	3·01	1,729	2·63	1,143	1·72	1,685	2·47	842	2·03	8,485	2·53
Fractures, Fracture-Dislocations and Dislocations	213	3·62	965	3·30	1,690	2·89	1,759	2·67	1,588	2·40	2,476	3·62	980	2·36	9,671	2·88
Amputations	2	0·03	15	0·05	26	0·05	—	—	—	—	—	—	—	—	43	0·01
Missile Wounds	6	0·10	222	0·76	178	0·30	167	0·25	136	0·20	232	0·34	97	0·24	1,038	0·31
Burns and Scalds	3	0·05	49	0·17	67	0·11	94	0·14	83	0·13	275	0·40	80	0·19	651	0·19
Multiple Fractures of Whole Lower Limb	1	0·02	27	0·09	69	0·12	4	0·01	1	0·001	10	0·02	1	0·002	113	0·03
Missile Wounds of Whole Lower Limb	1	0·02	25	0·08	40	0·07	—	—	10	0·02	9	0·01	10	0·02	95	0·03
Totals	630	10·71	3,378	11·54	5,384	9·21	5,300	8·05	4,153	6·27	6,610	9·67	2,939	7·08	28,394	8·46
Total of All Injuries	2,696	45·82	16,912	57·79	27,005	46·17	30,927	46·98	37,162	56·09	48,033	70·24	18,727	45·13	181,462	54·07
UNCLASSIFIED CONDITIONS																
Heat Exhaustion and Heat Hyperpyrexia	2	0·03	54	0·18	114	0·19	51	0·08	73	0·11	70	0·10	50	0·12	414	0·12
Surgical Amputations and Fitting of Artificial Appliances	—	—	—	—	—	—	87	0·13	113	0·17	190	0·28	136	0·33	526	0·16
Late Complications of Trauma	—	—	—	—	—	—	21	0·03	21	0·03	47	0·07	19	0·05	108	0·03
Prolonged Loss of Senses immediately following Injury	—	—	—	—	—	—	—	—	1	0·001	1	0·001	11	0·02	13	0·003
Totals	2	0·03	54	0·18	114	0·19	159	0·24	208	0·31	308	0·45	216	0·52	1,061	0·31
Grant Total of All Disabilities	17,004	289·01	122,853	419·77	201,684	344·80	226,632	344·25	261,137	394·11	302,839	442·87	151,602	367·32	1,283,751	382·50

* Figures for 1939 and 1945 are for the war periods of the years only *viz.* 1939—from September 3 to December 31; 1945—from January 1 to August 15.

TABLE 3(c)

R.A.F. Nosological Table for Forces Abroad
Period of Second World War, September 3, 1939 to August 15, 1945

	1939*		1940		1941		1942		1943		1944		1945*		Totals	
	Number of Cases	Incidence per 1,000 per annum	Number of Cases	Incidence per 1,000 per annum	Number of Cases	Incidence per 1,000 per annum	Number of Cases	Incidence per 1,000 per annum	Number of Cases	Incidence per 1,000 per annum	Number of Cases	Incidence per 1,000 per annum	Number of Cases	Incidence per 1,000 per annum	Number of Cases	Incidence per 1,000 per annum
INFECTIOUS DISEASES																
Amoebic Dysentery	1	0·20	25	0·79	105	1·35	994	4·91	2,663	8·62	4,129	12·95	1,588	8·40	9,505	8·38
Bacillary Dysentery	26	5·14	258	8·13	1,880	24·15	5,947	29·38	7,990	25·87	8,354	26·21	5,643	29·83	30,098	26·55
Enteric Group	4	0·79	10	0·32	104	1·34	354	1·75	400	1·30	543	1·70	294	1·55	1,709	1·51
Enteritis	203	40·13	1,044	32·90	4,215	54·14	4,919	24·30	1,071	3·47	1,473	4·62	1,020	5·39	13,945	12·30
Malaria	140	27·67	883	27·83	3,244	41·67	12,148	60·02	23,580	76·35	23,744	74·49	5,901	31·20	69,640	61·42
Other Tropical Infections	249	49·22	655	20·64	3,630	46·63	8,700	42·98	9,396	30·42	8,821	27·67	3,823	20·21	35,274	31·11
Bacillary Infections (Other than Typhoid and Dysentery)	2	0·39	27	0·85	100	1·28	379	1·87	490	1·59	811	2·54	251	1·33	2,060	1·82
Staphylococcal and Streptococcal Infections	5	0·99	45	1·42	100	1·28	535	2·65	998	3·23	655	2·06	56	0·30	2,394	2·11
Virus Infections	3	0·59	405	12·76	235	3·02	1,087	5·37	1,098	3·55	1,109	3·48	532	2·81	4,469	3·94
Metazoan Parasite Infections	8	1·58	21	0·66	36	0·46	146	0·72	367	1·19	433	1·36	340	1·80	1,351	1·19
Infections of Unknown or Doubtful Origin	80	15·81	212	6·68	956	12·28	3,482	17·20	9,311	30·15	10,358	32·49	2,641	13·96	27,040	23·85
Central Nervous System Infections	12	2·37	76	2·40	135	1·74	378	1·87	736	2·38	1,121	3·52	381	2·01	2,839	2·50
Totals	733	144·88	3,661	115·38	14,740	189·34	39,069	193·02	58,100	188·12	61,551	193·09	22,470	118·79	200,324	176·68

INFECTIONS OF RESPIRATORY TRACT																
Common Cold, Nasopharyngitis and Sore Throat	290	57·32	1,548	48·78	3,289	42·25	10,118	49·99	15,914	51·53	16,535	51·87	7,060	37·32	54,754	48·29
Influenza	109	21·54	1,174	37·00	1,615	20·74	4,017	19·85	4,710	15·25	3,145	9·87	540	2·86	15,310	13·51
Tonsillitis	232	45·86	1,080	34·04	3,928	50·46	10,751	53·11	14,079	45·58	13,720	43·04	6,190	32·72	49,980	44·08
Vincent's Angina	9	1·78	31	0·98	168	2·16	494	2·44	512	1·66	462	1·45	210	1·11	1,886	1·66
Upper Respiratory Tract Infections—Totals	640	126·50	3,833	120·80	9,000	115·61	25,380	125·39	35,215	114·02	33,862	106·23	14,000	74·01	121,930	107·45
PNEUMONIA	22	4·35	96	3·03	319	4·10	886	4·38	1,059	3·43	1,519	4·77	919	4·86	4,820	4·25
PULMONARY TUBERCULOSIS	14	2·77	30	0·94	112	1·44	364	1·80	481	1·56	225	0·71	252	1·33	1,478	1·30
TUBERCULOSIS OTHER THAN PULMONARY	—	—	8	0·25	24	0·31	68	0·34	95	0·31	118	0·37	26	0·14	339	0·30
VACCINIA AND POST-INOCULATION EFFECTS	8	1·58	46	1·45	116	1·49	287	1·42	796	2·58	888	2·79	360	1·90	2,501	2·21
CARRIERS	1	0·20	7	0·22	5	0·06	22	0·11	50	0·16	115	0·36	190	1·00	390	0·34
CONTACTS	2	0·39	16	0·51	39	0·50	71	0·35	168	0·54	192	0·60	20	0·11	508	0·45
VENEREAL DISEASES																
Gonorrhoea	294	58·11	662	20·86	1,133	14·55	3,149	15·56	4,779	15·48	7,441	23·34	3,843	20·31	21,301	18·78
Syphilis	26	5·14	92	2·90	169	2·17	551	2·72	822	2·66	1,466	4·60	753	3·98	3,879	3·42
Syphilis with Gonorrhoea	—	—	—	—	—	—	3	0·01	41	0·13	104	0·32	20	0·11	168	0·15
Others	35	6·92	97	3·06	216	2·78	433	2·14	679	2·20	2,173	6·82	1,160	6·13	4,793	4·23
Totals	355	70·17	851	26·82	1,518	19·50	4,136	20·43	6,321	20·47	11,184	35·08	5,776	30·53	30,141	26·58
SEPTIC CONDITIONS (Areolar Tissues, Lymphatic Channels and Breasts)																
Conditions due to Pyogenic Organisms	307	60·68	948	29·88	3,112	39·97	8,302	41·02	11,506	37·25	14,010	43·95	6,391	33·79	44,576	39·32
Other Conditions	6	1·19	30	0·95	146	1·88	462	2·28	715	2·32	952	2·99	471	2·49	2,782	2·45
Breasts	—	—	2	0·06	13	0·17	32	0·16	48	0·16	59	0·18	10	0·05	164	0·14
Totals	313	61·87	980	30·89	3,271	42·02	8,796	43·46	12,269	39·73	15,021	47·12	6,872	36·33	47,522	41·91

* Figures for 1939 and 1945 are for the war periods of the years only *viz.* 1939—from September 3 to December 31; 1945—from January 1 to August 15.

TABLE 3(c)—(*contd.*)

R.A.F. Nosological Table for Forces Abroad
Period of Second World War, September 3, 1939 to August 15, 1945

	1939*		1940		1941		1942		1943		1944		1945*		Totals	
	Number of Cases	Incidence per 1,000 per annum	Number of Cases	Incidence per 1,000 per annum	Number of Cases	Incidence per 1,000 per annum	Number of Cases	Incidence per 1,000 per annum	Number of Cases	Incidence per 1,000 per annum	Number of Cases	Incidence per 1,000 per annum	Number of Cases	Incidence per 1,000 per annum	Number of Cases	Incidence per 1,000 per annum
ALIMENTARY SYSTEM DISEASES																
Dental Conditions	33	6·52	75	2·36	286	3·67	624	3·08	818	2·65	857	2·69	390	2·06	3,083	2·72
Mouth, Pharynx and Oesophagus	8	1·58	41	1·29	122	1·57	297	1·47	303	0·98	532	1·67	302	1·60	1,605	1·42
Gastric Ulcer and its Complications	22	4·35	37	1·17	44	0·57	61	0·30	66	0·21	88	0·28	18	0·09	336	0·30
Other Gastric Conditions	95	18·78	252	7·94	683	8·77	1,769	8·74	2,607	8·44	3,442	10·80	1,584	8·37	10,432	9·20
Duodenal Ulcer and its Complications	31	6·13	38	1·20	88	1·13	248	1·23	406	1·31	442	1·39	201	1·06	1,454	1·28
Duodenitis	4	0·79	3	0·09	15	0·19	32	0·16	60	0·19	40	0·12	10	0·05	164	0·14
Appendicitis, all types	61	12·06	216	6·81	664	8·53	1,530	7·56	2,001	6·48	2,127	6·67	815	4·31	7,414	6·54
Other Intestinal Conditions	49	9·68	175	5·51	429	5·51	6,413	31·68	14,782	47·86	13,458	42·22	8,993	47·54	44,299	39·07
Rectum and Anus	42	8·30	165	5·20	409	5·25	1,250	6·18	1,912	6·19	2,296	7·20	1,250	6·61	7,324	6·46
Hernia, all types	38	7·51	90	2·84	218	2·80	600	2·97	936	3·03	1,290	4·05	461	2·44	3,633	3·21
Liver and Gall Bladder	8	1·58	25	0·79	106	1·36	296	1·46	728	2·36	883	2·77	217	1·15	2,263	2·00
Pancreas	—	—	1	0·03	2	0·03	1	0·004	3	0·01	11	0·03	10	0·05	28	0·02
Peritoneum	1	0·20	4	0·13	7	0·09	35	0·17	32	0·10	79	0·25	28	0·15	186	0·16
Totals	392	77·48	1,122	35·36	3,073	39·47	13,156	65·00	24,654	79·83	25,545	80·14	14,279	75·48	82,221	72·52

CIRCULATORY SYSTEM DISEASES																
Pericardium	—	—	1	0·03	3	0·04	10	0·05	10	0·03	11	0·03	—	—	35	0·03
Endocarditis and Valvular Diseases of the Heart	8	1·58	4	0·13	24	0·31	110	0·54	119	0·38	140	0·44	22	0·12	427	0·38
Myocardium	9	1·78	12	0·38	21	0·27	43	0·21	73	0·24	86	0·27	10	0·05	254	0·22
Cardiac Arrhythmias	5	0·99	30	0·94	33	0·42	72	0·36	78	0·25	98	0·31	64	0·34	380	0·34
Disordered Action of the Heart	8	1·58	25	0·79	60	0·77	164	0·81	216	0·70	307	0·96	151	0·80	931	0·82
Totals	30	5·93	72	2·27	141	1·81	399	1·97	496	1·60	642	2·01	247	1·31	2,027	1·79
Blood Vessels	34	6·72	70	2·21	222	2·85	693	3·42	1,179	3·82	1,358	4·26	758	4·00	4,314	3·80
Circulatory System—Totals	64	12·65	142	4·48	363	4·66	1,092	5·39	1,675	5·42	2,000	6·27	1,005	5·31	6,341	5·59
BLOOD, BLOOD-FORMING ORGANS, SPLEEN, AND RETICULO-ENDOTHELIAL SYSTEM																
Anaemias	2	0·39	12	0·38	33	0·43	83	0·41	129	0·42	115	0·36	27	0·14	401	0·35
Leukaemias	—	—	4	0·13	1	0·01	2	0·01	3	0·01	5	0·01	—	—	15	0·01
Purpuras	2	0·39	1	0·03	1	0·01	12	0·06	17	0·05	41	0·13	10	0·05	84	0·08
Other Diseases of the Blood	2	0·39	3	0·09	3	0·04	8	0·04	22	0·07	25	0·08	14	0·08	77	0·07
Lymphatic Glands	—	—	—	—	7	0·09	27	0·13	10	0·03	44	0·14	10	0·05	98	0·09
Spleen and Reticulo-Endothelial System	1	0·20	2	0·06	7	0·09	21	0·10	45	0·15	58	0·18	3	0·02	137	0·12
Totals	7	1·38	22	0·69	52	0·67	153	0·75	226	0·73	288	0·90	64	0·34	812	0·72
RESPIRATORY SYSTEM DISEASES																
Larynx and Trachea	—	—	1	0·03	4	0·05	74	0·37	256	0·83	184	0·58	140	0·74	659	0·58
Bronchi	96	18·97	310	9·77	615	7·90	2,081	10·28	4,060	13·15	4,397	13·79	2,336	12·35	13,895	12·26
Lungs	10	1·98	13	0·41	44	0·56	183	0·90	323	1·05	464	1·45	74	0·39	1,111	0·98
Pleura	11	2·17	62	1·95	197	2·53	603	2·98	715	2·31	904	2·84	371	1·96	2,863	2·53
Mediastinum	—	—	—	—	—	—	2	0·01	3	0·01	—	—	—	—	5	0·004
Totals	117	23·12	386	12·16	860	11·04	2,943	14·54	5,357	17·35	5,949	18·66	2,921	15·44	18,533	16·35
ALLERGY, DISEASES OF																
Asthma	14	2·77	31	0·98	120	1·54	251	1·24	257	0·83	320	1·00	134	0·71	1,127	0·99
Hay Fever	—	—	—	—	4	0·05	13	0·06	12	0·04	28	0·09	10	0·05	67	0·06
Urticaria	7	1·38	39	1·23	107	1·38	267	1·32	375	1·21	414	1·30	210	1·11	1,419	1·26
Others	1	0·20	2	0·06	11	0·14	46	0·23	57	0·19	78	0·24	10	0·05	205	0·18
Totals	22	4·35	72	2·27	242	3·11	577	2·85	701	2·27	840	2·63	364	1·92	2,818	2·49

* Figures for 1939 and 1945 are for the war periods of the years only *viz.* 1939—from September 3 to December 31; 1945—from January 1 to August 15.

TABLE 3(c)—(*contd.*)

R.A.F. Nosological Table for Forces Abroad
Period of Second World War, September 3, 1939 to August 15, 1945

	1939*		1940		1941		1942		1943		1944		1945*		Totals	
	Number of Cases	Incidence per 1,000 per annum	Number of Cases	Incidence per 1,000 per annum	Number of Cases	Incidence per 1,000 per annum	Number of Cases	Incidence per 1,000 per annum	Number of Cases	Incidence per 1,000 per annum	Number of Cases	Incidence per 1,000 per annum	Number of Cases	Incidence per 1,000 per annum	Number of Cases	Incidence per 1,000 per annum
URINARY SYSTEM DISEASES																
Anomalies of Urinary Secretion	15	2·96	44	1·39	115	1·48	400	1·98	620	2·01	720	2·26	331	1·75	2,245	1·98
Nephritis, all Forms	4	0·79	13	0·41	30	0·39	88	0·44	97	0·31	101	0·32	46	0·24	379	0·33
Kidney	14	2·77	41	1·29	96	1·23	234	1·16	390	1·26	423	1·33	285	1·51	1,483	1·31
Urinary Calculi and Urinary Colic	10	1·98	60	1·89	175	2·25	434	2·14	712	2·31	900	2·82	472	2·49	2,763	2·44
Bladder	10	1·98	33	1·04	100	1·28	266	1·31	405	1·31	474	1·49	242	1·28	1,530	1·35
Others	2	0·39	1	0·03	5	0·06	9	0·04	11	0·04	40	0·12	1	0·01	69	0·06
Totals	55	10·87	192	6·05	521	6·69	1,431	7·07	2,235	7·24	2,658	8·34	1,377	7·28	8,469	7·47
GENERATIVE SYSTEM DISEASES																
Prostate	2	0·39	6	0·19	16	0·21	100	0·50	134	0·43	156	0·49	70	0·37	484	0·43
Urethra	53	10·48	246	7·75	467	6·00	885	4·37	1,006	3·26	981	3·08	280	1·48	3,918	3·45
Penis	60	11·86	183	5·77	432	5·55	1,073	5·30	1,434	4·64	1,459	4·58	900	4·76	5,541	4·89
Spermatic Cord, Testis and Epididymis	16	3·16	62	1·95	125	1·60	438	2·16	817	2·65	939	2·94	560	2·96	2,957	2·61
Totals	131	25·89	497	15·66	1,040	13·36	2,496	12·33	3,391	10·98	3,535	11·09	1,810	9·57	12,900	11·38

LOCOMOTOR SYSTEM DISEASES																
Muscles	3	0·59	10	0·31	38	0·49	72	0·36	126	0·41	128	0·40	80	0·43	457	0·40
Rheumatic Group	68	13·44	183	5·77	327	4·20	972	4·80	1,566	5·07	2,143	6·72	986	5·21	6,245	5·51
Deformities	19	3·76	46	1·45	120	1·54	285	1·41	320	1·04	448	1·41	197	1·04	1,435	1·27
Joints	37	7·31	106	3·34	341	4·38	1,165	5·75	2,066	6·69	1,595	5·00	738	3·90	6,048	5·33
Internal Derangement of Knee Joint	5	0·99	17	0·54	58	0·74	200	0·99	400	1·29	537	1·69	162	0·86	1,379	1·22
Bones and Cartilages	10	1·98	8	0·25	55	0·71	142	0·70	195	0·63	176	0·55	118	0·62	704	0·62
Ligaments and Tendons	7	1·38	32	1·01	125	1·61	211	1·04	111	0·36	115	0·36	101	0·53	702	0·62
Effects of Old Injuries	—	—	—	—	—	—	—	—	—	—	820	2·57	335	1·77	1,155	1·02
Totals	149	29·45	402	12·67	1,064	13·67	3,047	15·05	4,784	15·49	5,962	18·70	2,717	14·36	18,125	15·99
NERVOUS SYSTEM AND MENTAL DISEASES																
Psychoneuroses	63	12·45	183	5·77	471	6·05	1,083	5·35	1,647	5·33	2,427	7·61	1,230	6·50	7,104	6·27
Psychoses	20	3·95	42	1·32	58	0·74	174	0·86	250	0·81	392	1·23	70	0·37	1,006	0·89
Psychopathic Personality	6	1·19	11	0·35	29	0·37	120	0·59	177	0·57	213	0·67	172	0·91	728	0·64
Mental Defect	—	—	—	—	8	0·10	13	0·06	27	0·09	8	0·02	35	0·18	91	0·08
Epilepsies	12	2·37	21	0·66	48	0·62	113	0·56	137	0·44	152	0·48	73	0·39	556	0·49
Indefinite Etiology	22	4·35	71	2·24	160	2·06	390	1·93	696	2·26	678	2·13	176	0·93	2,193	1·93
Totals	123	24·31	328	10·34	774	9·94	1,893	9·35	2,934	9·50	3,870	12·14	1,756	9·28	11,678	10·30
ORGANIC NERVOUS DISEASES																
Brain, Diseases of	1	0·20	8	0·25	25	0·32	65	0·32	102	0·33	156	0·49	46	0·24	403	0·36
Organic Diseases Indefinite	3	0·59	4	0·13	18	0·23	38	0·19	38	0·12	77	0·24	9	0·05	187	0·17
Cranial Nerves	5	0·99	11	0·35	26	0·33	74	0·37	96	0·31	150	0·47	73	0·39	435	0·38
Spinal Cord	3	0·59	2	0·06	10	0·13	12	0·06	31	0·10	4	0·01	6	0·03	68	0·06
Spinal and Peripheral Nerves	21	4·15	53	1·67	135	1·74	330	1·63	587	1·90	835	2·62	355	1·88	2,316	2·04
Others	—	—	—	—	1	0·01	—	—	—	—	—	—	—	—	1	0·0008
Totals	33	6·52	78	2·46	215	2·76	519	2·57	854	2·76	1,222	3·83	489	2·59	3,410	3·01
Nervous System and Mental Diseases—Totals	156	30·83	406	12·80	989	12·70	2,412	11·92	3,788	12·26	5,092	15·97	2,245	11·87	15,088	13·31
EYE DISEASES																
Defects of Vision	2	0·39	15	0·47	55	0·71	131	0·65	257	0·83	245	0·77	279	1·48	984	0·87
Inflammatory Conditions	27	5·34	78	2·46	212	2·72	561	2·77	827	2·68	1,192	3·74	680	3·59	3,577	3·15
Others	10	1·98	44	1·39	101	1·30	365	1·80	584	1·89	720	2·26	292	1·54	2,116	1·87
Totals	39	7·71	137	4·32	368	4·73	1,057	5·22	1,668	5·40	2,157	6·77	1,251	6·61	6,677	5·89

* Figures for 1939 and 1945 are for the war periods of the years only *viz.* 1939—from September 3 to December 31; 1945—from January 1 to August 15.

TABLE 3(c)—(*contd.*)

R.A.F. Nosological Table for Forces Abroad
Period of Second World War, September 3, 1939 to August 15, 1945

	1939*		1940		1941		1942		1943		1944		1945*		Totals	
	Number of Cases	Incidence per 1,000 per annum	Number of Cases	Incidence per 1,000 per annum	Number of Cases	Incidence per 1,000 per annum	Number of Cases	Incidence per 1,000 per annum	Number of Cases	Incidence per 1,000 per annum	Number of Cases	Incidence per 1,000 per annum	Number of Cases	Incidence per 1,000 per annum	Number of Cases	Incidence per 1,000 per annum
EAR DISEASES																
Deafness	—	—	—	—	—	—	31	0·15	80	0·26	121	0·38	59	0·31	291	0·26
Otitis Media, Acute	18	3·56	138	4·35	493	6·33	1,335	6·60	1,445	4·68	1,276	4·00	580	3·06	5,285	4·66
Otitis Media, Chronic	12	2·38	41	1·29	86	1·11	320	1·58	803	2·60	1,010	3·17	421	2·22	2,693	2·38
Otitis, Externa	52	10·28	136	4·29	270	3·47	745	3·68	1,459	4·72	1,782	5·59	1,131	5·98	5,575	4·92
Perforated Tympanic Membrane	2	0·39	9	0·28	19	0·24	29	0·15	14	0·04	10	0·03	20	0·11	103	0·09
Mastoiditis, Acute	—	—	11	0·35	84	1·08	65	0·32	79	0·26	151	0·47	30	0·16	420	0·37
Mastoiditis, Chronic	2	0·39	1	0·03	6	0·08	22	0·11	18	0·06	21	0·07	14	0·08	84	0·06
Others	7	1·38	4	0·13	19	0·24	41	0·20	66	0·21	39	0·12	60	0·32	236	0·21
Totals	93	18·38	340	10·72	977	12·55	2,588	12·79	3,964	12·83	4,410	13·83	2,315	12·24	14,687	12·95
NOSE AND THROAT DISEASES																
Nasal Passages	—	—	—	—	—	—	—	—	893	2·89	979	3·07	520	2·75	2,392	2·11
Sinuses	34	6·72	200	6·31	525	6·74	1,570	7·76	1,456	4·72	1,742	5·46	827	4·37	6,354	5·60
Naso-Pharynx	—	—	—	—	—	—	—	—	1,088	3·52	1,108	3·48	330	1·75	2,526	2·23
Throat	9	1·78	61	1·92	280	3·60	843	4·16	3	0·01	—	—	—	—	1,196	1·06
Totals	43	8·50	261	8·23	805	10·34	2,413	11·92	3,440	11·14	3,829	12·01	1,677	8·87	12,468	11·00

SKIN DISEASES																
Scabies	25	4·94	164	5·17	1,011	12·99	2,834	14·00	2,000	6·48	1,476	4·63	750	3·97	8,260	7·29
Impetigo	50	9·88	198	6·24	694	8·92	2,047	10·11	2,636	8·54	3,234	10·15	2,040	10·78	10,899	9·61
Pediculosis and Pediculitis	13	2·57	22	0·69	73	0·94	164	0·81	83	0·27	80	0·25	60	0·32	495	0·44
Tinea Cruris	18	3·56	65	2·05	239	3·07	354	1·75	412	1·33	682	2·14	413	2·18	2,183	1·93
Tinea, Others	32	6·33	94	2·96	351	4·51	1,030	5·09	1,619	5·24	1,839	5·77	1,331	7·04	6,296	5·55
Dermatitis and Eczema	46	9·09	157	4·95	473	6·07	1,742	8·61	2,662	8·62	3,140	9·85	1,552	8·20	9,772	8·62
Pityriasis and Erythemata	10	1·98	50	1·57	170	2·18	364	1·80	245	0·79	316	0·99	200	1·06	1,355	1·19
Psoriasis	3	0·59	12	0·38	36	0·46	95	0·47	152	0·49	186	0·58	52	0·27	536	0·47
Ingrowing Toenail	10	1·98	32	1·01	152	1·95	454	2·24	713	2·31	613	1·92	340	1·80	2,314	2·04
Other Conditions	24	4·74	91	2·87	272	3·49	1,022	5·05	1,819	5·89	2,733	8·57	1,765	9·33	7,726	6·81
Totals	231	45·66	885	27·89	3,471	44·58	10,106	49·93	12,341	39·96	14,299	44·85	8,503	44·95	49,836	43·95
ENDOCRINE DISEASES																
General Endocrine Disturbances	—	—	1	0·03	2	0·03	1	0·004	6	0·02	—	—	10	0·05	20	0·02
Male Gonads	—	—	—	—	11	0·14	17	0·08	27	0·09	63	0·20	38	0·20	156	0·14
Parathyroid	—	—	—	—	—	—	1	0·004	1	0·003	10	0·03	—	—	12	0·01
Pituitary	1	0·20	1	0·03	1	0·01	1	0·004	8	0·03	9	0·03	1	0·01	22	0·02
Suprarenal	—	—	1	0·03	—	—	—	—	6	0·02	10	0·03	3	0·02	20	0·02
Thymus	—	—	—	—	—	—	—	—	1	0·003	—	—	—	—	1	0·0008
Thyroid	1	0·20	7	0·22	16	0·21	52	0·26	53	0·17	27	0·08	42	0·22	198	0·17
Totals	2	0·39	10	0·31	30	0·39	72	0·36	102	0·33	119	0·37	94	0·50	429	0·38
DISEASES OF METABOLISM	5	0·99	8	0·25	16	0·21	49	0·24	58	0·19	37	0·12	36	0·19	209	0·18
DEFICIENCY DISEASES	—	—	5	0·16	3	0·04	28	0·14	189	0·61	436	1·37	199	1·05	860	0·76
EFFECTS OF TOXIC SUBSTANCES†	—	—	—	—	—	—	88	0·43	92	0·30	88	0·28	170	0·90	438	0·39
PHYSICAL AGENTS, EFFECTS OF†	—	—	—	—	—	—	4	0·02	12	0·04	—	—	—	—	16	0·01
CYSTS AND TUMOURS																
Cysts	6	1·19	21	0·66	59	0·76	245	1·21	449	1·46	599	1·88	440	2·33	1,819	1·61
Tumours, Benign	3	0·59	9	0·28	50	0·64	147	0·73	179	0·58	184	0·58	170	0·90	742	0·65
Tumours, Malignant	4	0·79	10	0·32	14	0·18	39	0·19	63	0·20	61	0·19	16	0·08	207	0·18
Tumours, Unspecified	—	—	1	0·03	3	0·04	19	0·09	63	0·20	87	0·27	16	0·08	189	0·17
Totals	13	2·57	41	1·29	126	1·62	450	2·22	754	2·44	931	2·92	642	3·39	2,957	2·61

* Figures for 1939 and 1945 are for the war periods of the years only *viz* 1939—from September 3 to December 31; 1945—from January 1 to August 15.

† *See* p. 481.

TABLE 3(c)—(*contd.*)

R.A.F. Nosological Table for Forces Abroad
Period of Second World War, September 3, 1939 to August 15, 1945

	1939*		1940		1941		1942		1943		1944		1945*		Totals	
	Number of Cases	Incidence per 1,000 per annum	Number of Cases	Incidence per 1,000 per annum	Number of Cases	Incidence per 1,000 per annum	Number of Cases	Incidence per 1,000 per annum	Number of Cases	Incidence per 1,000 per annum	Number of Cases	Incidence per 1,000 per annum	Number of Cases	Incidence per 1,000 per annum	Number of Cases	Incidence per 1,000 per annum
INDEFINITE AND GENERAL CONDITIONS																
Observation and No Apparent Disease	61	12·05	324	10·21	1,030	13·23	2,766	13·67	3,915	12·68	3,657	11·47	1,930	10·20	13,683	12·07
Debility	12	2·37	36	1·14	121	1·56	285	1·41	372	1·21	281	0·88	390	2·06	1,497	1·32
Pyrexia of Uncertain Origin	18	3·56	127	4·00	383	4·92	809	4·00	2,855	9·24	3,142	9·85	2,470	13·06	9,804	8·64
Accidental Contamination from Noxious Gases**	—	—	—	—	4	0·05	5	0·02	13	0·04	9	0·03	—	—	31	0·03
Others	1	0·20	48	1·51	46	0·59	195	0·96	600	1·94	815	2·56	415	2·20	2,120	1·87
Totals	92	18·18	535	16·86	1,584	20·35	4,060	20·06	7,755	25·11	7,904	24·79	5,205	27·52	27,135	233·9
Total All Diseases	3,699	731·11	14,991	472·46	44,728	574·55	127,301	628·92	191,740	620·84	210,754	661·13	97,759	516·79	690,972	609·42

GENERAL INJURIES																
Multiple Injuries with Fractures	27	5·35	220	6·93	522	6·71	1,254	6·19	1,146	3·71	1,163	3·65	590	3·12	4,922	4·34
Multiple Injuries with Burns	4	0·79	43	1·35	109	1·40	217	1·07	329	1·06	304	0·95	186	0·98	1,192	1·05
Multiple Wounds	—	—	10	0·32	22	0·28	88	0·43	109	0·35	55	0·17	56	0·30	340	0·30
Fractured Skull with Other Injuries	2	0·39	27	0·85	61	0·78	70	0·35	102	0·33	25	0·08	19	0·10	306	0·27
Missile Wounds, Multiple	2	0·39	33	1·04	94	1·21	101	0·50	81	0·26	29	0·09	7	0·04	347	0·30
Minor Injuries	14	2·77	64	2·02	197	2·53	315	1·56	321	1·04	299	0·94	170	0·90	1,380	1·22
Burns Generalised	13	2·57	61	1·92	113	1·45	220	1·09	390	1·26	406	1·27	169	0·89	1,372	1·21
Burns of Face and Hands	4	0·79	21	0·66	31	0·40	63	0·31	71	0·23	72	0·22	41	0·22	303	0·27
Scalds	—	—	4	0·13	10	0·13	12	0·06	13	0·04	—	—	—	—	39	0·03
Frostbite in Aircrew during Flight**	2	0·39	4	0·13	9	0·12	18	0·09	24	0·08	—	—	10	0·05	67	0·06
Exposure to Natural Elements	2	0·39	—	—	3	0·04	41	0·20	58	0·19	21	0·07	20	0·11	145	0·13
Drowning including Effects of Immersion	6	1·19	17	0·54	36	0·46	72	0·36	96	0·31	77	0·24	54	0·28	358	0·32
Injuries to Tissues and Specialised Structures†	—	—	—	—	—	—	374	1·85	1,288	4·17	1,795	5·63	831	4·39	4,288	3·78
Chemical Agents, Effects of Contact with††	—	—	—	—	—	—	18	0·09	55	0·18	57	0·18	20	0·11	150	0·13
Other Injuries	3	0·59	29	0·91	51	0·65	477	2·36	1,302	4·22	1,717	5·39	686	3·63	4,265	3·76
Missing, Presumed Dead	17	3·36	753	23·73	908	11·66	1,124	5·55	1,543	5·00	1,740	5·46	683	3·61	6,768	5·97
Totals	96	18·97	1,286	40·53	2,166	27·82	4,464	22·06	6,928	22·43	7,760	24·34	3,542	18·73	26,242	23·14
LOCALISED INJURIES:																
CRANIUM																
Contusions and Wounds	15	2·97	37	1·17	106	1·36	306	1·51	410	1·33	500	1·57	290	1·53	1,664	1·46
Fractures of Skull, Vault	—	—	17	0·54	51	0·66	144	0·71	168	0·54	200	0·62	5	0·03	585	0·52
Fractures of Skull, Base	4	0·79	—	—	—	—	466	2·30	—	—	—	—	37	0·20	507	0·45
Concussion	48	9·49	119	3·75	232	2·98	36	0·18	695	2·25	568	1·78	300	1·58	1,998	1·76
Missile Wounds	3	0·59	19	0·60	22	0·28	1	0·004	41	0·13	40	0·13	19	0·10	145	0·13
Burns and Scalds	—	—	1	0·03	1	0·01	16	0·08	3	0·01	—	—	—	—	21	0·02
Others	3	0·59	2	0·06	13	0·17	—	—	—	—	—	—	—	—	18	0·02
Totals	73	14·43	195	6·15	425	5·46	969	4·78	1,317	4·26	1,308	4·10	651	3·44	4,938	4·36
FACE AND MOUTH																
Contusions and Wounds	9	1·78	37	1·17	75	0·96	217	1·07	279	0·90	291	0·91	170	0·90	1,078	0·95
Fractures, Fracture-Dislocations and Dislocations	8	1·58	29	0·92	69	0·89	194	0·96	272	0·88	449	1·41	210	1·11	1,231	1·09
Missile Wounds	—	—	1	0·03	5	0·06	3	0·01	7	0·03	—	—	11	0·06	27	0·02
Tooth Injuries	—	—	2	0·06	2	0·03	4	0·02	1	0·003	20	0·06	10	0·05	39	0·03
Burns and Scalds	2	0·39	15	0·47	13	0·17	29	0·15	68	0·22	108	0·34	90	0·48	325	0·29
Totals	19	3·76	84	2·65	164	2·11	447	2·21	627	2·03	868	2·72	491	2·60	2,700	2·38

* Figures for 1939 and 1945 are for the war periods of the years only *viz.* 1939—from September 3 to December 31; 1945—from January 1 to August 15.
** *See* p. 483.
† *See* p. 483.
†† *See* p. 483.

TABLE 3(c)—(*contd.*)

R.A.F. Nosological Table for Forces Abroad
Period of Second World War. September 3, 1939 to August 15, 1945

	1939*		1940		1941		1942		1943		1944		1945*		Totals	
	Number of Cases	Incidence per 1,000 per annum	Number of Cases	Incidence per 1,000 per annum	Number of Cases	Incidence per 1,000 per annum	Number of Cases	Incidence per 1,000 per annum	Number of Cases	Incidence per 1,000 per annum	Number of Cases	Incidence per 1,000 per annum	Number of Cases	Incidence per 1,000 per annum	Number of Cases	Incidence per 1,000 per annum
EYES																
Eyelids, Injuries of	3	0·59	9	0·28	17	0·22	52	0·26	42	0·14	57	0·18	10	0·05	190	0·17
Eye Substance, Superficial Wounds of	4	0·79	14	0·44	40	0·51	100	0·50	115	0·37	175	0·55	80	0·43	528	0·47
Eye Substance, Injury to Eyeball	—	—	16	0·51	14	0·18	60	0·30	143	0·46	136	0·43	112	0·59	481	0·42
Eye Substance, Injuries resulting in Removal of Eye	—	—	3	0·09	7	0·09	4	0·02	9	0·03	9	0·03	4	0·02	36	0·03
Missile Wounds	—	—	3	0·09	2	0·03	9	0·04	5	0·02	—	—	—	—	19	0·02
Burns and Scalds of Eyelids and Eyes	—	—	4	0·13	11	0·14	20	0·10	20	0·07	19	0·06	10	0·05	84	0·07
Chemical Injuries of Eyelids and Eyes	—	—	—	—	—	—	3	0·01	17	0·05	17	0·05	20	0·11	57	0·05
Totals	7	1·38	49	1·54	91	1·17	248	1·23	351	1·14	413	1·30	236	1·25	1,395	1·23
EARS																
Pinna, Injuries to	—	—		0·03	5	0·06	8	0·04	5	0·02	10	0·03	—	—	29	0·03
Rupture of Tympanic Membranes	1	0·20		0·13	7	0·09	20	0·10	13	0·04	40	0·13	30	0·16	115	0·10
Burns and Scalds	—	—	—	—	—	—	1	0·004	—	—	—	—	—	—	1	0·0008
Totals	1	0·20	5	0·16	12	0·15	29	0·14	18	0·06	50	0·16	30	0·16	145	0·13

NECK																
Contusions and Wounds	3	0·59	5	0·16	4	0·05	16	0·08	18	0·06	50	0·16	20	0·11	116	0·10
Cut Throat	—	—	—	—	1	0·01	—	—	2	0·01	2	0·01	1	0·01	6	0·01
Missile Wounds	—	—	3	0·09	8	0·11	7	0·03	4	0·01	2	0·01	—	—	24	0·02
Burns and Scalds, Internal and External	—	—	—	—	1	0·01	4	0·02	1	0·003	—	—	—	—	6	0·01
Others	2	0·39	3	0·09	3	0·04	14	0·07	2	0·01	10	0·03	—	—	34	0·02
Totals	5	0·99	11	0·34	17	0·22	41	0·20	27	0·09	64	0·21	21	0·11	186	0·16
CHEST																
Contusion and Superficial Wounds	5	0·99	24	0·75	36	0·47	99	0·49	113	0·36	106	0·33	30	0·16	413	0·36
Compression and Blast Injury	—	—	—	—	3	0·04	8	0·04	13	0·04	14	0·04	1	0·01	39	0·03
Penetrating Wounds	—	—	1	0·03	—	—	11	0·05	6	0·02	23	0·08	21	0·11	62	0·05
Fractures, Fracture-Dislocations and Dislocations	10	1·98	17	0·54	32	0·41	70	0·35	80	0·26	66	0·21	51	0·27	326	0·29
Missile Wounds	—	—	10	0·32	22	0·28	32	0·16	45	0·15	6	0·02	15	0·08	130	0·12
Burns and Scalds	—	—	1	0·03	5	0·06	7	0·03	11	0·04	20	0·06	10	0·05	54	0·05
Totals	15	2·97	53	1·67	98	1·26	227	1·12	268	0·87	235	0·74	128	0·68	1,024	0·90
BACK AND VERTEBRAL COLUMN																
Contusions and Superficial Wounds	17	3·36	38	1·20	89	1·14	165	0·82	154	0·50	215	0·67	40	0·21	718	0·63
Contusions and Wounds involving Viscera	—	—	9	0·28	11	0·14	3	0·01	29	0·09	—	—	—	—	52	0·05
Wounds involving Spinal Cord	—	—	—	—	—	—	—	—	—	—	—	—	—	—	—	—
Spinal Concussion	—	—	—	—	—	—	1	0·004	8	0·03	10	0·03	10	0·05	29	0·02
Fractures, Fracture-Dislocation and Dislocations Body of Vertebrae	3	0·59	12	0·38	37	0·48	96	0·48	150	0·48	136	0·43	92	0·48	526	0·46
Fractures of Process and Coccyx	—	—	—	—	—	—	—	—	—	—	—	—	20	0·11	20	0·02
Missile Wounds involving Vertebral Column	—	—	—	—	—	—	20	0·10	8	0·03	3	0·01	—	—	31	0·03
Burns and Scalds	—	—	—	—	3	0·04	9	0·04	10	0·03	10	0·03	20	0·11	52	0·05
Totals	20	3·95	59	1·86	140	1·80	294	1·45	359	1·16	374	1·17	182	0·96	1,428	1·26

* Figures for 1939 and 1945 are for the war periods of the years only *viz.* 1939—from September 3 to December 31; 1945—from January 1 to August 15.

TABLE 3(c)—(*contd.*)

R.A.F. Nosological Table for Forces Abroad
Period of Second World War, September 3, 1939 to August 15, 1945

	1939*		1940		1941		1942		1943		1944		1945*		Totals	
	Number of Cases	Incidence per 1,000 per annum	Number of Cases	Incidence per 1,000 per annum	Number of Cases	Incidence per 1,000 per annum	Number of Cases	Incidence per 1,000 per annum	Number of Cases	Incidence per 1,000 per annum	Number of Cases	Incidence per 1,000 per annum	Number of Cases	Incidence per 1,000 per annum	Number of Cases	Incidence per 1,000 per annum
ABDOMEN																
Contusion and Superficial Wounds . . .	1	0·20	9	0·28	11	0·14	41	0·21	27	0·09	31	0·10	60	0·31	180	0·16
Contusion and Wounds involving Viscera . .	1	0·20	—	—	5	0·06	8	0·04	22	0·07	21	0·07	1	0·01	58	0·05
Wounds . . .	—	—	—	—	—	—	—	—	—	—	—	—	—	—	—	—
Missile Wounds . .	—	—	5	0·16	10	0·13	22	0·11	23	0·07	16	0·05	5	0·03	81	0·07
Burns and Scalds . .	—	—	1	0·03	—	—	3	0·01	6	0·02	30	0·09	30	0·16	70	0·06
Totals .	2	0·39	15	0·47	26	0·33	74	0·37	78	0·25	98	0·31	96	0·51	389	0·34
BUTTOCKS AND PELVIS																
Contusions and Wounds .	1	0·20	10	0·32	6	0·07	28	0·14	34	0·11	39	0·12	10	0·05	128	0·11
Contusions and Wounds of Generative Organs .	1	0·20	9	0·28	17	0·22	31	0·15	63	0·20	38	0·12	10	0·05	169	0·15
Contusions and Wounds of Other Organs . .	2	0·39	—	—	2	0·03	3	0·01	11	0·04	—	—	20	0·11	38	0·03
Fractures, Fracture-Dislocations and Dislocations . . .	1	0·20	2	0·06	17	0·22	25	0·13	34	0·11	102	0·32	10	0·05	191	0·17
Missile Wounds . .	—	—	2	0·06	4	0·05	21	0·10	21	0·06	—	—	10	0·05	58	0·05
Burns and Scalds . .	—	—	1	0·03	—	—	8	0·04	8	0·03	10	0·03	10	0·05	37	0·03
Totals .	5	0·99	24	0·75	46	0·59	116	0·57	171	0·55	189	0·59	70	0·37	621	0·55

UPPER LIMB, HAND AND WRIST																
Contusions and Wounds	22	4·35	46	1·45	103	1·33	325	1·60	457	1·48	560	1·76	280	1·48	1,793	1·58
Sprains	7	1·38	19	0·60	13	0·17	42	0·21	57	0·18	69	0·22	10	0·05	217	0·19
Fractures, Fracture-Dislocations and Dislocations	9	1·78	32	1·01	68	0·87	269	1·33	428	1·39	541	1·70	321	1·70	1,668	1·47
Amputations	2	0·39	4	0·13	22	0·28	23	0·11	50	0·16	—	—	—	—	101	0·09
Missile Wounds	1	0·20	19	0·60	24	0·31	34	0·17	222	0·72	14	0·04	—	—	314	0·28
Burns and Scalds	5	0·99	23	0·72	33	0·42	127	0·63	—	—	215	0·67	90	0·47	493	0·43
Totals	46	9·09	143	4·51	263	3·38	820	4·05	1,214	3·93	1,399	4·39	701	3·70	4,586	4·04
UPPER LIMB, REST OF LIMB																
Contusions and Wounds	6	1·19	20	0·63	83	1·06	196	0·97	207	0·67	129	0·41	122	0·64	763	0·67
Sprains and Strains, Traumatic Synovitis Muscle Fibre Tears	1	0·20	12	0·38	13	0·17	34	0·17	14	0·05	30	0·09	—	—	104	0·09
Fractures, Fracture-Dislocations and Dislocations	45	8·90	106	3·34	246	3·16	607	3·00	899	2·91	1,196	3·75	576	3·04	3,675	3·24
Amputations	—	—	1	0·03	1	0·01	—	—	—	—	—	—	—	—	2	0·002
Missile Wounds	3	0·59	28	0·88	44	0·57	63	0·31	81	0·26	48	0·15	20	0·11	287	0·26
Burns and Scalds	2	0·39	5	0·16	24	0·31	61	0·30	123	0·40	128	0·40	60	0·32	403	0·36
Multiple Fractures of Whole Upper Limb	—	—	—	—	1	0·01	1	0·004	3	0·01	—	—	—	—	5	0·004
Multiple Missile Wounds of Whole Upper Limb	—	—	6	0·19	11	0·14	—	—	2	0·01	—	—	—	—	19	0·02
Totals	57	11·27	178	5·61	423	5·43	962	4·75	1,329	4·31	1,531	4·80	778	4·11	5,258	4·64
LOWER LIMB, FOOT AND ANKLE																
Contusions and Wounds	17	3·36	59	1·86	136	1·75	367	1·81	515	1·67	568	1·78	310	1·64	1,972	1·74
Sprains and Strains	57	11·27	147	4·63	296	3·80	792	3·91	1,000	3·24	1,069	3·35	730	3·86	4,091	3·61
Fractures, Fracture-Dislocations and Dislocations	8	1·58	52	1·64	110	1·41	277	1·37	478	1·55	563	1·77	254	1·34	1,742	1·54
Amputations	—	—	1	0·03	3	0·04	—	—	—	—	—	—	—	—	4	0·004
Missile Wounds	—	—	13	0·41	24	0·31	59	0·28	48	0·15	15	0·05	10	0·05	169	0·15
Burns and Scalds	3	0·59	17	0·54	88	1·13	197	0·97	221	0·71	185	0·58	70	0·37	781	0·69
Totals	85	16·80	289	9·11	657	8·44	1,692	8·36	2,262	7·32	2,400	7·53	1,374	7·26	8,759	7·73

* Figures for 1939 and 1945 are for the war periods of the years only *viz.* 1939—from September 3 to December 31; 1945—from January 1 to August 15.

TABLE 3(c)—(*contd.*)

R.A.F. Nosological Table for Forces Abroad
Period of Second World War, September 3, 1939 to August 15, 1945

	1939*		1940		1941		1942		1943		1944		1945*		Totals	
	Number of Cases	Incidence per 1,000 per annum	Number of Cases	Incidence per 1,000 per annum	Number of Cases	Incidence per 1,000 per annum	Number of Cases	Incidence per 1,000 per annum	Number of Cases	Incidence per 1,000 per annum	Number of Cases	Incidence per 1,000 per annum	Number of Cases	Incidence per 1,000 per annum	Number of Cases	Incidence per 1,000 per annum
LOWER LIMB, REST OF LIMB																
Contusions and Wounds	28	5·53	79	2·49	283	3·63	730	3·61	692	2·24	850	2·67	323	1·71	2,985	2·63
Sprains and Strains	30	5·93	59	1·86	123	1·58	168	0·83	160	0·52	219	0·69	100	0·53	859	0·76
Internal Derangement of Knee Joint	74	14·63	160	5·04	258	3·31	630	3·11	529	1·71	1,025	3·21	390	2·06	3,066	2·71
Fractures, Fracture-Dislocations and Dislocations	24	4·74	97	3·06	227	2·92	556	2·75	717	2·32	1,125	3·53	404	2·14	3,150	2·78
Amputations	1	0·20	2	0·06	6	0·08	—	—	—	—	—	—	—	—	9	0·01
Missile Wounds	3	0·59	62	1·96	112	1·44	124	0·61	102	0·33	48	0·15	61	0·32	512	0·45
Burns and Scalds	2	0·40	19	0·60	86	1·10	239	1·18	364	1·18	371	1·16	120	0·63	1,201	1·06
Multiple Fractures of Whole Lower Limb	—	—	2	0·06	10	0·13	—	—	3	0·01	—	—	—	—	15	0·01
Missile Wounds of Whole Lower Limb	—	—	8	0·25	—	—	—	—	18	0·06	—	—	—	—	26	0·02
Totals	162	32·02	488	15·38	1,105	14·19	2,447	12·09	2,585	8·37	3,638	11·41	1,398	7·39	11,823	10·43
Totals of All Injuries	593	117·21	2,879	90·73	5,633	72·36	12,830	63·38	17,534	56·77	20,327	63·77	9,698	51·27	69,494	61·29
UNCLASSIFIED CONDITIONS																
Heat Exhaustion and Heat Hyperpyrexia	—	—	50	1·58	273	3·51	1,551	7·66	1,099	3·56	839	2·63	1,235	6·53	5,047	4·45
Surgical Amputations and Fitting of Artificial Appliances	—	—	—	—	—	—	46	0·23	67	0·22	28	0·09	31	0·16	172	0·15
Late Compications of Trauma	—	—	—	—	—	—	1	0·004	9	0·03	—	—	2	0·01	12	0·01
Prolonged Loss of Senses Immediately following Injury	—	—	—	—	—	—	4	0·02	2	0·01	—	—	21	0·11	27	0·03
Totals	—	—	50	1·58	273	3·51	1,602	7·91	1,177	3·82	867	2·72	1,289	6·81	5,258	4·64
Grand Total of All Disabilities	4,292	848·32	17,920	564·77	50,634	650·42	141,733	700·22	210,451	681·41	231,948	727·62	108,746	574·87	765,724	675·35

* Figures for 1939 and 1945 are for the war periods of the years only *viz.* 1939—from September 3 to December 31; 1945—from January 1 to August 15.

In Table 4 below the disease groups are arranged in order of incidence and for each group the number of cases, the incidence per 1,000 of strength and the percentage of the total diseases are shown. This table is for the total force over the whole war period and summarises the relative importance of the various disease groups according to the number of cases but does not, of course, compare the number of man-hours lost from each cause.

TABLE 4

R.A.F. Disease Groups in Order of Incidence

Disease Group	No. of Cases	Incidence per 1,000 of strength per annum	Percentage of all diseases
Upper Respiratory Tract Infections	465,063	103·6	25·95
Other Infectious Diseases	272,603	60·7	15·21
Alimentary System	222,643	49·6	12·42
Skin	120,538	26·8	6·73
Septic Conditions	112,737	25·1	6·29
Indefinite and General	80,341	17·9	4·48
Respiratory System (trachea, bronchi, lungs, pleura)	79,228	17·6	4·42
E.N.T.	79,165	17·6	4·42
Locomotor System	73,398	16·4	4·10
Nervous and Mental Diseases	67,157	15·0	3·75
Venereal Diseases	59,396	13·2	3·31
Generative System	32,702	7·3	1·82
Circulatory System	27,921	6·2	1·56
Urinary System	23,100	5·1	1·29
Eye	20,509	4·6	1·14
Pneumonia	19,553	4·4	1·09
Allergy	11,136	2·5	0·62
Cysts and Tumours	9,455	2·1	0·53
Tuberculosis (Pulmonary)	7,652	1·7	0·43
Tuberculosis (Other Sites)	1,963	0·4	0·11
Endocrine, Blood and Metabolism	5,940	1·3	0·33
Totals	1,792,200	399·1	100·00

INFECTIOUS DISEASES

The diseases at the head of this group which are chiefly of importance in tropical countries (amoebic dysentery, bacillary dysentery, enteric fever, enteritis and malaria) are dealt with in Section D relating to the tables of diseases caused by infection in certain Commands abroad (Tables 7(a), (b), (c), (d)).

Of the remainder, the incidences of the more important infections are shown in Table 6—'Certain Infectious Diseases in the Total Force 1939–45'. These diseases are discussed in the narrative attached to that table.

BACILLARY INFECTIONS, other than typhoid and dysentery, include diphtheria, tetanus, whooping cough and anthrax. These diseases never assumed great importance during the war.

VIRUS INFECTIONS refer to the common diseases of measles, rubella, mumps and chicken pox and others such as smallpox, herpes and psittacosis. The high incidence of 24 per 1,000 of strength in 1940 is largely accounted for by an epidemic of rubella which affected the whole country at that time.

The heading INFECTIONS OF UNKNOWN OR DOUBTFUL ORIGIN covers such diseases as rheumatic fever, glandular fever, infective hepatitis and Weil's disease.

CENTRAL NERVOUS SYSTEM INFECTIONS includes cerebro-spinal fever, anterior poliomyelitis and the various forms of encephalitis.

INFECTIONS OF THE UPPER RESPIRATORY TRACT

Infections of the Upper Respiratory Tract were responsible for more than 25 per cent. of sickness due to disease. The common cold heads the list with an average incidence of 44 per 1,000 of strength and peak incidences in 1940 at 58 per 1,000 of strength and in 1943 at 53 per 1,000 of strength. It must be remembered that these figures refer only to cases sufficiently severe to require admission for 48 hours or more and are no measure of the true incidence of the common cold. In 1944 the average duration of treatment before return to duty at home and abroad was six days compared with an average of eight days for influenza.

It was feared that war-time conditions would favour the development of influenza epidemics but these expectations were belied by experience. There was moderate epidemicity in the United Kingdom in 1940 and again in 1943 but in 1944 the number of influenza deaths in the country was the lowest since 1919. The incidence of influenza in the R.A.F., too, was highest in 1940 and 1943. Although the lowest incidence is recorded for 1945 this does not refer to a complete year; the lowest incidence in any complete year was in 1944. The incidence of influenza was slightly higher at home than abroad.

PNEUMONIA

This term includes all forms of pneumonia—those of bacterial origin and those due to non-bacterial agents, known or unknown. The chief point of interest is the high incidence in the force at home in 1944 when it was over 7 per 1,000 of strength or roughly double the incidence for other years. During that year there were 6,542 cases with 30 deaths. The average period of treatment before return to duty was 26 days. This may possibly be regarded as the aftermath of the influenza epidemic which occurred in the December quarter of 1943.

Apart from 1944 the incidence of pneumonia abroad did not differ significantly from the incidence at home.

TUBERCULOSIS

The Registrar General's reports show that during the pre-war years from 1935 there had been a progressive decline in tuberculosis morbidity. In 1939 there was an arrest of this downward trend, a considerable increase in 1940–41, a return to the 1938–39 level in 1942–43 and a resumption of the downward trend thereafter.

R.A.F. experience of tuberculosis did not parallel that of the community at large. Pulmonary tuberculosis shows an incidence which gradually rises to its highest level of 2·1 per 1,000 of strength in 1943. There was a fall to 1·4 per 1,000 in 1944 but the incidence again rose to 1·8 per 1,000 in 1945. The incidence for types other than pulmonary remained fairly steady throughout with an average incidence of 0·4 per 1,000. The mortality rates were highest in 1940 and 1942. (*See* Table 17.)

Probably the chief reason for the difference between R.A.F. and civilian figures was the increasing use made by the R.A.F. of mass chest radiography during the war. (*See R.A.F. Medical Services* Vol. I, Chap. 6, p. 288 ff.) Chest radiography for recruits was not a routine procedure in the R.A.F. at the start of the war. The first mass radiography unit was presented by the British Red Cross in 1941 and gradually other units were acquired. This meant that in the later years of the war the majority of recruits and many serving personnel had routine chest X-rays. Many cases of active tuberculosis were brought to light and its importance in eliminating foci of infection and in avoiding the expense and danger of training unfit and potentially infective men was obvious.

There was no significant difference between the incidence of tuberculosis at home and abroad. In 1939 and 1940 there were too few men abroad for the figures to be strictly comparable. In 1941 and 1942 the incidence was practically the same at home and abroad. In later years the incidence was higher at home than abroad—this was probably due to the discovery of cases by mass radiography prior to posting overseas.

VACCINIA AND POST-INOCULATION EFFECTS

During the war every recruit was offered vaccination against smallpox and inoculation against the typhoid and paratyphoid group and against tetanus. Efforts were made to maintain this immunity by re-vaccination at specified intervals and by yearly booster doses of T.A.B.C. and A.T.T. Protection against yellow fever and cholera was given to personnel posted to or passing through districts in which these diseases were endemic. The constitutional upset from T.A.B.C. inoculation was often severe enough to lead to admission to sick quarters. Vaccination against smallpox carried with it the risk of generalised vaccinia and the occasional risk of post-vaccinial encephalitis. In the early years of the war a number of cases of inoculation jaundice were caused by yellow fever inoculation with a vaccine prepared from pooled serum. Reactions to tetanus toxoid and cholera vaccine were rare.

CARRIERS AND CONTACTS

Treatment of carriers and contacts of infectious diseases caused a small but steady wastage during the war years. A measure of their importance is given in the 1945 statistics when 200 carriers spent an average of 24 days under treatment and 120 contacts an average of 17 days. The important diseases likely to be spread by symptomless carriers are cerebro-spinal fever, diphtheria, the dysenteries, cholera and enteric fevers. Diseases requiring the isolation of contacts included those mentioned above and others such as anterior poliomyelitis, smallpox and the common infectious fevers.

SEPTIC CONDITIONS

This group includes boils, carbuncles, abscesses, cellulitis, finger infections and lymphadenitis. As would be expected, the incidence abroad was about double the incidence at home—residents in tropical countries are particularly prone to septic infections.

VENEREAL DISEASES*

The peace-time incidence of venereal diseases in the R.A.F. at home was low and had fallen steadily since 1921. This low incidence has been attributed very largely to improved education, ample facilities for sport and frequent and regular home leave and to the fact that the bulk of R.A.F. personnel consisted of healthy, well-educated artisans with interesting work to occupy them.

It was anticipated at the outbreak of the war, with its rapid recruitment of men from all walks and conditions of life, that the incidence of venereal diseases would rise steeply. The lack of recreational facilities at many stations, the uncertain and reduced periods of leave and the irregular and increased hours of work would all tend to be factors leading to an increased incidence. In fact, the incidence of venereal diseases for the force at home does not show any marked rise until 1944, when the increase was almost entirely due to the inclusion of the Allied Expeditionary Air Force and the Air Forces of Occupation as

* *See R.A.F. Medical Services* Vol. I, Chap. 7, p. 399 and Vol. III, Chap. 11, p. 670.

home commands. Table 5 summarises all venereal diseases from 1921–45.

Gonorrhoea

The figures represent all cases of gonorrhoea treated during each year and include all relapses and all sequelae of gonococcal infections. At

CHART 4(a)
R.A.F. GONORRHOEA—AVERAGE DURATION OF TREATMENT IN DAYS, 1937–45

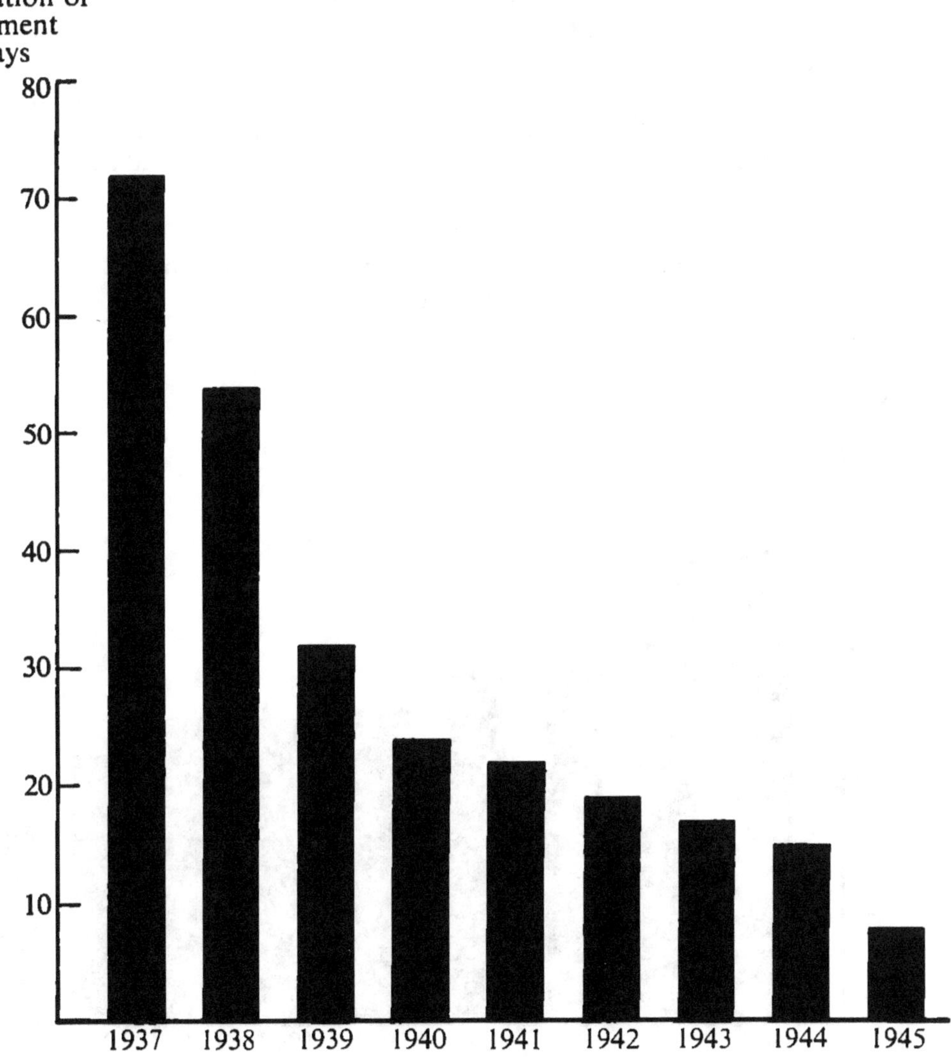

home, the incidence of gonorrhoea rose but slightly between the years 1939–43 but thereafter showed a marked increase. Overseas the incidence was always considerably higher than at home. The highest rate was in the small force overseas in 1939 when many men were serving in France. The lowest rate in the overseas forces was in 1941 when a large part of the force was in the Western Desert and opportunities for contracting venereal disease were limited. Thereafter there was a steady increase in incidence.

Venereal disease incidence is always higher abroad than at home and several factors play a part in this difference; the greater opportunities for sexual intercourse, the high rate of infection of the local populations, the absence of home moral ties, separation from family and the knowledge that diagnosis and treatment can easily be concealed from families at home.

The most dramatic fact about gonorrhoea was the reduction in the average duration of treatment of each case (Chart 4(a)). In 1937 this was 74 days for the R.A.F. as a whole. By 1943 with the rapid advances

CHART 4(b)

R.A.F. SYPHILIS—AVERAGE DURATION OF TREATMENT IN DAYS, 1937–45

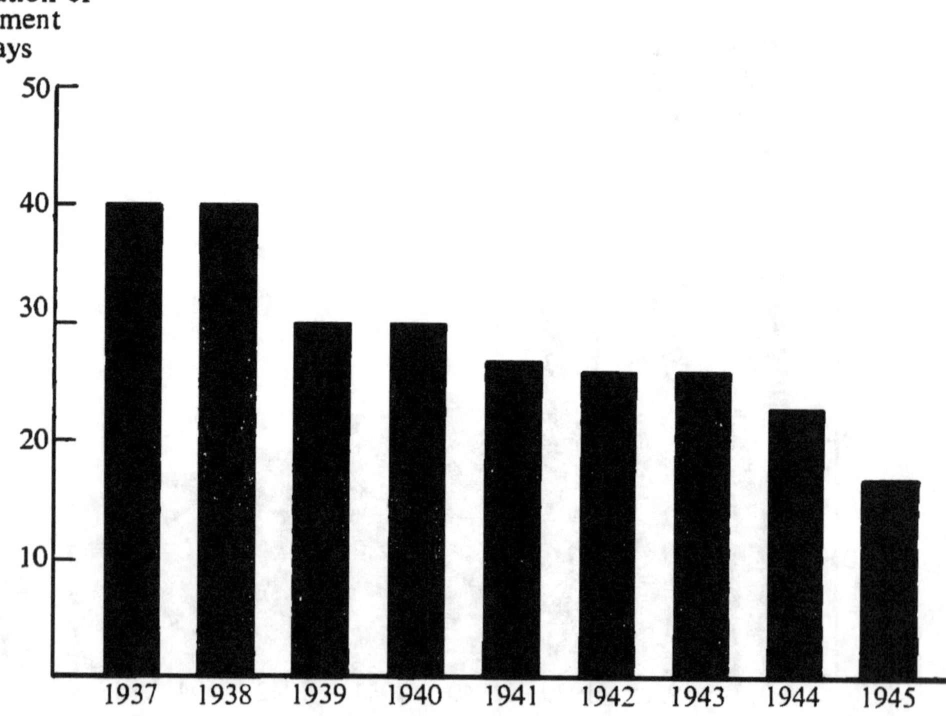

in the use of sulpha drugs in the treatment of gonorrhoea this figure dropped to 18 days. With the advent of penicillin the average duration of treatment was further reduced to 16 days in 1944 and 10 days in 1945.

Syphilis

Syphilis showed the same general trend in incidence as gonorrhoea—at home, a slowly increasing incidence up to 1943 and then a more rapid jump. Overseas the incidence was always higher than at home, with the lowest rate in 1941. The average duration of treatment is shown in Chart 4(b).

ALIMENTARY SYSTEM DISEASES

Diseases of the alimentary system showed a marked increase in incidence from 30 per 1,000 of strength in 1939 to 61 per 1,000 in 1944. This compares with an incidence of 27 per 1,000 in the five years before the war. The group 'other intestinal conditions' is mainly responsible for this increase. This miscellaneous group includes colitis in its various forms, diverticulosis and diverticulitis, the non-specific diarrhoeas and intestinal obstruction. The increase in incidence occurred mainly in the force abroad in the years 1943–45 but was also noticeable in the home force.

Peptic ulceration

In the civilian population of this country it has been estimated that some ten per cent. of the male population suffer or have suffered from peptic ulcers; of these, however, comparatively few appear to be chronic invalids and most manage to carry on, many probably settling into sheltered occupations. It was generally agreed before the war that peptic ulceration was a bar to service in the Armed Forces and most cases of proved ulceration were invalided. During the war this policy was modified and a larger proportion of cases returned to duty. This proportion was largest in the R.A.F., for two reasons; firstly, because the proportion of skilled technicians is high and every attempt was made to keep these valuable men; secondly, because the possibility of placing these men in sheltered appointments and even allowing them to live in their own homes was greater in the R.A.F. than in the other Services.

Peptic ulceration was not a major problem in aircrew before the war because of the care with which they were selected. A history suggestive of peptic ulceration or of recurring indigestion was a cause of rejection of candidates for flying duties.

Before the war the invaliding rate for peptic ulceration in the R.A.F. was just over 3 per cent. of those discharged for all diseases. By 1943 this figure had risen to 17 per cent.

The return to duty of pilots who have had peptic ulceration is gradual and many months with complete freedom from symptoms must elapse before a full flying category can be regained. Before the war, after a full course of treatment and convalescence, the patient was kept on ground duty, usually for nine months. After this period, which was nearly a year from the original illness, limited flying was allowed, the limitations usually being for height and duration of flight. A ceiling of 8,000 feet and flights of not more than two hours' duration were the limitations usually imposed. A full flying category was allowed after a further 6–12 months. During the war these periods were often cut down but in every case a gradual return to flying duty was recommended.

A survey was made in 1943 of the prognosis of cases of peptic ulcer returned to duty in the R.A.F. (Air Cdre. Rook, *Lancet*, June 12, 1943). Included in the survey were 26 members of aircrew. After roughly two years about half of them had returned to some form of flying duty, nine of them having regained full flying category. One of these was an officer whose gastric ulcer had perforated while he was flying alone; he managed to land safely and, after treatment, returned to flying duties.

There were 17,775 cases of peptic ulceration and their complications admitted during the war period, 1939–45. It is simpler to discuss these conditions as a whole under the heading 'peptic ulcers and their complications' than to discuss gastric ulcers and duodenal ulcers separately. Of these cases, 128 died and 9,279 were invalided from the Service. The average incidence over the period was 4 per 1,000 of strength per annum and the incidence rose steadily from 2·8 per 1,000 in 1939 to 4·4 per 1,000 in 1945. The average number of persons under treatment each day during the whole period was 265 with the peaks at 36 in 1939 and 404 in 1944. The average number of days under treatment was 34 so that the total man-power lost during the period was 692,988 days. This figure takes no account of the number of days off duty for sick leave or convalescence.

No valid comparison can be made between the incidence at home and abroad as personnel with a history of gastric symptoms would be unlikely to be posted abroad.

Duodenitis

This was a diagnosis based on radiological findings. It was chiefly an irregularity of the rugae and spasm without a detectable ulcerative lesion.

CIRCULATORY SYSTEM DISEASES

Heart disease is a much smaller problem in Service medicine than in civilian practice because of the selection of fit people from a limited age group. Inevitably, some case of congenital and rheumatic heart disease are missed at the initial medical boards but the numbers are never large. Degenerative vascular disease is also comparatively infrequent.

In the light of the experience of the First World War extensive preparations had been made to receive cases of disordered action of the heart and the relatively small numbers encountered came as a surprise. In 1944, the peak year, there were 765 cases of a total strength of over a million. It is probable that very much less overt attention was paid to the cardiac manifestations of psychoneurosis in 1939–45 than in 1914–18 and this avoided the development of cardiac fixations. Symptoms such as headache, depression and amnesia became more common. A rough estimation has shown that for the Services as a whole casualties from cardio-vascular causes, organic and functional, in the Second World War were approximately one-fiftieth of the numbers in the War of 1914–18.

DISEASES OF BLOOD VESSELS

Two important but quite unrelated conditions *viz.* hypertension and varicose veins, have unfortunately been classified under this heading and account for the vast majority of cases of diseases of the circulatory system. There was a progressive rise in incidence during the war years and in 1945 the incidence reached 5 per 1,000 of strength.

RESPIRATORY SYSTEM DISEASES

This group does not include pulmonary tuberculosis, the pneumonias or bronchial asthma. Diseases of the lung refer to such conditions as lung abscess, pulmonary collapse, emphysema, pulmonary embolus, pneumokoniosis, etc. Diseases of the pleura include all forms of pleurisy, pleural effusion and empyema and also pneumothorax and haemothorax.

The incidence of respiratory system diseases for the total force rose gradually to a peak in 1944, when there were 25 cases per 1,000 in the force at home and 18 per 1,000 abroad. In 1939 the incidence in the force abroad was 23 per 1,000 but this was out of a relatively small number of just over fifteen thousand personnel, many of whom had to live through the very severe winter in France.

A large proportion of diseases of the respiratory system is accounted for by bronchitis. The increase in the incidence of bronchitis is paralleled by the increase in the incidence of pneumonia. The unsuitability of the chronic bronchitic for service in tropical climates was often demonstrated during the war. Eventually such cases nearly always break down even if free of symptoms for a long period.

All cases of pleural effusion have been placed in this group without regard to aetiology. It is certain that many of these later proved to be due to pulmonary tuberculosis.

DISEASES OF ALLERGY

Bronchial asthma never proved a serious problem and the annual incidence never rose above 2 per 1,000 of strength. The incidence was rather higher at home than abroad. Urticaria, in common with other skin affections, was commoner abroad.

URINARY SYSTEM DISEASES

The classification 'Anomalies of urinary secretion' refers to conditions such as albuminuria, haematuria, glycosuria, etc. in which abnormal constituents are found in the urine. Uraemia is classified under nephritis. Kidney diseases distinct from the nephritic group include hydronephrosis, perinephric abscess, pyelitis and amyloid disease.

The investigation of symptomless cases of albuminuria, particularly in selection for aircrew, involved a considerable amount of wasted time. Often in the early years of the war men were admitted to hospital and submitted to a series of unnecessary and time-consuming investigations when simple tests as out-patients for orthostatic albuminuria would have proved sufficient.

Nephritis was uncommon and no particular correlation with streptococcal infection can be recorded.

Urinary calculi and urinary colic were more common in those serving abroad. Relative dehydration from excessive sweating in hot climates and often a diminished fluid intake were probably the chief factors in this higher incidence. Renal complications of the less soluble sulphonamides were occasionally seen when these drugs were first introduced.

GENERATIVE SYSTEM DISEASES

Urethritis in the War of 1939–45 presented a considerable problem in the number of cases that were frequently called non-venereal but were more correctly non-gonococcal. These are included here. Clinically these cases ranged from a mild anterior urethritis to severe purulent infections often involving the posterior urethra and prostate. Pathologically, the causes were believed to include ordinary mixed organisms such as staphylococci and streptococci, trichomonas infection, Ritter's syndrome and possibly pleuropneumonia organisms.

Diseases of the penis were more common abroad than at home. As in other skin diseases, service in the Tropics with excessive sweating and under poor hygienic conditions would lead one to expect an increased likelihood of balanitis.

LOCOMOTOR SYSTEM DISEASES

Diseases of muscles are an unimportant group and include myositis, dermatomyositis, the myopathies and myositis ossificans.

The diseases classified under the rheumatic group are fibrositis, myalgia, pleurodynia, lumbago, muscular rheumatism, torticollis and lumbosacral strain.

Deformities include malformations of the spinal column, deformities of feet and toes and conditions such as Dupuytren's contracture.

Diseases of joints include all forms of arthritis, acute and chronic, and prolapse of intervertebral discs.

Internal derangement of the knee joint refers only to tears of the menisci; this, however, caused a considerable wastage of man-power, chiefly due to the length of time spent in hospital or convalescent unit following meniscectomy. The injuries were normally contracted when playing football.

Articular rheumatism

The chronic 'rheumatic' diseases proved a steady form of wastage in the R.A.F. during the war as, indeed, they do in any medical practice nowadays. Acute varieties of articular rheumatism and rheumatoid arthritis were uncommon, but the vague categories of chronic rheumatic disorders had a high nuisance value. There were, of course, wide disparities in nomenclature, diagnosis and treatment and a detailed breakdown of the group would serve no useful purpose. The general opinion is that the precipitating factors were febrile illness, trauma and severe cold, but there is no doubt that the persistence of symptoms was often an expression of an underlying anxiety state. There existed a psychological problem very similar to that seen in peptic ulcer patients; physical examination was often not sufficient in doubtful cases and further investigation sometimes showed the patient's belief in the organic basis of his complaint to be unfounded.

NERVOUS SYSTEM AND MENTAL DISEASES

In the First World War all the emphasis was placed on physical fitness as the essential attribute of the pilot. Flack's tests and similar methods controlled the selection of candidates. Although the nature of fear and anxiety was recognised undue emphasis was placed on material factors; it was always regarded as important to discover an organic cause and such unfortunate terms as 'shell shock' and 'disordered action of the heart' were coined. In the period between the wars we had begun to learn the lesson that too much stress was being laid on physical efficiency and not enough on the psychological aspect. It is incredible what disabilities a man can overcome if he has the right temperament for a war pilot; men have flown while undergoing treatment with artificial pneumothorax or after thoracoplasty. At the same time there are many apparently fit men who have been quite unable to stand up to the strain of flying.

Psychoneuroses ranged from cases of severe depressive states admitted to hospital to those with milder anxiety states and the psychosomatic group with peptic ulcers, low back pain or asthma. Headaches and 'blackouts' were also common. Psychoneurosis which could be attributed to fear and flying stress was found among aircrew and the incidence was, not surprisingly, greatest among the operational commands. It was highest in night bombers and lowest in Flying Training Command; emotional tension proved more important than physical fatigue. (*See R.A.F. Medical Services* Vol. II, pp. 122–36 and *Medicine and Pathology* Chapter XV.) But the number of psychoneuroses which could be directly attributed to combatant conditions or fear was small and there was no significant difference in total incidence of psychoneuroses between aircrew and ground personnel. The precipitating cause was obvious enough—the dislocation of normal life, separation from wife and family, Service discipline and the learning of new occupations. Many of the men had long histories of previous instability but did not break down until removed from the shelter and seclusion of home life.

The incidence of psychoses showed little significant change from year to year. Although the onset in a number of cases was accelerated by war conditions the true causes were found in the patients' past histories.

The incidence of psychopathic personalities showed a progressive rise during the war years, presumably correlated with the urgent need for expansion and the consequent less strict selection of recruits. The heading includes emotional instability, immature personality and psychological inferiority as well as the more obvious behaviour disorders.

Nervous system diseases of indefinite aetiology included airsickness, headache, migraine, enuresis, tic and vertigo.

In their investigations into *Psychological Disorders in Flying Personnel of the R.A.F.* (H.M.S.O. 1947) Air Vice Marshal Sir Charles Symonds and Wing Commander Denis Williams included an investigation of the Psychological Aspects of Airsickness. Their broad general conclusion was as follows:

> 'When a man is suspended for airsickness at any stage of training the cause is usually motion sickness uncomplicated by psychological factors. Psychological factors—either neurosis, neurotic predisposition or faulty morale—may contribute by lowering the physiological threshold for tolerance of motion or by reducing a man's ability or

willingness to endure symptoms, but psychological abnormality may co-exist with airsickness without contributing to it. As a cause of suspension for airsickness psychological factors are seldom of major importance. Psychological factors are never the direct cause of true airsickness which should be clearly distinguished from visceral reactions to anxiety occurring in the air.'*

ORGANIC NERVOUS DISEASES

As would be expected there is little variation in the incidence from year to year.

The heading 'indefinite organic diseases' includes disseminated sclerosis, the muscular dystrophies, myasthenia gravis and Parkinson's disease.

EYE DISEASES

Inflammatory conditions of the eye were more common abroad than at home. Conjunctivitis was sometimes apparently due to non-specific causes and was not uncommon in the desert, owing largely to exposure to sun, wind and sand. In the humid climates of the Far East much of the conjunctival trouble was due to sweat, dirt and dandruff.

EAR DISEASES (*See* Section on Oto-Rhino-Laryngology in the 'Surgery' volume in this series)

Chronic suppurative otitis media constituted the chief cause of aural morbidity. In the majority of cases the condition was present prior to entry into the R.A.F. and very often little or no comment on the aural condition was made by the National Service Medical Boards. Personnel already in the Service and trained or partly trained were treated on conservative lines and kept under close specialist supervision. These men were a liability when sent overseas and although efforts were made to grade them for home service only many were still posted to Commands abroad.† Untrained men were usually invalided. Flying personnel with active C.S.O.M. were taken off flying. Following treatment they were allowed to fly in a non-operational capacity as long as the condition remained inactive.

Otitis externa was more common overseas than at home. In the Middle East irritation by wind and sand was a potent cause. In the Far East otitis externa or 'tropical ear' was a considerable problem and often proved intractable to treatment.

* *See* also *R.A.F. Medical Services* Vol. II, pp. 120–22.

† It was considered by many medical officers that such men should have been debarred from serving even in certain United Kingdom Units, where conditions aggravated their complaint. (*See*, for example, the section on the Outer Hebrides, in the *R.A.F. Medical Services* Vol. II, p. 240.)

Surprisingly few ear injuries resulted from non-fatal flying accidents.

Otitic barotrauma was an important cause of non-effectiveness among flying personnel. This is the syndrome resulting from inability to adjust intratympanic pressure on descent from higher altitudes. The outstanding contributory factor was found to be an upper respiratory infection giving rise to Eustachian tube insufficiency. The condition was responsible for loss of 'man-flying hours', recategorisation, limitation in flying category and often cessation of flying.

SKIN DISEASES

Statistics for cases of skin diseases requiring admission for 48 hours or more do not give a true picture of the incidence of these conditions. Most cases of skin diseases are treated as out-patients and only a few of the more serious call for admission.

Scabies was the most common skin disease and rose to an incidence of 11 per 1,000 of strength in 1941–42. In 1943 there was a considerable fall in incidence to 5 per 1,000 and in 1945 the incidence was only 2 per 1,000. The incidence was higher abroad than at home. Treatment with benzyl benzoate came into general use in 1942 and this probably accounted for the fall in incidence; treatment with sulphur had been attended by a high rate of relapse and complications. It is interesting to note that scabies had shown a progressive rise in incidence in the pre-war years:*

	1935	1936	1937	1938	1939†	1940
Scabies	1·1	2·0	2·8	3·0	4·2	6·5
Impetigo	4·4	4·8	5·1	5·3	5·2	4·0
Tinea, all types	4·4	5·5	7·4	3·9	2·5	1·8

(Incidences are shown as rates per 1,000 of strength.)

In warm climates echthymatous sores were a constant source of trouble and caused a serious loss of efficiency. They were variously described—desert sores in the Middle East, jungle sores in the Far East. The aetiological factor appeared to be loss of resistance of skin devitalised by exposure to sun, wind and dust, frequently coupled with inadequate ablution facilities.

Tinea and other fungus infections were very common in tropical countries due to excessive sweating and irritation by clothing. There was a great tendency to diagnose tinea without adequate proof, clinical or

* *See* also *R.A.F. Medical Services* Vol. II, p. 580, 'Free from Infection Inspections'.

† These figures, of course, do not coincide with those shown in Table 3(a) which refer only to the one period rather than the complete year.

microscopical, and many harmless skin conditions were converted into chemical dermatoses by over-enthusiastic fungicidal therapy.

Pediculosis was never very prevalent in the R.A.F. during the war. The conditions which made infestation almost universal in the trenches in the First World War rarely occurred in the War of 1939–45.

Impetigo was another serious form of wastage, particularly overseas. It is a disease which often occurs in epidemic forms in communities of men living together.

Seborrhoeic dermatitis is a common and troublesome condition in war-time. Nervous and anxiety states, limitation of protein and protective foods and restricted facilities for personal hygiene are the aggravating factors.

TABLE 5. *R.A.F. Venereal Disease, 1921–45*

Year	Total Force				Home				Abroad			
	Number of cases	Incidence of cases per 1,000 of strength	Averages		Number of cases	Incidence of cases per 1,000 of strength	Averages		Number of cases	Incidence of cases per 1,000 of strength	Averages	
			Number sick daily	Number of days treatment before return to duty			Number sick daily	Number of days treatment before return to duty			Number sick daily	Number of days treatment before return to duty
1945	21,456	23·0	562·2	9	11,920	18·6	290·0	10	9,536	32·4	272·2	9
1944	18,676	18·6	807·9	16	7,105	10·4	249·2	12	11,571	36·3	558·7	18
1943	11,264	11·6	565·9	18	4,680	7·1	186·3	14	6,884	21·3	379·6	21
1942	8,763	10·2	476·0	20	4,626	7·0	221·9	18	4,137	20·4	254·1	23
1941	5,556	8·4	336·5	22	4,038	6·9	237·9	21	1,518	19·5	98·6	23
1940	2,637	8·1	174·1	24	1,786	6·1	112·9	23	851	26·8	61·2	26
1939	1,300	9·2	110·4	31	685	5·5	58·5	31	615	35·3	51·9	31
1938	629	8·3	84·1	49	338	5·3	45·4	49	291	24·5	38·6	48
1937	548	9·2	96·5	64	294	6·0	54·5	68	254	24·1	42·0	60
1936	435	9·0	74·5	63	183	5·1	32·5	65	252	21·0	42·0	61
1935	333	9·5	59·7	65	141	5·6	25·2	65	192	19·5	34·5	66
1934	303	9·9	53·5	65	141	6·6	22·8	59	162	17·6	30·7	69
1933	355	11·5	57·0	59	158	7·2	27·2	63	197	21·9	29·8	53
1932	360	11·3	59·9	61	169	7·3	28·7	62	191	21·6	31·2	60
1931	476	14·7	76·7	59	245	10·4	42·0	63	231	25·8	34·7	55
1930	517	16·1	80·6	57	293	12·7	50·6	63	224	25·4	30·2	49
1929	466	15·0	70·7	55	250	11·0	37·8	55	216	25·5	32·9	56
1928	556	18·2	79·0	52	302	13·5	44·6	54	254	31·3	34·4	50
1927	528	17·5	72·4	50	269	12·5	40·8	55	259	30·1	31·6	45
1926	565	17·1	91·3	59	357	14·9	59·5	61	208	23·0	31·8	56
1925	656	19·9	93·4	52	400	16·8	57·0	52	256	27·9	36·4	52
1924	704	22·3	103·3	54	432	19·2	59·3	50	272	30·0	44·0	59
1923	781	26·2	107·2	50	482	23·8	64·8	49	299	31·4	42·3	52
1922	788	27·2	110·5	51	525	24·9	76·1	53	263	33·5	34·4	48
1921	1,023	36·1	146·4	52	709	32·3	94·2	48	314	49·2	52·2	61

CERTAIN INFECTIOUS DISEASES IN THE TOTAL FORCE, 1939–45

Table 6 shows the incidence per 1,000 of strength of the more important infectious diseases other than the tropical diseases.

TABLE 6

R.A.F. Certain Infectious Diseases in the Total Force, 1939–45

DISEASES	Incidence per 1,000 of strength							
	1939	1940	1941	1942	1943	1944	1945	5 years average 1940–44
Acute anterior poliomyelitis	0·1	0·1	0·05	0·08	0·2	0·3	0·1	0·1
Acute rheumatism	2·3	2·1	1·6	1·2	0·8	1·2	0·5	1·4
Infective hepatitis (catarrhal jaundice)	1·5	1·2	2·4	5·1	11·6	12·1	7·0	6·5
Cerebro-spinal fever	0·1	1·1	0·7	0·3	0·2	0·2	0·1	0·5
Chicken-pox	1·0	0·9	0·9	0·8	0·9	1·3	0·8	1·0
Diphtheria	0·3	0·5	0·6	0·7	0·8	1·3	0·5	0·8
Encephalitis lethargica	0·03	0·03	0·02	0·02	0·006	0·05	0·002	0·03
German measles	13·7	20·6	3·1	1·8	1·8	4·2	0·6	6·3
Measles	1·8	2·1	1·7	0·7	1·1	0·6	0·5	0·2
Mumps	1·3	1·1	1·5	2·9	1·4	1·3	2·5	1·6
Scarlet Fever	2·3	2·2	1·1	1·0	1·8	1·8	0·4	1·6
Smallpox	Nil	0·01	0·01	0·02	0·07	0·2	0·09	0·06
Tetanus	0·01	Nil	0·005	0·005	Nil	Nil	Nil	0·002
Typhus	0·01	0·01	0·01	0·03	0·08	0·1	0·2	0·05

ACUTE ANTERIOR POLIOMYELITIS

This disease never proved a great problem in the R.A.F. during the war and there were only small epidemics.* The highest incidence was in 1944 when there were 0·3 cases per 1,000 of strength.

ACUTE RHEUMATISM

A study of Acute Rheumatic Fever in the R.A.F. in 1940 and 1941 has been published (Barber, H. S., 1946, *Brit. Med. J.* 2. 83). Rheumatic fever has for long shown a decline both in incidence and severity. The War of 1939–45 caused no increase in its incidence but it is still an important cause of morbidity in large communities of young adults. The disease is traditionally associated with exposure to damp and chill but when these conditions are met with in great severity in war-time they cause no noticeable increase in the incidence of the disease unless associated with upper respiratory infections. In the R.A.F. Apprentice Schools the condition has always been a source of anxiety and in 1940 the incidence among boy entrants and apprentices rose to over 10 cases per 1,000 of strength. This can be related to the epidemic of upper respiratory infections in the winter of 1940. The incidence in the total force in 1940 was 2·1 per 1,000 of strength, the highest recorded for the war period. (*See Medicine and Pathology* Chapter IV.)

* *See R.A.F. Medical Services* Vol. II, p. 320.

INFECTIVE HEPATITIS

This was of chief importance in the overseas theatres and is discussed in the narrative relating to Tables 7(a), (b), (c), (d)—'Diseases Caused by Infection in Certain Commands Abroad'.

CEREBRO-SPINAL FEVER

During the War of 1914–18 cerebro-spinal fever assumed epidemic proportions throughout the country but rapidly abated after the end of the war. Towards the end of 1939, with the concentrations of recruits, mass movement of population and the problems of overcrowding and poor ventilation, it was expected that similar or even greater outbreaks would occur. In 1940 there was, in fact, a severe epidemic in Great Britain and it appeared that the disease would be a major problem in subsequent years. But happily, although prevalence remained higher than in peace-time, there were no further serious outbreaks. The incidence in the R.A.F. in 1940 was 1·1 per 1,000 of strength. (*See Medicine and Pathology* Chapter VI.)

GERMAN MEASLES

The high incidence of rubella in 1940 corresponded with a nation-wide epidemic.

SCARLET FEVER

The Registrar General's report shows that for the country as a whole the incidence of scarlet fever declined in the period 1939–41; it then increased to epidemic proportions in 1943, with some regression in 1944. This experience was not paralleled in the R.A.F., where the highest incidence was 2·2 per 1,000 of strength in 1940. There was a fall in incidence in 1941 and 1942, but a further rise in 1943 and 1944.

SMALLPOX

There were only 27 cases of smallpox in the United Kingdom during the war and all R.A.F. cases occurred abroad. The highest incidence was in 1944 when there were 0·2 cases per 1,000 of strength. Most cases occurred in India where, in certain areas such as Bengal, the disease is endemic.

MEASLES

There was a severe epidemic in the United Kingdom during 1940 and 1941, followed by a decline in 1942 and a recrudescence in 1943. A similar trend is observed in the R.A.F. figures.

TYPHUS

There was a severe outbreak of epidemic louse-borne typhus fever in Egypt in 1942 among the civilian population. About 22,000 cases with some 5,000 deaths were recorded but this certainly does not represent the true extent of the epidemic. Only seven cases with three deaths occurred among R.A.F. personnel.

DISEASES CAUSED BY INFECTION IN CERTAIN COMMANDS ABROAD, 1939–45

The principal diseases caused by infection in certain Commands abroad are recorded in Tables 7(a), (b), (c) and (d). The Commands are India and A.C.S.E.A. (Air Command South-East Asia, formed in 1943), Middle East, Iraq and West Africa. Diseases in other important areas overseas, such as South Africa and Canada, have not been analysed as conditions there more closely resembled those at home.

AMOEBIC DYSENTERY

Amoebic dysentery is endemic in many tropical and sub-tropical countries and is especially common in districts where sanitation is deficient. Its control is essentially one of efficient hygienic measures. Epidemics of the disease have occurred, notably in the British Army in Gallipoli in 1915.

There were 870 cases of amoebic dysentery recorded for the force at home during the war years, and it may be assumed that many of these infections were contracted during service abroad, but it is of interest to note that a small epidemic of amoebic dysentery has been recorded in an R.A.F. station in this country since the war, many of the victims never having served abroad.*

Altogether, over 10,000 cases of amoebic dysentery were recorded in the total force and as the disease often runs a protracted course this represented a very considerable wastage. In 1943, for instance, the average period of treatment before return to duty was 36 days. In 1944 there was an incidence of 13 per 1,000 of strength in the force abroad. The R.A.F. in India and South-East Asia suffered most heavily, and there the incidence rose steeply to 36 per 1,000 in 1944. The year 1944 was also the peak year in Iraq (25 per 1,000) and in the Middle East (8 per 1,000). 1945 saw a considerable fall in incidence in all three Commands.

BACILLARY DYSENTERY

Bacillary dysentery has always been a common cause of wastage in armies in the field. Out of 30,000 British soldiers who fought in the Crimea 7,883 suffered from dysentery and of these 2,143 died. In the South African War there were 38,108 cases with 1,342 deaths. In the R.A.F. in the Second World War improved hygienic measures and the discovery that sulphonamide drugs have a marked action on dysentery bacilli made it possible to avert major outbreaks of the disease and to bring about rapid cure of most cases which came under early treatment.

* *See B.M.J.*, 19th July, 1952, p. 114–16. *Indigenous Amoebiasis, a Recent Outbreak in England* by Morton, T. C., Stamm, W. P. and Seidelin, R.

There were nearly 32,000 cases altogether but the mortality was very low.

A distinction is made in Table 7(a), (b), (c) and (d), between cases where the Shigella organism had been isolated from the faeces and cases which were diagnosed on clinical grounds alone. The ease of treatment with sulphaguanidine enabled medical officers to treat dysentery without the necessity for pathological investigation of the faeces. Indeed, very many mild cases treated early must have gone unrecorded. It is safe to say that the diagnosis was less frequently made and less regularly controlled by laboratory studies than in the First World War. This was largely due to the necessity for treating operational personnel in forward areas immediately and the almost invariable lack of microscopes to examine faeces.

In the R.A.F. at home there were sporadic outbreaks of a minor nature but the fact that only 1,764 cases were recorded for the war period is a tribute to the standard of hygiene. Abroad, where hygienic control was so much more difficult and where the disease is so widespread among the local populations, bacillary dysentery presented a serious problem.* The R.A.F. in India and South-East Asia suffered heavily and in 1942 the incidence rose to 53 per 1,000 of strength. There was a fall in 1943 to 40 per 1,000 but again in 1944 a rise to 53 per 1,000. Sulphaguanidine first began to be used in 1942 and this probably explains the decreased incidence in 1943. 1944 saw a considerable expansion in the Far East Air Force and many units had to live under unsatisfactory sanitary conditions in forward areas.

In the Middle East the incidence rose sharply to a peak of 44 per 1,000 in 1941 but had fallen to 27 per 1,000 in 1943. In 1944 there was a slight rise to 33 per 1,000 but 1945 saw a big drop to 12 per 1,000.

ENTERIC FEVERS

Prophylactic inoculation and improved standards of hygiene have greatly reduced the importance of typhoid and paratyphoid fevers. In the R.A.F. there were only 1,845 cases during the Second World War and this provides a remarkable contrast to the British Army in the South African War when there were 57,684 cases with 8,022 deaths.

The majority of cases occurred abroad and there were only 136 at home. A few outbreaks occurred in India in units close to villages where typhoid was endemic. Isolated cases were contracted by drinking water from unauthorised supplies and by eating in local cafés.

ENTERITIS

This term was used to cover a wide variety of acute episodes of diarrhoea and vomiting and such conditions as 'Gippy tummy'. Isolated

* *See R.A.F. Medical Services* Vol. III, pp. 100, 104, 666–68.

attacks of gastro-enteritis accompanied by profuse diarrhoea with passing of blood and mucus, lasting 24–48 hours, often occurred in the desert. Such attacks were considered inevitable among new arrivals. In many cases the attacks had little effect on general well-being but in others there was marked prostration.

At home the highest incidences were in 1940 and 1941 at 6 per 1,000 of strength, while after 1942 the incidence was always less than 1 per 1,000. Abroad the incidence was high from 1939–42 and then fell sharply for the remaining years. It is possible that the introduction of sulphaguanidine accounts for this fall in incidence in 1943; many mild cases of enteritis previously requiring admission would be effectively treated with sulphaguanidine. This enormous drop in incidence is reflected in the figures for the four Commands overseas.

MALARIA*

Owing to its world-wide distribution and endemicity in most warm countries malaria is the most common of human diseases in peace and war. The clinical effect of malaria in war-time is no more severe than in peace-time and no new aetiological factor is introduced, but various factors tend to increase the morbidity from the disease. The introduction of large numbers of non-immunes into endemic areas frequently gives rise to serious epidemics. Personal protection and preventive measures are often difficult in the mobile conditions of war. Air transport and the movement of large bodies of men may introduce malaria into previously non-malarious areas.

In the War of 1914–18 of all the diseases responsible for non-effectiveness malaria easily took first place. In the British Army alone the admissions to hospital for malaria were almost half a million. Although a greater measure of control was possible in the R.A.F. during the Second World War there was still a total of nearly 75,000 cases. In India and the Far East in 1944 malaria accounted for 17 per cent. of all diseases, in the Middle East in 1940 for 10 per cent. of all diseases and in West Africa in 1942 for 55 per cent. of all diseases. Much of this wastage was preventable and was due in no small measure to the failure of the executive in the early stages of the war to realise that malaria discipline required their active co-operation. It was often difficult for the R.A.F. to select camp sites of low malaria risk because the primary consideration was to find a level stretch of ground for a landing strip and the best of such sites were often in low lying, marshy districts. In many instances dress discipline was poor, officers and men bathed after dusk and failed to carry out other precautions such as the use of repellents and mosquito nets. Prophylactic mepacrine was often not taken consistently. The work of malaria control squads was not

* *See R.A.F. Medical Services* Vol. III, Chaps. 7 and 11.

regarded with the importance which it should have been accorded and men of low grade and poor intelligence were usually assigned to such work. Eventually, malaria control was made the direct responsibility of the unit commander and the considerable fall in incidence in 1945 was due to the subsequent close attention to every detail of malaria control.

The use of mepacrine was one of the greatest steps forward during the war. It permitted campaigns to be fought and won which could not have been fought successfully without it and malaria came to be regarded in forward areas as less of a major hazard.

At home 5,077 cases of malaria were recorded but these refer to men who contracted their infections, primary or recurrent, when serving abroad.

For the force overseas as a whole the worst years were 1943 (76 per 1,000) and 1944 (75 per 1,000). There was a considerable fall in 1945 to 31 per 1,000. In India and South-East Asia the peak was in 1944 with 157 per 1,000, in the Middle East in 1940 and 1941 with 60 cases per 1,000 and in Iraq in 1944 with 83 per 1,000. In West Africa in 1942 there was an incidence of 844 cases per 1,000 of strength in a force just over 5,000 strong.

In the Far East benign tertian malaria was consistently more common than malignant tertian malaria whereas in the Middle East in 1940 and 1941 the malignant form was the commoner of the two.

In the later years in the Middle East benign tertian malaria showed a slightly higher incidence. *P. falciparum*, the parasite of malignant tertian malaria, is confined to the warmer regions of the earth and is found especially in the hot, dry desert countries with a limited water supply. In North Africa it was the commonest form encountered. In West Africa the infections were predominantly malignant tertian. Quartan malaria, as has always been the experience, was rare in all commands.

INFECTIVE HEPATITIS

Epidemics of jaundice have occurred in every war but it is impossible to decide whether the epidemics in earlier compaigns were due to infective hepatitis, Weil's disease or other factors. Many of the cases of jaundice which occurred in the armies in France and Flanders in the War of 1914–18 were due to Weil's disease but there was no epidemic of this disease during 1939–1945. Infective hepatitis reached epidemic proportions in some units of the British Army in the Middle East during the War of 1914–18. During the Second World War infective hepatitis became extremely widespread among forces in the Mediterranean region and caused an enormous wastage of man-power. In the Northern Hemisphere epidemics start in the late summer, reach their peak in mid-winter and die down in the spring. This seasonal swing was seen in the Mediterranean where there were four large epidemics—two in the Middle East Forces at the end of 1942 and 1943 and two in the Central Mediterranean Forces at the end of 1943 and 1944. In India the seasonal incidence appears to vary on the two sides of the country in keeping with the monsoons.

The Army experienced its heaviest outbreaks in the Mediterranean region and there particularly among the front line troops. Although the R.A.F. experienced a high incidence in the Middle East the rate was actually higher in India and the Far East. Both areas had peak incidences in 1944 when there were 44 cases per 1,000 of strength in the Far East and 35 cases per 1,000 of strength in the Middle East. Iraq shows a parallel rate with the highest incidence in 1944. In West Africa the highest rate was 35 per 1,000 in 1943. (*See Medicine and Pathology* Chapter IX and Appendix p. 267 and *R.A.F. Medical Services* Vol. III, pp. 101, 127, 134, 190, 285, 425, 509, 680.)

PHLEBOTOMUS FEVER

Phlebotomus fever or Sandfly fever is widely distributed in Africa and Asia and in the Tropics it may break out at any time as an epidemic among new arrivals; in the sub-tropics it occurs principally during the summer and early autumn. Natives of endemic areas appear to be immune.

In the Far East Forces the highest incidence was in the early years of the war and there was a notable falling off in later years. The force in Iraq suffered heavily and in 1941 the incidence there was 317 per 1,000 of strength. Here, too, there was a fall in incidence in the later years of the war and in 1944 there were 42 cases per 1,000.

UPPER RESPIRATORY TRACT INFECTIONS AND INFLUENZA

Upper respiratory tract infections were no less important abroad than at home and even in tropical areas a consistently high sickness rate was recorded.

TABLE 7(a)

R.A.F. Diseases Caused by Infection, India and A.C.S.E.A., 1939–45*
Incidence per 1,000 per annum

	1939	1940	1941	1942	1943	1944	1945
DISEASES							
Dysentery:							
Clinical primary	3·0	6·3	15·6	23·8	14·30	16·63	15·69
Bacillary primary	9·6	10·6	18·3	29·2	25·45	36·60	29·97
Amoebic primary	0·5	1·6	2·4	17·1	23·62	35·58	17·94
Recurrent	—	0·5	0·7	1·1	0·51	0·97	0·41
Totals	13·1	19·0	37·0	71·2	63·88	89·78	64·00
Enteric group:							
Typhoid fever	1·0	0·5	—	1·5	0·92	1·59	0·86
Paratyphoid (A. B. and C.)	—	0·5	—	0·4	0·14	0·54	0·17
Clinical enteric	0·5	—	—	1·3	1·00	1·10	0·35
Totals	1·5	1·0	—	3·2	2·07	3·23	1·38
Enteritis	23·7	38·1	57·9	30·7	1·89	3·11	5·52
Malaria:							
Clinical	5·0	4·2	3·0	23·1	20·78	19·64	7·25
Quartan	—	0·5	0·3	0·7	0·36	0·11	0·08
Benign tertian	26·3	21·1	21·7	53·1	61·14	74·90	18·95
Malignant tertian	4·0	6·9	6·4	33·2	25·68	30·37	7·77
Recurrent	4·0	13·3	2·4	8·6	26·45	30·37	4·97
Blanket treatment	—	—	—	—	—	1·72	1·18
Totals	39·3	46·0	33·8	118·7	134·41	157·11	40·20
Infective hepatitis (catarrhal jaundice)	—	—	—	23·2	32·10	44·14	19·67
Pyrexia of uncertain origin	—	1·6	3·4	6·0	5·24	4·93	8·04
Phlebotomus fever	28·3	40·7	44·0	21·9	10·26	10·51	5·44
Influenza	—	14·3	8·5	16·6	6·40	4·83	1·73
Upper respiratory tract infections	67·5	72·5	72·2	80·5	77·04	102·88	68·43
Tuberculosis, all types	2·5	1·6	1·4	2·2	1·75	1·74	2·42
Venereal diseases	15·2	16·4	18·6	36·0	31·70	38·34	32·19
Other infections	11·6	30·7	27·1	94·5	56·97	69·83	38·50
All diseases caused by infection and pyrexia of uncertain origin	202·7	281·9	303·9	504·7	423·71	530·43	287·52
All other diseases and unclassified conditions	202·2	205·1	212·0	351·7	314·55	407·46	322·29
Totals of all diseases	404·9	487·0	515·9	856·4	738·26	937·89	609·81
INJURIES							
General injuries	8·6	8·5	7·8	12·9	14·04	24·01	19·35
Local injuries	58·5	56·9	48·1	38·6	28·54	38·19	34·18
Totals of all injuries	67·1	65·4	55·9	51·5	42·58	62·20	53·53
Totals of all diseases and injuries	472·0	552·4	571·8	907·9	780·84	1,000·09	663·34

* A.C.S.E.A. was formed in November 1943.

TABLE 7(b)

R.A.F. Diseases Caused by Infection, Middle East, 1939–45
Incidence per 1,000 per annum

	1939	1940	1941	1942	1943	1944	1945
DISEASES							
Dysentery:							
Clinical primary	1·3	5·1	17·5	14·9	6·62	7·54	3·20
Bacillary primary	4·7	11·6	26·2	22·7	20·49	25·34	9·04
Amoebic primary	—	1·0	2·4	2·8	5·23	8·43	2·55
Recurrent	—	0·1	0·3	0·5	0·12	0·14	0·14
Totals	6·0	17·8	46·4	40·9	32·46	41·45	14·93
Enteric group:							
Typhoid fever	0·2	0·1	1·4	1·6	1·23	1·94	1·99
Paratyphoid (A. B. and C.)	0·2	—	0·4	0·2	0·40	0·85	0·14
Clinical enteric	0·5	0·3	0·3	0·3	0·43	0·85	0·97
Totals	0·9	0·4	2·1	2·1	2·06	3·64	3·10
Enteritis	39·4	50·4	69·8	26·2	6·28	7·97	5·15
Malaria:							
Clinical	2·5	16·8	13·8	6·3	6·76	4·98	1·81
Quartan	0·4	0·1	0·4	0·2	0·09	—	—
Benign tertian	14·2	15·6	13·3	20·4	17·86	15·38	5·29
Malignant tertian	3·5	17·6	26·9	9·1	16·11	11·70	4·59
Recurrent	2·1	10·1	6·0	1·5	6·23	9·11	2·24
Blanket treatment	—	—	—	—	—	—	0·55
Totals	22·7	60·2	60·4	37·5	47·05	41·17	14·48
Infective hepatitis (catarrhal jaundice)	—	5·5	16·2	22·1	24·94	34·88	11·30
Pyrexia of uncertain origin	3·9	8·4	8·7	4·9	15·61	22·07	20·17
Phlebotomus fever	20·5	24·6	48·9	42·2	29·07	28·04	9·18
Influenza	—	25·2	11·8	12·2	8·20	9·68	1·67
Upper respiratory tract infections	100·1	95·4	96·8	85·5	85·73	107·19	67·76
Tuberculosis, all types	1·1	1·1	1·1	1·8	3·28	3·00	1·84
Venereal diseases	31·0	26·3	21·3	13·8	12·31	22·99	18·94
Other infections	7·6	27·6	35·4	17·7	20·52	31·55	13·24
All diseases caused by infection and pyrexia of uncertain origin	233·2	342·9	418·9	306·9	287·51	353·63	181·76
All other diseases and unclassified conditions	246·5	256·1	278·5	266·3	277·78	328·00	209·01
Totals of all diseases	479·7	599·0	697·4	573·2	565·29	681·63	390·77
INJURIES							
General injuries	6·4	29·0	34·6	25·7	28·37	28·38	16·12
Local injuries	54·9	51·5	48·0	40·9	37·14	55·79	29·04
Totals of all injuries	61·3	80·6	82·6	66·6	65·51	84·17	45·16
Totals of all diseases and injuries	541·0	679·6	780·0	639·8	630·80	765·80	435·93

TABLE 7(c)

R.A.F. Diseases caused by Infection, Iraq, 1939–45
Incidence per 1,000 per annum

	1939	1940	1941	1942	1943	1944	1945
DISEASES							
Dysentery:							
Clinical primary	—	0·5	3·6	20·4	17·56	24·93	36·88
Bacillary primary	1·4	2·0	3·0	34·1	24·90	47·09	52·24
Amoebic primary	1·0	4·0	0·9	6·1	8·90	24·93	6·15
Recurrent	—	—	—	0·5	0·72	—	—
Totals	2·4	6·5	7·5	61·1	52·08	96·96	95·27
Enteric group:							
Typhoid fever	1·9	—	0·3	1·2	0·48	—	—
Paratyphoid (A. B. and C.)	0·5	0·5	0·3	0·9	0·24	—	6·15
Clinical enteric	—	—	—	0·6	0·72	—	—
Totals	2·4	0·5	0·6	2·7	1·44	—	6·15
Enteritis	84·8	54·0	53·5	38·8	1·32	22·16	9·22
Malaria:							
Clinical	18·5	9·0	6·6	5·0	6·02	16·62	15·36
Quartan	—	—	—	0·3	0·12	—	—
Benign tertian	14·6	22·0	21·7	22·4	25·26	30·47	6·15
Malignant tertian	9·3	6·5	5·1	9·9	16·00	30·75	0·31
Recurrent	8·3	5·5	5·1	1·0	9·74	5·54	3·07
Blanket treatment	—	—	—	—	—	—	3·07
Totals	50·7	43·0	38·5	38·6	57·14	83·38	27·96
Infective hepatitis (catarrhal jaundice)	—	—	—	20·0	22·98	33·24	12·29
Pyrexia of uncertain origin	2·4	1·0	1·2	4·7	7·46	24·93	73·75
Phlebotomus fever	136·9	79·6	317·4	155·6	68·69	41·55	55·32
Influenza	—	—	1·5	1·6	1·92	2·77	6·15
Upper respiratory tract infections	103·3	67·1	83·3	106·4	105·86	146·82	156·73
Tuberculosis, all types	2·4	3·5	2·7	2·0	3·13	1·11	6·76
Venereal diseases	15·1	18·0	34·0	26·3	21·17	52·63	39·95
Other infections	14·1	18·5	23·8	19·2	23·46	38·78	36·88
All diseases caused by infection and pyrexia of uncertain origin	414·5	291·7	564·0	477·1	366·65	544·32	526·43
All other diseases and unclassified conditions	206·5	213·6	229·6	361·2	367·50	508·31	487·71
Totals of all diseases	621·0	505·3	793·6	838·3	734·15	1,052·63	1,014·14
INJURIES							
General injuries	9·7	5·5	22·3	9·0	15·40	30·75	16·59
Local injuries	50·2	36·5	49·0	32·7	35·73	58·45	43·33
Totals of all injuries	59·9	42·0	71·3	41·7	51·13	89·20	59·92
Totals of all diseases and injuries	680·9	547·3	864·9	880·0	785·28	1,141·83	1,074·06

TABLE 7(d)

R.A.F. Diseases Caused by Infection, West Africa, 1942–45
Incidence per 1,000 per annum

	1942	1943	1944	1945
DISEASES				
Dysentery:				
Clinical primary	28·5	10·68	1·21	1·95
Bacillary primary	32·7	28·25	21·83	13·61
Amoebic primary	19·4	5·61	6·07	1·95
Recurrent	0·8	0·11	—	—
Totals	81·4	44·65	29·11	17·51
Enteric group:				
Typhoid fever	—	—	—	—
Paratyphoid (A. B. and C.)	0·2	—	—	—
Clinical enteric	0·2	0·11	—	—
Totals	0·4	0·11	—	—
Enteritis	64·6	2·33	4·85	3·89
Malaria:				
Clinical	338·4	161·46	94·60	48·62
Quartan	—	—	—	—
Benign tertian	9·4	3·60	3·64	—
Malignant tertian	487·6	219·13	111·58	27·62
Recurrent	8·1	8·36	2·43	1·95
Blanket treatment	—	—	—	—
Totals	843·5	392·55	212·25	78·19
Infective hepatitis (catarrhal jaundice)	4·5	34·49	8·49	—
Pyrexia of uncertain origin	6·8	7·30	2·42	1·95
Phlebotomus fever	0·9	0·11	—	—
Influenza	3·8	0·53	—	1·95
Upper respiratory tract infections	75·1	75·02	89·75	44·74
Tuberculosis, all types	3·4	2·01	0·85	3·69
Venereal diseases	42·8	29·84	44·88	44·74
Other infections	23·0	17·56	15·89	9·92
All diseases caused by infection and pyrexia of uncertain origin	1,150·2	606·50	408·49	206·58
All other diseases and unclassified conditions	393·2	300·60	335·35	261·62
Totals of all diseases	1,543·4	907·10	743·84	468·20
INJURIES				
General injuries	19·1	21·69	22·68	11·48
Local injuries	42·3	33·12	39·42	23·92
Totals of all injuries	61·4	54·81	62·10	35·40
Totals of all diseases and injuries	1,604·8	961·91	805·94	503·60

Injuries

In Tables 3(a), (b) and (c), injuries are analysed according to the part of the body affected, no distinction being made between fatal and non-fatal cases. The table below, which is extracted from the above-mentioned tables, shows the number of injuries in the various anatomical sites in descending order of frequency.

TABLE 8

R.A.F. Anatomical Sites of Injury

Anatomical Region	Total Injuries	Percentage of All Injuries
Generalised, including missing, presumed dead	105,131	41·9
Lower limb, excluding ankle and foot	40,217	16·0
Ankle and Foot	28,433	11·3
Head and Scalp	20,169	8·0
Arm, excluding hand and wrist	16,844	6·7
Hand and Wrist	13,739	5·5
Face and Mouth	9,248	3·7
Back and Vertebral Column	4,906	2·0
Eyes and Eyelids	4,806	1·9
Chest and Neck	3,983	1·6
Buttocks and Pelvis	1,983	0·8
Abdomen	1,172	0·5
Ears	325	0·1
Totals	250,956	100·0

Table 10 is a fuller analysis of injuries for 1944, the year in which there was the greatest number of injuries, and Table 11 shows aircrew injuries for the same year.

Although these statistics apply to both aircrew and ground personnel, the dominating problem in the R.A.F. is the care of aircrew. These carefully selected and highly trained young men were fighting either alone, as in the case of fighter pilots, or in small units of a few men. They lived and worked in exceptional circumstances; they were submitted to the special risks of flying at high speeds, to the hazards of weather, altitude and cold, and to the perils of exposure to enemy action. Ground personnel were exposed to a much lesser degree to risks attributable to war.

FATAL INJURIES

In certain circumstances loss of life results from a multiplicity of injuries. In no other Service, and in no other conditions, was this such a common event—mid-air collisions, diving into the ground at high speed, fierce and rapid fires in aircraft. Such accidents result in injuries which allow of no survival.

Analysis of these cases of fatal injury shows that they fall into three main groups. The first results in a pulverisation of the whole body where the force of impact on crashing or the severity of an explosion causes complete disintegration of the whole body. The second and more common group results in multiple injuries with fractures; most of the bones in the body may be fractured and the skull splintered into small fragments. Associated visceral injuries are severe and extensive and death is usually instantaneous. The third group of cases comprises severe burns which result in incineration of the body.

COMMON NON-FATAL INJURIES

Certain characteristic injuries were found to occur in flying personnel. Burns, frostbite, immersion injuries, head injuries and certain types of fracture all presented problems to R.A.F. surgeons.

BURNS

Burns (Table 9) were responsible for an important number of injuries to R.A.F. flying personnel. There was often a characteristic distribution of burns in those who survived, particularly in fighter pilots, involving the face, hands and wrists. The area affected was small and the associated mortality slight but the morbidity from these burns was very great. It was found that protection by gloves, helmets and clothing was of the greatest value and the wearing of gloves and helmets did, in fact, give complete protection in many instances. It will be noted that there was a higher percentage of burns of the leg in men serving abroad and an

TABLE 9

R.A.F. Burns, 1939–45

Site of Burn	Total Force		Home		Abroad	
	No. of Cases	Percentage of Total	No. of Cases	Percentage of Total	No. of Cases	Percentage of Total
Generalised	2,526	20·8	1,154	16·6	1,372	26·4
Face and Hands	1,170	9·6	867	12·5	303	5·8
Head and Neck, Eyes and Ears	1,560	12·8	1,123	16·2	437	8·4
Hand and Wrist	1,918	15·8	1,425	20·5	493	9·5
Arm	922	7·6	519	7·5	403	7·7
Foot and Ankle	1,871	15·4	1,090	15·7	781	15·0
Leg	1,852	15·3	651	9·4	1,201	23·1
Trunk	327	2·7	114	1·6	213	4·1
Totals	12,146	100·0	6,943	100·0	5,203	100·0
Percentage of Total Injuries	4·8%		3·8%		7·5%	

important factor in this was the habit of working and flying in shorts. Obviously, under prevailing conditions, it was impossible to wear many clothes, but the small loss of comfort in wearing gloves, long sleeves and long trousers often meant the difference between a minor and a severe burn.

Shortly after the outbreak of the war it was realised that improved forms of treatment for burns were required in the R.A.F. At this time the treatment of burns consisted mainly of the use of coagulants, chiefly tannic acid. A Burns Sub-Committee was set up and in 1941 four Burns Centres were formed at the R.A.F. Hospitals at Halton, Ely, Cosford and Rauceby. The primary object of these centres was to establish uniform and recognised treatment of burns in the R.A.F. These specialised R.A.F. Centres made considerable contributions to the advances in the knowledge of the treatment of burns. (*See R.A.F. Medical Services* Vol. I, p. 302.)

HEAD INJURIES

Aircraft crashes result in a large number of severe head injuries. A study of head injuries in aircrews in the first two years of the war was made in 1942 (Stanford Cade, *Brit. J. of Surgery*, 1944, 32, 125). The report dealt with a period of 25 months, September 3, 1939 to September 30, 1941, and consisted of an analysis of 1,545 cases in which the predominant injury was to the cranium. The number of head injuries over this period was only slightly less than the number of multiple injuries; it is apparent that head injuries were a very important cause of loss of trained flying personnel. The conclusions drawn from this investigation were:

(1) The vast majority of fractures of the skull were fatal. The fatality rate was 99·4 per cent. for cases of fractured skull associated with other injuries and 93·7 per cent. for cases of fractured skull only. Of the 56 cases of fracture of the skull who survived, the majority were simple fractures of the vault. The majority of fatal cases had fractures of both the vault and the base of the skull.

(2) Death was instantaneous in 83 per cent. of the fatal cases; 13 per cent. died within the first twenty-four hours so that of the fatal cases only 4 per cent. lived more than one day.

(3) All cases of concussion survived.

(4) The end result of head injuries in aircraft accidents can be expressed by the 'all or nothing' principle. If a case of head injury escapes death, the injury is such that return to full flying duties can be confidently anticipated; 74 per cent. of survivors returned to full flying duties.

(5) Crash landing on return from operational flights accounted for 44 per cent. of the total of cases.

(6) There were very few fatal cases due to missile wounds of the head. Of those who returned, there are only 18 cases recorded in the entire R.A.F. for the first 25 months of the war.

MAXILLO-FACIAL INJURIES (*See* Inter Allied Conferences on War Medicine, Sqn.-Ldr. T. Cradock Henry)

The typical deceleration injury in aircrew is fracture of the middle third of the face. Three types commonly occur.

(1) The malar-maxillary fracture which may result in loss of malar floor, enophthalmos and by direct injury to one of the muscles may cause permanent diplopia.

(2) The naso-maxillary fracture in which displacement or crumpling of the septum will obstruct the airway—a matter of great significance in flying.

(3) Fracture of the tooth-bearing segments with resultant mal-occlusion.

The mandible is rarely fractured in comparison with the middle third of the face; of 487 injuries of the middle third and the mandible, only 34 were fractures of the mandible. Where fracture of the mandible has been recorded comminution has usually been severe.

As injuries to the face were usually due to flying accidents and not to missile wounds they did not as a rule present large tissue losses and the associated problems of these rarely arose.

The combination of burns with other maxillo-facial injuries necessitated special provision for treatment and accommodation. Each maxillo-facial unit was self-contained at a base hospital and under unified control.

SPINAL INJURIES

Spinal injuries were common as a result of aircraft crashes. Two main causes of fracture of the spine are recognised.

(1) Vertical compression. A fall in the standing or sitting position may cause telescopic compression and simple crush fracture of the vertebrae, usually in the lumbar region. This is the commonest cause of spinal fracture in civil life and is a common injury in heavy parachute landings.*

(2) Forcible flexion. Violent bending movements which double up the spine like a clasp knife cause a more severe fracture, again in the lumbar region because this is the site of greatest bending movement.

* *See R.A.F. Medical Services* Vol. II, pp. 478, 483–84.

Both types of fracture may occur in aircrew. When an aircraft makes a crash landing, the pilot may strike the ground violently in a sitting position and sustain a simple vertical compression fracture of the first type. There is no efficient form of protection against this injury. More frequently, however, the pilot's feet, hips and lower spine are relatively fixed, the upper spine and head travel forward with considerable momentum and a forcible flexion fracture of the second type is

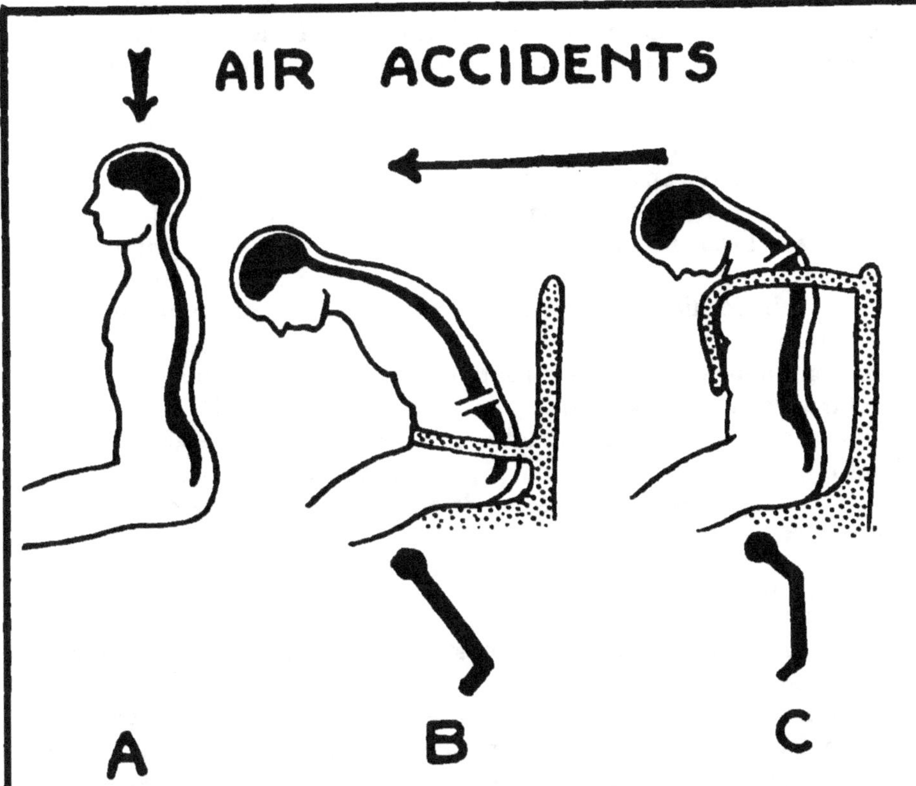

Diagrammatic representation of Crash Fractures of Spine.

A—*Compression fracture as may occur on heavy landing by parachute.*

B—*Dorso-lumbar flexion fracture of spine in aircraft when wearing lap-type safety belt.*

C—*Cervico-dorsal flexion fracture of spine when wearing shoulder-type safety harness during an aircraft crash.*

sustained. If this forward movement is unrestricted the fracture is likely to be of a severe type occurring in the lumbar region and often with a crushing of the nerves and paralysis. A much more severe type of fracture was usual in bomber crews, where certain crew members, owing to the nature of their duties, wore less effective restrictive harness. The harness,* however, although undoubtedly responsible for preventing a number of fractures of the spine, may also be held responsible for causing some fractures of the upper dorsal vertebrae—since the trunk is held it cannot double up at the waist and as only the head travels forward with momentum the level of the fracture is raised. (*See* diagram on previous page.)

OTHER ORTHOPAEDIC INJURIES

A fairly large number of fractures due to air crashes and road accidents has always been a feature of R.A.F. surgery. A special orthopaedic service was instituted during the war to deal with the large numbers of severe orthopaedic injuries which could be expected from intensive air warfare.

Certain injuries were more common than in other Services. Multiple fractures were common; three or more distinct injuries were often found in the same person. Fractures of the talus with associated ankle joint injuries were seen particularly in pilots; they were caused by the mid-tarsal region of the foot being driven forcibly downwards on to the rudder bar.

FROSTBITE

The danger of frostbite was constantly present for R.A.F. bomber crews operating over Germany, where for most of the year extremely low temperatures were met. Flying at altitudes between 20,000 and 25,000 feet the external air temperature varied between −30°C and −55°C. Means of protection against cold and frostbite had to be devised by the development of suitable clothing, including electrically heated flying suits, waistcoats, gloves and boots. It was necessary to find out where applied heat would be most effective, either peripherally or centrally to limbs or body, particularly over the course of blood vessels. The main lessons learned were that crew discipline regarding clothing and adequate oxygen intake is a potent factor in preventing frostbite and that for this purpose reliance should not be placed on cabin heating for war planes, particularly as they may be holed in combat. (*See R.A.F. Medical Services* Vol. II, p. 109 ff.)

It is of interest to note that during 1944–45 frostbite only occurred at a rate of ·08 per 1,000 individuals engaged in bomber sorties.

* *See R.A.F. Medical Services* Vol. III, Chap. 10, pp. 520, 521.

IMMERSION INJURIES

These injuries occurred in aircrew who were forced to spend long periods in rubber dinghies after crashes at sea. A full account of these conditions is given in *Medicine and Pathology* in this series.

INJURIES, 1944

A more detailed analysis of injuries is presented for 1944, the year which had the highest injury rate. Table 10 gives the injuries for the total force in 1944 and shows the number of cases (including those remaining from 1943), the number of deaths, the number finally invalided or returned to duty, the number remaining in hospital on December 31, 1944, the incidence of cases per 1,000 of strength, the average number of sick daily and the average number of days treatment before return to duty. Table 11 is an analysis of injuries among all personnel with aircrew qualifications in 1944; the majority of these injuries were sustained in flying accidents or through enemy action but some were due to other causes and there were men with aircrew qualifications who rarely flew but whose duties were purely administrative. Of the 491 cases of internal derangement of the knee recorded it is fair to suppose that the majority were athletic injuries unconnected with flying.

General injuries in the whole force were responsible for 31,257 cases or 44·3 per cent. of the total injuries and 18,349 or 97·1 per cent. of the total deaths from injuries. Those listed as missing, presumed dead accounted for 13,015 cases and of these 10,868 were aircrew. As would be expected both the categories Multiple Injuries with Fractures and Multiple Injuries with Burns show high fatality rates—71·2 per cent. and 82·3 per cent. for the total force and 87·4 per cent. and 88·6 per cent. for aircrew. Cases of Fractured Skull with other Fractures had a fatality rate of 79·8 per cent. for the total force and 100 per cent. among aircrew.

The figure of 128 cases of general injuries finally invalided cannot be regarded as a true picture since a number of the more severe cases were still in R.A.F. hospitals at the end of the year and were eventually invalided, while a number of those invalided during 1944 had been injured in the previous year. But even taking these factors into consideration a remarkably high proportion (39·0 per cent.) of cases were able to return to duty.

TABLE 10

R.A.F. Injuries, 1944. Total Cases*

Injury	Total Force							
							Averages	
	Number of cases	Number of deaths	Number finally invalided	Number of cases returned to duty	Number of cases remaining in hospital on December 31	Incidence of cases per 1,000 of strength	Number sick daily	Number of days treatment before return to duty
GENERAL INJURIES:								
Multiple injuries with fractures	5,041	3,589	72	1,150	230	5·03	226·67	50
Multiple injuries with burns	1,510	1,242	8	200	60	1·51	56·42	75
Multiple wounds	223	19	4	170	30	0·22	22·13	30
Fractured skull with other fractures	104	83	1	10	10	0·10	3·07	8
Missile wounds, multiple	123	26	7	80	10	0·12	12·02	38
Minor injuries	1,030	—	—	1,030	—	1·03	25·01	9
Burns, generalised	759	134	15	570	40	0·77	69·98	32
Burns of face and hands	280	—	10	260	10	0·28	18·36	23
Scalds	—	—	—	—	—	—	—	—
Frostbite in Aircrew during flight**	42	—	2	40	—	0·04	5·34	41
Exposure to natural elements	115	14	1	100	—	0·11	3·74	13
Drowning, including effects of immersion	187	157	—	30	—	0·19	2·70	33
Injuries to tissues and specialised structures†	4,907	—	7	4,770	130	4·89	202·04	15
Chemical agents, effects of contact with††	118	8	—	110	—	0·12	4·18	14
Other injuries	3,803	62	1	3,670	70	3·79	108·73	10
Missing, presumed dead	13,015	13,015	—	—	—	12·98	—	—
Totals	31,257	18,349	128	12,190	590	31·18	760·39	19

LOCALISED INJURIES:								
CRANIUM								
Contusions and wounds	1,616	75	11	1,460	70	1·61	73·34	17
Fractures of skull, vault	299	75	4	190	30	0·30	27·97	45
Fractures of skull, base	334	173	1	140	20	0·33	14·12	33
Concussion	2,524	2	2	2,480	40	2·52	111·69	16
Missile wounds	123	80	3	30	10	0·12	3·08	8
Burns and scalds	—	—	—	—	—	—	—	—
Totals	4,896	405	21	4,300	170	4·88	230·20	18
FACE AND MOUTH:								
Contusions and wounds	1,250	—	—	1,220	30	1·25	29·86	9
Fractures, fracture-dislocations and dislocations	1,101	—	1	1,050	50	1·10	57·92	19
Missile wounds	11	1	—	10	—	0·01	0·20	7
Tooth injuries	20	—	—	20	—	0·02	0·30	5
Burns and scalds	321	—	1	310	10	0·32	10·04	11
Totals	2,703	1	2	2,610	90	2·70	98·32	13
EYES:								
Eyelids, injuries of	140	—	—	140	—	0·14	4·30	11
Eye substance, superficial wounds of	580	—	—	550	30	0·58	16·52	10
Eye substance, injury to eyeball	442	—	2	420	20	0·44	26·68	21
Eye substance, injuries resulting in removal of eye	54	—	4	50	—	0·05	12·71	88
Missile wounds	22	1	1	20	—	0·02	1·59	25
Burns and scalds of eyelids and eyes	70	—	—	70	—	0·07	2·66	14
Chemical injuries of eyelids and eyes	80	—	—	80	—	0·08	2·69	12
Totals	1,388	1	7	1,330	50	1·38	67·15	17
EARS:								
Pinna, injuries to	10	—	—	10	—	0·01	0·33	12
Rupture of tympanic membrane	80	—	—	70	10	0·08	2·55	13
Burns and scalds	—	—	—	—	—	—	—	—
Totals	90	—	—	80	10	0·09	2·88	13

TABLE 10—(*contd.*)

R.A.F. Injuries, 1944. Total Cases*

Injury	Total Force						Averages	
	Number of cases	Number of deaths	Number finally invalided	Number of cases returned to duty	Number of cases remaining in hospital on December 31	Incidence of cases per 1,000 of strength	Number sick daily	Number of days treatment before return to duty
NECK:								
Contusions and wounds	131	1	—	130	—	0·13	2·88	8
Cut throat	3	3	—	—	—	0·003	0·03	—
Missile wounds	6	6	—	—	—	0·006	—	—
Fractures	—	—	—	—	—	—	—	—
Burns and scalds (internal and external)	30	—	—	30	—	0·03	0·44	5
Totals	170	10	—	160	—	0·17	3·35	7
CHEST:								
Contusions and superficial wounds	372	2	—	370	—	0·37	6·58	6
Compression and blast injury	26	6	—	10	10	0·03	1·29	3
Penetrating wounds	28	7	1	20	—	0·03	1·28	20
Fractures, fracture-dislocations and dislocations	221	1	—	210	10	0·22	13·18	21
Missile wounds	74	33	1	30	10	0·07	3·40	35
Burns and scalds	20	—	—	20	—	0·02	0·47	9
Totals	741	49	2	660	30	0·74	26·20	13

BACK AND VERTEBRAL COLUMN:								
Contusions and superficial wounds	620	—	—	620	—	0·62	19·04	11
Contusions and wounds involving viscera	10	—	—	10	—	0·01	1·07	39
Spinal concussion	20	—	—	10	10	0·02	1·10	31
Fractures, fracture-dislocations and dislocations body of vertebrae	402	24	18	310	50	0·40	49·26	39
Fractures of process and coccyx	71	—	1	70	—	0·07	4·05	19
Missile wounds	25	5	—	20	—	0·02	1·32	23
Missile wounds involving vertebral column	1	1	—	—	—	0·001	—	—
Burns and scalds	10	—	—	10	—	0·01	0·22	8
Totals	1,159	30	19	1,050	60	1·16	76·06	21
ABDOMEN:								
Contusions and superficial wounds	87	4	3	80	—	0·08	3·12	12
Contusions and wounds involving viscera	70	9	1	50	10	0·07	7·04	39
Missile wounds	58	18	—	40	—	0·06	3·11	27
Burns and scalds	30	—	—	30	—	0·03	0·99	12
Totals	245	31	4	200	10	0·24	14·26	22
BUTTOCKS AND PELVIS:								
Contusions and wounds	122	2	—	110	10	0·12	1·73	5
Contusions and wounds of generative organs	180	—	—	180	—	0·18	7·32	15
Contusions and wounds of other organs	1	1	—	—	—	0·001	0·02	—
Fractures, fracture-dislocations and dislocations	235	1	4	220	10	0·24	24·45	37
Missile wounds	34	—	4	10	20	0·03	5·29	58
Burns and scalds	30	—	—	30	—	0·03	1·45	18
Totals	602	4	8	550	40	0·60	40·26	23

TABLE 10—(*contd.*)

R.A.F. Injuries, 1944. Total Cases*

Injury	Total Force							
							Averages	
	Number of cases	Number of deaths	Number finally invalided	Number of cases returned to duty	Number of cases remaining in hospital on December 31	Incidence of cases per 1,000 of strength	Number sick daily	Number of days treatment before return to duty
UPPER LIMB, HAND AND WRIST:								
Contusions and wounds	1,582	1	1	1,560	20	1·58	74·60	17
Sprains	120	—	—	110	10	0·12	2·63	8
Fractures, fracture-dislocations and dislocations	1,544	—	4	1,490	50	1·54	80·08	18
Missile wounds	116	1	5	100	10	0·12	10·27	34
Burns and scalds	710	—	—	680	30	0·70	26·60	14
Totals	4,072	2	10	3,940	120	4·06	194·18	17
UPPER LIMB, REST OF LIMB:								
Contusions and wounds	514	1	3	500	10	0·51	19·62	12
Sprains and strains	60	—	—	60	—	0·06	1·40	8
Fractures, fracture-dislocations and dislocations	3,406	—	16	3,220	170	3·40	248·41	26
Missile wounds	197	2	5	180	10	0·19	13·32	25
Burns and scalds	310	—	—	280	30	0·31	12·46	14
Multiple fractures of whole upper limb	10	—	—	10	—	0·01	5·01	183
Multiple missile wounds of whole upper limb	—	—	—	—	—	—	—	—
Totals	4,497	3	24	4,250	220	4·48	300·22	23

LOWER LIMB, FOOT AND ANKLE:								
Contusions and wounds	1,400	—	—	1,370	30	1·40	40·49	11
Sprains and strains	3,761	—	1	3,750	10	3·75	89·95	9
Fractures, fracture-dislocations and dislocations	2,176	—	6	2,100	70	2·17	127·98	21
Missile wounds	93	—	3	80	10	0·09	11·76	22
Burns and scalds	490	—	—	470	20	0·49	22·66	16
Totals	7,920	—	10	7,770	140	7·90	292·84	13
LOWER LIMB, REST OF LIMB:								
Contusions and wounds	2,409	5	—	2,320	80	2·40	98·30	15
Sprains and strains	650	—	4	620	30	0·65	22·47	12
Internal derangement of knee joint	2,832	—	2	2,740	90	2·83	206·07	26
Fractures, fracture-dislocations and dislocations	3,969	8	31	3,650	280	3·96	431·22	37
Missile wounds	310	3	7	280	20	0·31	20·04	23
Burns and scalds	662	—	2	660	—	0·66	53·32	29
Multiple fractures of whole lower limb	11	1	—	—	10	0·01	3·84	—
Missile wounds of whole lower limb	13	—	3	10	—	0·01	1·31	39
Totals	10,856	17	49	10,280	510	10·83	836·57	27
Total of All Injuries	70,596	18,902	284	49,370	2,040	70·41	2,942·88	19

* It should be noted that this table includes a number of cases remaining from 1943; the figures do not agree therefore with those given in Table 3(a).

** *See* p. 483.

† See p. 483.

†† *See* p. 483.

TABLE 11

Aircrew Injuries, 1944—G.D. Officers and Airman Aircrew

CAUSE OF DISABILITY	Number of Cases Returned to Duty or Remaining in Hospital at end of Year	Number of Deaths	Number Finally Invalided During Year	Totals
GENERAL INJURIES				
Multiple Injuries and Fractures	390	2,953	35	3,378
Multiple Injuries and Burns	190	1,535	8	1,733
Multiple Wounds	60	5	—	65
Fractured Skull with other fractures	—	58	—	58
Missile wounds, multiple	40	13	2	55
Minor Injuries	250	—	—	250
Generalised Burns	240	88	7	335
Burns of face and hands	50	—	8	58
Frostbite in Aircrew during Flight*	40	—	2	42
Exposure to natural elements	20	13	1	34
Drowning, including effects of Immersion	10	91	—	101
Injuries to Tissues and Specialised Structures*	770	—	—	770
Chemical agents, effects of contact with*	—	2	—	2
Other Injuries	820	22	—	842
Missing, Presumed dead	—	10,868	—	10,868
Totals	2,880	15,648	63	18,591
LOCALISED INJURIES				
Cranium:				
Contusions and Wounds	410	34	5	449
Fractures of Skull, Vault	50	44	2	96
Fractures of Skull, Base	—	89	—	89
Concussion	450	1	1	452
Missile wounds	—	31	2	33
Totals	910	199	10	1,119
Face and Mouth:				
Contusions and Wounds	260	—	—	260
Fractures and Fracture dislocations	120	—	1	121
Missile wounds	10	—	—	10
Tooth Injuries	10	—	—	10
Burns and Scalds	60	—	1	61
Totals	460	—	2	462
Eyes:				
Eyelids	40	—	—	40
Eye Substance—Superficial wounds	50	—	—	50
Eye Substance—Injury to Eyeball	110	—	1	111
Eye Substance—Removal of eye	30	—	—	30
Missile wounds	—	—	1	1
Burns and Scalds	10	—	—	10
Totals	240	—	2	242
Ears:				
Pinna, injuries to	10	—	—	10
Rupture of Tympanic membrane	40	—	—	40
Totals	50	—	—	50
Neck:				
Contusions and Wounds	10	1	—	11
Missile wounds	—	2	—	2
Burns and Scalds	10	—	—	10
Totals	20	3	—	23

* *See* p. 483.

TABLE 11 (*contd.*)

Aircrew Injuries, 1944—G.D. Officers and Airman Aircrew

CAUSE OF DISABILITY	Number of Cases Returned to Duty or Remaining in Hospital at end of Year	Number of Deaths	Number Finally Invalided During Year	Totals
Chest:				
Contusions and Wounds	20	1	—	21
Penetrating wounds	—	2	—	2
Fractures	60	1	—	61
Missile wounds	30	16	1	47
Burns and Scalds	10	—	—	10
Totals	120	20	1	141
Back and Vertebral Column:				
Contusions and Wounds	130	—	—	130
Fractures	130	16	9	155
Fracture of Coccyx	40	—	1	41
Missile wounds	—	1	—	1
Totals	300	17	10	327
Abdomen:				
Contusions and Wounds	20	2	1	23
Wounds involving viscera	10	3	—	13
Missile wounds	10	8	—	18
Totals	40	13	1	54
Buttocks and Pelvis:				
Contusions and Wounds	10	—	—	10
Wounds of Generative Organs	10	—	—	10
Fractures	20	—	—	20
Missile wounds	10	—	1	11
Burns and Scalds	10	—	—	10
Totals	60	—	1	61
Upper Limb—hands and wrists:				
Contusions and Wounds	140	—	—	140
Fractures	190	—	1	191
Missile wounds	30	1	—	31
Burns and Scalds	40	—	—	40
Totals	400	1	1	402
Upper Limb—rest of limb:				
Contusions and wounds	100	—	—	100
Sprains and Strains	30	—	—	30
Fractures	760	—	5	765
Missile wounds	60	1	4	65
Totals	950	1	9	960
Lower Limb—foot and ankle:				
Contusions and Wounds	170	—	—	170
Sprains and Strains	680	—	1	681
Fractures	270	—	2	272
Missile wounds	30	—	1	31
Burns and Scalds	30	—	—	30
Totals	1,180	—	4	1,184
Lower Limb—rest of limb:				
Contusions and Wounds	390	3	2	395
Sprains and Strains	170	—	—	170
Fractures	610	4	7	621
I.D.K.	490	—	1	491
Missile wounds	150	3	3	156
Missile wounds, Multiple	10	—	—	10
Burns and Scalds	50	—	—	50
Totals	1,870	10	13	1,893
Total Injuries	9,480	15,912	117	25,509
Amputations	70	—	22	92
Effects of Heat	40	1	—	41
Late complications of trauma	—	—	5	5
GRAND TOTALS	9,590	15,913	144	25,647

FATALITY RATES FOR CASES OF SKULL INJURY, 1944

Skull injuries were the most important cause of death among localised injuries.

NATURE OF INJURY	Fatality Rates per cent.	
	Total Force	Aircrew
Contusions and Wounds .	4·6	7·6
Fractures of Skull:		
Vault	25·1	45·8
Base	51·8	98·9
Concussion . . .	0·07	0·2
Missile Wounds . .	65·0	100·0

A comparison of the figures for fractured skull for the total force over the period 1939–45 (Table 3(a)) reveals one of the difficulties of statistical classification. It might be supposed that the number of cases of fractured skull would bear some direct relationship to the total number of injuries. Thus, it is natural to expect that in 1944, when there was a total of 68,360 injuries, there would be more cases of fractured skull than in 1941 when there were 32,638 injuries. This is indeed borne out in the figures for fractured skull without other injuries as shown below; but there were many more cases of fractured skull with other injuries in 1941 than in 1944.

Year	Fractured Skull with other fractures		Fractured Skull	
	No. of Cases*	Deaths	No. of Cases*	Deaths
1939	140	122	101	59
1940	382	360	298	196
1941	640	516	419	280
1942	463	405	497	314
1943	232	205	462	247
1944	104	83	633	248
1945	85	61	424	174

* Fresh cases and cases remaining from previous year.

In fact the differences are largely due to varying nomenclature which makes exact comparison impossible—for example, in 1944 many cases of fractured skull with other fractures were classified under the heading Multiple Injuries with Fractures; these cases cannot now be identified.

FACE AND MOUTH

In the investigation of head injuries in aircrew carried out for the first two years of the war there were 162 maxillo-facial injuries out of a total of 545 cases. None of the maxillo-facial injuries was fatal. With the exception of fractures of the lower jaw, maxillo-facial injuries recover very quickly; thus most fractures of the nose returned to duty within a few days.

EYE INJURIES

Eye injuries were an important cause of morbidity. The average period of treatment was 17 days and for injuries resulting in removal of the eye the average period of treatment before return to duty was 88 days.

INJURIES—CAUSES

Table 12 is an analysis of injuries according to the more common causes and shows the number of fatal and non-fatal cases from each cause for the war years. The anatomical distribution of injuries from the various causes is also shown but this does not differentiate between fatal and non-fatal cases.

Little comment is necessary on injuries due to ENEMY AIR ACTION. All missing persons presumed to be dead are included in this group. This column reflects the rising scale of operations against the enemy and the tremendous cost in human life involved. The peak casualty figures due to enemy air action were in 1943 when 12,179 were killed and in 1944 when 13,928 were killed.

The casualties from ENEMY GROUND ACTION show a steady rise in numbers up to 1944. This can be correlated with the steadily increasing size of the force abroad exposed to enemy ground activities and the development of close fighter-bomber support for the Army with the necessity of establishing airfields as near to the front line as possible.

As would be expected, AIR-RAID casualties were greatest in the years 1940 and 1941 when the enemy was still in a position to carry out heavy bombing attacks on this country.

FLYING ACCIDENTS took a heavy toll of life and the number of fatalities from this cause was nearly half the number of fatalities from enemy air action. There must, inevitably, have been some confusion in the classification of accidents as due to enemy air action or flying accidents; accidents which occurred on take-off or landing on operational flights were sometimes recorded as flying accidents and sometimes as due to enemy air action.

PROPELLER ACCIDENTS caused a relatively small but avoidable series of accidents. The increased amount of flying as the R.A.F. expanded, which is reflected in the increased flying accident figures over the years 1941–44, would have been expected to cause a commensurate rise in propeller accidents. In point of fact, the number of propeller accidents varied only slightly over the years 1941–43 and this may be attributed to stricter precautions against such accidents.

Injuries in the column headed MECHANICAL TRANSPORT represents injuries suffered both by occupants of various vehicles involved in accidents and by pedestrians. It includes a large number of people who were injuried in off-duty hours. In 1944, for instance, of the 5,221 casualties due to mechanical transport accidents 1,362, of which 56 were fatal, occurred off-duty.

ATHLETIC INJURIES provided the greatest single cause of non-fatal injuries and over half of these were injuries to the lower limb. The seemingly large number of deaths from athletic injuries is due to the inclusion of deaths from drowning while bathing. In 1943 there were 49 deaths from athletic injuries, of which 45 were due to drowning, one to a fractured cervical spine from diving and three to football injuries.

TABLE 12

R.A.F. Causes of Injuries, 1939–45
Total Cases in Each Year

	Enemy Air Action	Enemy Ground Action	Air Raid Casualties	Flying	Propeller	Mechanical Transport	Starting-Motor Engines	Workshop Accidents	Accidental Explosions	Athletic	Self-Inflicted Injuries	Other Causes	Totals
1939 Non-Fatal .	27	2	—	259	34	1,054	60	22	18	1,493	3	2,638	5,610
Fatal . .	219	4	—	473	7	78	—	—	7	7	13	58	866
Totals . .	246	6	—	732	41	1,132	60	22	25	1,500	16	2,696	6,476
1940 Non-Fatal .	694	5	734	1,086	95	2,147	133	83	156	2,299	10	6,300	13,742
Fatal . .	3,191	9	449	1,686	20	180	—	—	83	12	40	403	6,073
Totals . .	3,885	14	1,183	2,772	115	2,327	133	83	239	2,311	50	6,703	19,815
1941 Non-Fatal .	451	33	744	1,958	213	3,419	191	73	276	4,341	21	11,645	23,365
Fatal . .	4,751	2	499	3,173	37	298	—	1	87	38	65	413	9,364
Totals . .	5,202	35	1,243	5,131	250	3,717	191	74	363	4,379	86	12,058	32,729
1942 Non-Fatal .	501	59	598	2,422	205	2,572	130	52	643	6,798	22	17,959	31,961
Fatal . .	6,916	18	314	4,027	48	144	—	—	91	30	81	529	12,198
Totals . .	7,417	77	912	6,449	253	2,716	130	52	734	6,828	103	18,488	44,159
1943 Non-Fatal .	633	125	367	2,839	204	2,705	153	47	731	8,990	25	22,246	39,065
Fatal . .	12,179	31	147	4,489	47	104	—	—	107	49	72	485	17,710
Totals . .	12,812	156	514	7,328	251	2,809	153	47	838	9,039	97	22,731	56,775
1944 Non-Fatal .	772	368	304	2,538	185	4,998	460	131	529	11,677	72	29,660	51,694
Fatal . .	13,928	136	142	3,889	33	223	1	—	54	12	71	413	18,902
Totals . .	14,700	504	446	6,427	218	5,221	461	131	583	11,689	143	30,073	70,596
1945 Non-Fatal .	439	154	178	1,396	91	4,382	230	50	224	7,626	41	20,387	35,198
Fatal . .	3,874	48	60	2,297	12	229	—	—	45	—	66	403	7,034
Totals . .	4,313	202	238	3,693	103	4,611	230	50	269	7,626	107	20,790	42,232

The Strength of the Royal Air Force by Age Groups, 1939–45

The figures given in Table 13 are derived from returns provided by the Manning Branch of the Air Ministry, which give the numbers of men for different age groups at January 1 and July 1 each year. The figures shown for each year have been calculated by adding the strengths on January 1 and July 1 of the year and January 1 of the following year and dividing by three. It should be noted that the figures obtained may mislead if the force either increased or decreased in a particular year as the R.A.F. did in 1939. Returns for shorter intervals (months, for example) would be required to give a more accurate assessment of the average yearly strengths, but the returns at intervals of six months are the only ones available. For the first two years, 1939 and 1940, the totals for all R.A.F. personnel are known but the frequencies for age groups are available only for airmen. The relative frequencies for different age groups for airmen must have been close to those for the total force.

The changing constitution of a force is the result of a number of factors—the intake of recruits, the loss of men falling out for various reasons and ageing of personnel in the Service.

The main changes from 1939–43 must have depended on the influx of recruits and in 1945 on the outflow of demobilised men. Under the 1939 Military Training Act 16,000 men aged 20 expressed preference for service in the R.A.F. and they were called up in October and November of that year. However, the reservists recalled outnumbered the younger recruits.

The National Service Act of 1939 made all men between the ages of 18 and 41 liable for service in the Armed Forces and the first registration under this Act was on October 21, 1939. In 1940 age groups 20 to 35 were registered and in the first six months of 1941 registration was extended up to the age of 40. In 1941 the lower age of registration was reduced to 19 and in 1942 to 18. The National Service Act of 1941 extended the liability for service up to the age of 51 but men over the age of 40 were never, in fact, called upon to register. During 1940 and until April 1941 many younger men were in reserved civilian occupations but from that date they were combed out and the policy thereafter was to grant few reservations to fit men below the age of 35. The ages of reservation for various occupations were gradually raised throughout 1942. These circumstances are reflected in the age distribution for the years 1939–42. In 1941 the R.A.F. was beginning to show signs of 'ageing' but the balance was largely restored by 1942 as the younger men previously reserved were called up.

In 1943 and 1944 deferment of service was more and more restricted, being cancelled in stages, and the closest approach to total mobilisation of fit men up to the age of 40 was reached at the end of 1944. Coal miners, agricultural workers and some others were still reserved. The proportion of men between the ages of 20 and 24 remained practically constant from 1942–44 but the average age of the force was still increasing. The maximum size of the force had now been reached and the trend must have been due principally to the ageing of men in the Service.

If full mobilisation had been required throughout 1945 it would have been expected that the average age of the force would be about one year higher than in 1944. Actually the average age for 1945 was only 0·07 years greater than that for 1944. This was due, of course, to the beginning of demobilisation leading to a relatively greater reduction in the older age groups. Changes in the maximum age of men called up was another factor; the maximum age was reduced to 35 on October 1, 1944, and to 30 on May 1, 1945.

TABLE 13

R.A.F. Average Yearly Strengths for Specified Age Groups, 1939–45

Years	Age														Totals*	Average Age
	Under 20		20–24		25–29		30–34		35–39		40–44		Over 44			
	No.	Percentage	No.	Percentage	No.	Percentage	No.	Percentage	No.	Percentage	No.	Percentage	No.	Percentage		
	AIRMEN ONLY															
1939	13,894	10·71	58,584	45·17	25,188	19·42	13,054	10·06	9,081	7·00	6,171	4·76	3,729	2·88	129,701	26·80
1940	32,073	10·54	140,023	45·99	65,347	21·46	28,492	9·36	18,936	6·22	12,509	4·11	7,072	2·32	304,452	27·26
	OFFICERS AND AIRMEN															
1941	38,179	5·76	244,851	36·94	164,227	24·78	122,519	18·49	58,989	8·90	21,114	3·19	12,893	1·94	662,772	27·47
1942	28,465	3·31	347,916	40·42	166,404	19·33	160,617	18·66	106,477	12·37	34,952	4·06	15,916	1·85	860,747	28·23
1943	48,376	4·98	391,690	40·32	160,398	16·51	173,454	17·86	131,238	13·51	49,729	5·12	16,554	1·70	971,439	28·55
1944	29,922	2·98	385,566	38·46	170,804	17·04	177,392	17·69	146,656	14·63	68,590	6·84	23,663	2·36	1,002,593	28·75
1945	19,928	2·13	316,987	33·94	225,769	24·18	159,237	17·05	126,862	13·58	64,546	6·91	20,593	2·21	933,922	28·82

* The Total Force (Officers and Airmen) was 140,862 in 1939 and 324,398 in 1940.

DISEASE AND INJURY ANALYSED BY AGE GROUPS

Tables 14(a) and 14 (b) show sickness of over 48 hours' duration as rates per 1,000 of strength per annum for each age group; important individual diseases, disease groups and injuries are shown separately.

For the first two years (1939 and 1940) the incidence of sickness by age groups is available for airmen only. From 1941 data are available for officers as well as airmen.

As would be expected, the highest incidence of disease was in the under 20 age group. The problems caused by herding together young recruits, the vast majority of whom are new to communal life, are well known. The exertion and fatigue of the unaccustomed life, the rigours of service conditions compared with home life and the overcrowding in almost every phase of their activities all played their part in producing this high incidence. Sickness rates tend to be much higher among young recruits to the Services than in comparable groups of young men in schools and colleges where conditions would also tend to favour the spread of infections; the important factor in this difference between recruit camps and schools appears to be the more rapid change over in the personnel of the former,* where, as soon as one community has become adapted to its bacteriological environment, another group of non-immunes is introduced.

There is a considerable drop in the incidence of all disabilities in the 20–24 age group but this group does show a consistently higher sickness rate than the older age groups. There is little difference in the sickness rates for all age groups between 25 and 44, but a rise in incidence occurs in the over 45 age group which, under war-time conditions, contained many men over 60.

UPPER RESPIRATORY TRACT infections provided a true reflection of the susceptibility of recruits and the incidence was much higher in this category throughout the war years. In 1944 the rate in the under 20 age group reached the very high level of 448 cases per 1,000 of strength whereas the incidence in the other age groups was no higher than the average for the other war years. In the December quarter of 1943 there was an epidemic of influenza in the civilian population; the full force of this epidemic was not felt in the recruit centres until the early months of 1944 and this would account for the high incidence of upper respiratory tract infections for this year.

PNEUMONIA showed its highest incidence in the under 20 age group; this is in keeping with the higher rate of upper respiratory tract infections in this group. The incidence in the over 45 age group is consistently slightly greater than in the age groups 20–44. In 1944 all age groups showed an increased incidence of pneumonia but this was most

* *R.A.F. Medical Services* Vol. II, p. 577.

apparent in the under 20 age group where the incidence rose to 42 per 1,000 of strength compared with 13 per 1,000 in the previous year. The incidence in the over 45 age group was 12 per 1,000 compared with 7 per 1,000 in the previous year. Most cases occurred in March and April following the season of upper respiratory tract infections. There was no increase in notifications of, or deaths from, pneumonia in the civilian population in 1944.

The highest incidence of PULMONARY TUBERCULOSIS was in the under 20 age group and reached a peak of 10 cases per 1,000 in 1944 and 1945 when the average incidence for the whole force was 2·1 per 1,000 in 1944 and 2·4 per 1,000 in 1945. The explanation must lie partly in the greater use made of mass radiography in R.A.F. recruit centres in the later years of the war; this revealed many cases of unsuspected tuberculosis which swelled the notification figures in that group. (*See R.A.F. Medical Services* Vol. I, p. 288.) There was no significant difference in the incidence of tuberculosis in the age groups other than that of the under 20.

TUBERCULOSIS IN OTHER SITES also showed a predilection for the under 20 age group and reached a peak incidence of 4 per 1,000 in 1945. There was a steady fall in incidence with increasing age and the lowest incidence was in the 40–44 age group.

VENEREAL DISEASE was most prevalent in the age group 20–24. All age groups showed a tendency to increased incidence as the war progressed. It is not surprising to find the maximum incidence in the 20–24 group; the majority were unmarried and for many it was the first experience of being away from the moral ties and influence of home life. There would still be an element of bravado in their lives and many would be over-indulging in drinking for the first time.

The table for INFECTIVE HEPATITIS shows that the young are much more susceptible than the old and this bears out the experience of the Army. The peak incidence was in 1943 and 1944, corresponding with the major epidemics in the Middle East.

POST INOCULATION EFFECTS showed a heavy incidence in the under 20 age group. There is a considerable fall in incidence in the 20–24 age group and then, on the whole, a very slight decrease with increasing age. An attempt was made to provide every recruit with vaccination against smallpox and inoculation against the enteric fevers. This meant that nearly every man in the under 20 age group experienced inoculation against the typhoid group for the first time in his life and many were vaccinated for the first time. In the older age groups, although the aim was to maintain a man's immunity, a much smaller proportion were inoculated and vaccinated each year. Booster doses of T.A.B.C. and revaccination seldom produced as severe a reaction as the initial doses.

TABLE 14(a)

R.A.F. Incidence of Sickness and Injury Analysed by Age Groups, 1939–45

		Incidence per 1,000 per annum							
		Under 20	20 to 24	25 to 29	30 to 34	35 to 39	40 to 44	45 and Over	Average Whole Force
DISEASES									
Upper Respiratory Tract Infections	1939	—	—	—	—	—	—	—	116·1
	1940	—	—	—	—	—	—	—	146·3
	1941	211·8	103·4	105·9	81·1	59·9	75·9	89·9	101·1
	1942	317·2	97·2	95·0	72·5	57·9	50·2	56·8	91·9
	1943	280·9	136·4	119·9	92·5	82·2	75·3	92·8	121·9
	1944	447·8	119·0	94·9	82·3	64·4	59·9	57·9	104·7
	1945	237·9	98·3	60·1	65·1	52·9	41·5	32·1	74·8
Pneumonia	1939	—	—	—	—	—	—	—	2·1
	1940	—	—	—	—	—	—	—	3·7
	1941	11·4	3·9	3·8	4·0	3·8	3·6	5·4	4·3
	1942	13·1	3·3	3·3	3·2	3·2	4·2	3·8	3·6
	1943	12·6	3·5	3·3	3·1	3·4	4·5	6·5	3·9
	1944	42·0	5·6	5·3	4·9	7·1	6·4	12·3	6·9
	1945	17·2	3·7	2·8	3·2	3·5	2·9	4·1	3·6
Tuberculosis, Pulmonary	1939	—	—	—	—	—	—	—	1·0
	1940	—	—	—	—	—	—	—	1·4
	1941	3·2	1·4	1·6	1·6	1·4	1·9	1·5	1·6
	1942	8·9	1·9	2·2	1·8	2·0	2·4	1·6	2·2
	1943	8·0	2·4	2·4	1·9	1·9	2·3	3·1	2·5
	1944	9·6	2·1	1·8	2·0	1·5	1·4	2·6	2·1
	1945	9·6	2·4	1·8	2·6	2·0	2·1	3·1	2·4

Tuberculosis, other than Pulmonary	1939	—	—	—	—	—	—	—	0·3
	1940	—	—	—	—	—	—	—	0·3
	1941	1·1	0·6	0·4	0·4	0·3	0·1	0·1	0·5
	1942	1·9	0·5	0·5	0·4	0·4	0·2	0·3	0·5
	1943	0·8	0·5	0·5	0·4	0·3	0·1	0·2	0·5
	1944	2·6	0·7	0·6	0·7	0·3	0·7	0·1	0·7
	1945	3·7	0·5	0·3	0·4	0·2	0·1	—	0·4
Venereal Disease .	1939	—	—	—	—	—	—	—	9·2
	1940	—	—	—	—	—	—	—	8·1
	1941	10·7	10·3	9·2	5·8	4·7	4·6	1·9	8·4
	1942	14·6	12·3	13·1	7·0	5·1	4·5	2·4	10·2
	1943	6·4	15·1	14·8	9·1	5·8	5·1	3·7	11·6
	1944	14·0	26·0	20·9	15·6	9·5	6·0	4·6	18·6
	1945	22·6	33·2	22·3	20·0	12·6	8·2	6·6	23·0
Infective Hepatitis (Catarrhal Jaundice)	1939	—	—	—	—	—	—	—	1·5
	1940	—	—	—	—	—	—	—	1·2
	1941	4·4	3·0	2·6	1·3	1·2	1·2	1·2	2·4
	1942	11·0	7·0	5·3	3·2	2·0	1·3	0·9	5·1
	1943	9·7	16·1	13·1	8·1	5·7	3·7	3·0	11·6
	1944	10·7	17·9	12·8	8·3	6·4	4·0	2·2	12·1
	1945	15·1	11·3	5·2	5·8	4·4	2·2	1·0	7·2
Post Inoculation Effects .	1939	—	—	—	—	—	—	—	6·3
	1940	—	—	—	—	—	—	—	7·4
	1941	16·5	3·1	2·6	3·6	2·7	0·9	0·3	3·7
	1942	9·6	1·3	1·2	0·9	1·0	1·3	0·7	1·4
	1943	13·3	3·0	2·4	2·3	1·8	1·6	0·1	3·0
	1944	30·8	2·7	2·2	1·5	1·8	1·8	1·3	3·0
	1945	28·1	1·5	0·9	0·9	1·0	0·9	0·5	1·7
Dysentery, Amoebic .	1939	—	—	—	—	—	—	—	0·1
	1940	—	—	—	—	—	—	—	0·1
	1941	0·1	0·2	0·2	0·2	0·2	0·1	0·3	0·2
	1942	1·4	1·3	1·3	1·2	0·8	0·9	0·3	1·2
	1943	1·4	3·2	3·6	3·0	2·4	2·1	1·2	2·9
	1944	3·0	5·0	5·2	4·4	4·9	2·5	3·8	4·7
	1945	1·0	4·1	2·8	3·5	4·3	3·6	1·5	3·6

TABLE 14(a)—(contd.)

R.A.F. Incidence of Sickness and Injury Analysed by Age Groups, 1939–45

		Incidence per 1,000 per annum							
		Under 20	20 to 24	25 to 29	30 to 34	35 to 39	40 to 44	45 and Over	Average Whole Force
Dysentery, Bacillary	1939	—	—	—	—	—	—	—	0·5
	1940	—	—	—	—	—	—	—	0·9
	1941	4·3	4·1	3·0	1·7	1·4	1·2	0·6	3·0
	1942	14·3	8·7	7·5	5·6	4·3	2·7	1·6	7·2
	1943	6·7	11·0	9·3	7·7	6·7	4·6	2·7	8·9
	1944	12·7	11·9	8·8	7·7	7·0	3·9	1·3	9·1
	1945	22·6	11·8	6·0	7·9	8·1	4·2	2·4	8·7
Malaria	1939	—	—	—	—	—	—	—	2·8
	1940	—	—	—	—	—	—	—	2·9
	1941	7·9	7·6	5·7	2·7	2·3	2·1	1·9	5·5
	1942	23·6	18·5	16·4	10·4	7·3	5·0	3·5	14·5
	1943	11·2	33·6	27·9	20·5	16·9	10·6	7·0	25·3
	1944	13·0	38·0	24·9	22·6	19·2	9·8	5·1	26·8
	1945	10·4	15·0	9·9	8·8	9·2	6·2	3·5	10·9
Enteric Group	1939	—	—	—	—	—	—	—	0·1
	1940	—	—	—	—	—	—	—	0·1
	1941	0·7	0·3	0·2	0·1	0·1	0·1	—	0·2
	1942	1·2	0·5	0·6	0·3	0·2	0·1	0·1	0·5
	1943	0·3	0·6	0·6	0·4	0·4	0·2	0·2	0·5
	1944	1·0	0·7	0·7	0·5	0·6	0·5	0·4	0·6
	1945	0·1	1·0	0·2	0·3	0·4	0·2	—	0·5

Enteritis	1939	—	—	—	—	—	—	—	7·3
	1940	—	—	—	—	—	—	—	8·2
	1941	18·6	13·3	11·3	8·1	6·1	8·7	9·7	11·3
	1942	15·2	8·5	8·3	6·0	5·3	4·6	6·8	7·6
	1943	1·2	1·7	1·4	1·3	1·1	0·7	0·9	1·4
	1944	2·0	2·3	1·2	1·5	1·6	1·2	0·4	1·7
	1945	3·5	2·5	1·2	1·4	1·9	1·1	—	1·8
Other Infections	1939	—	—	—	—	—	—	—	28·7
	1940	—	—	—	—	—	—	—	34·5
	1941	50·6	21·2	19·3	11·9	7·4	9·5	7·6	18·8
	1942	95·8	27·3	23·1	18·8	12·8	10·2	10·4	24·4
	1943	52·4	25·8	21·8	16·3	12·5	10·2	7·8	21·9
	1944	131·2	29·5	22·0	18·2	15·7	9·7	6·6	25·3
	1945	64·3	23·0	11·6	12·2	10·2	8·2	6·9	16·2
Septic Conditions	1939	—	—	—	—	—	—	—	18·3
	1940	—	—	—	—	—	—	—	20·3
	1941	38·3	20·4	17·9	15·8	15·4	16·3	14·4	19·3
	1942	61·3	25·4	22·9	20·4	19·7	19·1	17·7	24·1
	1943	34·9	29·8	26·6	22·4	21·4	19·7	18·1	26·4
	1944	85·6	36·8	27·1	28·0	28·4	19·3	20·7	32·2
	1945	51·2	32·0	19·3	24·1	22·3	16·5	12·8	25·2
Alimentary System Gastric and Duodenal Ulcers and their Complications	1939	—	—	—	—	—	—	—	2·8
	1940	—	—	—	—	—	—	—	3·7
	1941	2·1	1·7	4·3	6·8	9·1	11·7	11·5	4·5
	1942	2·1	1·5	3·9	5·5	7·3	9·1	10·0	3·9
	1943	0·9	1·5	3·9	5·0	6·6	8·3	12·6	3·8
	1944	1·5	2·2	4·6	6·2	7·4	8·9	12·0	4·7
	1945	1·1	2·3	3·2	5·6	8·0	6·9	9·6	3·8
Other Conditions	1939	—	—	—	—	—	—	—	24·1
	1940	—		—	—	—	—	—	28·3
	1941	45·0	24·4	27·9	31·1	34·6	39·9	39·2	29·4
	1942	90·4	37·7	43·1	43·4	49·5	51·4	52·7	43·8
	1943	60·7	50·7	53·4	47·9	51·0	52·1	55·6	51·3
	1944	127·2	59·3	48·1	53·7	57·0	55·2	53·3	57·7
	1945	110·0	56·4	33·9	49·3	54·2	48·3	44·2	49·8

TABLE 14(a)—(*contd.*)

R.A.F. Incidence of Sickness and Injury Analysed by Age Groups, 1939–45

		Incidence per 1,000 per annum							
		Under 20	20 to 24	25 to 29	30 to 34	35 to 39	40 to 44	45 and Over	Average Whole Force
Circulatory System	1939	—	—	—	—	—	—	—	3·9
	1940	—	—	—	—	—	—	—	5·2
	1941	5·4	3·6	5·5	7·2	7·6	8·1	18·3	5·6
	1942	9·1	3·9	6·7	8·0	9·1	10·6	19·7	6·6
	1943	4·6	4·2	5·9	7·6	8·5	9·8	25·1	6·3
	1944	7·8	5·0	5·6	7·1	8·5	10·6	26·0	6·9
	1945	6·7	4·8	4·5	7·8	9·0	11·3	18·7	6·6
Respiratory System Plenrisy with Effusion	1939	—	—	—	—	—	—	—	0·3
	1940	—	—	—	—	—	—	—	0·5
	1941	1·8	0·6	0·4	0·3	0·3	—	0·5	0·5
	1942	3·0	0·8	0·6	0·3	0·3	0·2	0·2	0·6
	1943	1·9	0·7	0·7	0·3	0·3	0·2	0·2	0·6
	1944	6·8	0·9	0·8	0·6	0·2	0·5	0·5	0·9
	1945	2·1	0·8	0·3	0·3	0·3	0·4	0·1	0·5
Other Conditions	1939	—	—	—	—	—	—	—	9·8
	1940	—	—	—	—	—	—	—	14·1
	1941	19·4	8·2	10·1	11·5	12·9	21·6	32·1	11·3
	1942	47·2	11·3	14·0	14·5	19·6	25·0	43·9	15·8
	1943	30·8	14·4	16·6	17·1	21·2	30·8	60·8	18·6
	1944	71·2	18·5	20·5	19·3	24·8	32·5	52·4	23·3
	1945	40·8	15·8	10·4	15·5	17·5	23·7	43·3	16·4
Allergy	1939	—	—	—	—	—	—	—	2·1
	1940	—	—	—	—	—	—	—	2·4
	1941	4·8	2·3	2·5	2·4	2·6	2·9	1·9	2·6
	1942	6·8	2·2	2·3	2·4	2·0	2·7	2·5	2·4
	1943	3·7	2·4	2·2	2·0	1·9	1·7	2·4	2·3
	1944	8·4	3·1	1·9	3·7	2·2	2·0	2·6	2·9
	1945	4·3	3·0	2·3	2·2	2·5	1·8	1·7	2·5

Urinary System .	1939	—	—	—	—	—	—	—	4·4
	1940	—	—	—	—	—	—	—	4·2
	1941	5·0	3·3	5·0	5·3	4·8	5·6	6·1	4·5
	1942	9·3	4·3	5·7	4·7	4·9	4·6	6·5	4·9
	1943	4·5	4·3	6·1	6·2	6·3	7·1	8·9	5·5
	1944	6·4	5·1	6·1	7·0	8·5	5·3	11·5	6·3
	1945	6·4	5·1	4·6	5·3	6·4	7·0	6·7	5·4
Generative System .	1939	—	—	—	—	—	—	—	5·1
	1940	—	—	—	—	—	—	—	6·0
	1941	10·2	7·5	6·8	4·7	4·5	5·0	3·7	6·5
	1942	14·0	8·2	8·1	5·8	5·0	5·6	6·3	7·4
	1943	6·8	9·7	9·3	6·0	5·2	5·0	6·1	7·9
	1944	11·1	10·2	7·8	7·1	6·3	6·5	8·2	8·4
	1945	13·1	9·4	4·8	5·6	6·2	3·7	5·8	6·8
Locomotor System									
Rheumatic Group of Diseases .	1939	—	—	—	—	—	—	—	3·5
	1940	—	—	—	—	—	—	—	5·0
	1941	4·0	2·6	4·8	5·6	6·9	13·5	13·6	4·7
	1942	4·9	2·4	4·4	5·6	8·0	11·2	15·0	4·8
	1943	2·5	2·6	4·9	5·7	8·5	12·3	15·4	5·1
	1944	8·1	4·2	5·2	8·9	10·5	13·7	16·1	7·2
	1945	4·5	3·8	3·6	5·7	9·4	11·4	17·3	5·7
Other Conditions .	1939	—	—	—	—	—	—	—	6·8
	1940	—	—	—	—	—	—	—	8·5
	1941	11·8	7·1	9·7	11·3	12·2	14·6	19·1	9·7
	1942	15·7	7·7	11·8	11·6	13·5	14·4	18·2	10·7
	1943	9·8	8·5	12·0	12·2	13·8	15·6	23·2	11·2
	1944	17·9	10·0	14·1	14·6	15·9	16·9	25·6	13·5
	1945	10·7	10·0	8·3	12·2	14·1	17·3	24·5	11·3
Nervous System and Mental Diseases									
Psychoneurosis	1939	—	—	—	—	—	—	—	2·8
	1940	—	—	—	—	—	—	—	5·3
	1941	6·8	5·0	6·6	7·2	8·3	12·6	14·3	6·6
	1942	9·2	4·9	7·8	8·0	9·8	11·3	12·9	7·2
	1943	5·7	5·2	8·3	8·4	9·1	12·4	16·1	7·4
	1944	10·7	7·9	9·4	9·8	10·2	11·9	16·1	9·4
	1945	8·9	8·5	6·1	8·7	11·2	10·1	11·2	8·5

TABLE 14(a)—(*contd.*)

R.A.F. Incidence of Sickness and Injury Analysed by Age Groups, 1939–45

		Incidence per 1,000 per annum							
		Under 20	20 to 24	25 to 29	30 to 34	35 to 39	40 to 44	45 and Over	Average Whole Force
Psychoses	1939	—	—	—	—	—	—	—	0·9
	1940	—	—	—	—	—	—	—	0·9
	1941	1·3	0·7	0·7	0·9	1·1	1·5	1·1	0·8
	1942	1·3	0·6	0·8	0·7	0·8	0·9	1·5	0·7
	1943	1·0	0·7	0·8	0·7	0·6	0·9	1·6	0·8
	1944	1·8	1·2	1·2	0·9	0·7	0·6	0·9	1·1
	1945	1·3	1·1	0·8	0·8	1·1	0·4	1·9	1·0
Psychopathic Personality	1939	—	—	—	—	—	—	—	0·6
	1940	—	—	—	—	—	—	—	0·8
	1941	1·4	0·8	0·7	0·9	0·8	1·0	0·5	0·8
	1942	2·6	0·8	0·7	0·8	0·9	1·0	1·0	0·9
	1943	1·8	1·1	1·1	1·0	1·1	1·4	1·0	1·1
	1944	4·5	1·9	2·0	1·8	1·8	2·7	1·9	2·0
	1945	5·4	2·0	1·2	1·6	1·9	2·4	1·0	1·8
Mental Defects	1939	—	—	—	—	—	—	—	0·1
	1940	—	—	—	—	—	—	—	0·1
	1941	0·8	0·2	0·2	0·3	0·3	0·3	0·1	0·3
	1942	0·9	0·2	0·2	0·2	0·3	0·2	0·1	0·2
	1943	0·5	0·2	0·1	0·1	0·2	0·4	0·1	0·2
	1944	0·5	0·1	0·1	0·1	0·3	0·2	0·3	0·2
	1945	0·4	0·2	0·1	0·2	0·2	0·1	0·1	0·2
Epilepsies	1939	—	—	—	—	—	—	—	1·0
	1940	—	—	—	—	—	—	—	1·0
	1941	3·4	1·0	0·8	0·8	1·4	0·7	1·1	1·1
	1942	3·1	0·8	0·8	0·7	0·8	0·2	0·6	0·8
	1943	1·6	0·7	0·6	0·6	0·6	0·6	0·9	0·7
	1944	3·2	0·6	0·6	0·4	0·7	0·2	0·3	0·6
	1945	1·1	0·6	0·4	0·3	0·5	0·6	0·3	0·5

Indefinite aetiology	1939	—	—	—	—	—	—	—	1·7
	1940	—	—	—	—	—	—	—	1·7
	1941	3·3	1·8	1·5	1·4	1·2	1·7	1·8	1·7
	1942	4·3	1·5	2·0	2·1	1·7	1·3	1·2	1·8
	1943	2·3	1·8	2·0	1·6	1·5	1·6	1·8	1·8
	1944	3·7	1·7	2·0	1·4	1·6	1·5	3·2	1·7
	1945	2·6	1·7	0·6	1·2	1·3	1·3	2·4	1·3
Organic Nervous System	1939	—	—	—	—	—	—	—	2·3
	1940	—	—	—	—	—	—	—	2·5
	1941	2·1	1·6	2·3	3·4	4·6	6·5	9·6	2·7
	1942	4·2	1·5	2·6	3·2	4·0	5·2	6·9	2·7
	1943	1·9	1·8	2·9	3·4	4·5	6·1	11·4	3·0
	1944	4·2	2·7	2·9	4·3	6·4	6·3	12·1	4·0
	1945	2·2	2·4	2·1	4·0	3·9	6·0	6·4	3·1
Eye	1939	—	—	—	—	—	—	—	3·3
	1940	—	—	—	—	—	—	—	3·6
	1941	6·8	3·5	3·8	3·3	3·9	4·3	3·9	3·8
	1942	9·1	3·6	4·2	3·9	4·4	3·7	4·1	4·1
	1943	5·3	4·4	4·9	4·0	5·1	4·9	6·5	4·6
	1944	11·9	5·6	5·3	5·7	5·5	5·6	8·2	5·8
	1945	10·4	5·8	4·1	5·2	4·7	6·8	7·3	5·3
Ear, Nose and Throat	1939	—	—	—	—	—	—	—	11·0
	1940	—	—	—	—	—	—	—	13·0
	1941	28·5	15·2	14·7	11·7	9·3	9·6	8·9	14·4
	1942	50·9	18·0	18·7	13·2	11·4	9·7	7·9	17·0
	1943	31·4	21·3	20·3	15·0	12·7	12·4	11·4	18·7
	1944	68·2	26·2	19·9	19·3	13·6	12·9	11·6	22·1
	1945	30·8	24·2	14·8	14·3	13·1	12·6	11·3	17·8
Skin	1939	—	—	—	—	—	—	—	19·5
	1940	—	—	—	—	—	—	—	20·3
	1941	58·2	30·2	24·9	20·3	16·8	17·6	12·6	26·7
	1942	98·9	33·3	28·0	23·3	21·9	19·7	14·0	30·3
	1943	41·5	31·0	25·4	21·5	20·6	18·4	15·1	26·6
	1944	71·1	34·8	23·8	26·0	25·0	19·7	17·4	29·6
	1945	52·3	35·1	17·9	21·6	23·1	19·2	15·3	25·9

TABLE 14(a)—(*contd.*)

R.A.F. Incidence of Sickness and Injury Analysed by Age Groups, 1939–45

		Incidence per 1,000 per annum							
		Under 20	20 to 24	25 to 29	30 to 34	35 to 39	40 to 44	45 and Over	Average Whole Force
All Other Diseases and Effects of Heat	1939	—	—	—	—	—	—	—	10·6
	1940	—	—	—	—	—	—	—	11·5
	1941	22·8	13·2	13·2	13·2	13·8	18·3	24·8	14·2
	1942	34·4	17·1	18·7	16·8	16·7	17·8	23·7	18·0
	1943	18·8	21·2	22·6	17·9	17·6	18·4	23·4	20·1
	1944	36·2	26·1	20·9	21·7	20·7	20·6	26·7	23·6
	1945	41·4	30·5	20·3	26·5	23·4	23·8	25·6	26·0
Totals of All Diseases	1939	—	—	—	—	—	—	—	311·0
	1940	—	—	—	—	—	—	—	374·1
	1941	624·5	327·3	330·1	287·9	263·9	323·2	359·5	332·7
	1942	1,010·5	376·0	385·8	326·4	313·9	312·5	355·8	379·0
	1943	677·7	471·3	451·6	372·9	359·5	360·9	446·9	439·6
	1944	1,288·3	525·3	430·8	417·9	395·9	361·1	426·2	480·5
	1945	843·2	463·8	288·7	349·6	344·7	313·0	331·7	380·6
INJURIES	1939	—	—	—	—	—	—	—	46·0
	1940	—	—	—	—	—	—	—	61·1
	1941	75·7	58·5	51·5	35·2	28·9	29·9	30·9	49·4
	1942	98·4	57·2	60·5	40·9	31·8	29·0	27·9	51·3
	1943	74·9	65·7	63·8	50·8	43·5	39·2	43·3	58·4
	1944	145·4	79·8	69·0	65·8	53·2	46·4	43·9	70·4
	1945	76·9	61·1	38·5	37·4	34·2	29·5	22·2	45·2
Totals of All Disabilities	1939	—	—	—	—	—	—	—	356·9
	1940	—	—	—	—	—	—	—	435·2
	1941	700·2	385·8	381·6	323·1	292·8	353·1	390·4	382·1
	1942	1,108·9	433·2	446·3	367·3	345·7	341·5	383·7	430·3
	1943	752·6	537·0	515·4	423·8	403·0	400·1	490·2	498·0
	1944	1,433·7	605·1	499·8	483·7	449·0	407·5	470·1	550·9
	1945	920·1	524·9	327·2	386·9	378·9	342·5	353·9	425·8

TABLE 14(b)

R.A.F. Incidence of Diseases and Injuries by Age Groups
1939–1945
Rates per 1000 of Strength per annum

AGE GROUPS		under 20	20–24	25–29	30–34	35–39	40–44	45 and over	Average whole Force
*1939	All diseases	1049·3	242·3	230·5	193·7	226·3	176·9	241·4	317·3
	All injuries	106·0	39·9	37·1	31·6	27·7	25·9	32·4	43·9
	All disabilities	1155·3	282·2	267·6	225·3	254·0	202·8	273·8	361·2
*1940	All diseases	630·9	325·1	343·6	378·3	362·5	345·4	397·5	371·1
	All injuries	72·3	53·6	57·5	49·1	39·7	39·4	40·2	54·3
	All disabilities	703·2	378·7	401·1	427·4	402·2	384·8	437·7	425·4
1941	All diseases	624·5	327·3	330·1	287·9	263·9	323·2	359·5	332·7
	All injuries	75·7	58·5	51·5	35·2	28·9	29·9	30·9	49·4
	All disabilities	700·2	385·8	381·6	323·1	292·8	353·1	390·4	382·1
1942	All diseases	1010·5	376·0	385·8	326·4	313·9	312·5	355·8	379·0
	All injuries	98·4	57·2	60·5	40·9	31·8	29·0	27·9	51·3
	All disabilities	1108·9	433·2	446·3	367·3	345·7	341·5	383·7	430·3
1943	All diseases	677·7	471·3	451·6	372·9	359·5	360·9	446·9	439·6
	All injuries	74·9	65·7	63·8	50·8	43·5	39·2	43·3	58·4
	All disabilities	752·6	537·0	515·4	423·7	403·0	400·1	490·2	498·0
1944	All diseases	1288·3	525·3	430·8	417·9	395·9	361·1	426·2	480·5
	All injuries	145·4	79·8	69·0	65·8	53·1	46·4	43·9	70·4
	All disabilities	1433·7	605·1	499·8	483·7	449·0	407·5	470·1	550·9
1945	All diseases	843·2	463·8	288·7	349·6	344·7	313·0	331·7	380·6
	All injuries	76·9	61·1	38·5	37·4	34·2	29·5	22·2	45·2
	All disabilities	920·1	524·9	327·2	386·9	378·9	342·5	353·9	425·8

* Figures for 1939 and 1940 are for airmen only. Strengths for officers in the different age groups were not available.

There is an interesting contrast between the age distributions of AMOEBIC and BACILLARY DYSENTERIES; amoebic dysentery shows its greatest incidence in the middle age groups and its least at the extremes whereas bacillary dysentery has its highest incidence in the under 20 age group and steadily and progressively decreases with increasing age. Amoebic dysentery is almost entirely confined to tropical countries and as a smaller percentage of men under 20 and men over 45 were sent abroad than men in the middle age groups the higher incidence in the latter is not unexpected. Similarly, although bacillary dysentery occurs in all climates its greater prevalence in local populations abroad and the poor hygienic conditions existing abroad, would also lead one to expect a higher incidence in the middle age groups. An attack of bacillary dysentery does not confer immunity to further attacks. Following an attack, there is an increase in specific antibodies in the blood but, unlike the enteric fevers, the site of infection is local in the intestinal mucosa and antibodies can play little part in preventing infection. Only in B. *Shiga* infections do antibodies play any part in reducing the severity of the disease. It is probable that the explanation of the decreasing incidence with age lies in the improved hygienic standards which normally accompany experience of life abroad. Amoebic dysentery, on the other hand, shows a tendency to relapse and many cases recorded in the older age groups must represent recurrences.

MALARIA shows its greatest incidence in the 20–24 age group with a progressive decrease in incidence with age. The lower incidence in the under 20 age group is because relatively fewer of this group were sent abroad. Immunity in malaria, unlike bacterial infections, is dependent on the continued presence of the malaria parasite in the body. This type of immunity is called premunition; once the parasites have left the body premunition gradually disappears. The immunity is specific for homologous strains and fresh infection can occur with heterologous strains. Increasing experience of tropical conditions and of the value of prophylactic measures would also be factors in the decreasing incidence with age.

The incidence of ENTERIC FEVER remained at a very low level in all age groups and in only one instance did the rate rise above 1 per 1,000 of strength—in 1942 in the under 20 age group when the incidence was 1·2 per 1,000.

ENTERITIS showed a high incidence in all age groups in the early years of the war but fell considerably from 1943 onwards. There is a general tendency to increased incidence in the younger age groups.

The miscellaneous group OTHER INFECTIONS follows the general trend in showing the highest incidence in the under 20 age group and then decreasing incidence with age. This applies also to the group of SEPTIC INFECTIONS.

The usual history of PEPTIC ULCER was not belied by the experience of the R.A.F. and there was a steadily increasing incidence with age. It must be remembered, however, that peptic ulcers are very rarely cured and as no distinction is made between fresh cases and recurrent cases, the older age groups would tend to show a far greater proportion of recurrent cases than the younger age groups. In other words, the figures for the different age groups do not represent the absolute incidence of new cases of peptic ulcer in any one year but are made up of new and recurrent cases. (*See* also under 'Sickness as a Whole', p. 526.)

The heading OTHER CONDITIONS OF THE ALIMENTARY TRACT covers a vast number of different diseases and includes such common conditions as appendicitis and hernia. There is a high incidence in the under 20 age group but the other groups show a fairly constant rate.

The lowest incidence of CIRCULATORY SYSTEM DISORDERS is in the age group 20–24. The higher incidence in the age group under 20 is possibly due largely to two factors:

(a) A not inconsiderable number of men with organic disease of the heart may have been passed fit by the National Service Medical Boards and their disability not discovered until later when they developed symptoms or on routine medical examination by R.A.F. medical officers.

(b) The after-effects of rheumatic fever. Rheumatic fever is primarily a disease of recruits, apprentices and boy entrants.

After the age of 30 there was a rapid increase in the incidence of circulatory system disorders with increasing age.

PLEURISY WITH EFFUSION is classified with no reference to aetiology. It is probable that most of the cases with no evident underlying pathology at the time were, in fact, due to pulmonary tuberculosis. The highest incidence is in the under 20 age group.

OTHER CONDITIONS OF THE RESPIRATORY TRACT have their highest incidence in the under 20 age group and in the over 45 group. These two groups represent the chief sufferers from acute respiratory conditions in the first instance and chronic conditions in the second.

Apart from a slightly higher incidence in the under 20 age group DISEASES OF ALLERGY show no special predilection for any particular age group.

The groups of diseases of the URINARY SYSTEM and the GENERATIVE SYSTEM contain a large number of common conditions and there is little to be gained by attempting to relate them to age, for there are no considerable differences between the age groups.

The RHEUMATIC GROUP OF DISEASES are all conditions which, in common experience, are more prevalent in the older age groups and this is borne out by the R.A.F. figures. These remarks apply also to the LOCOMOTOR SYSTEM conditions.

War-time conditions provided a fruitful breeding ground for the PSYCHONEUROSES. Incidence was highest in 1943 and 1944 and there is an increasing incidence with age. This may be correlated with the increasing stress and strain associated with the greater responsibility of higher rank and with the added worries of home and family.

Cases of PSYCHOSES AND PSYCHOPATHIC PERSONALITY showed no increase in incidence with age. In the development of psychoses a man's predisposition and past history are more important than psychological factors such as harrowing emotional experiences or heavy responsibilities.

The higher incidences of MENTAL DEFECTS and EPILEPSY in the under 20 age group probably represent the unavoidable number of such men who, withholding any history, are passed as fit by the entry medical boards and are detected soon after enrolment.

Organic NERVOUS DISEASES show their highest incidence in the over 45 age group and there is a progressive increase in incidence with age.

EAR, NOSE AND THROAT conditions show a decreasing incidence with increasing age. In common with other infections, there is a markedly higher incidence in the under 20 age group. Here again, large numbers of recruits were found to be suffering from chronic ear conditions which had not been commented on by the National Service Medical Boards.

SKIN CONDITIONS follow the trend of infections in general and show a decreasing incidence with age.

INJURIES were most common in the under 20 age group and there is a progressive decrease with age.

Incidence of Sickness and Injury among Officers, Airman Aircrew and Ground Personnel, 1939–45

Tables 15(a) and 15(b) record the incidence of sickness and injury among General Duties officers, non-flying officers, airman aircrew and airman ground personnel. For the years 1939 to 1941 disease and injury among airmen were analysed by trade groups and these years are shown in Table 15(a). The practice of separating the trade groups ceased in 1941 and from then on the only distinction was between airman aircrew and airman ground personnel (Table 15(b)).

The General Duties (G.D.) branch of officers includes all those officers with aircrew qualifications. The majority of officers in this branch were engaged in active flying duties during the war but there were G.D. officers whose duties were mainly administrative. Among airman aircrew, a smaller proportion were confined to ground duties.

These tables are not reliable for a comparison of sickness rates in the various groups as they cannot be standardised for age. Many of the apparent differences are due to differences in the age structures of the groups.

The stress of flying, the long hours involved, the physical hardship and the extremes of heat and cold make it not surprising that there was a higher sickness rate among flying personnel than among ground personnel. This is particularly evident in the incidence of UPPER RESPIRATORY TRACT INFECTIONS where aircrew show a persistently higher sickness rate than ground personnel. One factor which must be taken into account here is that far more attention was paid to upper respiratory tract infections in flying personnel than in ground personnel. Squadron medical officers would forbid men with colds to fly, often against the man's own wishes, and this policy tended to swell disproportionately the sickness rates in flying personnel. (*See R.A.F. Medical Services* Vol. II, p. 71.) The highest rate of upper respiratory tract infections was in airman aircrew, and in 1943 this rose to 203 cases per 1,000 of strength.

The distinction between flying and ground personnel is less clear cut in PNEUMONIA rates. Airman aircrew showed a consistently higher incidence than airman ground personnel, particularly in 1944 when the ratio was 10 per 1,000 for airman aircrew to 6 per 1,000 for ground personnel. There was virtually no difference between the incidences for G.D. officers and officers of other branches.

There was little difference in the TUBERCULOSIS incidence in the four groups. The highest incidence again was in airman aircrew and in this group there were nearly 5 cases per 1,000 of strength in 1943.

VENEREAL DISEASE rates were higher among airmen than among officers. All groups showed a rising incidence as the war progressed.

TABLE 15(a)

R.A.F. Incidence of Diseases in the Various Trade Groups, 1939–41

		Officers		Airman aircrew	Aircraft-hands	Apprentices and boys	Clerks and office workers	Domestic, medical and welfare trades and instructors	Drivers and open air workers	Fitters	Metal workers	Wireless operators, riggers and armourers	Workshop workers	Average, Total Force
		General duties	Non-Flying											
DISEASES:														
Upper respiratory tract infections	1939	99·2	82·2	55·5	131·2	339·4	89·6	109·7	75·9	79·3	68·2	159·7	73·4	116·1
	1940	209·1	168·9	153·0	118·5	564·8	132·8	160·3	167·4	135·0	99·7	249·8	111·7	146·3
	1941	158·1	111·8	96·8	90·8	163·8	99·1	116·4	108·6	110·8	78·6	165·4	80·0	101·1
Pneumonia, acute primary	1939	0·9	2·0	1·2	2·3	4·0	2·5	2·2	2·3	1·7	0·8	3·6	1·2	2·1
	1940	3·1	4·1	2·6	3·7	8·6	3·3	3·8	3·4	2·9	2·4	7·7	2·2	3·7
	1941	5·3	5·0	3·5	4·8	5·0	3·7	5·7	3·3	3·7	2·4	7·1	3·3	4·3
Tuberculosis, all types	1939	0·5	0·6	0·5	1·5	0·9	1·1	1·2	1·9	1·3	1·6	2·1	1·7	1·3
	1940	1·0	1·1	0·9	1·8	0·4	1·4	2·9	2·6	1·4	0·9	3·4	1·6	1·7
	1941	2·0	2·0	0·4	2·4	1·4	2·4	1·9	1·5	2·0	1·6	3·1	1·5	2·1
Venereal diseases	1939	6·5	1·4	7·9	8·6	0·5	9·8	7·0	12·7	12·7	9·8	12·5	11·3	9·2
	1940	9·1	1·3	7·3	6·7	—	8·1	7·6	14·7	11·8	6·0	10·2	6·7	8·1
	1941	15·0	2·2	6·9	7·2	0·9	6·0	9·1	12·9	11·3	6·6	13·6	6·7	8·4
Other infections	1939	43·2	28·4	23·3	55·7	118·2	36·7	40·6	32·7	36·2	19·9	68·9	31·6	47·9
	1940	102·9	49·2	72·9	48·2	150·3	60·4	61·2	47·0	47·0	28·0	88·7	45·7	55·8
	1941	90·3	45·6	40·3	33·4	42·6	56·1	50·4	43·6	55·0	21·8	101·8	50·8	45·1
Septic conditions	1939	11·7	12·8	7·4	18·6	28·7	16·0	17·0	17·6	21·3	13·0	25·3	15·2	18·3
	1940	13·6	11·4	14·7	18·0	31·4	15·9	30·0	24·0	26·3	16·4	34·0	18·1	20·3
	1941	19·6	13·2	12·6	16·3	13·3	17·7	26·0	23·8	26·8	18·0	30·9	17·9	19·3
Alimentary system														
Gastric and duodenal ulcers and their complications	1939	1·3	3·4	0·5	3·3	—	2·3	3·8	8·2	3·1	3·3	3·3	3·9	3·0
	1940	3·2	6·6	1·3	3·6	0·9	2·7	5·9	7·4	3·3	6·1	7·7	3·5	4·0
	1941	3·6	6·2	0·9	5·0	—	4·9	4·7	6·6	3·7	6·5	6·2	3·0	4·5
Other conditions	1939	22·3	19·0	10·0	26·3	22·4	21·7	28·6	28·7	23·3	21·1	31·7	22·4	23·9
	1940	26·9	27·4	17·7	27·2	27·6	23·2	37·8	35·6	28·8	24·1	41·9	24·6	28·0
	1941	35·3	27·8	13·9	29·0	16·0	29·5	36·3	34·8	31·0	32·1	47·6	26·3	29·4
Circulatory system	1939	1·8	2·8	0·8	4·6	3·3	2·5	6·2	6·1	3·9	2·8	4·7	4·6	3·9
	1940	1·7	5·6	1·9	5·5	8·2	4·1	6·0	8·4	4·3	6·4	8·6	3·9	5·2
	1941	2·9	5·6	1·8	6·1	0·5	6·2	7·5	6·4	5·2	8·0	8·8	4·1	5·6
Respiratory system	1939	5·4	13·4	3·7	13·7	9·1	7·8	12·4	16·0	6·9	7·3	11·0	7·7	10·1
	1940	12·1	22·3	10·4	14·2	14·6	11·3	17·8	21·6	11·8	15·1	25·1	10·0	14·6
	1941	13·3	13·6	7·5	12·5	5·9	11·3	14·0	11·9	9·7	13·7	19·8	9·9	11·8
Allergy, diseases of	1939	0·7	1·7	0·3	2·6	0·4	3·0	2·0	4·1	1·7	3·2	2·8	2·3	2·1
	1940	2·1	1·7	1·1	2·6	1·6	2·4	2·1	3·1	2·3	1·8	3·5	1·9	2·4
	1941	3·3	1·8	1·6	2·4	0·5	3·2	2·7	3·2	2·3	2·7	5·1	2·3	2·6
Urinary system	1939	3·0	7·3	2·4	4·5	4·5	4·5	6·0	5·0	4·8	3·2	5·0	3·2	4·4
	1940	4·3	3·9	3·1	3·5	5·3	4·4	6·7	5·8	4·9	3·7	6·5	3·4	4·2
	1941	5·9	5·1	3·1	4·0	1·8	5·3	6·0	5·1	4·5	4·5	7·5	4·5	4·5
Generative system	1939	4·2	2·5	2·7	5·2	1·9	4·8	5·0	6·4	6·0	4·1	8·5	5·4	5·1
	1940	8·6	3·3	5·0	4·8	2·7	5·5	6·8	8·1	8·1	5·7	9·0	5·3	6·0
	1941	13·9	4·8	4·7	5·6	1·8	6·2	6·3	7·9	8·3	5·0	12·3	5·7	6·5
Locomotor system														
Rheumatic group of diseases	1939	2·5	5·0	1·0	3·3	1·8	3·5	4·6	4·3	3·6	4·1	5·2	5·2	3·5
	1940	3·6	7·3	1·8	4·6	3·1	4·8	6·8	8·6	4·3	4·9	8·9	4·2	5·0
	1941	7·4	6·7	2·1	4·3	0·9	4·5	5·9	7·2	4·6	8·2	6·2	4·1	4·7
Others	1939	6·2	3·9	3·4	7·1	6·8	5·0	4·2	8·8	8·4	8·1	7·5	6·6	6·8
	1940	6·9	7·5	5·3	8·3	6·6	6·2	9·7	13·0	8·6	11·3	11·8	7·6	8·5
	1941	13·3	7·4	7·7	9·7	4·6	8·1	11·2	13·6	10·4	14·4	7·5	7·8	9·7

Nervous system and mental diseases														
Psychoneuroses	1939	2·9	5·9	1·1	3·0	0·4	3·3	3·0	5·5	1·9	0·8	3·6	2·9	2·8
	1940	9·5	11·7	4·1	5·1	2·4	4·4	4·5	8·1	3·4	4·9	7·9	3·1	5·3
	1941	18·8	12·2	6·6	6·7	0·5	6·6	7·2	7·0	4·8	8·6	6·4	4·2	6·6
Psychoses	1939	0·3	2·2	0·1	1·2	0·3	0·9	0·4	1·1	0·9	0·4	1·6	0·6	0·9
	1940	0·2	2·1	1·3	1·1	—	0·8	1·0	1·1	0·5	0·6	0·1	0·9	0·9
	1941	0·9	0·9	0·1	1·1	—	0·9	0·7	0·7	0·7	0·9	0·8	0·8	0·8
Psychopathic personality	1939	0·3	0·3	0·1	1·2	0·5	0·5	0·6	0·3	0·3	—	0·3	—	0·6
	1940	1·0	1·7	0·3	1·1	0·2	0·4	1·4	0·8	0·4	0·4	0·9	0·4	0·8
	1941	0·2	0·6	0·2	1·1	0·5	0·9	1·0	0·8	0·6	2·8	0·8	0·5	0·8
Mental defect	1939	—	—	—	0·1	—	—	—	—	0·1	—	—	—	0·1
	1940	—	—	—	0·2	—	—	—	—	—	—	0·1	—	0·1
	1941	—	—	—	0·6	—	—	0·1	0·1	0·02	0·2	0·03	—	0·3
Epilepsies	1939	0·3	0·3	0·3	1·7	0·4	0·7	1·2	0·1	0·9	1·2	0·8	0·5	1·0
	1940	0·2	0·1	0·5	1·5	—	0·6	1·1	0·9	0·8	0·2	0·1	1·1	1·0
	1941	1·2	0·3	0·3	1·7	—	0·7	1·0	0·6	0·7	1·0	1·1	1·0	1·1
I ndefinite aetiology	1939	0·8	1·1	0·7	1·5	1·5	1·1	1·6	1·6	1·3	2·4	1·9	1·4	1·4
	1940	2·1	1·3	1·4	1·5	1·1	1·4	1·7	1·8	1·3	1·5	2·2	1·1	1·5
	1941	1·2	0·9	1·5	1·8	1·8	2·0	1·3	1·7	1·6	1·8	2·3	1·2	1·7
Organic Nervous diseases	1939	2·2	4·5	1·2	2·7	1·3	2·8	3·6	4·3	2·7	2·0	2·7	2·9	2·6
	1940	2·6	5·6	1·8	2·3	0·9	2·6	3·3	4·5	2·6	3·1	3·6	2·5	2·7
	1941	3·7	5·2	1·2	2·5	0·5	2·3	3·2	4·8	2·6	4·3	3·0	2·1	2·7
Eye	1939	2·0	1·4	2·3	4·2	4·1	1·8	2·6	4·5	3·6	2·4	2·9	2·1	3·3
	1940	4·2	2·3	3·2	3·5	4·9	3·0	4·3	4·4	4·0	2·8	5·0	2·9	3·6
	1941	4·6	2·6	3·2	3·5	2·3	5·4	3·9	4·0	3·8	3·9	6·6	3·2	3·8
Ear, Nose and Throat	1939	14·6	8·7	5·4	10·2	26·3	9·5	11·2	10·6	10·2	6·9	13·9	6·3	11·0
	1940	21·9	11·3	12·0	10·7	38·7	10·0	15·0	12·3	12·4	8·2	31·3	9·1	13·1
	1941	34·9	13·2	12·3	13·0	12·8	13·9	16·0	14·8	15·8	13·3	25·5	11·1	14·4
Skin	1939	6·3	2·8	5·9	23·8	34·5	15·8	14·4	18·5	19·8	16·3	27·1	15·5	19·5
	1940	8·2	5·8	10·9	21·1	29·6	16·8	25·3	24·4	22·3	20·1	33·6	17·0	20·3
	1941	16·7	8·1	16·0	27·7	12·4	22·6	25·2	33·6	29·9	24·2	46·4	24·6	26·7
All other diseases and effects of heat	1939	5·8	7·3	4·8	11·2	14·2	11·3	9·8	11·4	9·9	4·9	12·6	8·3	10·0
	1940	9·7	11·7	8·9	10·2	13·9	10·5	17·6	13·5	10·7	9·3	17·1	7·9	11·0
	1941	19·0	14·8	9·1	13·4	4·6	16·3	18·8	15·3	15·4	13·4	21·6	12·5	14·2
Total of all diseases	1939	244·9	220·9	142·5	349·3	625·4	258·5	298·9	288·6	265·8	207·8	419·2	236·2	310·9
	1940	467·8	375·1	342·4	329·5	917·8	337·0	440·7	442·5	359·3	283·6	620·8	296·4	374·1
	1941	490·4	317·6	255·3	306·6	294·4	335·8	382·5	373·8	365·2	296·5	557·4	289·1	332·7
INJURIES	1939	91·0	27·6	64·0	35·3	37·8	31·2	35·4	51·0	49·6	35·3	72·0	35·6	46·0
	1940	303·9	36·2	188·1	32·1	27·2	27·8	49·2	69·7	55·3	35·6	76·2	39·0	61·1
	1941	338·0	29·9	144·4	26·8	22·9	25·6	36·0	59·3	47·8	32·9	62·8	30·5	49·4
Total of all Disabilities	1939	335·9	248·5	206·5	384·6	663·2	289·7	334·3	339·6	315·4	243·1	491·2	271·8	356·9
	1940	771·7	411·3	530·5	361·6	945·0	364·8	489·9	512·2	414·6	319·2	697·0	335·4	435·2
	1941	828·4	347·5	399·7	333·4	317·3	361·4	418·5	433·1	413·0	329·4	620·2	319·6	382·1

TABLE 15(b)

R.A.F. Incidence of Sickness and Injury among Officers, Airman Aircrew and Ground Personnel, 1942–45

		OFFICERS		AIRMEN		
		General duties branch	Other branches	Aircrew	Ground personnel	Average, Total Force
DISEASES						
Upper respiratory tract infections	1942	116·5	75·8	135·2	86·9	91·9
	1943	130·9	109·9	202·6	110·7	121·9
	1944	103·0	70·6	181·5	95·0	104·7
	1945	79·9	68·0	88·1	73·4	74·8
Pneumonia	1942	4·5	4·1	4·3	3·5	3·6
	1943	3·6	3·9	5·8	3·6	3·9
	1944	6·5	5·6	10·1	6·5	6·9
	1945	3·2	3·5	3·9	3·6	3·6
Tuberculosis, all types	1942	1·9	1·8	3·5	2·6	2·7
	1943	1·6	2·7	4·7	2·8	3·0
	1944	2·3	3·0	3·5	2·7	2·8
	1945	3·1	3·1	2·8	2·8	2·8
Venereal diseases	1942	11·9	2·4	10·9	10·4	10·2
	1943	8·6	2·6	12·2	12·1	11·6
	1944	11·4	5·2	17·7	20·0	18·6
	1945	14·1	10·7	23·4	24·3	23·0
Other infections	1942	74·4	59·6	58·1	62·2	61·9
	1943	77·3	77·5	68·6	76·3	75·5
	1944	75·2	85·6	82·0	83·9	83·4
	1945	36·6	49·8	32·8	44·7	43·4
Septic conditions	1942	18·7	13·3	22·4	24·9	24·1
	1943	14·0	15·7	24·4	27·6	26·4
	1944	17·7	21·3	28·0	34·3	32·2
	1945	13·9	18·0	18·6	27·2	25·2
Alimentary system						
Gastric and duodenal ulcers and their complications	1942	2·4	5·5	1·5	4·2	3·9
	1943	3·0	5·1	1·8	4·0	3·8
	1944	5·1	8·9	1·7	4·9	4·7
	1945	3·5	8·6	2·6	4·4	4·4
Other conditions	1942	41·8	41·4	35·4	45·0	43·8
	1943	45·0	50·0	44·4	52·6	51·3
	1944	48·6	53·9	54·2	58·9	57·7
	1945	42·4	56·3	42·3	50·7	49·8
Circulatory System	1942	3·5	5·9	3·3	7·1	6·6
	1943	3·1	7·5	3·2	6·8	6·3
	1944	3·0	10·3	3·3	7·5	6·9
	1945	4·4	9·7	3·1	7·0	6·6
Respiratory system	1942	15·8	17·9	14·6	16·6	16·4
	1943	14·9	21·5	19·3	19·2	19·2
	1944	19·5	19·7	28·2	24·0	24·1
	1945	8·6	19·5	14·7	17·5	16·9
Allergy, diseases of	1942	2·3	2·0	1·8	2·5	2·4
	1943	1·7	2·3	1·7	2·3	2·3
	1944	1·5	2·7	2·7	3·1	2·9
	1945	1·7	2·3	2·2	2·7	2·5
Urinary system	1942	5·1	3·6	4·6	5·0	4·9
	1943	3·7	6·5	3·4	5·8	5·5
	1944	4·5	7·1	3·4	6·8	6·3
	1945	2·7	6·2	4·1	5·7	5·4
Generative system	1942	6·2	7·6	6·0	7·5	7·4
	1943	10·0	4·6	7·7	8·1	7·9
	1944	7·0	4·2	7·7	8·8	8·4
	1945	4·7	6·2	5·2	7·2	6·8

TABLE 15(b)—(*contd.*)

R.A.F. Incidence of Sickness and Injury among Officers, Airman Aircrew and Ground Personnel, 1942–45

		OFFICERS		AIRMEN		
		General duties branch	Other branches	Aircrew	Ground personnel	Average, Total Force
Locomotor system						
Rheumatic group of diseases	1942	4·2	6·0	2·2	5·0	4·8
	1943	3·3	7·0	2·5	5·4	5·0
	1944	3·7	8·1	4·0	7·8	7·2
	1945	2·7	7·7	3·1	6·0	5·7
Other conditions .	1942	8·9	9·1	6·4	11·3	10·7
	1943	8·1	9·1	7·5	11·9	11·2
	1944	9·2	12·1	9·0	14·4	13·5
	1945	8·2	14·0	9·7	11·6	11·3
Nervous system and mental diseases						
Psychoneurosis . .	1942	12·6	9·5	5·8	7·2	7·2
	1943	9·7	9·5	6·9	7·3	7·4
	1944	15·0	14·4	9·3	8·8	9·4
	1945	8·5	11·7	9·1	8·2	8·5
Psychoses . .	1942	1·1	0·7	0·3	0·8	0·7
	1943	0·5	0·5	0·4	0·9	0·8
	1944	1·2	0·9	0·7	1·1	1·1
	1945	0·8	1·2	0·7	1·0	1·0
Psychopathic personality .	1942	0·6	0·8	0·4	0·9	0·9
	1943	0·7	1·0	0·7	1·2	1·1
	1944	0·1	1·3	1·3	2·3	2·0
	1945	0·1	0·7	1·2	2·1	1·8
Mental defect . .	1942	—	—	—	0·3	0·2
	1943	—	—	0·02	0·2	0·2
	1944	0·03	0·02	—	0·2	0·2
	1945	0·2	—	0·2	0·2	0·2
Epilepsies . .	1942	0·5	0·3	0·7	0·9	0·8
	1943	0·3	0·2	0·6	0·8	0·7
	1944	0·2	0·1	0·5	0·7	0·6
	1945	0·3	0·4	0·4	0·5	0·5
Indefinite aetiology .	1942	2·4	1·4	1·6	1·9	1·8
	1943	1·3	1·4	1·8	1·8	1·8
	1944	0·8	2·0	2·5	1·7	1·8
	1945	0·7	1·0	1·6	1·3	1·3
Organic nervous diseases .	1942	3·0	4·7	1·5	2·7	2·7
	1943	2·1	4·7	1·9	3·1	3·0
	1944	3·6	7·5	2·1	4·2	4·0
	1945	2·5	5·5	1·4	3·2	3·1
Eye .	1942	2·9	2·8	3·4	4·2	4·1
	1943	2·6	3·2	3·9	4·9	4·6
	1944	3·2	2·6	5·3	6·2	5·8
	1945	3·2	4·2	3·0	5·8	5·3
Ear, nose and throat . .	1942	30·5	13·0	23·3	16·1	17·0
	1943	26·7	16·3	27·5	17·3	18·7
	1944	30·9	18·7	35·0	19·8	22·1
	1945	22·7	14·6	19·1	17·4	17·8
Skin . . .	1942	14·5	10·9	27·6	31·9	30·3
	1943	12·0	11·8	23·5	28·3	26·6
	1944	15·7	14·3	27·0	31·6	29·6
	1945	14·3	16·1	22·2	27·7	25·9

TABLE 15(b)—(*contd.*)

R.A.F, Incidence of Sickness and Injury among Officers, Airman Aircrew and Ground Personnel, 1942–45

		OFFICERS		AIRMEN		
		General duties branch	Other branches	Aircrew	Ground personnel	Average, Total Force
All other diseases and unclassified conditions .	1942	24·0	18·2	13·6	18·4	18·0
	1943	18·9	21·0	15·9	20·7	20·1
	1944	20·2	22·5	19·9	24·4	23·6
	1945	31·1	24·7	25·0	25·9	26·0
Total of All Diseases . .	1942	410·2	318·3	388·4	380·0	379·0
	1943	403·7	395·4	492·7	435·7	439·6
	1944	408·8	402·5	540·5	479·6	480·5
	1945	322·3	373·3	349·4	388·6	380·6
INJURIES	1942	224·8	25·5	145·7	37·0	51·3
	1943	196·4	25·7	164·8	40·2	58·4
	1944	186·3	41·7	159·3	52·5	70·4
	1945	84·9	26·1	86·4	38·9	45·2
Total of All Disabilities .	1942	635·0	343·8	534·1	417·0	430·3
	1943	600·1	421·1	657·4	475·9	498·0
	1944	595·1	444·2	699·8	532·0	550·9
	1945	407·1	399·4	435·7	427·5	425·8

There was little difference between the rates for airman aircrew and airman ground personnel, but G.D. officers showed a considerably higher incidence than ground officers. The younger average age of G.D. officers, the 'devil-may-care' attitude engendered by the risks involved in their duties, the element of hero worship, the longer duty-free periods and the absence of marital ties were all factors in the greater incidence of venereal disease among G.D. officers. (*See R.A.F. Medical Services* Vol. II, p. 74.) The sudden rise in incidence among ground officers towards the end of the war is probably explained by the greater number serving abroad. In operational units, even those at home, ground staff showed a higher rate than in non-operational ones. It is hard to know why this should have been so, but it may have been due to the kind of example of the aircrews with whom they were working.

The composite table OTHER INFECTIONS shows little significant variation among the four groups. There was a considerable fall in incidence in all groups in 1945.

SEPTIC CONDITIONS were consistently lower among the officers but there was no significant difference between aircrew and ground personnel.

PEPTIC ULCER was most prevalent among officers on ground duties. The average age of these officers was greater than that of the G.D.

officers and furthermore any man who gave a past history suggestive of dyspepsia was never accepted for aircrew duties. Similarly, the incidence was higher among airman ground personnel than among airman aircrew. G.D. officers showed a consistently higher incidence than airman aircrew.

Other conditions of the ALIMENTARY SYSTEM showed little variation among the four groups.

Again correlated with average age, the incidence of CIRCULATORY DISTURBANCES was higher in ground personnel than in flying personnel. Diseases of the RESPIRATORY SYSTEM, URINARY SYSTEM, GENERATIVE SYSTEM, LOCOMOTOR SYSTEM and diseases of ALLERGY show no significant variations among the four groups except in so far as accounted for by age differences.

The incidence of PSYCHONEUROSES was higher among officers than among airmen and in the two officer groups the G.D. officers generally had the higher rate. There was little difference between airman aircrew and airman ground personnel. Flying stress accounts for the high incidence in G.D. officers and it was found that emotional tension was more important than physical fatigue. Exhaustion, air-sickness, cold, injury and the effects of altitude were subsidiary factors. The incidence was highest in operational commands and highest of all in Bomber Command. The subject of 'Flying Stress' is discussed more fully in R.A.F. Vol. II in this series, Chapter 1 (p. 122 ff.), while details of the relative incidence by crew category and by Commands is given in *Medicine and Pathology* (pp. 384–5).

PSYCHOSES occurred at a fairly constant rate of from 0·5–1·0 per 1,000 of strength for all groups.

PSYCHOPATHIC PERSONALITIES were found chiefly among the airman ground personnel. Men in the other groups had all been selected and medically screened and this tended to lower the number with such disorders in these groups. Similarly, men with mental defect are unlikely to progress beyond the airman ground personnel category.

EPILEPSY occurred slightly more frequently in airman ground personnel than in the other groups.

ORGANIC NERVOUS DISEASES are directly related to the average ages of the group; the highest rate is in the officers engaged on ground duties, followed by airman ground personnel, G.D. officers and airman aircrew.

EAR, NOSE AND THROAT conditions showed a consistently higher incidence among aircrew than among ground personnel. The importance of efficient hearing in aircrew is obvious and there was a tendency for aircrew to report sick (quite rightly) with ear complaints which would not have troubled ground personnel unduly. The same factors which led to a higher incidence of upper respiratory tract infections in aircrew also led to a high incidence of ear infections and sinusitis. The necessity for the constant wearing of earphones in aircraft was shown to be an important factor in causing and aggravating otitis externa. Otitic barotrauma—the effect on the eardrum of rapidly altering altitude without adequate compensation by the Eustachian apparatus—was a considerable cause of aural morbidity among aircrew.

Airmen in both groups had a higher incidence of SKIN DISEASE than officers. This is related to the poorer living conditions of airmen and the greater prevalence of such conditions as impetigo, scabies, tinea and pediculosis.

The INJURY RATE among aircrew was several times that of ground personnel. The highest incidence was among G.D. officers.

Final Invalidings in the R.A.F., 1939–45

Table 16 records the final invalidings from the R.A.F. during the war and shows the causes leading to invaliding, the total number of cases, the total number of invalidings, the invaliding rate per cent. of cases and the invaliding incidence per 1,000 of strength for each year. The figures refer to the total force. Any man serving overseas who required invaliding from the Service was first transferred to the United Kingdom before invaliding action could be taken.

The number of men invalided from the R.A.F. during the war years was 73,868. Of this number 72,459 or 98 per cent. were invalided as a result of disease and 1,140 or 1·5 per cent. as a result of injury.

The group of NERVOUS SYSTEM AND MENTAL DISEASES led to 24,807 invalidings or about one third of all invalidings. PSYCHONEUROSES were the most important cause of invaliding and were responsible for 16 per cent. of total invalidings due to disease. The invaliding incidence per 1,000 of strength due to psychoneuroses showed a considerable rise in 1941 and maintained this higher level for the remainder of the war. All psychiatric conditions had a high invaliding rate per cent. of cases.

ALIMENTARY SYSTEM DISEASES were responsible for 11,267 invalidings or 15 per cent. of the total invalidings due to disease. The majority of these were cases of PEPTIC ULCER.

Diseases of the LOCOMOTOR SYSTEM were also responsible for a large number of invalidings—8,252, representing 11 per cent. of the total invalidings due to disease. DEFORMITIES and DISEASES OF JOINTS were the most prominent conditions.

There were 6,362 invalidings due to PULMONARY TUBERCULOSIS and this represents an invaliding rate per cent. of cases of 83·1. TUBERCULOSIS IN OTHER SITES was responsible for 862 invalidings with an invaliding rate per cent. of cases of 43·9.

There were 5,025 invalidings due to diseases of the RESPIRATORY SYSTEM. BRONCHITIS was responsible for the majority of these cases.

The incidence of total invalidings due to disease rose from 7·9 per 1,000 of strength in 1939 to 14·9 per 1,000 of strength in 1941. It then remained fairly steady until 1945 when there was a further rise to 18·8 per 1,000 of strength. The end of the war against Germany (May 1945) and Japan (August 1945) undoubtedly influenced standards adopted by medical boards.

TABLE 16

Final Invalidings R.A.F., 1939–45 (War Period)

CAUSES OF INVALIDING	Number of Cases	Number of Invalidings	Invaliding Rate Per Cent. of Cases	INVALIDING INCIDENCE PER 1,000 OF STRENGTH						
				1939	1940	1941	1942	1943	1944	1945
DISEASES:										
Acute Infections	272,603	598	0·21	0·1	0·12	0·13	0·09	0·11	0·14	0·14
Tuberculosis, Pulmonary	7,652	6,362	83·14	0·6	1·01	1·00	1·42	1·50	1·39	1·28
Tuberculosis, Other Sites	1,963	862	43·91	0·2	0·18	0·21	0·19	0·16	0·16	0·18
Venereal Diseases	59,396	147	0·24	0·06	0·03	0·03	0·02	0·01	0·04	0·05
Septic Conditions	112,737	95	0·08	0·01	0·01	0·02	0·02	0·02	0·01	0·03
Alimentary System	222,643	11,267	5·06	0·8	1·60	2·84	2·58	1·98	1·99	2·79
Circulatory System	27,921	3,336	11·94	0·7	0·81	0·59	0·63	0·63	0·67	0·81
Blood, Blood-forming Organs, R.E. System	2,208	237	10·73	0·04	0·04	0·04	0·05	0·05	0·05	0·07
Respiratory System	79,228	5,025	6·34	0·7	0·91	0·83	0·94	0·92	1·16	1·30
Allergy	11,136	896	8·04	0·2	0·22	0·27	0·15	0·13	0·15	0·24
Urinary System	23,100	1,049	4·54	0·2	0·18	0·21	0·22	0·17	0·22	0·27
Generative System	32,702	155	0·47	0·04	0·02	0·01	0·04	0·02	0·03	0·05
Locomotor System	73,398	8,252	11·24	0·5	0·92	1·25	1·44	1·59	1·75	2·68
Other Minor Diseases and Conditions	501,671	—	—	—	—	—	—	—	—	—
Nervous System and Mental Diseases										
Psychoneuroses	33,201	12,065	36·33	0·6	1·23	2·59	2·59	2·28	2·38	3·24
Psychoses	3,146	2,375	75·49	0·5	0·49	0·48	0·45	0·43	0·50	0·55
Psychopathic Personality	5,556	4,531	81·55	0·5	0·55	0·61	0·59	0·66	1·30	1·52
Mental Defect	860	747	86·86	0·04	0·06	0·24	0·19	0·15	0·15	0·11
Epilepsies	3,304	1,995	60·38	0·7	0·60	0·68	0·44	0·34	0·30	0·26
Indefinite Aetiology	7,521	1,315	17·48	0·3	0·19	0·31	0·31	0·22	0·27	0·28
Organic Nervous Diseases	13,569	1,779	13·11	0·3	0·22	0·34	0·35	0·34	0·39	0·45
Total Nervous System and Mental Diseases	67,157	24,807	36·93	2·9	3·34	5·25	4·92	4·42	5·29	6·41

Eye	20,509	1,225	5·97	0·3	0·35	0·32	0·27	0·21	0·20	0·24
E.N.T.	79,165	4,677	5·90	0·4	0·53	1·40	1·19	0·77	0·66	1·17
Skin	120,538	1,335	1·10	0·1	0·07	0·15	0·21	0·24	0·29	0·54
Endocrine	2,407	408	16·95	0·06	0·08	0·08	0·05	0·06	0·09	0·13
Metabolism	1,325	527	39·77	0·1	0·07	0·08	0·11	0·10	0·11	0·14
Cysts and Tumours	9,455	595	6·29	0·06	0·08	0·11	0·13	0·11	0·14	0·13
Indefinite and General Conditions	63,286	604	0·96	0·05	0·05	0·05	0·07	0·13	0·22	0·16
Total Invaliding due to Disease	1,792,200	72,459	4·04	7·9	10·62	14·87	14·74	13·33	14·76	18·81
INJURIES:										
Multiple Injuries with Fractures	18,551	225	1·21	—	0·02	0·02	0·05	0·06	0·07	0·04
Multiple Burns	9,410	38	0·40	—	0·01	0·01	0·01	0·01	0·02	0·004
Other General Injuries	77,170	153	0·19	0·06	0·02	0·03	0·02	0·02	0·04	0·04
Eye	4,806	41	0·85	0·01	0·003	0·01	0·002	0·004	0·007	0·02
Other Head and Neck Injuries	30,298	107	0·35	—	0·03	0·03	0·02	0·01	0·02	0·03
Trunk	11,488	101	0·87	—	0·01	0·02	0·01	0·02	0·03	0·03
Upper Limbs	30,583	154	0·50	0·01	0·02	0·04	0·01	0·03	0·03	0·04
Lower Limbs	68,650	321	0·46	0·05	0·05	0·09	0·07	0·06	0·06	0·07
Total Invalidings due to Injury	250,956	1,140	0·45	0·13	0·15	0·25	0·19	0·21	0·28	0·28
UNALLOCATED CONDITIONS	6,319	269	4·25	—	—	—	0·03	0·03	0·09	0·13
Grand Total of Invalidings	2,049,475	73,868	3·60	8·3	10·77	15·12	14·96	13·57	15·13	19·22

Deaths in the Royal Air Force, 1939–45

Table 17 is an analysis of deaths over the war period by disease and injury groups for the total force. The number of cases, the number of deaths and the fatality rate per cent. of cases are shown and the incidence of deaths per 1,000 of strength for each year. The number of deaths from all causes in the various geographical areas are shown in Tables 1 and 2.

There were 74,797 deaths during the war, 71,093 being caused by injuries and 3,704 by disease.

Of the ACUTE INFECTIONS, the enteric fevers had the highest fatality rate; the 150 deaths from this cause represented a death rate of 8·1 per cent. of cases. There were only 125 deaths from malaria out of 74,717 cases.

TUBERCULOSIS caused more deaths than any other single disease—a total of 413 deaths from pulmonary tuberculosis and from tuberculosis in other sites. It must be remembered that most cases of tuberculosis were invalided from the Service after six months so that the mortality rate recorded here is not the true mortality rate.

As would be expected, diseases of the MYOCARDIUM had a high fatality rate of 23·2 per cent.

The number of deaths due to disease of the BLOOD VESSELS, a group which includes hypertension and varicose veins, is only 57. This is a misleading figure, however, as all deaths due to vascular lesions of the brain are included under Organic Nervous Diseases; many of these deaths must have been due primarily to hypertension.

The deaths recorded under diseases of the URINARY SYSTEM were mainly due to the various forms of nephritis.

The group CYSTS AND TUMOURS includes all malignant growths and was responsible for 388 deaths.

Deaths due to INJURIES are discussed on pages 549 et seq.

TABLE 17

R.A.F. Deaths During War Period

CAUSES OF DEATH	Number of Cases	Number of Deaths	Fatality Rate Per Cent. of Cases	INCIDENCE OF DEATHS PER 1,000 OF STRENGTH						
				1939	1940	1941	1942	1943	1944	1945
DEATHS DUE TO DISEASES:										
Acute Infections										
Enteric Group	1,845	150	8·13	—	0·003	0·02	0·06	0·05	0·02	0·02
Malaria	74,717	125	0·16	—	0·009	0·01	0·05	0·05	0·02	0·01
Staphylococcal and Streptococcal Infections	7,469	75	1·00	—	0·02	0·02	0·02	0·02	0·01	0·01
C.N.S. Infections	11,394	176	1·54	—	0·06	0·05	0·04	0·04	0·04	0·02
Other Infections	177,178	227	0·12	—	0·02	0·03	0·05	0·09	0·05	0·02
Pneumonia	19,553	232	1·18	0·01	0·09	0·07	0·05	0·06	0·03	0·03
Tuberculosis										
Pulmonary	7,652	296	3·86	—	0·07	0·05	0·08	0·06	0·06	0·06
Other Sites	1,963	117	5·96	0·01	0·03	0·03	0·03	0·02	0·02	0·03
Alimentary System										
Peptic Ulcer and Complications	17,775	128	0·72	0·03	0·05	0·03	0·03	0·02	0·02	0·02
Appendicitis	24,407	115	0·47	0·01	0·02	0·04	0·03	0·02	0·02	0·01
Others	180,461	331	0·18	0·03	0·07	0·07	0·09	0·08	0·07	0·04
Circulatory System										
Endocarditis and Valvular Disease	1,885	50	2·65	0·01	0·02	0·01	0·01	0·01	0·01	0·01
Myocardium	1,342	312	23·24	0·03	0·06	0·07	0·06	0·07	0·07	0·05
Others	4,717	35	0·74	—	0·02	0·01	0·01	0·01	0·004	0·001
Blood Vessels	19,977	57	0·28	0·02	0·03	0·01	0·005	0·01	0·01	0·01
Blood, Blood-forming Organs, Spleen and Reticulo-Endothelial System	2,208	129	5·84	0·01	0·02	0·03	0·02	0·03	0·03	0·03
Respiratory System	79,228	150	0·18	0·01	0·04	0·03	0·03	0·04	0·03	0·03
Urinary	23,100	100	0·43	0·01	0·009	0·03	0·02	0·02	0·02	0·02
Organic Nervous Diseases	13,569	336	2·47	—	0·08	0·07	0·08	0·08	0·08	0·05
Nervous System and Mental Diseases	53,588	31	0·05	—	0·02	0·02	0·003	0·01	0·002	0·003

TABLE 17—(*contd.*)

R.A.F. Deaths During War Period

CAUSES OF DEATH	Number of Cases	Number of Deaths	Fatality Rate Per Cent. of Cases	INCIDENCE OF DEATHS PER 1,000 OF STRENGTH						
				1939	1940	1941	1942	1943	1944	1945
Cysts and Tumours	9,455	388	4·10	0·01	0·07	0·06	0·07	0·09	0·10	0·08
All Other Diseases	1,049,717	144	0·01	0·04	0·02	0·21	0·21	0·21	0·02	0·02
Totals All Diseases	1,792,200	3,704	0·20	0·22	0·82	0·79	0·86	0·92	0·75	0·53
DEATHS DUE TO INJURIES:										
Missing, Presumed Dead	43,536	43,536	100·00	1·81	9·81	7·45	8·05	12·47	12·98	3·33
Multiple Injuries with Fractures	18,551	14,149	76·27	0·89	4·09	2·99	2·98	2·86	3·58	1·92
Multiple Injuries with Burns	6,884	6,256	90·87	0·58	1·51	1·42	1·52	1·63	1·24	0·65
Fractured Skull with Other Fractures	1,929	1,694	87·81	0·50	1·11	0·78	0·47	0·21	0·08	0·06
Multiple Missile Wounds	974	249	25·56	0·01	0·11	0·10	0·07	0·05	0·03	0·02
Generalised Burns	2,526	758	30·00	0·11	0·33	0·16	0·13	0·17	0·13	0·11
Drowning, Including Effect of Immersion	1,208	915	75·74	0·14	0·30	0·25	0·20	0·21	0·16	0·11
Others	29,523	406	1·37	0·04	0·11	0·08	0·08	0·09	0·10	0·06
Total General Injuries	105,131	67,963	64·64	4·07	17·43	13·22	13·49	17·68	18·30	6·26
Sites of Injury Causing Death										
Head	34,548	2,084	6·03	0·23	0·82	0·55	0·47	0·39	0·41	0·24
Neck	556	46	8·27	0·01	0·02	0·01	0·02	0·002	0·01	0·004
Chest	3,427	310	9·04	0·01	0·16	0·11	0·07	0·05	0·05	0·03
Back and Vertebral Column	4,906	187	3·81	0·01	0·07	0·05	0·04	0·05	0·03	0·02
Abdomen	1,172	199	16·97	—	0·10	0·06	0·05	0·03	0·03	0·02
Buttocks and Pelvis	1,983	43	2·16	0·01	0·02	0·03	0·005	0·01	0·004	0·003
Upper Limbs	30,583	24	0·07	—	0·01	0·02	0·001	0·003	0·005	0·001
Lower Limbs	68,650	152	0·22	0·02	0·10	0·08	0·03	0·01	0·02	0·01
Total of Injuries	250,956	71,008	28·29	4·37	18·72	14·13	14·17	18·23	18·85	6·58
UNALLOCATED CONDITIONS	6,319	85	1·34	—	0·01	0·005	0·04	0·02	0·01	0·02
Grand Totals—Diseases and Injury	2,049,475	74,797	3·64	4·59	19·55	14·92	15·07	19·17	19·61	7·12

II. THE WOMEN'S AUXILIARY AIR FORCE

Before the Women's Auxiliary Air Force was formed, a nucleus known as the Royal Air Force Companies existed in the Auxiliary Territorial Service and was identified by a blue shoulder flash. On June 28, 1939, the Women's Auxiliary Air Force was formed with the object of releasing man-power in the Royal Air Force wherever practicable by substituting women. Service was for a period of four years, but the personnel were not subject to military law and could, if they chose, resign from the Service. At the end of the four years they were allowed to take their discharge or enrol for the duration of the war, having declared their willingness to serve in any part of the United Kingdom or overseas. There was no medical examination on enrolment but recruits were required to furnish a satisfactory health certificate from their regular doctors. Age limits were from 18–43 years but individuals with service in the War of 1914–18 were eligible up to the age of 50.

At the beginning of the war all volunteers were embodied into the Service and were medically examined by Royal Air Force medical officers. The medical standards were the same as for airman recruits with appropriate modifications, that is, the standards accepted were Grade I, Grade II general service and Grade II home service only. All new volunteers were examined by Service medical officers at the Women's Auxiliary Air Force Centres opened for the purpose.

In the early years of the war W.A.A.F. personnel were accommodated in married quarters on stations or were billeted out. Further information may be obtained from the R.A.F. Vol. I in this Series, Chapter 9.

The average strength of the Women's Auxiliary Air Force during the war months of 1939 was 2,300, but the Force expanded rapidly and by 1943 the average strength was 178,689. Thereafter, there was a slight decrease in numbers to 173,066 in 1944 and a fall to an average strength of 142,045 in 1945.

Sickness in the W.A.A.F., 1939–45

Table 18 is an analysis of sickness in the W.A.A.F. during the war; the rates per 1,000 are also shown in diagram form in Chart 5. The table is constructed on the same lines as Table 1 and the R.A.F. figures are shown here for ease of comparison between the two forces; it should be noted, however, that in the war period of 1939 the numbers involved were so small that true comparison is not possible.

In 1940 there was a higher incidence of sickness in the W.A.A.F. than during any other war year and both the incidence of total sickness and that of sickness over 48 hours' duration were roughly double the corresponding figures for the R.A.F. However, the average number of days' treatment before return to duty was appreciably less in the W.A.A.F.

CHART 5

SICKNESS IN THE WOMEN'S AUXILIARY AIR FORCE, 1939–45

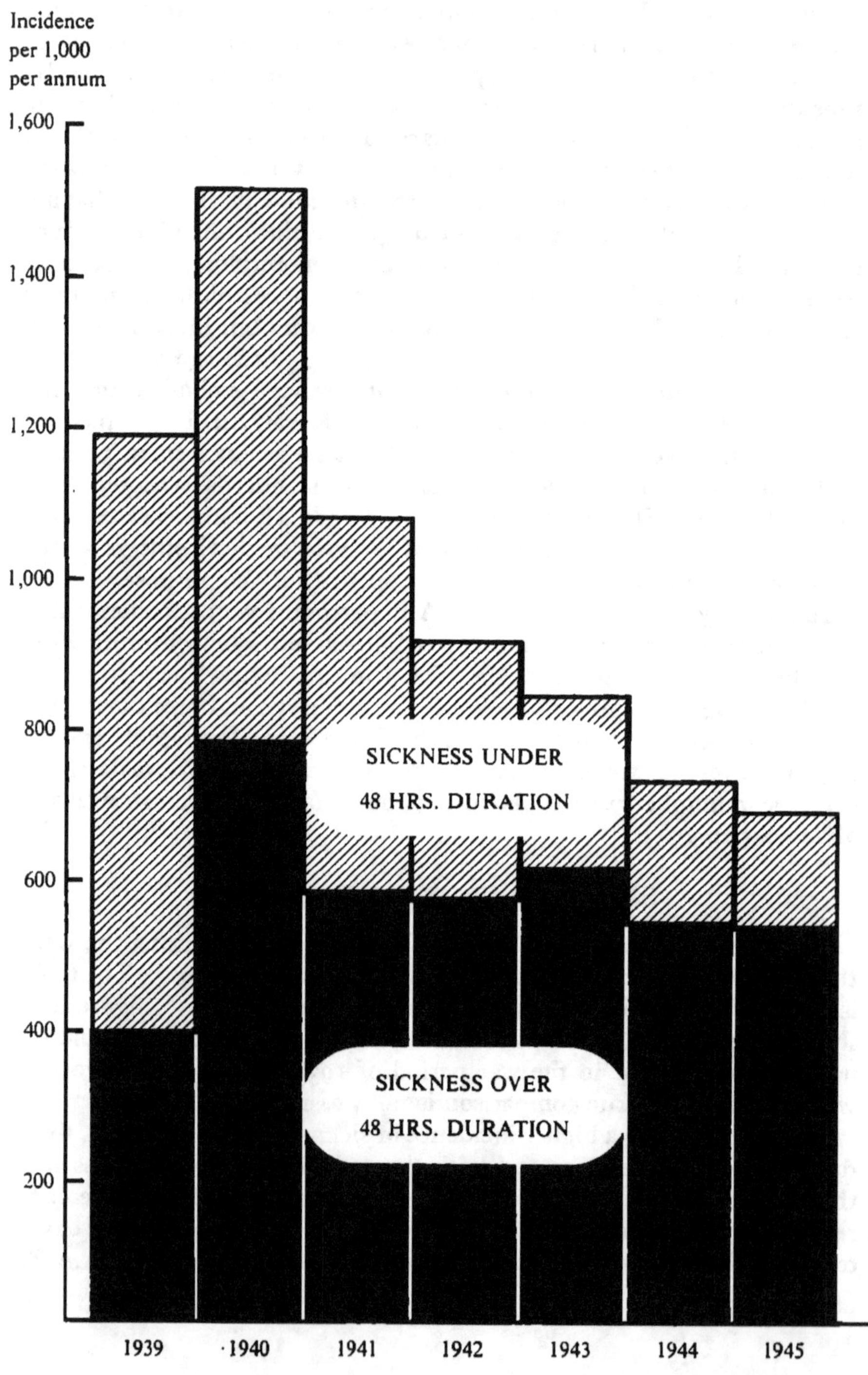

CHART 6

WOMEN'S AUXILIARY AIR FORCE.—NUMBER OF SICK DAILY PER 1,000 OF STRENGTH, 1939–45

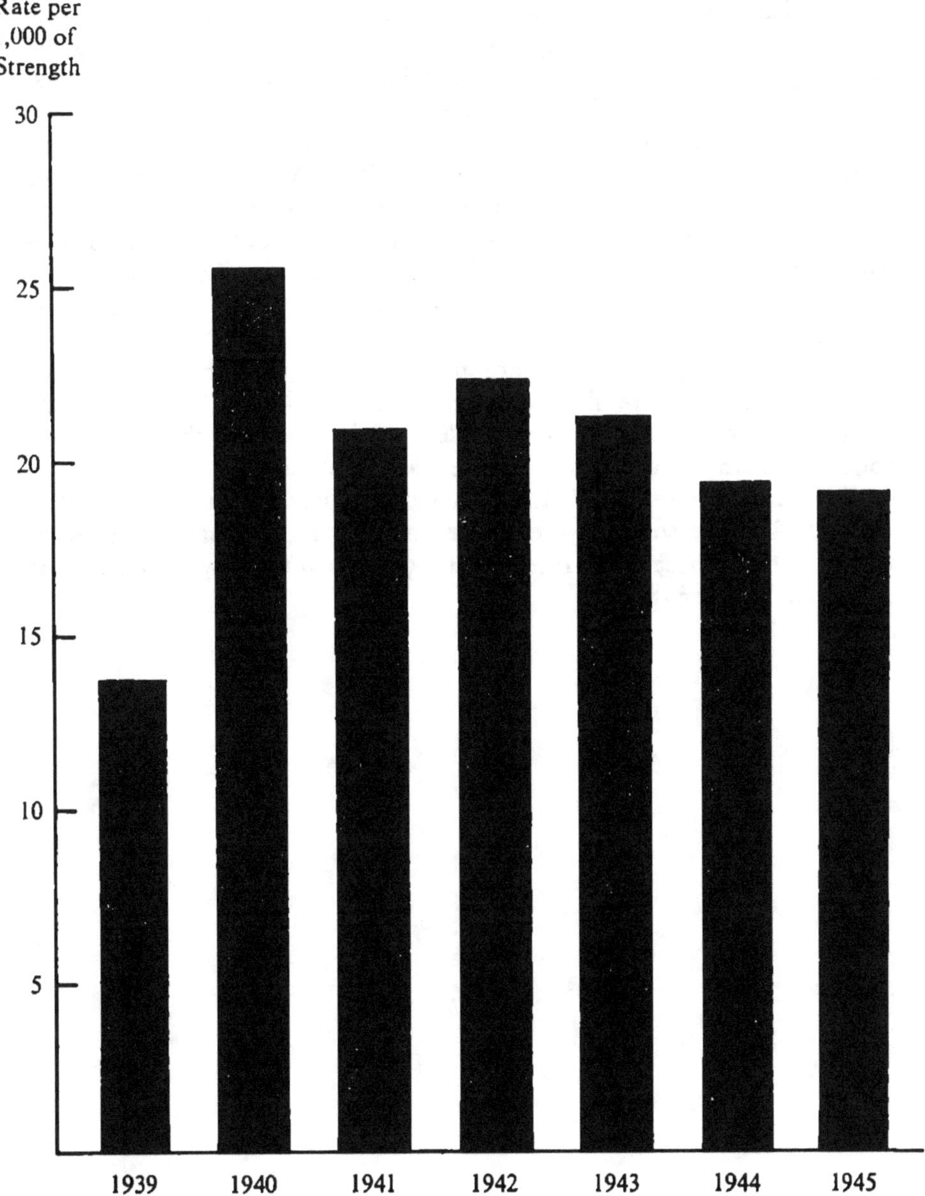

than in the R.A.F. and this may indicate a greater proportion of minor ailments in the W.A.A.F.

In 1941 there was a considerable fall in the incidence of total sickness and in the incidence of sickness over 48 hours' duration. This decrease in the incidence of total sickness was maintained throughout the remaining years of the war and in 1945 was 692 per 1,000 of strength compared with 1,512 per 1,000 in 1940. The incidence of sickness over 48 hours' duration showed little difference over the years 1941–45 and averaged 566 per 1,000 of strength. Although the incidence of sickness is consistently higher in the W.A.A.F. than in the R.A.F. the actual wastage as measured by the average number of days' sickness per head and by the number of sick daily (*see* also Chart 6) per 1,000 of strength was greater in the R.A.F. in 1943 and 1944. These were the years when a large proportion of the R.A.F. was serving overseas and when injuries tended to swell the sickness rates.

Final invaliding incidences are also shown in this table. The causes of final invaliding are shown separately in Table 23. Until 1941 the incidence of final invalidings was below the incidence in the R.A.F. but for the remaining war years the rate was higher than in the R.A.F.

The death rate in the W.A.A.F. never approached that in the R.A.F. as W.A.A.F. personnel were never engaged in primarily combatant duties. The highest death rate was in 1942 when there were 0·9 deaths per 1,000 of strength.

TABLE 18

Sickness in the Royal Air Force and the Women's Auxiliary Air Force, 1939–45

		1939	1940	1941	1942	1943	1944‡	1945‡
Average Strength	R.A.F.	140,862*	324,398	662,772	860,747	971,439	1,002,593	933,922
	W.A.A.F.	2,300*	13,085	48,182	127,781	178,689	173,066	142,045
TOTAL SICKNESS:								
Number of Cases	R.A.F.	96,649	259,015	421,576	568,130	708,494	766,079	572,212
	W.A.A.F.	2,731	19,788	51,813	117,097	148,807	125,468	98,274
Incidence per 1,000 of strength	R.A.F.	686	798	636	660	729	764	613
	W.A.A.F.	1,187	1,512	1,075	916	833	725	692
Average number of days' treatment before return to Duty	R.A.F.	8·2	9·5	9·5	9·5	9·5	10·8	10·0
	W.A.A.F.	4·3	6·3	6·5	8·0	8·6	8·9	10·3
Average number of days' sickness per head	R.A.F.	5·6	6·8	6·5	6·9	7·9	8·8	6·8
	W.A.A.F.	5·1	9·5	7·7	8·2	7·8	7·1	7·1
Number of sick daily per 1,000 of strength	R.A.F.	15·4	18·7	17·8	19·0	21·5	24·2	18·7
	W.A.A.F.	13·8	25·9	21·1	22·5	21·4	19·4	19·4
SICKNESS EXCLUDING CASES OF 48 HOURS AND UNDER:†								
Number of Cases	R.A.F.	50,276	141,170	253,225	370,388	483,813	552,303	397,644
	W.A.A.F.	910	10,286	27,961	73,127	107,909	93,170	75,794
Incidence per 1,000 of strength	R.A.F.	357	435	382	430	498	551	426
	W.A.A.F.	396	786	580	572	604	538	534
Average number of days' treatment before return to Duty	R.A.F.	14·4	14·5	15·1	14	14	15	14
	W.A.A.F.	10	11	11	12	12	12	12
Average number of days' sickness per head	R.A.F.	5·1	6·3	6·1	6·6	7·5	8·6	6·6
	W.A.A.F.	3·8	8·3	6·9	7·6	7·5	6·8	6·9
Number of sick daily per 1,000 of strength	R.A.F.	14·1	17·3	16·8	18·1	20·7	23·5	18·1
	W.A.A.F.	10·4	22·8	18·8	20·9	20·6	18·8	18·9
CASES OF SICKNESS OF 48 HOURS AND UNDER:	R.A.F.	46,373	117,845	168,351	197,742	224,681	213,776	174,568
	W.A.A.F.	1,821	9,502	23,852	43,970	40,898	32,298	22,480

TABLE 18—(*contd.*)

Sickness in the Royal Air Force and the Women's Auxiliary Air Force, 1939–45

		1939	1940	1941	1942	1943	1944‡	1945‡
FINAL INVALIDINGS:								
Numbers	R.A.F.	1,173	3,497	10,017	12,875	13,181	15,177	17,946
	W.A.A.F.	9	141	549	3,006	3,777	3,727	2,863
Incidence per 1,000 of strength	R.A.F.	8·3	10·8	15·1	15·0	13·6	15·1	19·2
	W.A.A.F.	3·9	10·8	11·4	23·5	21·1	21·5	20·2
DEATHS:								
Numbers	R.A.F.	950	6,343	9,892	12,973	18,625	19,665	7,758
	W.A.A.F.	3	8	34	119	129	138	104
Incidence per 1,000 of strength	R.A.F.	6·7	19·6	14·9	15·1	19·2	19·6	8·3
	W.A.A.F.	1·3	0·6	0·7	0·9	0·7	0·8	0·7

* Calculated strength for the year. † Includes cases resulting in death or invaliding, irrespective of duration.
‡ In 1944 and 1945 every case which resulted in death or invaliding was coded as usual. The statistics for all other cases were calculated from a ten per cent. random sample.

SICKNESS AS A WHOLE IN THE W.A.A.F., 1939–45

Table 19(a) is the main nosological table analysing the incidence of disease and injury for the war period. The number of W.A.A.F. personnel who served abroad was small and no separate table has been prepared for those who did go overseas. The arrangement of the table is similar to that of the nosological table for the Royal Air Force (Table (3a)) but an additional section relating to conditions peculiar to women has been included. The nosological table does not record cases of disease or injury of less than 48 hours' duration, except where these resulted in death or invaliding.

The disease groups shown in Table 19(b) have been extracted from the main nosological table and are arranged in descending order of incidence. The percentage contribution which each group makes to the total of all diseases is also shown.

As in the Royal Air Force, INFECTIONS OF THE UPPER RESPIRATORY TRACT form the largest single group. The highest incidence was in 1940 when there were 244 cases per 1,000 of strength. The winter of 1940 was severe. The two mild epidemics of influenza which affected the country as a whole in 1940 and 1943 are reflected in the influenza figures for the W.A.A.F.

OTHER INFECTIOUS DISEASES do not figure so largely in the W.A.A.F. tables as in the R.A.F. tables because so few W.A.A.F. personnel were called upon to serve abroad. Thus only a relatively insignificant number of tropical diseases are recorded. More than half the total of infectious diseases is made up of virus infections, mumps, measles, chicken pox and rubella being the common ones. (*See* Table 20, Certain Infectious Diseases in the W.A.A.F., 1939–45.)

PNEUMONIA was consistently less prevalent in the W.A.A.F. than in the R.A.F. The lowest incidence of all was in 1944 when the R.A.F. incidence was very high.

The incidence of TUBERCULOSIS tended to be higher than the incidence in the R.A.F. The average incidence of pulmonary tuberculosis in the W.A.A.F. over the whole war period was 2·46 cases per 1,000 of strength as against 1·8 cases per 1,000 in the R.A.F. The highest incidence was in 1942 when there were 3·22 cases per 1,000 of strength.

TABLE 19(a)

W.A.A.F. Nosological Table
Period of Second World War, September 3, 1939 to August 15, 1945—Fresh Cases

	1939*		1940		1941		1942		1943		1944		1945*		Totals	
	Number of Cases	Incidence per 1,000 per annum	Number of Cases	Incidence per 1,000 per annum	Number of Cases	Incidence per 1,000 per annum	Number of Cases	Incidence per 1,000 per annum	Number of Cases	Incidence per 1,000 per annum	Number of Cases	Incidence per 1,000 per annum	Number of Cases	Incidence per 1,000 per annum	Number of Cases	Incidence per 1,000 per annum
INFECTIOUS DISEASES:																
Amoebic Dysentery	—	—	—	—	—	—	6	0·05	4	0·02	—	—	30	0·31	40	0·06
Bacillary Dysentery	—	—	1	0·08	8	0·17	58	0·45	92	0·51	159	0·92	340	3·47	658	1·03
Enteric group	—	—	—	—	7	0·15	3	0·02	3	0·01	11	0·06	—	—	24	0·04
Enteritis	—	—	3	0·23	7	0·15	81	0·63	19	0·11	40	0·23	170	1·74	320	0·50
Malaria	1	0·4	1	0·08	2	0·04	5	0·04	10	0·05	10	0·06	10	0·10	39	0·06
Other Tropical Infections	1	0·4	—	—	5	0·10	14	0·11	29	0·16	49	0·28	141	1·44	239	0·37
Bacillary Infections (other than Typhoid and Dysentery)	2	0·9	12	0·92	79	1·64	152	1·19	213	1·19	138	0·80	100	1·02	696	1·09
Staphylococcal and Streptococcal Infections	3	1·3	21	1·60	118	2·45	254	1·99	362	2·03	311	1·80	100	1·02	1,169	1·82
Virus Infections	74	32·2	1,721	131·53	2,200	45·66	1,793	14·03	1,861	10·41	3,176	18·35	750	7·66	11,575	18·06
Metazoan Parasite Infections	1	0·4	1	0·08	4	0·08	42	0·33	50	0·28	19	0·11	20	0·20	137	0·21
Infections of Unknown or Doubtful Origin	5	2·2	31	2·37	128	2·66	1,019	7·97	874	4·89	544	3·14	313	3·20	2,914	4·55
Central Nervous System Infections	6	2·6	51	3·90	169	3·51	379	2·96	594	3·32	551	3·18	170	1·74	1,920	3·00
Totals	93	40·4	1,842	140·77	2,727	56·60	3,806	29·79	4,111	23·01	5,008	28·94	2,144	21·89	19,731	30·78
INFECTIONS OF RESPIRATORY TRACT:																
Common Cold, Nasopharyngitis and Sore Throat	114	49·6	1,227	93·77	3,259	67·64	10,506	82·22	16,333	91·40	10,937	63·20	6,280	64·12	48,656	75·90
Influenza	81	35·2	1,291	98·66	1,935	40·16	3,555	27·82	10,561	59·10	2,752	15·90	1,840	18·79	22,015	34·34
Tonsillitis	45	19·6	663	50·67	2,088	43·34	6,229	48·75	9,222	51·61	8,813	50·92	4,800	49·01	31,860	49·70
Vincent's Angina	2	0·8	16	1·22	181	3·76	652	5·10	732	4·10	539	3·11	230	2·35	2,352	3·67
Upper Respiratory Tract Infections—Totals	242	105·2	3,197	244·33	7,463	154·89	20,942	163·89	36,848	206·21	23,041	133·14	13,150	134·26	104,883	163·61

PNEUMONIA	4	1·7	23	1·77	137	2·84	446	3·49	441	2·47	204	1·18	185	1·89	1,440	2·25
PULMONARY TUBERCULOSIS	1	0·4	13	0·99	73	1·52	411	3·22	484	2·71	405	2·34	188	1·92	1,575	2·46
TUBERCULOSIS, OTHER THAN PULMONARY	—	—	13	0·99	39	0·81	118	0·92	189	1·06	99	0·57	49	0·50	507	0·79
VACCINIA AND POST-INOCULATION EFFECTS	—	—	64	4·89	216	4·48	198	1·55	392	2·19	358	2·07	50	0·51	1,278	1·99
CARRIERS	—	—	1	0·08	1	0·02	17	0·13	30	0·17	51	0·29	10	0·10	110	0·17
CONTACTS	2	0·9	16	1·22	17	0·35	71	0·56	111	0·62	59	0·34	10	0·10	286	0·45
VENEREAL DISEASES:																
Gonorrhoea	1	0·4	14	1·07	99	2·05	335	2·62	236	1·32	199	1·15	121	1·24	1,005	1·57
Syphilis	—	—	1	0·08	21	0·44	121	0·95	133	0·74	109	0·63	70	0·71	455	0·71
Syphilis with Gonorrhoea	—	—	—	—	9	0·19	—	—	23	0·13	10	0·06	6	0·06	48	0·07
Others	—	—	—	—	—	—	—	—	2	0·01	—	—	1	0·01	3	0·01
Totals	1	0·4	15	1·15	129	2·68	456	3·57	394	2·20	318	1·84	198	2·02	1,511	2·36
SEPTIC CONDITIONS, AREOLAR TISSUES, LYMPHATIC CHANNELS AND BREASTS:																
Conditions due to Pyogenic Organisms	34	14·8	378	28·89	1,477	30·65	3,965	31·03	5,339	29·88	5,300	30·62	2,612	26·67	19,105	29·80
Other Conditions	1	0·4	10	0·76	36	0·75	224	1·75	129	0·72	88	0·51	30	0·31	518	0·81
Totals	35	15·2	388	29·65	1,513	31·40	4,189	32·78	5,468	30·60	5,388	31·13	2,642	26·98	19,623	30·61
ALIMENTARY SYSTEM DISEASES:																
Dental Conditions	11	4·8	63	4·81	185	3·84	521	4·08	720	4·03	811	4·69	470	4·80	2,781	4·34
Mouth, Pharynx and Oesophagus	—	—	17	1·30	100	2·08	234	1·83	391	2·19	420	2·43	241	2·46	1,403	2·19
Gastric Ulcer and its Complications	25	10·9	5	0·38	5	0·10	52	0·41	32	0·18	10	0·06	36	0·37	165	0·26
Other Gastric Conditions	—	—	180	13·76	576	11·95	3,285	25·71	2,098	11·74	2,080	12·02	1,420	14·50	9,639	15·04
Duodenitis	—	—	—	—	6	0·12	12	0·09	9	0·05	3	0·02	12	0·12	42	0·06
Duodenal Ulcer and its Complications	—	—	—	—	20	0·42	41	0·32	110	0·62	51	0·29	53	0·54	275	0.43
Appendicitis, All types	43	18·6	247	18·80	839	17·41	2,010	15·73	2,356	13·18	1,705	9·85	1,310	13·38	8,510	13·28
Other Intestinal Conditions	19	8·3	243	18·57	886	18·39	1,470	11·50	3,923	21·95	4,423	25·56	3,684	37·61	14,648	22·85
Rectum and Anus	2	0·9	18	1·38	81	1·68	276	2·16	324	1·81	325	1·88	240	2·45	1,266	1·97
Hernia, All types	2	0·9	8	0·61	17	0·35	63	0·49	83	0·46	94	0·54	60	0·61	327	0·51
Liver and Gall Bladder	4	1·7	35	2·68	48	1·00	81	0·63	243	1·36	154	0·89	82	0·84	647	1·01
Peritoneum	—	—	1	0·08	1	0·02	20	0·16	12	0·07	4	0·02	42	0·43	80	0·12
Totals	106	46·1	817	62·44	2,764	57·37	8,065	63·12	10,301	57·65	10,080	58·24	7,650	78·11	39,783	62·06

* Figures for 1939 and 1945 are for the war periods of the years only *viz.* 1939—from September 3 to December 31; 1945—from January 1 to August 15.

TABLE 19(a)—(*contd.*)

W.A.A.F. Nosological Table
Period of Second World War, September 3, 1939 to August 15, 1945—Fresh Cases

	1939*		1940		1941		1942		1943		1944		1945*		Totals	
	Number of Cases	Incidence per 1,000 per annum	Number of Cases	Incidence per 1,000 per annum	Number of Cases	Incidence per 1,000 per annum	Number of Cases	Incidence per 1,000 per annum	Number of Cases	Incidence per 1,000 per annum	Number of Cases	Incidence per 1,000 per annum	Number of Cases	Incidence per 1,000 per annum	Number of Cases	Incidence per 1,000 per annum
CIRCULATORY SYSTEM DISEASES:																
Pericardium	—	—	—	—	1	0·02	1	0·01	1	0·01	2	0·01	—	—	5	0·01
Endocarditis and Valvular Diseases of the Heart	3	1·3	13	0·99	35	0·73	110	0·86	113	0·63	99	0·57	15	0·15	388	0·61
Myocardium	—	—	6	0·46	17	0·35	36	0·28	21	0·12	6	0·03	1	0·01	87	0·14
Cardiac Arrhythmias	—	—	9	0·69	24	0·49	53	0·41	63	0·35	30	0·17	12	0·12	191	0·30
Disordered Action of the Heart	2	0·9	24	1·83	115	2·39	310	2·43	324	1·81	298	1·72	173	1·77	1,246	1·94
Totals	5	2·2	52	3·97	192	3·98	510	3·99	522	2·92	435	2·51	201	2·05	1,917	2·99
Blood Vessels	4	1·7	40	3·06	129	2·68	297	2·32	674	3·77	721	4·17	544	5·55	2,409	3·76
Circulatory System Totals	9	3·9	92	7·03	321	6·60	807	6·32	1,196	6·69	1,156	6·68	745	7·61	4,326	6·75
BLOOD, BLOOD-FORMING ORGANS, SPLEEN AND RETICULO-ENDOTHELIAL SYSTEM:																
Anaemias	6	2·6	25	1·91	104	2·17	327	2·56	460	2·57	500	2·89	265	2·71	1,687	2·63
Leukaemias	—	—	—	—	—	—	1	0·01	11	0·06	—	—	2	0·02	14	0·02
Purpuras	—	—	1	0·08	3	0·06	7	0·05	9	0·05	3	0·02	1	0·01	24	0·04
Other Diseases of the Blood	—	—	1	0·08	—	—	5	0·04	10	0·06	1	0·01	1	0·01	18	0·03
Lymphatic Glands	—	—	1	0·08	6	0·12	14	0·11	21	0·12	30	0·17	22	0·22	94	0·15
Spleen and Reticulo-Endothelial System	1	0·4	—	—	1	0·02	6	0·04	9	0·05	2	0·01	11	0·11	30	0·05
Totals	7	3·0	28	2·14	114	2·37	360	2·82	520	2·91	536	3·10	302	3·08	1,867	2·91

RESPIRATORY SYSTEM DISEASES:																
Larynx and Trachea	24	10·4	247	18·88	435	9·03	4	0·03	1,515	8·48	1,366	7·89	770	7·86	4,361	6·80
Bronchi	84	36·5	560	42·80	1,344	27·89	2,003	15·68	4,189	23·44	3,995	23·08	2,613	26·68	14,788	23·07
Lungs	2	0·9	8	0·61	43	0·89	118	0·92	211	1·18	160	0·92	139	1·42	681	1·06
Pleura	3	1·3	31	2·37	93	1·93	296	2·32	301	1·68	252	1·46	181	1·85	1,157	1·80
Totals	113	49·1	846	64·65	1,915	39·75	2,421	18·95	6,216	34·79	5,773	33·36	3,703	37·81	20,987	32·74
ALLERGY, DISEASES OF:																
Asthma	3	1·3	21	1·60	118	2·45	419	3·28	428	2·40	446	2·58	198	2·02	1,633	2·55
Hay Fever	—	—	4	0·31	2	0·04	13	0·10	22	0·12	10	0·06	31	0·32	82	0·12
Urticaria	1	0·4	27	2·06	92	1·91	239	1·87	308	1·72	323	1·87	152	1·55	1,142	1·78
Others	3	1·3	11	0·84	31	0·64	21	0·16	42	0·24	61	0·35	11	0·11	180	0·28
Totals	7	3·0	63	4·81	243	5·04	692	5·42	800	4·48	840	4·85	392	4·00	3,037	4·74
URINARY SYSTEM DISEASES:																
Anomalies of Urinary Secretion	—	—	8	0·61	55	1·14	110	0·86	205	1·15	162	0·94	113	1·15	653	1·02
Nephritis, All Forms	—	—	4	0·31	24	0·50	81	0·63	57	0·32	67	0·39	20	0·20	253	0·39
Kidney	7	3·1	46	3·52	238	4·94	708	5·54	926	5·18	727	4·20	487	4·97	3,139	4·90
Urinary Calculi and Urinary Colic	3	1·3	7	0·53	24	0·50	83	0·65	42	0·24	107	0·62	72	0·74	338	0·53
Bladder	9	3·9	38	2·90	208	4·32	649	5·08	951	5·32	1,030	6·30	766	7·82	3,711	5·79
Ureter	—	—	3	0·23	11	0·23	15	0·12	18	0·10	—	—	—	—	47	0·07
Others	—	—	1	0·08	—	—	—	—	—	—	50	0·29	30	0·31	81	0·13
Totals	19	8·3	107	8·18	560	11·62	1,646	12·88	2,199	12·31	2,203	12·73	1,488	15·19	8,222	12·83

* Figures for 1939 and 1945 are for the war periods of the years only *viz.* 1939—from September 3 to December 31; 1945—from January 1 to August 15.

TABLE 19(a)—(*contd.*)

W.A.A.F. Nosological Table

Period of Second World War, September 3, 1939 to August 15, 1945—Fresh Cases

	1939*		1940		1941		1942		1943		1944		1945*		Totals	
	Number of Cases	Incidence per 1,000 per annum	Number of Cases	Incidence per 1,000 per annum	Number of Cases	Incidence per 1,000 per annum	Number of Cases	Incidence per 1,000 per annum	Number of Cases	Incidence per 1,000 per annum	Number of Cases	Incidence per 1,000 per annum	Number of Cases	Incidence per 1,000 per annum	Number of Cases	Incidence per 1,000 per annum
LOCOMOTOR SYSTEM DISEASES:																
Muscles	—	—	13	0·99	12	0·25	67	0·53	61	0·34	70	0·40	80	0·82	303	0·47
Fibrositis, Myalgia, Lumbago and Rheumatic Group	13	5·7	130	9·94	385	7·99	1,275	9·98	1,571	8·79	1,335	7·71	919	9·38	5,628	8·78
Deformities	3	1·3	33	2·52	87	1·81	334	2·61	314	1·76	300	1·73	121	1·24	1,192	1·86
Joints	6	2·6	83	6·34	219	4·55	485	3·80	991	5·55	688	3·98	366	3·74	2,838	4·43
Internal Derangement of Knee Joint	—	—	4	0·31	29	0·60	53	0·41	84	0·47	107	0·62	62	0·63	339	0·53
Bones and Cartilages	4	1·7	5	0·38	91	1·89	71	0·56	144	0·81	82	0·47	73	0·75	470	0·73
Ligaments and Tendons	3	1·3	10	0·76	53	1·09	322	2·52	167	0·93	206	1·19	104	1·06	865	1·35
Effects of Old Injuries	—	—	—	—	—	—	—	—	—	—	150	0·87	192	1·96	342	0·53
Others	—	—	—	—	14	0·29	—	—	—	—	—	—	—	—	14	0·02
Totals	29	12·6	278	21·25	890	18·47	2,607	20·40	3,332	18·65	2,938	16·98	1,917	19·57	11,991	18·71
NERVOUS SYSTEM AND MENTAL DISEASES																
Psychoneuroses	7	3·0	126	9·63	460	9·55	1,708	13·37	2,601	14·56	2,367	13·68	1,346	13·74	8,615	13·44
Psychoses	3	1·3	5	0·38	65	1·35	194	1·52	108	0·60	66	0·38	49	0·50	490	0·76
Psychopathic Personality	—	—	6	0·46	52	1·08	268	2·10	475	2·66	745	4·30	439	4·48	1,985	3·10
Mental Defect	—	—	2	0·15	10	0·21	75	0·59	83	0·46	55	0·32	13	0·13	238	0·37
Epilepsies	2	0·9	17	1·30	55	1·14	203	1·59	165	0·92	162	0·94	70	0·71	674	1·05
Indefinite Aetiology	2	0·9	44	3·36	146	3·03	469	3·67	532	2·98	531	3·07	233	2·38	1,957	3·05
Totals	14	6·1	200	15·28	788	16·35	2,917	22·83	3,964	22·18	3,926	22·69	2,150	21·95	13,959	21·78
ORGANIC NERVOUS DISEASES																
Brain, Inflammatory Lesions	—	—	—	—	—	—	—	—	—	—	4	0·02	3	0·03	7	0·01
Brain, Diseases of	1	0·4	2	0·15	17	0·35	36	0·28	40	0·22	18	0·10	13	0·13	127	0·20
Organic Diseases, Indefinite	—	—	—	—	—	—	—	—	—	—	28	0·16	29	0·30	57	0·09
Cranial Nerves	—	—	3	0·23	17	0·35	25	0·20	39	0·22	60	0·35	30	0·31	174	0·27
Spinal Cord	1	0·4	—	—	—	—	25	0·20	4	0·02	3	0·02	10	0·10	43	0·07
Spinal and Peripheral Nerves	10	4·4	36	2·75	120	2·49	253	1·98	365	2·04	348	2·01	211	2·15	1,343	2·10
Neuromuscular System	—	—	1	0·08	1	0·02	1	0·01	35	0·19	—	—	—	—	38	0·06
Unplaced and General Headache, Sequelae of Concussion	—	—	—	—	7	0·15	50	0·39	—	—	—	—	—	—	57	0·09
Totals	12	5·2	42	3·21	162	3·36	390	3·05	483	2·70	461	2·66	296	3·02	1,846	2·88

Nervous System and Mental Diseases Totals	26	11·3	242	18·49	950	19·72	3,307	25·88	4,447	24·89	4,387	25·35	2,446	24·97	15,805	24·66
EYE DISEASES																
Defects of Vision	1	0·4	8	0·61	40	0·83	87	0·68	121	0·68	107	0·62	86	0·88	450	0·70
Inflammatory Conditions	—	—	39	2·98	116	2·41	308	2·41	389	2·18	403	2·33	241	2·46	1,496	2·33
Others	2	0·9	8	0·61	55	1·14	141	1·10	181	1·01	121	0·70	94	0·96	602	0·94
Totals	3	1·3	55	4·20	211	4·38	536	4·19	691	3·87	631	3·65	421	4·30	2,548	3·97
EAR DISEASES																
Deafness	—	—	—	—	—	—	—	—	22	0·12	36	0·21	18	0·18	76	0·12
Otitis Media, Acute	6	2·6	48	3·67	204	4·23	566	4·43	722	4·04	498	2·88	340	3·47	2,384	3·72
Otitis Media, Chronic	1	0·4	14	1·07	38	0·79	109	0·85	176	0·98	134	0·77	74	0·76	546	0·85
Otitis Externa	—	—	5	0·38	31	0·64	72	0·56	154	0·86	194	1·12	205	2·09	661	1·03
Perforated Tympanic Membrane	—	—	—	—	1	0·02	23	0·18	1	0·01	—	—	—	—	25	0·04
Mastoiditis, Acute	—	—	3	0·23	14	0·29	48	0·38	55	0·31	19	0·11	10	0·10	149	0·23
Mastoiditis	1	0·4	2	0·15	6	0·12	3	0·02	10	0·06	—	—	3	0·03	25	0·04
Others	—	—	4	0·31	15	0·31	17	0·13	39	0·22	7	0·04	—	—	82	0·13
Totals	8	3·4	76	5·81	309	6·41	838	6·56	1,179	6·60	888	5·13	650	6·64	3,948	6·16
NOSE AND THROAT DISEASES																
Nasal Passages	15	6·5	251	19·18	759	15·75	689	5·39	543	3·04	495	2·86	263	2·69	4,597	7·17
Sinuses									671	3·76	489	2·83	422	4·31		
Naso-Pharynx	4	1·8	3	0·23	9	0·19	997	7·80	1,624	9·09	1,112	6·43	800	8·17	4,549	7·10
Throat																
Totals	19	8·3	254	19·41	768	15·94	1,686	13·19	2,838	15·88	2,096	12·11	1,485	15·16	9,146	14·27

* Figures for 1939 and 1945 are for the war periods of the years only *viz.* 1939—from September 3 to December 31; 1945—from January 1 to August 15.

TABLE 19(a)—(*contd.*)

W.A.A.F. Nosological Table
Period of Second World War, September 3, 1939 to August 15, 1945—Fresh Cases

	1939*		1940		1941		1942		1943		1944		1945*		Totals	
	Number of Cases	Incidence per 1,000 per annum	Number of Cases	Incidence per 1,000 per annum	Number of Cases	Incidence per 1,000 per annum	Number of Cases	Incidence per 1,000 per annum	Number of Cases	Incidence per 1,000 per annum	Number of Cases	Incidence per 1,000 per annum	Number of Cases	Incidence per 1,000 per annum	Number of Cases	Incidence per 1,000 per annum
SKIN DISEASES:																
Scabies	14	6·1	144	11·00	791	16·42	2,541	19·89	1,652	9·25	789	4·56	300	3·06	6,231	9·72
Impetigo	5	2·2	31	2·37	204	4·23	868	6·79	1,132	6·36	776	4·48	500	5·11	3,516	5·48
Pediculosis and Pediculitis	4	1·7	26	1·99	89	1·85	—	—	78	0·44	20	0·12	10	0·10	227	0·35
Tinea Cruris	—	—	—	—	—	—	12	0·09	1	0·01	—	—	—	—	13	0·02
Tinea, Others	2	0·9	4	0·31	20	0·42	41	0·32	110	0·61	60	0·35	70	0·71	307	0·48
Dermatitis and Eczema	8	3·5	52	3·97	184	3·82	595	4·66	828	4·63	674	3·89	392	4·00	2,733	4·26
Pityriasis and Erythemata	—	—	27	2·06	65	1·35	333	2·61	333	1·86	418	2·42	146	1·49	1,322	2·06
Psoriasis	—	—	4	0·31	17	0·35	62	0·49	87	0·49	39	0·23	55	0·56	264	0·41
Ingrowing Toenail	—	—	10	0·76	30	0·62	77	0·60	118	0·66	59	0·34	70	0·71	364	0·57
Other Conditions	6	2·6	30	2·29	123	2·55	494	3·87	482	2·70	703	4·06	455	4·65	2,293	3·58
Totals	39	17·0	328	25·07	1,523	31·61	5,023	39·31	4,821	26·98	3,538	20·44	1,998	20·40	17,270	26·94
ENDOCRINE DISEASES:																
General Endocrine Disturbances	—	—	2	0·15	13	0·27	22	0·17	62	0·35	55	0·32	11	0·11	165	0·26
Parathyroid	—	—	—	—	2	0·04	1	0·01	2	0·01	—	—	—	—	5	0·01
Pituitary	—	—	—	—	4	0·08	13	0·10	16	0·09	5	0·03	2	0·02	40	0·06
Suprarenal	—	—	—	—	—	—	11	0·09	1	0·01	41	0·24	1	0·01	54	0·08
Thyroid	1	0·4	19	1·45	48	1·00	128	1·00	155	0·87	123	0·71	68	0·67	542	0·85
Totals	1	0·4	21	1·60	67	1·39	175	1·37	236	1·32	224	1·29	82	0·84	806	1·26
DISEASES OF METABOLISM	—	—	4	0·31	9	0·19	19	0·15	34	0·19	42	0·24	7	0·07	115	0·18
DIABETES MELLITUS	3	1·3	—	—	—	—	3	0·02	—	—	—	—	—	—	6	0·01
DEFICIENCY DISEASES	—	—	2	0·15	5	0·10	1	0·01	38	0·21	19	0·11	21	0·21	86	0·13
EFFECTS OF TOXIC SUBSTANCES**	—	—	—	—	—	—	—	—	36	0·20	29	0·17	20	0·20	85	0·13
CYSTS AND TUMOURS:																
Cysts	—	—	7	0·54	35	0·73	71	0·56	192	1·07	238	1·38	231	2·36	774	1·21
Tumours, Benign	3	1·3	16	1·22	41	0·85	91	0·71	100	0·56	127	0·73	124	1·27	502	0·78
Tumours, Malignant	—	—	8	0·61	11	0·23	20	0·16	26	0·15	50	0·29	33	0·34	148	0·23
Tumours, Unspecified	—	—	—	—	15	0·31	4	0·03	49	0·27	67	0·39	13	0·13	148	0·23
Totals	3	1·3	31	2·37	102	2·12	186	1·46	367	2·05	482	2·79	401	4·09	1,572	2·45

DISEASES PECULIAR TO WOMEN:																
Disorders of Menstruation	15	6·5	115	8·80	452	9·38	1,694	13·26	2,322	12·99	2,749	15·88	1,341	13·69	8,688	13·55
Generative Organs	4	1·7	87	6·63	417	8·65	614	4·81	540	3·02	540	3·12	316	3·23	2,518	3·93
Inflammatory Conditions of Pelvic Organs	5	2·2	26	1·99	74	1·54	942	7·37	1,814	10·15	1,951	11·27	956	9·76	5,768	9·00
Pregnancy and Disorders of Pregnancy	3	1·3	49	3·74	235	4·88	1,085	8·49	1,848	10·34	2,522	14·57	1,404	14·34	7,146	11·15
Breasts	—	—	1	0·08	17	0·35	123	0·96	128	0·72	86	0·50	72	0·74	427	0·67
Ill Defined Conditions	—	—	9	0·69	29	0·60	—	0·96	—	—	—	—	—	—	38	0·06
Totals	27	11·7	287	21·93	1,224	25·40	4,458	34·89	6,652	37·23	7,848	45·35	4,089	41·75	24,585	38·35
INDEFINITE AND GENERAL CONDITIONS:																
Observation and no Apparent Disease	10	4·3	180	13·76	1,063	22·06	1,767	13·83	2,119	11·86	2,552	14·75	1,350	13·78	9,041	14·10
Debility	11	4·8	198	15·13	505	10·48	1,143	8·94	1,431	8·01	1,940	11·21	803	8·20	6,031	9·41
Pyrexia of Uncertain Origin	2	0·9	—	—	—	—	197	1·54	210	1·18	463	2·68	231	2·36	1,103	1·72
Poisons	—	—	—	—	34	0·71	69	0·54	—	—	—	—	—	—	103	0·16
Accidental Contamination by Noxious Gases†	1	0·4	—	—	—	—	1	0·01	1	0·01	—	—	—	—	3	0·01
Rheumatism	4	1·7	—	—	—	—	8	0·06	—	—	—	—	—	—	12	0·01
Others	—	—	77	5·88	142	2·95	—	—	847	4·74	832	4·81	545	5·56	2,443	3·81
Totals	28	12·1	455	34·77	1,744	36·20	3,185	24·93	4,608	25·79	5,787	33·44	2,929	29·91	18,736	29·23
Totals All Diseases	825	358·3	9,558	730·46	26,034	540·33	66,669	521·74	98,979	553·92	84,428	487·84	49,372	504·10	335,865	523·94
GENERAL INJURIES:																
Multiple Injuries with Fractures	1	0·4	18	1·38	20	0·42	109	0·85	73	0·41	97	0·56	12	0·12	330	0·51
Multiple Injuries with Burns	—	—	—	—	8	0·17	18	0·14	15	0·08	1	0·01	1	0·01	43	0·07
Multiple Wounds	—	—	—	—	6	0·12	17	0·13	8	0·04	—	—	—	—	31	0·05
Fractured Skull with Other Injuries	—	—	—	—	2	0·04	14	0·11	6	0·03	3	0·02	1	0·01	26	0·04
Missile Wounds, Multiple	—	—	—	—	—	—	2	0·01	2	0·01	1	0·01	1	0·01	6	0·01
Minor Injuries	12	5·3	46	3·52	77	1·60	338	2·65	314	1·76	447	2·58	90	0·92	1,324	2·07
Burns Generalised	—	—	1	0·08	4	0·08	36	0·28	18	0·10	10	0·06	1	0·01	70	0·11
Burns of Face and Hands	—	—	—	—	2	0·04	24	0·19	10	0·06	9	0·05	10	0·10	55	0·09
Scalds	—	—	—	—	4	0·08	21	0·16	13	0·07	20	0·12	—	—	58	0·09
Frostbite	—	—	—	—	—	—	5	0·04	—	—	—	—	—	—	5	0·01
Exposure to Natural Elements	—	—	—	—	—	—	1	0·01	3	0·02	1	0·01	—	—	5	0·01
Drowning, including Effects of Immersion	—	—	—	—	—	—	8	0·06	—	—	3	0·02	4	0·04	15	0·02
Injuries to Tissues and Specialised Structures†	—	—	36	2·74	—	—	—	—	456	2·55	394	2·28	180	1·84	1,066	1·66
Chemical Agents, Effects of Contact with†	—	—	—	—	—	—	—	—	34	0·19	11	0·06	20	0·20	65	0·10
Other Injuries	—	—	60	4·58	181	3·76	67	0·52	461	2·58	325	1·88	390	3·98	1,484	2·31
Missing, Presumed Dead	—	—	—	—	—	—	—	—	—	—	1	0·01	3	0·03	4	0·01
Totals	13	5·7	161	12·30	304	6·31	660	5·17	1,413	7·91	1,323	7·64	713	7·28	4,587	7 16

* Figures for 1939 and 1945 are for the war periods of the years only *viz.* 1939—from September 3 to December 31; 1945—from January 1 to August 15.
** *See* p. 481.
† *See* p. 483.

TABLE 19(a)—(*contd.*)

W.A.A.F. Nosological Table

Period of Second World War, September 3, 1939 to August 15, 1945—Fresh Cases

	1939*		1940		1941		1942		1943		1944		1945*		Totals	
	Number of Cases	Incidence per 1,000 per annum	Number of Cases	Incidence per 1,000 per annum	Number of Cases	Incidence per 1,000 per annum	Number of Cases	Incidence per 1,000 per annum	Number of Cases	Incidence per 1,000 per annum	Number of Cases	Incidence per 1,000 per annum	Number of Cases	Incidence per 1,000 per annum	Number of Cases	Incidence per 1,000 per annum
LOCALISED INJURIES:																
CRANIUM																
Contusions and Wounds	4	1·7	14	1·07	65	1·35	132	1·04	249	1·39	254	1·47	120	1·23	838	1·31
Fractures of Skull	2	0·9	4	0·31	15	0·31	16	0·13	37	0·21	29	0·17	42	0·43	145	0·23
Concussion	17	7·4	61	4·66	130	2·70	406	3·18	395	2·21	268	1·55	250	2·55	1,527	2·38
Burns and Scalds	—	—	—	—	1	0·02	4	0·03	6	0·03	—	—	—	—	11	0·02
Others	—	—	14	1·07	—	—	62	0·48	—	—	—	—	—	—	76	0·12
Totals	23	10·0	93	7·11	211	4·38	620	4·85	687	3·84	551	3·18	412	4·21	2,597	4·05
FACE AND MOUTH:																
Contusions and Wounds of Face	2	0·9	10	0·76	36	0·75	103	0·81	165	0·92	276	1·59	50	0·51	642	1·00
Burns of Face	1	0·4	1	0·08	12	0·25	27	0·21	51	0·29	60	0·35	20	0·20	172	0·27
Fractures, Fracture-Dislocations and Dislocations	—	—	5	0·39	14	0·29	24	0·19	66	0·37	97	0·56	10	0·10	216	0·34
Totals	3	1·3	16	1·22	62	1·29	154	1·21	282	1·58	433	2·50	80	0·82	1,030	1·61
EYES:																
Eyelids, Injuries of	1	0·4	4	0·31	5	0·10	31	0·24	22	0·12	20	0·12	10	0·10	93	0·14
Eye Substance, Superficial Wounds of	—	—	—	—	5	0·10	16	0·13	22	0·12	19	0·11	30	0·31	92	0·14
Eye Substance, Injury to Eyeball	1	0·4	2	0·15	5	0·10	8	0·06	11	0·06	—	—	10	0·10	37	0·06
Eye Substance, Injuries Resulting in Removal of Eye	—	—	—	—	—	—	—	—	—	—	10	0·06	—	—	10	0·02
Missile Wounds	—	—	—	—	—	—	—	—	—	—	—	—	—	—	—	—
Burns and Scalds of Eyelids and Eyes	—	—	—	—	1	0·02	10	0·08	8	0·05	—	—	10	0·10	29	0·04
Chemical Injuries	—	—	—	—	—	—	—	—	5	0·03	—	—	—	—	5	0·01
Totals	2	0·8	6	0·46	16	0·32	65	0·51	68	0·38	49	0·28	60	0·61	266	0·41

EARS:																
Pinna, Injuries to	—	—	—	—	1	0·02	1	0·01	1	0·01	—	—	—	—	3	0·01
Rupture of Tympanic Membranes	—	—	—	—	—	—	2	0·02	5	0·02	—	—	—	—	7	0·01
Burns and Scalds	—	—	—	—	—	—	—	—	—	—	—	—	—	—	—	—
Totals	—	—	—	—	1	0·02	3	0·03	6	0·03	—	—	—	—	10	0·02
NECK:																
Contusions and Wounds	—	—	—	—	1	0·02	7	0·05	4	0·02	—	—	—	—	12	0·02
Muscle Sprains and Strains	—	—	—	—	—	—	4	0·03	—	—	—	—	—	—	4	0·01
Burns and Scalds	—	—	—	—	1	0·02	1	0·01	4	0·02	—	—	—	—	6	0·01
Totals	—	—	—	—	2	0·04	12	0·09	8	0·04	—	—	—	—	22	0·03
CHEST:																
Contusions and Superficial Wounds	—	—	4	0·31	8	0·17	46	0·36	31	0·17	35	0·20	—	—	124	0·19
Compression and Blast Injury	—	—	1	0·08	2	0·04	4	0·03	—	—	—	—	4	0·04	11	0·02
Penetrating Wounds, Fractures, Fracture-Dislocations and Dislocations	3	1·3	3	0·23	6	0·12	11	0·08	17	0·10	10	0·06	10	0·10	60	0·09
Missile Wounds	—	—	—	—	1	0·02	2	0·02	1	0·01	1	0·01	—	—	5	0·01
Burns and Scalds	1	0·4	—	—	3	0·06	2	0·02	6	0·03	—	—	—	—	12	0·02
Totals	4	1·7	8	0·61	20	0·42	65	0·51	55	0·31	46	0·27	14	0·14	212	0·33
BACK AND VERTEBRAL COLUMN:																
Contusions and Superficial Wounds	1	0·4	12	0·92	48	0·99	126	0·99	124	0·69	127	0·73	100	1·02	538	0·84
Contusions and Wounds Involving Viscera	—	—	3	0·23	1	0·02	5	0·04	2	0·01	—	—	—	—	11	0·02
Wounds Involving Spinal Cord	—	—	—	—	—	—	3	0·02	1	0·01	—	—	—	—	4	0·01
Spinal Concussion	—	—	—	—	—	—	2	0·02	3	0·01	10	0·06	—	—	15	0·02
Fractures, Fracture-Dislocations and Dislocations, Body of Vertebrae	—	—	5	0·38	8	0·17	28	0·22	48	0·27	16	0·09	20	0·10	125	0·19
Burns and Scalds	—	—	—	—	1	0·02	2	0·02	6	0·03	—	—	10	0·10	19	0·03
Totals	1	0·4	20	1·53	58	1·18	167	1·31	184	1·03	153	0·88	130	1·33	712	1·11
ABDOMEN:																
Contusions and Wounds	1	0·4	1	0·08	3	0·06	30	0·24	18	0·10	21	0·12	—	—	74	0·12
Missile Wounds	—	—	—	—	1	0·02	—	—	—	—	10	0·06	—	—	11	0·02
Burns and Scalds	—	—	—	—	—	—	2	0·02	1	0·01	—	—	—	—	3	0·01
Totals	1	0·4	1	0·08	4	0·08	32	0·26	19	0·11	31	0·18	—	—	88	0·14

* Figures for 1939 and 1945 are for the war periods of the years only *viz.* 1939—from September 3 to December 31; 1945—from January 1 to August 15.

TABLE 19(a)—(*contd.*)

W.A.A.F. Nosological Table
Period of Second World War, September 3, 1939 to August 15, 1945—Fresh Cases

	1939*		1940		1941		1942		1943		1944		1945*		Totals	
	Number of Cases	Incidence per 1,000 per annum	Number of Cases	Incidence per 1,000 per annum	Number of Cases	Incidence per 1,000 per annum	Number of Cases	Incidence per 1,000 per annum	Number of Cases	Incidence per 1,000 per annum	Number of Cases	Incidence per 1,000 per annum	Number of Cases	Incidence per 1,000 per annum	Number of Cases	Incidence per 1,000 per annum
BUTTOCKS AND PELVIS:																
Contusions and Wounds	1	0·4	5	0·36	11	0·23	22	0·17	29	0·16	46	0·27	10	0·10	124	0·19
Contusions and Wounds of Generative Organs	—	—	—	—	6	0·12	—	—	23	0·13	40	0·23	—	—	69	0·11
Fractures, Fracture-Dislocations and Dislocations	—	—	1	0·08	7	0·15	7	0·05	16	0·09	—	—	1	0·01	32	0·05
Burns and Scalds	1	0·4	—	—	—	—	2	0·02	9	0·05	—	—	—	—	12	0·02
Totals	2	0·8	6	0·44	24	0·50	31	0·24	77	0·43	86	0·50	11	0·11	237	0·37
UPPER LIMB, HAND AND WRIST:																
Contusions and Wounds	1	0·4	12	0·92	45	0·93	138	1·08	218	1·27	205	1·18	70	0·71	689	1·07
Sprains	1	0·4	—	—	—	—	16	0·13	14	0·08	20	0·12	10	0·10	61	0·10
Fractures, Fracture-Dislocations and Dislocations	—	—	6	0·45	3	0·48	52	0·41	83	0·46	28	0·16	30	0·31	222	0·35
Burns and Scalds	1	0·4	4	0·31	26	0·54	90	0·70	105	0·59	96	0·55	40	0·41	362	0·56
Totals	3	1·2	22	1·68	94	1·95	296	2·32	420	2·35	349	2·02	150	1·53	1,334	2·08
UPPER LIMB, REST OF LIMB:																
Contusions and Wounds	2	0·8	6	0·45	28	0·58	107	0·84	75	0·42	88	0·51	30	0·31	336	0·52
Sprains and Strains, Traumatic Synovitis, Muscle Fibre Tears	—	—	—	—	1	0·02	45	0·35	4	0·02	—	—	—	—	50	0·08
Fractures, Fracture-Dislocations and Dislocations	1	0·4	27	2·06	80	1·66	263	2·06	302	1·69	205	1·18	200	2·04	1,078	1·68
Burns and Scalds	1	0·4	5	0·38	23	0·48	95	0·74	138	0·77	156	0·90	10	0·10	428	0·67
Totals	4	1·7	38	2·90	132	2·74	510	3·99	519	2·90	449	2·59	240	2·45	1,892	2·95

LOWER LIMB, FOOT AND ANKLE:																
Contusions and Wounds	2	0·9	28	2·14	57	1·18	147	1·15	205	1·15	113	0·65	70	0·71	622	0·97
Sprains and Strains	5	2·2	76	5·81	239	4·96	698	5·46	767	4·29	704	4·07	420	4·29	2,909	4·54
Fractures, Fracture-Dislocations and Dislocations	2	0·9	14	1·07	48	1·00	101	0·79	138	0·77	59	0·34	31	0·32	393	0·61
Burns and Scalds	—	—	6	0·46	28	0·58	188	1·47	283	1·58	368	2·13	170	1·74	1,043	1·63
Totals	9	4·0	124	9·48	372	7·72	1,134	8·87	1,393	7·80	1,244	7·19	691	7·06	4,967	7·75
LOWER LIMB, REST OF LIMB:																
Contusions and Wounds	8	3·4	41	3·13	102	2·12	446	3·49	440	2·46	299	1·73	160	1·63	1,496	2·33
Sprains and Strains	5	2·2	6	0·46	13	0·27	115	0·90	41	0·23	19	0·11	10	0·10	209	0·33
Internal Derangement, Knee Joint	2	0·9	16	1·22	29	0·60	177	1·38	112	0·63	133	0·77	50	0·51	519	0·81
Fractures, Fracture-Dislocations and Dislocations	3	1·3	32	2·44	88	1·83	277	2·17	298	1·67	238	1·38	91	0·93	1,027	1·79
Missile Wounds	—	—	2	0·15	2	0·02	1	0·01	2	0·01	—	—	—	—	7	0·01
Burns and Scalds	2	0·9	13	0·99	53	1·10	191	1·49	327	1·83	303	1·75	140	1·43	1,029	1·60
Totals	20	8·7	110	8·41	287	5·96	1,207	9·44	1,220	6·83	992	5·73	451	4·60	4,287	6·69
Totals of All Injuries	85	36·7	605	46·24	1,587	32·92	4,955	38·78	6,351	35·54	5,706	32·97	2,952	30·14	22,241	34·70
UNCLASSIFIED CONDITIONS:																
Heat Exhaustion and Heat Hyperpyrexia	—	—	2	0·15	25	0·52	20	0·15	45	0·25	9	0·05	70	0·71	171	0·27
Surgical Amputations and Fitting of Artificial Appliances	—	—	—	—	—	—	38	0·30	26	0·15	2	0·01	—	—	66	0·10
Late Complications of Trauma	—	—	—	—	—	—	—	—	8	0·04	—	—	—	—	8	0·01
Prolonged Loss of Senses immediately following Injury	—	—	—	—	—	—	—	—	—	—	—	—	—	—	—	—
Totals	—	—	2	0·15	25	0·52	58	0·45	79	0·44	11	0·06	70	0·71	245	0·38
Grand Total of All Disabilities	910	395·7	10,165	776·85	27,646	573·76	71,682	560·98	105,409	589·90	90,145	520·88	52,394	534·95	358,351	559·01

*Figures for 1939 and 1945 are for the war periods of the years only *viz.* 1939—from September 3 to December 31; 1945—from January 1 to August 15.

The VENEREAL DISEASE incidence in the W.A.A.F. was considerably lower than in the R.A.F. at home—the average incidence for all venereal diseases over the whole war period was 2·36 per 1,000 as compared with 8·7 per 1,000 in the R.A.F. The highest rate was recorded in 1942 when there were 3·57 cases per 1,000.

The incidence of ALIMENTARY SYSTEM DISEASES was higher than in the R.A.F. and the relative importance of the conditions making up this group was different. Both GASTRIC and DUODENAL ULCER figured less prominently than in the R.A.F. tables; thus the incidence of duodenal ulcer averaged 0·43 cases per 1,000 compared with 3·9 cases per 1,000 in the R.A.F. APPENDICITIS, on the other hand, was more common in the W.A.A.F.—an average of 13·28 cases per 1,000 as opposed to 5 per 1,000 in the R.A.F. As would be expected cases of HERNIA were very much less common in the W.A.A.F. than in the R.A.F. The biggest difference between the two sexes was in the Group of OTHER INTESTINAL CONDITIONS which is largely made up of cases of enteritis—the average incidence in the W.A.A.F. was 23 per 1,000 compared with 9 per 1,000 in the R.A.F.

There was a high incidence of diseases of the RESPIRATORY SYSTEM, particularly of bronchitis. In 1940 the incidence of bronchitis was 42·8 per 1,000 compared with a R.A.F. figure of 11·5 per 1,000. The incidence of diseases of the respiratory system was at its lowest in 1942 but rose again in 1943 and remained high until the end of the war.

The incidence of URINARY SYSTEM DISEASES was much higher than in the R.A.F., chiefly due to a considerably higher incidence of cystitis and pyelitis.

The incidence of DISEASES OF THE LOCOMOTOR SYSTEM differed little from year to year and was slightly higher than the incidence in the R.A.F. at home. Diseases of the rheumatic group were more prominent than in the R.A.F., but joint conditions, and particularly internal derangement of the knee joint, were less common.

There was a high incidence of PSYCHONEUROSIS throughout with a peak in 1943 of 14·56 cases per 1,000. The incidence of PSYCHOPATHIC PERSONALITY, too, was high with a peak of 4·48 cases per 1,000 in 1945. The incidence of PSYCHOSES did not differ significantly from the incidence in the R.A.F.

The total incidence of EAR DISEASES was roughly the same as in the R.A.F. but the relative importance of acute and chronic otitis media was different in the two sexes; acute otitis media was consistently more common in the W.A.A.F. whereas the R.A.F. showed a higher incidence of the chronic form.

SKIN DISEASES rose steadily in incidence to reach a peak in 1942 with an incidence of 40 per 1,000. There was a considerable fall in incidence in the succeeding years. It must be remembered that it is impossible to achieve a true picture of the incidence of skin diseases merely by considering those cases which were admitted for over forty-eight hours; most skin diseases are treated as out-patients and only the more serious cases require admission. Thus, although in 1942 more than half the admissions were due to SCABIES, the considerable reduction in incidence of scabies in 1943 may not reflect any reduction in the true incidence of scabies in that year but merely improved methods of treatment enabling more cases to be treated as out-patients. Actually, 1943 was the year in which benzyl benzoate first became generally adopted in the R.A.F. for treatment of scabies and its ease of application and absence of complications were certainly responsible for fewer admissions for scabies.

PEDICULOSIS was known to be very common in W.A.A.F. recruits and yet as its treatment is almost invariably possible in the out-patients' department the nosological table shows only a small number of cases.

INJURIES are classified on the same lines as the R.A.F. injuries. The numbers were relatively small as W.A.A.F. personnel were not employed on operational flights.

Table 20 shows the annual incidence of certain infectious diseases for the W.A.A.F. It is constructed on similar lines to the corresponding R.A.F. table (Table 4).

TABLE 19(b)

Number of Fresh Cases, Incidence and Percentage Distribution of Disease, W.A.A.F.

CAUSES	*Number of Cases*	*Incidence/ 1,000 per Annum*	*Percentage of all Diseases*
Upper Respiratory Tract Infections	104,883	163·61	31·2
Alimentary System	39,783	62·06	11·8
Diseases Peculiar to Women	24,585	38·35	7·3
Respiratory System	20,987	32·74	6·2
Infectious Diseases	19,731	30·78	5·9
Septic Conditions	19,623	30·61	5·8
Skin Diseases	17,270	26·94	5·1
Nervous and Mental Diseases	15,805	24·66	4·7
E.N.T. Conditions	13,094	20·43	3·9
Locomotor System	11,991	18·71	3·6
Urinary System	8,222	12·83	2·4
Circulatory System	4,326	6·75	1·3
Diseases of Allergy	3,037	4·74	0·9
Eye Conditions	2,548	3·97	0·8
Tuberculosis—Pulmonary	1,575	2·46	0·5
Tuberculosis—Other than Pulmonary	507	0·79	0·2
Blood and Blood-forming Organs, R.E. System	1,867	2·91	0·6
Cysts and Tumours	1,572	2·45	0·5
Pneumonia	1,440	2·25	0·4
Venereal Diseases	1,511	2·36	0·5
Indefinite and General	21,508	33·54	6·4
Totals	335,865	523·94	100·0

TABLE 20

Certain Infectious Diseases, W.A.A.F., 1939–45—Fresh Cases

DISEASES	Annual Incidence per 1,000 of Strength						
	1939	1940	1941	1942	1943	1944	1945
Acute anterior poliomyelitis	—	—	0·02	0·08	0·06	0·006	0·07
Acute rheumatism	1·7	2·2	1·6	5·21	2·0	1·07	0·70
Infective hepatitis	—	1·4	0·9	2·39	2·65	1·33	2·97
Cerebro-spinal fever	—	0·8	0·5	0·35	0·15	0·12	0·14
Chicken-pox	1·7	1·6	1·9	1·44	1·58	1·58	0·84
Diphtheria	0·9	0·8	1·4	1·14	1·12	0·58	0·66
Encephalitis lethargica	0·4	—	0·02	0·01	—	0·006	—
German measles	4·4	103·4	5·4	3·92	4·73	15·54	2·18
Measles	0·9	6·5	4·3	1·84	3·20	1·68	1·69
Mumps	0·4	2·1	2·6	4·95	2·54	1·33	1·62
Scarlet Fever	0·9	0·9	1·9	1·64	1·66	1·39	0·49
Smallpox	—	—	—	—	—	—	—
Tetanus	—	—	—	0·02	0·01	—	—
Typhus	—	—	—	—	0·01	—	—

ACUTE ANTERIOR POLIOMYELITIS had an even lower incidence in the W.A.A.F. than in the R.A.F.

The highest incidence of ACUTE RHEUMATISM was in 1942 when there were 666 cases with an incidence of 5·2 per 1,000 of strength. This was considerably higher than the R.A.F. incidence of 1·2 per 1,000 of strength but in other years the incidence in the two sexes was roughly equal.

The major epidemics of INFECTIVE HEPATITIS occurred overseas and it is not surprising that there is a higher incidence in the R.A.F. In 1945 there were 160 cases in W.A.A.F. personnel serving overseas and this represents an incidence of 32·4 per 1,000 of strength overseas.

CEREBRO-SPINAL FEVER had an incidence of 0·8 per 1,000 in 1940 and thereafter declined steadily.

RUBELLA reached the very high incidence of 103·4 per 1,000 in 1940, when there was a nation-wide epidemic of the disease. There was a smaller epidemic in 1944 when the incidence was 15·5 per 1,000.

MEASLES showed peak incidences of 6·5 per 1,000 in 1940 and 3·2 per 1,000 in 1943, corresponding with nation-wide epidemics.

There were no cases of SMALLPOX in the W.A.A.F.

INCIDENCE OF DISEASE AND INJURY ANALYSED BY AGE GROUPS, 1941–45

Table 21 is an analysis of disease and injury by age groups for the years 1941–45; data are not available for the years 1939 and 1940.

In all years the highest incidence of sickness is in the under 20 age group and in both 1943 and 1945 disease and injury in this age group were at an incidence of nearly 1,400 per 1,000 of strength. The lowest incidence of sickness was consistently in the age groups 25–29 and 30–34. There was always a jump in the incidence of sickness in the age group 40–44 and in most years the rate was higher in this group than in the over 45 age group. A possible explanation of this is that the menopause often occurs between the ages of 40 and 44 and this would have an effect on a woman's general well-being.

The greater liability of the under 20 age group to infection is well illustrated in the figures for INFECTIONS OF THE UPPER RESPIRATORY TRACT. The incidence in this group is usually greater than the incidence in any other age group.

PNEUMONIA, too, was generally more prevalent among those under 20 than in the other age groups, but in 1943 most cases occurred in those over the age of 45 and in 1944 and 1945 the 35–39 age group suffered most heavily.

The general picture of PULMONARY TUBERCULOSIS is of a high incidence in the under 20 age group with a rapid fall to a relatively low incidence round the age of 30 and a secondary but smaller peak in the late thirties or early forties. TUBERCULOSIS other than pulmonary shows a somewhat similar trend.

The age group distribution of VENEREAL DISEASE does not exactly parallel that of the R.A.F. In the W.A.A.F. the highest incidence is consistently in the under 20 age group whereas in the R.A.F. there is a tendency for the incidence to be highest in the next two age groups.

INFECTIVE HEPATITIS was most prevalent in the younger age groups with a progressive decrease in incidence with increasing age.

POST-INOCULATION EFFECTS, as in the R.A.F., were most common in the under 20 age group, when the majority of initial Service inoculations were carried out.

The groups OTHER INFECTIONS and SEPTIC CONDITIONS follow the general trend with a high incidence in the under 20 age group and a progressive fall in rates until the late thirties and early forties when there was a secondary rise.

Diseases of the CIRCULATORY SYSTEM had a very high incidence in the age groups over 40.

PLEURISY WITH EFFUSION has not been separated from other respiratory system diseases in the tables. In keeping with tuberculosis and respiratory tract infections its highest incidence was in the under 20 age group.

Diseases of the URINARY SYSTEM were generally most prevalent in those under 20 but showed no significant differences between the other age groups.

DISORDERS OF MENSTRUATION were most common in older women but also showed a high incidence in the under 20's. Other diseases peculiar to women showed similar trends.

PSYCHONEUROSES were least common between the ages of 20 and 30 and rose considerably in incidence in the higher age groups. There was also a high incidence in the under 20's.

There appears to be no consistent pattern in the incidence of PSYCHOSES in the different age groups.

PSYCHOPATHIC PERSONALITIES occurred least frequently between the ages of 20 and 30. In general, the highest incidences were in the under 20 age group but there was also a marked increase after the age of 30.

MENTAL DEFECT was most common under the age of 20. EPILEPSY showed a declining incidence with increasing age. ORGANIC NERVOUS DISEASES were more prominent in the older age groups.

LOCOMOTOR SYSTEM DISEASES, as in the R.A.F., were more prevalent in the older age groups.

EYE conditions showed no significant difference between the various age groups.

EAR, NOSE AND THROAT conditions were most common in the under 20 age group and declined steadily with age.

SKIN DISEASES, too, were more common in the younger age groups.

TABLE 21

W.A.A.F. Diseases and Injuries by Age Groups, 1941–45—Rates per 1,000 Strength

DISEASES:	Year	AGE GROUPS Under 20	20–24	25–29	30–34	35–39	40–44	45 and Over	Rate per 1,000 All Ages
Pneumonia	1941	4·90	2·20	2·60	3·60	2·30	2·60	—	2·90
	1942	7·00	2·80	3·60	3·90	5·40	2·00	6·00	3·70
	1943	7·69	2·13	2·34	1·88	1·99	6·32	9·42	2·65
	1944	4·66	1·60	0·27	—	5·31	—	—	1·46
	1945	2·74	1·40	2·63	1·97	6·08	—	—	1·94
Tuberculosis, Pulmonary	1941	1·60	1·60	1·60	0·70	2·30	2·60	3·40	1·60
	1942	6·10	3·20	2·60	1·90	2·20	4·70	—	3·50
	1943	8·20	2·98	2·34	1·50	2·24	2·10	—	3·15
	1944	8·96	2·52	1·22	2·50	4·78	1·21	1·32	2·67
	1945	6·22	2·78	1·37	1·38	2·03	1·42	1·37	2·32
Tuberculosis, other than Pulmonary	1941	0·60	1·00	0·70	—	1·50	4·00	—	0·80
	1942	2·30	0·80	0·80	1·30	1·00	0·70	—	1·00
	1943	2·68	1·08	0·88	1·22	0·50	0·53	—	1·15
	1944	0·56	0·92	0·29	0·19	0·80	—	—	0·70
	1945	1·99	0·54	0·36	0·10	—	0·71	—	0·48
Venereal Diseases	1941	3·10	3·00	2·60	2·20	1·50	4·00	—	2·80
	1942	7·10	3·70	2·40	3·90	1·30	3·30	—	3·90
	1943	6·82	2·10	1·69	1·97	2·49	0·53	1·18	2·37
	1944	4·94	2·12	1·20	1·48	2·92	0·61	—	2·05
	1945	9·45	2·25	1·37	1·38	1·16	2·83	1·37	2·11
Inefective Hepatitis	1941	1·50	0·70	1·00	—	—	—	—	0·80
	1942	5·00	2·00	2·50	1·10	0·60	0·70	—	2·40
	1943	6·97	2·50	1·88	1·41	2·49	1·05	1·18	2·65
	1944	—	1·59	1·33	0·93	—	—	—	1·33
	1945	—	3·65	1·90	3·94	2·90	—	—	2·97
Post-Inoculation Effects	1941	8·90	3·60	4·20	2·90	2·30	2·60	—	4·70
	1942	3·80	1·20	1·20	1·40	0·60	0·70	3·00	1·60
	1943	5·15	2·04	1·98	0·28	1·00	7·37	3·53	2·21
	1944	9·33	1·48	2·40	0·93	—	—	—	2·08
	1945	4·98	0·75	0·24	—	—	—	—	0·63

TABLE 21—(*contd.*)

W.A.A.F. Diseases and Injuries by Age Groups, 1941–45—Rates per 1,000 Strength

DISEASES:		AGE GROUPS							Rate per 1,000 All Ages
		Under 20	20–24	25–29	30–34	35–39	40–44	45 and Over	
Other Infections	1941	102·80	46·70	47·00	32·40	19·20	34·20	13·50	56·50
	1942	79·90	36·20	34·10	31·40	33·00	44·40	31·70	41·90
	1943	63·79	19·64	16·87	15·86	15·20	9·48	12·96	22·10
	1944	63·06	32·71	15·06	15·95	23·92	12·11	—	29·18
	1945	46·52	20·73	11·75	18·12	23·18	14·16	27·40	18·64
Septic Conditions	1941	52·20	26·20	27·40	24·50	24·50	42·10	13·50	31·80
	1942	70·60	28·30	26·90	26·60	30·10	28·50	28·70	34·20
	1943	91·58	27·59	22·00	24·40	27·67	27·38	11·78	31·29
	1944	63·44	35·57	18·15	16·69	23·92	24·21	—	31·82
	1945	52·24	35·88	15·40	26·59	8·69	21·25	—	28·60
Alimentary System	1941	91·70	47·90	45·50	54·40	61·40	77·60	60·80	58·00
	1942	102·80	43·90	38·60	33·30	43·60	50·40	39·20	51·00
	1943	146·81	53·76	47·19	42·60	49·85	52·66	65·96	59·10
	1944	118·01	59·98	45·42	54·88	42·52	62·35	29·10	59·60
	1945	199·25	81·79	51·66	57·21	73·00	44·62	43·83	73·62
Circulatory System	1941	7·70	5·40	4·50	10·10	22·20	15·80	20·30	6·70
	1942	8·70	5·00	6·60	8·80	11·20	17·90	28·70	6·50
	1943	14·00	5·57	6·53	7·88	9·22	18·96	37·69	6·90
	1944	8·96	6·03	6·25	7·69	9·30	32·69	59·52	6·92
	1945	11·69	7·72	7·56	7·68	9·85	9·91	17·81	7·91
Respiratory System	1941	44·70	32·00	41·80	59·40	74·40	103·90	118·20	40·50
	1942	30·20	15·90	19·50	23·20	28·80	47·70	37·70	19·90
	1943	75·25	30·50	30·81	35·37	60·07	58·45	73·03	35·46
	1944	56·44	34·81	24·77	37·91	47·30	69·61	46·30	34·82
	1945	112·19	38·74	28·63	37·91	18·83	46·03	30·14	37·30
Allergy, Diseases of	1941	5·90	4·50	4·50	6·50	8·40	5·30	10·10	5·10
	1942	8·40	5·10	4·30	4·70	7·40	6·00	12·10	5·50
	1943	8·71	4·44	3·51	3·47	4·49	3·69	8·24	4·56
	1944	12·69	4·80	1·86	9·45	5·85	0·61	1·32	4·91
	1945	26·12	4·76	2·20	3·25	5·79	—	—	4·45

Urinary System	1941	12·40	10·40	11·10	16·90	20·70	17·10	16·90	11·70
	1942	18·50	12·30	12·70	11·20	12·80	8·60	10·50	13·10
	1943	24·75	12·02	10·82	12·67	10·72	10·00	12·96	12·79
	1944	14·37	13·41	12·90	11·49	11·16	6·05	—	13·06
	1945	22·89	16·05	11·37	14·38	2·90	7·79	1·37	14·26
Diseases Peculiar to Women									
Disorders of Menstruation	1941	10·20	7·80	10·50	13·00	18·40	25·00	—	9·50
	1942	18·80	11·00	13·10	13·00	16·00	47·70	66·40	13·50
	1943	24·96	10·93	12·28	13·14	22·93	43·71	75·38	13·30
	1944	34·61	15·74	11·39	6·67	18·87	68·40	66·14	16·19
	1945	27·36	13·58	8·65	15·26	14·20	50·28	46·20	13·16
Other conditions	1941	17·80	12·80	19·20	21·60	25·30	40·80	40·50	16·20
	1942	26·30	18·00	24·10	25·00	32·30	37·20	31·70	21·30
	1943	44·05	22·28	24·24	29·18	29·66	35·28	20·02	25·00
	1944	35·82	33·47	23·07	28·64	20·46	19·98	—	30·50
	1945	44·78	29·69	19·26	21·96	37·66	22·66	54·79	26·72
Locomotor System									
Rheumatic Group of Diseases	1941	7·60	6·80	7·20	9·70	23·00	25·00	30·40	8·10
	1942	11·90	8·00	11·40	13·80	23·40	24·50	24·10	10·20
	1943	18·00	6·82	9·59	12·76	18·69	28·96	24·73	9·10
	1944	9·42	6·66	7·02	13·26	29·76	24·82	13·23	8·02
	1945	17·66	7·74	11·23	14·08	12·17	7·79	82·19	10·00
Other conditions	1941	13·20	8·30	12·20	13·70	11·50	21·10	23·70	10·60
	1942	15·80	8·80	9·30	12·60	17·30	19·20	36·20	10·60
	1943	18·87	8·50	9·13	13·60	14·71	24·75	38·87	10·17
	1944	12·50	8·51	9·66	10·85	23·12	24·21	22·49	9·68
	1945	41·79	9·47	8·81	9·85	7·53	29·75	10·96	10·38
Nervous System and Mental diseases									
Psychoneuroses	1941	12·30	6·90	12·10	10·10	23·80	15·80	13·50	9·60
	1942	18·50	10·60	15·40	18·40	25·30	35·10	28·70	13·80
	1943	27·00	11·93	14·43	22·52	28·41	40·55	47·11	15·00
	1944	9·98	13·96	13·46	20·67	20·99	22·40	29·10	14·32
	1945	25·87	12·51	11·89	15·75	15·93	8·50	23·29	13·04
Psychoses	1941	1·50	1·10	1·20	2·90	3·80	1·30	—	1·40
	1942	2·20	1·20	2·20	3·10	1·60	4·00	3·00	1·70
	1943	1·89	0·60	0·45	1·03	1·50	2·10	2·36	0·74
	1944	1·03	0·48	0·29	0·83	0·27	3·03	—	0·51
	1945	4·97	0·41	0·31	0·49	0·58	—	—	0·51

TABLE 21 (*contd.*)

W.A.A.F. Diseases and Injuries by Age Groups, 1941–45—Rates per 1,000 Strength

DISEASES:		AGE GROUPS							Rate per 1,000 All Ages
		Under 20	20–24	25–29	30–34	35–39	40–44	45 and Over	
Psychopathic Personality	1941	1·30	0·80	1·40	0·70	2·30	4·00	—	1·10
	1942	4·00	1·50	2·20	3·10	4·20	4·00	—	2·20
	1943	7·84	2·00	2·18	4·13	4·99	3·16	2·36	2·69
	1944	9·42	4·28	3·17	3·80	6·64	8·47	11·90	4·45
	1945	16·42	3·96	2·53	4·23	6·37	2·13	4·11	3·95
Mental Defect	1941	0·20	0·30	0·10	—	—	—	—	0·20
	1942	1·30	0·50	0·60	0·10	—	1·30	—	0·60
	1943	1·16	0·42	0·23	0·66	0·75	0·53	—	0·46
	1944	1·03	0·26	0·21	0·46	0·27	1·21	—	0·32
	1945	0·99	0·14	0·02	0·20	0·29	—	—	0·13
Epilepsies	1941	2·00	1·00	0·40	1·10	3·10	1·30	—	1·20
	1942	3·90	1·20	1·20	1·80	0·30	1·30	—	1·60
	1943	3·41	0·87	0·29	0·84	0·25	0·53	—	0·95
	1944	1·40	1·04	1·01	0·19	0·27	—	—	0·97
	1945	1·49	0·55	0·47	1·18	1·16	0·71	—	0·61
Indefinite Aetiology	1941	4·80	2·80	2·50	3·20	2·30	2·60	3·40	3·20
	1942	7·70	3·60	2·70	3·70	5·40	7·30	12·10	4·20
	1943	7·98	2·56	2·50	2·91	4·24	3·16	3·53	3·04
	1944	2·61	3·07	2·87	3·89	—	12·11	13·23	3·12
	1945	5·47	2·56	1·63	1·97	0·29	—	13·70	2·30
Organic Nervous Diseases	1941	3·00	2·30	4·30	5·00	10·00	7·90	13·50	3·20
	1942	3·50	2·20	3·10	3·40	3·50	11·90	9·00	2·80
	1943	3·77	2·26	3·44	4·97	5·48	6·85	2·36	2·87
	1944	6·25	2·48	2·21	3·43	7·97	1·21	3·97	2·83
	1945	2·74	2·76	2·39	3·35	7·24	7·79	16·44	2·92
Eye	1941	6·40	3·40	5·20	3·60	2·30	7·90	10·10	4·40
	1942	8·40	3·60	4·10	2·50	3·80	0·70	6·00	4·30
	1943	9·22	3·38	3·28	4·13	4·24	8·43	4·71	3·93
	1944	6·72	4·14	2·26	1·95	—	6·66	13·23	3·73
	1945	14·92	5·22	2·80	2·07	6·08	0·71	—	4·50

Ear Nose and Throat	1941	33·10	20·70	20·20	16·50	19·20	6·60	10·10	22·60
	1942	39·90	17·70	15·90	13·10	13·10	10·60	6·00	20·10
	1943	61·47	21·37	15·92	15·29	14·96	12·64	14·13	22·89
	1944	32·47	19·84	12·37	8·99	13·55	7·26	13·23	18·04
	1945	74·38	23·36	13·86	21·27	6·95	8·50	1·37	21·17
Skin	1941	63·40	26·90	18·50	12·90	14·60	18·40	6·80	31·90
	1942	97·60	33·70	25·00	19·20	12·80	17·90	12·10	39·90
	1943	95·57	24·16	18·04	13·42	11·96	13·16	12·96	27·53
	1944	62·23	22·33	9·63	11·40	6·38	18·16	13·23	20·93
	1945	63·68	26·45	8·91	16·35	8·98	21·95	—	20·97
All other Disorders and Unclassified conditions	1941	60·50	36·10	40·20	47·90	50·60	52·60	60·80	43·30
	1942	51·80	27·60	28·10	34·60	35·20	32·50	51·30	32·00
	1943	72·93	29·50	31·04	33·87	45·11	31·07	51·83	33·85
	1944	57·19	43·58	33·98	47·00	42·52	38·14	43·65	42·48
	1945	94·28	45·42	24·54	41·36	24·04	53·12	19·18	39·73
Totals of all Diseases	1941	798·80	449·10	505·90	540·00	643·40	739·50	645·20	546·60
	1942	969·40	455·60	447·90	436·30	511·80	614·70	564·10	532·30
	1943	1,360·52	506·26	458·84	492·12	575·27	655·61	681·98	567·10
	1944	909·32	521·81	364·02	418·52	456·55	586·56	420·64	503·86
	1945	1,385·82	460·24	338·07	453·57	353·13	440·51	463·01	503·23
INJURIES	1941	48·80	28·20	29·30	37·40	36·00	40·80	40·50	33·70
	1942	77·60	34·10	31·50	30·20	34·60	41·80	36·20	41·00
	1943	93·47	32·70	30·00	27·49	31·16	48·97	41·22	36·79
	1944	55·79	35·22	28·71	25·58	30·56	44·79	39·68	34·49
	1945	78·11	32·56	24·11	22·94	11·88	56·66	27·40	30·36
Totals of all Disabilities	1941	847·60	477·30	535·20	577·40	679·40	780·30	685·70	580·30
	1942	1,047·00	489·70	479·40	466·50	546·40	656·50	600·30	572·30
	1943	1,453·99	538·96	488·84	519·61	606·43	704·58	723·20	603·89
	1944	965·11	557·03	392·73	444·10	487·11	631·35	460·32	538·35
	1945	1,463·93	592·80	362·18	476·51	365·01	497·17	490·41	533·59

INCIDENCE OF DISEASE AMONG W.A.A.F. OFFICERS AND AIRWOMEN, 1942–45

Table 22 records the incidence of disease per 1,000 of strength for officers and airwomen for the years 1942–45. Comparisons between the two groups are of very little value as they have not been standardised for age.

In the early years of the war the incidence of sickness tended to be higher in airwomen, but in 1944 and 1945 there was a higher total incidence of disease among officers.

PSYCHONEUROSES tended to be more prevalent among officers and, as would be expected, PSYCHOPATHIC PERSONALITIES were more common among airwomen. VENEREAL DISEASE was much less common in officers than in airwomen.

FINAL INVALIDINGS, W.A.A.F.

There were 14,072 invalidings from the W.A.A.F. during the war years and all except 65 were due to disease. The conditions leading to invaliding are shown in Table 23, which gives the total number of cases of each condition, the total number invalided, the invaliding rate per cent. of cases and the invaliding incidence per 1,000 of strength for each year except 1939, when there were only 9 invalidings.

The total invaliding incidence in 1940 and 1941 was low and compared favourably with the incidence in the R.A.F.; in 1941, for instance, the invaliding rate due to disease in the R.A.F. was 14·9 per 1,000 of strength and in the W.A.A.F. 11·3 per 1,000 of strength. In 1942, however, there was a big jump in the W.A.A.F. invaliding rate and, although there was a slight fall in later years, the rate remained high for the rest of the war. In the early years of the war the W.A.A.F. was entirely a volunteer force and the increase in invaliding in 1942 may be in some degree attributed to the introduction of conscription.

DISEASES OF THE NERVOUS SYSTEM AND MENTAL DISEASES as a group were responsible for 7,247 invalidings, or just over half the total. PSYCHONEUROSES accounted for 3,856 of this number and the invaliding rate per 1,000 of strength for psychoneuroses was much higher than in the R.A.F. This difference was almost certainly due to the greater difficulty women experienced in adapting themselves to Service conditions. A considerable proportion of these women had never had a civilian job and tended to break down rapidly under conditions of community regimentation. They were usually solitary, shy individuals with few external interests and dependent on maternal decisions. They had a tendency to form strong emotional attachments.

TABLE 22

W.A.A.F.—Incidence of Diseases among Officers and Airwomen, 1942–45

	OFFICERS				AIRWOMEN			
	1942	1943	1944	1945	1942	1943	1944	1945
DISEASES:								
Upper Respiratory Tract	143·6	191·67	155·04	143·95	166·1	209·8	136·51	137·66
Pneumonia	3·8	3·20	—	3·47	3·7	2·63	1·51	1·87
Tuberculosis, all types	1·7	1·01	3·55	1·73	4·6	4·41	3·36	2·85
Venereal Diseases	—	0·17	0·16	—	4·0	2·45	2·12	2·19
Other Infections	56·2	39·11	37·31	45·27	45·6	26·54	32·43	21·26
Septic Conditions	20·5	15·34	22·61	15·61	34·8	31·84	32·16	29·15
Alimentary System	53·5	72·32	62·34	89·49	50·9	58·64	59·50	72·95
Circulatory System	2·5	5·23	6·94	12·66	6·6	6·96	6·92	7·70
Respiratory System	23·3	38·94	45·87	33·82	19·8	35·34	34·41	37·45
Allergy, Diseases of	4·9	3·71	0·16	—	5·5	4·59	5·08	4·64
Urinary System	15·2	15·51	11·31	9·02	13·0	12·70	13·13	14·48
Diseases Peculiar to Women:								
Disorders of Menstruation	14·4	18·38	13·40	19·77	13·4	13·13	16·29	12·89
Others	20·1	30·85	24·55	26·02	21·4	24·80	30·72	26·75
Locomotor System:								
Rheumatic Group of Diseases	12·9	11·80	17·93	10·75	10·1	9·01	7·66	9·97
Others	9·7	12·47	13·08	7·11	10·7	10·09	9·55	10·51
Nervous System and Mental Diseases:								
Psychoneuroses	13·9	18·04	29·88	28·79	13·8	14·89	13·75	12·37
Psychoses	1·3	0·34	0·48	0·17	1·7	0·76	0·51	0·53
Psychopathic Personality	1·5	0·84	1·45	3·47	2·2	2·76	4·56	3·97
Mental Defect	—	—	—	—	0·6	0·48	0·33	0·14
Epilepsies	0·4	0·17	—	0·17	1·7	0·97	1·01	0·63
Indefinite Aetiology	2·7	2·36	3·39	0·17	4·2	3·06	3·10	2·39
Organic Nervous Diseases	5·3	5·23	3·71	7·28	2·7	2·79	2·79	2·74
Eye	1·5	5·39	6·46	3·99	4·4	3·88	3·63	4·52
Ear, Nose and Throat	26·9	25·79	16·15	22·89	19·8	22·79	18·11	21·10
Skin	8·5	6·07	19·38	10·41	41·1	28·27	20·99	21·41
All Other Diseases and Unallocated Conditions	38·1	36·24	46·86	27·40	31·8	33·76	42·31	40·25
Totals of all Diseases	482·4	560·18	541·99	523·41	534·2	567·34	502·44	502·37
INJURIES	29·0	27·48	21·32	29·83	40·4	37·10	34·98	30·39
Totals of all Diseases and Injuries	511·4	587·66	563·31	553·24	574·6	604·44	537·42	532·76

TABLE 23

Final Invalidings, W.A.A.F., 1939–45

CAUSES OF INVALIDING	Number of Cases*	Number of Invalidings	Invaliding Rate per cent. of Cases	Invaliding incidence per 1,000 of strength					
				1940	1941	1942	1943	1944	1945*
DISEASES									
Acute Infections	22,088	141	0·63	0·31	0·10	0·41	0·24	0·13	0·20
Tuberculosis, Pulmonary	1,825	1,395	76·4	0·84	0·79	2·63	2·47	1·94	1·64
Tuberculosis (Other sites)	574	294	51·2	0·38	0·27	0·55	0·49	0·36	0·40
Septic Conditions	20,126	25	0·12	Nil	Nil	0·08	0·03	0·04	0·02
Alimentary System	38,971	419	1·07	0·23	0·44	0·77	0·62	0·68	0·48
Circulatory System	4,491	545	12·13	0·69	0·75	1·18	0·81	0·71	0·57
Venereal Diseases	1,661	17	1·02	0·08	0·04	0·07	0·03	Nil	Nil
Blood, Blood-forming Organs, Spleen and R.E. System	1,942	69	3·55	0·15	0·04	0·14	0·10	0·11	0·07
Respiratory System	21,746	623	2·86	0·69	0·37	0·67	0·89	1·19	1·02
Allergy	3,076	226	7·34	0·08	0·29	0·50	0·20	0·34	0·37
Urinary System	8,444	219	2·59	Nil	0·31	0·40	0·29	0·34	0·30
Locomotor System	12,427	901	7·25	0·76	0·37	1·24	1·27	1·46	1·65
Nervous System and Mental Diseases:									
Psychoneuroses	8,986	3,856	42·9	2·21	3·00	6·20	6·70	5·31	5·44
Psychoses	572	440	76·9	0·23	0·85	1·30	0·54	0·39	0·44
Psychopathic Personality	2,035	1,925	94·6	0·23	0·64	1·95	2·30	4·10	3·67
Mental Defect	240	231	96·25	0·08	0·17	0·56	0·43	0·32	0·13
Epilepsies	690	401	58·1	0·61	0·56	1·09	0·58	0·45	0·32
Indefinite Aetiology	1,988	216	10·9	0·23	0·21	0·44	0·28	0·34	0·26
Organic Nervous Diseases	1,873	177	9·45	0·15	0·15	0·30	0·20	0·29	0·30
Total Nervous System and Mental Diseases	16,384	7,247	44·1	3·74	5·58	11·84	11·03	11·20	10·56
Eye	2,607	108	4·14	Nil	0·04	0·27	0·15	0·15	0·13
E.N.T.	13,417	366	2·72	0·31	0·29	0·78	0·50	0·42	0·61
Skin	17,617	199	1·12	0·23	0·04	0·16	0·29	0·42	0·34
Endocrine	862	216	25·05	0·38	0·27	0·31	0·28	0·34	0·35
Metabolism	120	58	48·33	0·15	0·08	0·09	0·12	0·07	0·05
Cysts and Tumours	1,636	93	5·68	0·53	0·15	0·14	0·07	0·17	0·13
Diseases peculiar to women	25,241	620	2·45	0·53	0·66	0·99	0·08	1·03	0·85
Indefinite and General	19,261	226	1·17	0·69	0·39	0·27	0·27	0·35	0·39
Other Minor Sickness	110,383	—	—	—	—	—	—	—	—
Total Invalidings by Diseases	344,899	14,007	4·06	10·77	11·27	23·42	20·98	21·45	20·13
Other Conditions	211	—	—	—	—	—	—	—	—
INJURIES	23,162	65	0·28	Nil	0·12	0·11	0·16	0·08	0·02
Grand Total Invalidings by Disease and Injury	368,272	14,072	3·82	10·77	11·39	23·53	21·14	21·53	20·15

* September 1939—August 15, 1945.

As would be expected the invaliding rate per cent. of cases was very high for mental diseases, particularly for cases of PSYCHOPATHIC PERSONALITY and MENTAL DEFECT.

PULMONARY TUBERCULOSIS was second in order of frequency as a cause of invaliding; there were 1,395 invalidings due to this disease with an invaliding rate of 76·4 per cent. Tuberculosis in other sites was responsible for 294 invalidings.

Discharges from the Service due to PREGNANCY do not appear as invalidings.

DEATHS, W.A.A.F., 1939–45

Table 24 records the number of deaths from the specified causes and the fatality rate per cent. of cases.

There was a total of 496 deaths in the W.A.A.F. during the war, 287 due to disease and 209 due to injuries. TUBERCULOSIS was the most important cause of death and was responsible for 68 deaths. Conditions of the ALIMENTARY SYSTEM led to 46 deaths, of the NERVOUS SYSTEM and MENTAL DISEASES to 31 deaths, and ACUTE INFECTIONS to 30 deaths.

TABLE 24

Deaths, W.A.A.F., 1939–45

CAUSES	Number of Cases	Number of Deaths	Fatality Rate per cent. of Cases
DISEASES			
Acute Infections	22,088	30	0·13
Pneumonia	1,552	21	1·82
Pulmonary Tuberculosis	1,825	29	1·58
Tuberculosis (other sites)	574	39	6·8
Alimentary System	38,971	46	0·11
Circulatory System	4,491	12	0·26
Blood, Blood-forming Organs, Spleen and Reticulo-Endothelial System	1,942	16	0·82
Respiratory System	21,746	10	0·04
Nervous System and Mental Diseases	16,441	31	0·18
Urinary System	8,444	9	0·10
Cysts and Tumours	1,636	20	1·22
Diseases peculiar to women	25,241	10	0·03
All other Diseases	199,948	14	0·007
Total Diseases	344,899	287	0·08
INJURIES	23,162	209	0·90
Other Conditions	211		
Total Diseases and Injuries	368,272	496	0·13

The Emergency Medical Services

A WAR-TIME STUDY OF CAUSES OF ADMISSIONS TO HOSPITAL

An Analysis of the Records of E.M.S. In-Patients, 1940-47

by Eileen M. Brooke, M.Sc.

21*CMS

CONTENTS

INTRODUCTION

'Up to the present time the statistics of hospitals have been kept on no uniform plan. Every hospital has followed its own nomenclature and classification of diseases, and there has been no reduction on any uniform model of the vast amount of observations which have been made in these establishments. So far as relates either to medical or sanitary science, these observations in their present state bear exactly the same relation as an indefinite number of astronomical observations made without concert and reduced to no common standard, would bear to the progress of astronomy. The material exists, but it is inaccessible.'

Thus wrote Florence Nightingale, in presenting to the Fourth Session of the International Statistical Congress of 1860, a 'Proposal for an Uniform Plan of Hospital Statistics'. Her remarks were probably scarcely less applicable in 1939 at the outbreak of the Second World War than when they were written. Two problems were indicated by Miss Nightingale; firstly, the need for providing a uniform classification of diseases for use in hospitals, and secondly that for collecting observations in a uniform way. Although a uniform classification had existed for about eighty years, it related primarily to causes of death and was unsuitable for morbidity coding, while, with the possible exception of mental hospitals, there was a complete lack of uniformity in the keeping of medical records.

Early attempts at classifying diseases were made by de Lacroix (1706–77), Linnaeus (1707–78) and Cullen (1710–90). William Farr, first Medical Statistician to the General Register Office, was greatly impressed with the need for a classification of diseases for statistical purposes; and in 1853 at the First International Statistical Congress he laid down the principles which he considered should be followed in producing such a List. The Congress, recognising the value of a uniform classification, asked Farr and d'Espine of Geneva to prepare classifications for consideration at the Congress of 1855. D'Espine's grouping was based on the nature of diseases; for example, gouty, herpetic, haematic, etc. Farr's list contained five groups:

(1) epidemic diseases

(2) constitutional (or general) diseases

(3) local diseases according to anatomical site

(4) developmental diseases

(5) diseases which were the direct result of violence.

The Congress of 1855 adopted a list of 139 classes arranged in accordance with Farr's proposals. Subsequent congresses in 1864, 1874, 1880 and 1886 revised the original list, but without departing from the original structure. When the International Congress was replaced by the International Statistical Institute in 1891, a committee under the chairmanship of Dr. Bertillon was requested to prepare a classification of causes of death. The result, which was adopted in 1893, followed Farr's principle of separating general diseases from those which attacked an isolated organ. Subsequent revisions of the classification gradually began to come into international use, and in 1923, following Bertillon's death, it was agreed that responsibility for the classification should be shared by the International Statistical Institute and the Health Organisation of the League of Nations. While interest had centred on a classification of causes of death, the necessity had not been overlooked for extending the classification to diseases which cause disability, without usually being fatal. Two difficulties arose in this connexion, the lack of definition of what constitutes a sick person and the lack of a suitable body of material to classify, since except for certain infectious diseases, there has been no registration of sickness comparable with the registration of cause of death. In both 1900 and 1909 when the Classification of Causes of Death was revised, attempts were made to provide a parallel list for coding illnesses which are generally non-fatal, but they met with little success. In 1936 Canada published a 'Standard Morbidity Code' for use in the Dominion Council of Health, and in 1944 the Medical Research Council issued a 'Provisional Classification of Diseases and Injuries for use in compiling Morbidity Statistics'. This was the classification used to code causes of admission to Emergency Medical Service Hospitals—the subject matter of the present report.

The experience gained from using this list was subsequently helpful in the preparation by a specialist committee of the World Health Organisation of the Manual of the International Statistical Classification of Diseases, Injuries and Causes of Death (Sixth Revision of the International List of Diseases, Injuries and Causes of Death). This classification, which was adopted in 1948, came into use in 1950 for the preparation by Member States of the World Health Organisation of their official statistics of both mortality and morbidity.

The second need to which Miss Nightingale referred, namely that of obtaining a body of observations recorded and abstracted in a uniform way was largely overcome when the Emergency Medical Services were brought into operation in 1939. With the increasing tension in Europe during 1937–39, the possibility of a second European war could not be ignored. The experience of the Spanish Civil War showed the need for defending the civilian population against aerial attack and for providing treatment for casualties. Early in 1938 medical officers of the Ministry of Health surveyed the existing hospital accommodation in England and Wales, and recorded 3,128 hospitals and institutions containing 400,000–500,000 beds of which 130,000 were in mental hospitals. Hospitals were divided into two categories, voluntary and municipal. The former class comprised general and special hospitals run by voluntary contributions; the latter consisted of general hospitals, those for infectious diseases, tuberculosis hospitals and sanatoria and maternity and child welfare institutions, whose support was derived partly from Ministry grants and partly from local rates. Both classes co-operated fully in the Survey. Prior to June 1938, local authorities were required to provide accommodation for the treatment of casualties as part of their air-raid precautions, but in June 1938 the Ministry of Health assumed responsibility for the scheme.

It had been estimated that in the event of war immediate accommodation should be available for 300,000 civilian casualties, in addition to the possible requirements of the Fighting Services. This was to be done in three ways, by discharging all ambulant patients and those who could safely be sent home, thus clearing about 100,000 beds, by 'crowding' hospitals by introducing 110,000 extra beds and by building new hutted hospitals to hold 90,000 beds. When the war broke out the Emergency Medical Services had retained 2,370 hospitals with 492,570 beds, of which 309,354 were suitable for casualties, the rest being mostly in Infectious Diseases hospitals and sanatoria. Within a week 187,000 extra beds had been provided by 'crowding'.

As the expected aerial bombardment did not materialise a number of hospitals were released for the treatment of ordinary civilian sick, so that by January 1940 there were 1,207 hospitals remaining in the scheme, with 407,612 beds, of which 262,859 were for casualties. By the end of 1942 a further reduction had taken place, leaving 892 hospitals and institutions with 278,761 beds. The numbers then remained fairly constant, but from 1945 onwards there was a steady decline, so that by the end of 1947 329 hospitals were left in the service containing 18,000 beds, which were, however, available for ordinary civilian use when not required for E.M.S. patients. The Emergency Hospital Services were finally merged in the National Health Service in July 1948.

In addition to ordinary facilities for the treatment of casualties, a number of special centres were set up, either as separate hospitals or as wings of existing hospitals. These numbered about 120 in all, the main groups being for cases requiring orthopaedic surgery (20), for skin diseases (20), neurosis (14), maxillo-facial injuries (12), head injuries (11) and chest injuries (10).

The main classes of E.M.S. patients were:

(a) Civilians, including regular Police, suffering from war injuries and injuries incurred in the performance of Civil Defence duties.

(b) Service men and women, whether sick or injured, including repatriated prisoners-of-war, Dominion and Allied Forces, including their auxiliary medical personnel.

(c) Merchant Navy officers and men.

(d) Evacuee children, refugees from Gibraltar and the Channel Islands, sick civilians moved from target areas, transferred war workers and those in agricultural or forestry camps.

(e) Persons whom, in the interest of the war effort, it was necessary to restore to health and full working capacity as quickly as possible, notably cases of fractures and certain other types of injury occurring among manual workers in factories and full-time Civil Defence workers.

The medical records of most of these patients, whether Service or civilian, receiving in-patient treatment in E.M.S. hospitals were collected at the Ministry of Pensions either during or after the war. Where a patient was admitted to hospital once or several times, the case papers for each admission were put in a separate envelope, these being filed alphabetically according to surname. A one-fifth sample of admissions was made by taking the files in order, assigning serial numbers to the admissions occurring in each half-year, and extracting all whose serial number ended in 0 or 5. Three other methods of sampling suggested themselves, to select certain letters and take all cases filed under these, to take all admissions to hospital on certain days or to select a number of hospitals and take all their admissions. All these methods would have introduced a bias, the first because of the preponderance of certain initial letters in Welsh and Scotch surnames, the second because of the seasonal variation in disease incidence and the last because of the greater prevalence of some diseases in particular regions, as of jaundice in the eastern counties. If a patient, after discharge, re-entered hospital for further treatment of the same condition within a week of discharge, the second visit was not counted as a separate admission. In the comparatively rare event of the case papers not containing a definite diagnosis, the envelope next in the series was taken as a substitute. It may reasonably be claimed that, as far as the documents were concerned, the sample was a random one.

The information gained from the case papers was entered on a card, the following items being recorded:

Dates of admission and discharge.
Sex. Age. Service or Civilian case.
Branch of Service. Rank.
Civil Defence Service or other occupation, for civilian patients.
Name of Hospital and county in which situated.

Result of treatment, e.g., return to duty, regraded, discharged from the Forces, etc.

Number of days of in-patient treatment, including time spent in other hospitals and convalescent homes, and, in the case of men with injuries received abroad, the time from date of injury to discharge from hospital. Space was provided for showing the names of hospitals to which the patients were transferred.

The final diagnosis of the patient's condition was entered under four headings by inserting the appropriate code number from the M.R.C. Provisional Classification of Diseases, Injuries and Causes of Death.

(1) Principal disease or injury causing admission.
(2) Principal complications of (1).
(3) Principal accessory acute disease or injury.
(4) Principal chronic disease.

These four items, and any other pathological conditions mentioned in the case history, were recorded in words on the back of the card. For research purposes it was found desirable to record the theatre of war in which an injury was received and also whether or not a blood transfusion was given.

The work of reading the case papers, filling in cards and coding diseases was done by clerks with occasional recourse to medical advice. It was usually easy to find which was the principal cause of admission, but in cases where two acute conditions were given as joint causes, the rules for selection on page 9 of the M.R.C. Classification were followed. With coding rules established and a good medical dictionary available, lack of previous knowledge was not found to be an insuperable difficulty. An average coder could easily read and record fifty cases a day, while quicker or more experienced workers achieved a rate of seventy or over. This may have some bearing on problems of hospital administration, for if hospital records were designed to include a uniform front sheet to the case history it should be possible for statistical records to be abstracted at a sufficiently high rate to make feasible the collection of hospital statistics on a national scale. The form used in the Hospital In-patient Enquiry conducted as an experiment by the General Register Office was designed for use also as a front sheet for case histories with intention that the section dealing with diagnosis should be completed under the direction of a doctor. Expense is lessened and uniformity enhanced if coding is done at a central office.

The objection raised against hospital statistics of causes of admission is that they are biased because of the method of selection of cases for in-patient treatment. Under ordinary circumstances the more serious cases are sent to hospital, or those which for various reasons cannot be nursed at home. This results in an unduly high case-fatality rate for hospital cases. Also there may have been, at any rate in the past, a tendency for the wealthier sections of the community to be treated in nursing homes. Diseases showing a social class differential would, therefore, not be represented in their true proportions in hospital statistics. Conditions of life in the Forces were such, however, that the greater number of patients requiring treatment in bed for more than four days had to be sent to hospital; hence Service cases were more representative of varying degrees of severity.

It may be urged that the population from which the E.M.S. hospital cases were mainly drawn was a specially selected one, because those with certain chronic diseases would be excluded by the Medical Boards from entry to the Services at all. The methods of modern warfare, requiring a relatively large number of technicians, are such that it was not quite so essential to have all Service men of as high a standard of fitness as in previous wars, while reserved occupations had to retain a large number of those fit for service.

Most hospital statistics which have been presented in the past have been based on serial observations made over a number of years in a particular hospital. While the limitations of the E.M.S. data are fully appreciated it is considered useful to produce an analysis of the results obtained, firstly, because any conclusions which may be drawn are based on a larger number of cases than has been available to individual workers, secondly, because there has been a serious lack of knowledge of such matters as duration of hospitalisation both for sickness and injuries, and lastly, because information is available about conditions such as homologous serum jaundice, which the war brought into prominence.

PART I. Service Patients

CAUSES OF ADMISSION

In all, the records of 317,699 patients admitted during 1940–47 were examined, the constitution of the sample by sex and branch of Service being as follows:

	Army	*Navy*	*Air Force*	*Totals*
Males	234,809	13,313	40,465	288,587
Females	18,388	994	9,730	29,112

The numbers of males admitted were 12·8, 13·4 and 4·2 times those of females for the Army, Navy and Air Force respectively. The composition of the sample by sex and age is shown below.

	15–	25–	35–	45–	55–	All Ages
Males:						
Numbers	115,917	120,415	45,643	5,964	648	288,587
Proportions	402	417	158	21	2	1,000
Females:						
Numbers	22,048	5,720	1,147	191	6	29,112
Proportions	757	197	39	7	0	1,000

Whereas the population of the country at large varies continuously, so that it is possible to make a reasonably reliable estimate of its composition at intercensal periods, the number of Armed Forces at home was subject to sudden fluctuations, making it impossible to calculate a population at risk on which sickness rates could be based. The problem of calculating rates would be further complicated by the admission to E.M.S. Hospitals of cases returning from overseas theatres of war, and in the later years of sick ex-prisoners-of-war. While it seems probable that the number of Service cases treated in Military Hospitals was about double that in E.M.S. Hospitals, it is by no means certain that individual diseases were represented in the same proportions in the two types of institution; this applies particularly to venereal diseases which were mainly treated in Military Hospitals. For these reasons it has been judged best to present proportionate rates. Since the incidence of infective and respiratory diseases is subject to variation from year to year, while the number of injuries depend very much on varying external factors, the proportions have been based in each year on the total hospital admissions due to diseases not included in the 'infective' and 'respiratory' sections of the classification. For convenience in presentation the diagnoses of primary causes of admission have been condensed into a Short List of forty-two groups, the composition of which in terms of code numbers of the Medical Research Council's Classification, is as follows:

S.L.	M.R.C.	S.L.	M.R.C.	S.L.	M.R.C.
1	02, 03	17	38–42	30	60, 61
2	04, 05	18	43	31	56–59
3	070–073, 443	19	450–452	32	620, 650
4	096	20	445–448	33	621–646, 651–679
5	00, 01, 06, 076–095, 097, 098	21	440–442, 444, 449, 453–468	34	68, 69
6	10, 700–706	22	47	35	71, 72
7	11–20	23	481, 482	36	73–75
8	22	24	540, 541, 543, 7686	37	76 (except 7686)
9	270–274	25	520–525	38	800, 840
10	21, 23–26, 275–299	26	491–494	39	841–845
11	331–333	27	500–503	40	90–92
12	51	28	507	41	93
13	30, 32, 330, 34, 35	29	480, 483–490, 495–499, 504–506, 508, 509, 526–539, 542, 544–554	42	801–839, 846–898 94–96
14	36				
15	37				
16	31				

The names of diseases in the groups have now been put in under each section, for example, S.L.1. 02,03 Tuberculosis.

The non-infective and non-respiratory disease total on which proportions are based consists of Sections I-XI of the Abridged Classification in Table I of Nos. 6–18; 22–37, in the Short List.

Annual tabulations according to the forty-two Short List numbers, subdivided by ten yearly age groups for each sex are given in Appendix I, page 724. The principal causes of admission for each year at all ages are shown in Table 1.

The rheumatic diseases accounted for between one-twentieth and one-twenty-fifth of the basic total of admissions of male patients and a rather lower proportion of those of women. It was to be expected that, owing to exposure to unfavourable weather conditions, Service men would be more prone to rheumatic diseases than women, while at the same time the nature of their work would make it less possible for them to carry on their duties when suffering from such complaints.

The group of illnesses comprising psychoneuroses, functional digestive disorders, psychoses and other nervous diseases contributed their highest proportions in 1944 and 1945 among men, coinciding with the campaign in Western Europe. It may well be that to many with a neurotic disposition this was the precipitating factor. The proportionate rate for women was highest in 1944, while for both sexes the rates were comparatively low in 1943 and declined after 1945.

Eye and ear diseases showed fairly constant rates, varying for men between 3 per cent. and 5 per cent. of the basic total and for women between about 2½ per cent. and 3½ per cent. The rates for diseases of the

TABLE 1

Causes of Admission of Service Patients to E.M.S. Hospitals, 1940–47. Proportion per 1,000 Non-infective and Non-respiratory Illnesses.

	Disease Group	Males								Females							
		1940	1941	1942	1943	1944	1945	1946	1947	1940	1941	1942	1943	1944	1945	1946	1947
I	Rheumatic diseases	51	52	53	48	47	40	33	27	33	30	53	47	37	32	33	4
II	Psychoses, neuroses and other nervous diseases	92	98	116	109	125	142	107	78	74	89	89	78	91	88	46	49
III	Eye and ear diseases	33	38	38	40	48	43	45	48	29	29	32	30	26	37	27	16
IV	Diseases of veins	71	89	85	78	75	66	59	44	24	22	19	29	37	32	41	20
V	Acute sore throat	101	75	69	82	67	62	75	89	152	92	101	133	88	58	82	69
VI	Hernia	101	83	68	62	60	66	71	50	7	8	3	4	6	3	4	—
VII	Gastric and duodenal ulcers	43	42	36	32	40	55	47	28	7	4	3	3	4	16	8	—
VIII	Other digestive diseases	126	126	132	129	127	125	146	193	295	253	219	205	214	240	254	323
IX	Diseases of skin and cellular tissue	178	179	151	177	176	152	157	193	99	100	88	95	108	97	107	86
X	Diseases of bones, joints and muscles	73	75	73	69	64	53	59	58	17	33	30	37	33	28	45	57
XI	Other non-respiratory and non-infective diseases	131	143	179	174	171	196	201	192	263	340	363	339	356	369	353	376
	Total non-infective and non-respiratory	1,000	1,000	1,000	1,000	1,000	1,000	1,000	1,000	1,000	1,000	1,000	1,000	1,000	1,000	1,000	1,000
XII	Infective diseases	372	219	154	208	217	208	273	260	807	322	247	216	149	140	144	184
XIII	Respiratory diseases	128	122	132	134	114	120	122	159	112	120	95	82	73	69	85	77
XIV	Head injuries	46	39	42	40	58	30	40	73	28	28	23	20	19	11	21	16
XV	Fractures (except skull)	86	86	106	112	200	117	86	114	20	32	34	34	30	22	25	24
XVI	Other injuries	164	121	160	160	401	131	104	144	44	50	77	66	62	43	64	58
	Total diseases and injuries	1,796	1,587	1,594	1,654	1,990	1,606	1,625	1,750	2,011	1,552	1,476	1,418	1,333	1,285	1.339	1,359

veins were much higher for men than women, and this may be compared with the fact that in the Social Survey of Sickness enquiry in 1949, 1 per cent. of men and 6 per cent. of women between the ages of 16 and 64 interviewed, reported diseases of the veins. It is possible that the higher proportion of male admissions attributed to vein diseases may have been due to the active conditions of service necessitating treatment with which it had been possible to dispense in civilian life, while for aesthetic reasons women would be more likely to seek early treatment for such a condition as varicose veins.

Acute sore throat, which comprises acute tonsillitis and acute pharyngitis, showed high proportions in 1940. During the subsequent years both sexes followed the same trend, showing decline in 1941 and 1942, an increase in 1943, further decreases in 1944 and 1945 and a rise in 1946. The proportionate rates varied among men between 6 per cent. and 10 per cent. and between 6 per cent. and 15 per cent. among women. Hernia accounted for comparatively few of the women's admissions, while for men the rates were only a little less than those for diseases of the veins.

Gastric and duodenal ulcers showed relatively high proportions in 1945 and 1946 for both sexes. From 1942 to 1947 the men's rates showed a similar trend to that for nervous diseases; declining from 1942 to 1943, rising to a maximum in 1945, then declining again in 1946 and 1947. This similarity is understandable in view of the psychoneurotic underlay in ulcer cases. The high proportion of women's admissions attributed to other digestive diseases is due to a large number of cases of appendicitis. Both sexes show high proportions of admissions due to skin diseases, 15–19 per cent. of the basic total for men and 9–11 per cent. for women. It is possible that this may be due to some extent to the transmission of such diseases as impetigo or *sycosis barbae*. Among males, admissions for diseases of bones, joints and muscles included a considerable number attributable to internal derangement of the knee joint, often due to physical training or organised games. Of the remaining non-infective and non-respiratory causes, the higher proportions for women were due to child-bearing and diseases of the female genital organs, the proportions in the eight years due to these causes being 14·3, 14·1, 14·0, 13·9, 19·0, 19·3, 16·4 and 22·2 per cent.

The proportions of admissions due to the conditions classed as infective diseases were highest for both males and females in 1940. For men the rate decreased in 1941 and 1942, and then increased, while for women there was a steady decline up to 1945, after which the rate again increased. Venereal diseases in every year had proportionate rates of less than 1 per cent. The rate for respiratory conditions remained fairly steady for men, while for women it declined between 1941 and 1945. The proportionate rates for injuries of all kinds depended to a large extent on the number of war injuries. In 1940, the year of the Dunkirk evacuation, the rate was 296 admissions for injury to every 1,000 admissions for non-infective and non-respiratory diseases and declined to 246 in 1941; this was followed by an increase in 1942 and 1943, reaching the peak value of 659 in 1944, with the opening of the Western front.

Selected Causes of Admission by Disease Group

TUBERCULOSIS (Short List Number 1)

The ratios of the numbers of admissions for all forms of Tuberculosis to 1,000 admissions for non-infective and non-respiratory illnesses in the corresponding sex-age groups were as follows:

TABLE 2

Tuberculosis, all forms. Proportion per 1,000 Admissions for Non-infective and Non-respiratory Illnesses, by Sex and Age, 1940–47

Year	Males						Females			
	Age groups						Age groups			
	15–	25–	35–	45–	55 up	All	15–	25–	35–44	15–44
1940	13	13	13	23	47	13	8	25	—	11
1941	21	16	12	11	18	17	12	10	12	12
1942	30	21	16	23	29	23	26	36	12	27
1943	26	16	18	17	16	20	19	14	16	18
1944	29	26	13	19	13	24	16	16	6	15
1945	28	25	23	14	—	26	30	24	16	27
1946	38	38	43	28	—	38	15	38	—	18
1947	67	123	103	92	—	78	10	30	250	16

Among men, from 1941–45, tuberculosis cases showed a greater ratio to the basic total of causes of admission at ages 15–24 than at any other age. Subject to yearly variations, there was a generalised upward trend in the rates over the eight years at ages 15–44. Since those who showed signs of tuberculosis at their medical examination would have been excluded, there would be a lag between entering the Forces and developing a disease like tuberculosis, and hence an increase in the rate with time is to be expected. The rates for women do not show the same trend, but as they were based on small numbers, particularly during the earlier years, it is inadvisable to attach too much importance to them. It is possible that the increased tendency towards tuberculosis among men may have been partly aggravated by exposure to adverse weather, lack of drying facilities for wet clothes, or being of necessity crowded together on the lower decks of troopships, conditions which would not apply to women, while the retention in the Services of those with chronic disease during the demobilisation of 1946–47 and also the severe winter of 1947 would have contributed to the high rates in those years.

Many young women at the susceptible ages would have been leading much healthier lives, with more fresh air and exercise, a better diet and more regular hours than they would have led in civilian life.

TABLE 3

Ratio of Number of Admissions for Respiratory Tuberculosis to that for Other Forms

Year	Males				Females		
	Age groups				Age groups		
	15–	25–	35 up	All	15–	25 up	All
1940	2·9	3·1	7·7	3·5	2·0	1·5	1·7
1941	2·1	3·3	7·8	2·9	2·7	0·5	1·8
1942	3·5	4·1	7·1	4·1	1·7	2·3	1·9
1943	4·4	3·3	5·7	4·1	2·5	1·8	2·4
1944	4·0	4·4	13·8	4·7	2·6	0·9	2·0
1945	3·3	5·7	6·2	4·6	2·7	2·1	2·5
1946	4·4	9·3	18·0	6·4	1·2	5·0	1·8
1947	6·4	19·0	*	8·8	1·0	1·0	1·0

* Indeterminate

The ratio of the number of cases of respiratory tuberculosis (M.R.C. code numbers 020–029) to that of non-respiratory (030–039) increased for men of all ages from 2·9 in 1941 to 8·8 in 1947. This was primarily due to an increase in pulmonary tuberculosis and pleural tuberculosis with effusion, the former being over three times as frequent in 1944 as in 1940. The commonest sites of non-respiratory tuberculosis among both men and women were the lymphatic and genito-urinary systems. Cases of pleural tuberculosis with effusion for both sexes and all ages were 30 times as numerous as those without mention of effusion. This may be contrasted with pleurisy described as non-tuberculous, in which the proportion of cases with effusion to those without was 0·58. This supports the view that cases of pleurisy with effusion are more likely than not to be tuberculous, and in the International Statistical Classification of Diseases, Injuries and Causes of Death (1948) pleurisy with effusion without mention of cause is included in the group 'Pleural tuberculosis'.

Since a follow-up of tuberculosis cases after discharge from the Army was impracticable, it has not been possible to obtain accurate case-fatality rates. The following rates are based on such deaths as were known to have occurred, and therefore, particularly for some forms of respiratory tuberculosis, they are under-estimated.

The fatality rate for tuberculosis of the vertebral column was more than six times that for other bones and joints. A high case-fatality rate, 95 per cent., was recorded for tuberculosis of the meninges, but the introduction of streptomycin will have reduced by now the death rate

TABLE 4

Case-fatality Rates for certain forms of Tuberculosis, 1940–47

M.R.C. Code No.	Diagnoses	Cases	Recorded Deaths	Fatality Rate per cent.
0210	Pleural Tuberculosis with effusion . .	418	12	2·6
0220	Miliary Tuberculosis lungs; no evidence of generalised miliary Tuberculosis .	32	22	68·8
0221	Pulmonary Tuberculosis, bacilli sought but not found	817	14	1·7
0225	Pulmonary Tuberculosis, Ungraded, but bacilli found	1,757	130	7·4
0226	Pulmonary Tuberculosis, unqualified as to presence or absence of bacilli . .	257	12	4·7
023	Miliary Tuberculosis lungs, with evidence of generalised miliary Tuberculosis	15	8	53·3
030	Tuberculosis, meninges and central nervous system . .	42	40	95·2
031	,, intestines and peritoneum (including mesenteric lymph nodes) . .	108	9	8·3
032	,, vertebral column . .	92	5	5·4
033	,, other bones and joints .	118	1	0·8
035	,, lymphatic system . .	235	0	—
036	,, genito-urinary system .	196	3	1·5

from this disease. Most of the 40 deaths occurred within three weeks of admission to hospital, the median period between admission and death being 11 days. The distribution is shown below.

Tuberculosis of the Meninges and Central Nervous System. Period between Admission and Death

Days .	1–	3–	5–	7–	10–	14–	21–	28–	56–	91–	365 up
Deaths.	1	2	3	7	14	6	2	0	3	1	1

These deaths do not include cases of respiratory tuberculosis complicated by tuberculous meningitis in which the latter was probably the terminal cause of death.

In 121 cases, tuberculosis of more than one site was recorded. The frequencies with which such combinations occurred is shown below, without regard to the order in which the sites were affected.

Tuberculosis of lungs and trachea with
    Pulmonary tuberculosis . . . . 16 *cases*

Pleural tuberculosis with
    Pulmonary tuberculosis . . 7 ,,
    T.B. of meninges and C.N.S. . 1 ,,
    ,, ,, intestines and peritoneum 5 ,,

„ „ lymphatic system	1	„
„ „ genito-urinary system	2	„
„ „ other sites	1	„
Pulmonary tuberculosis with		
Miliary T.B. of lungs and evidence of generalised miliary	1	„
T.B. of meninges and C.N.S.	14	„
„ „ intestines and peritoneum	17	„
„ „ vertebral column	5	„
„ „ other bones and joints	13	„
„ „ skin	1	„
„ „ lymphatic system	8	„
„ „ genito-urinary system	8	„
„ „ other sites	4	„
Other disseminated tuberculosis	2	„
Miliary T.B. of the lungs and evidence of generalised miliary with		
T.B. of meninges and C.N.S.	1	„
„ „ intestines and peritoneum	1	„
„ „ other sites	1	„
Radiological evidence of T.B. lungs with		
T.B. of lymphatic system	1	„
T.B. of meninges and C.N.S. with		
Other disseminated T.B.	2	„
T.B. of intestines and peritoneum with		
T.B. of lymphatic system	1	„
Acute generalised miliary tuberculosis	1	„
T.B. of vertebral column with		
T.B. of other bones and joints	2	„
„ „ lymphatic system	1	„
„ „ genito-urinary system	1	„
Acute generalised miliary T.B.	1	„
T.B. of other bones and joints with		
T.B. of lymphatic system	1	„
„ „ genito-urinary system	1	„

In five cases out of every 1,000 with tuberculosis there was mention of pleural effusion which was not described as tuberculous. Gastric or duodenal ulcer was concurrent with tuberculosis in 3 cases per 1,000 and perirectal abscess in 2 per 1,000. In only one case was there mention of diabetes.

VENEREAL DISEASES (Short List Number 2)

Table 5 shows the ratio of admissions for venereal diseases per 1,000 non-infective and non-respiratory illnesses. There is little sex-age variation, probably due to only a small proportion of cases of venereal diseases being treated in E.M.S. hospitals.

TABLE 5

Venereal Diseases. Ratio per 1,000 Admissions for Non-infective and Non-respiratory Illnesses, 1940–47

Year	Males						Females				
	Age groups						Age groups				
	15–	25–	35–	45–	55 up	All ages	15–	25–	35–	45 up	All Ages
1940	6	2	5	14	12	5	8	—	—	—	6
1941	8	6	7	15	—	7	8	5	—	—	7
1942	4	4	5	6	—	4	4	4	—	37	4
1943	3	3	3	9	32	3	3	5	16	—	4
1944	3	3	4	5	13	3	2	7	—	—	3
1945	2	3	4	9	—	3	2	1	—	—	2
1946	2	5	5	28	—	4	3	6	—	—	3
1947	2	6	—	—	—	2	5	—	—	—	4

For 1943, the percentages of cases of gonorrhoea and syphilis among 100 sick military personnel treated in hospitals in the United Kingdom were 5·3 and 1·2 respectively. (*Statistical Report on the Health of the Army, 1943–45*, H.M.S.O., 1948.) The number of men treated in Military Hospitals for gonorrhoea was 55 times that in E.M.S. hospitals, and for syphilis, including toxic jaundice, 33 times.

TABLE 6

Venereal Diseases. Proportionate Age Distribution of Admissions. Males. 1940–47.

M.R.C. Code	Disease Group	Age Groups					
		15–	25–	35–	45–	55 up	All Ages
040–049	Syphilis and its sequelae.	296	328	247	115	14	1,000
050–057	Gonorrhoea and other venereal diseases .	423	416	144	17	—	1,000

It may be seen from Table 6 that cases of syphilis were spread fairly evenly over the age groups under 45, whereas gonorrhoea was more frequent in those under 35. This may be due to appearance of delayed manifestations of syphilis at older ages among those who had not been completely cured. The number of cases of congenital, primary and secondary syphilis in men under 35 was 5·1 times the number in men of 35 and over, while cases of cardio-vascular syphilis (including aneurysm of the aorta) locomotor ataxia, general paralysis of the insane and other forms of neurosyphilis were 2·8 times the number in those over 35.

INFLUENZA, COLDS AND LARYNGITIS (Short List Number 3)

These three diseases made a considerable contribution to the causes of admission to hospital, especially during 1940 and 1943, as appears from Table 7.

TABLE 7

Colds, Influenza and Laryngitis. Ratio per 1,000 Admissions for Non-infective and Non-respiratory Illnesses, 1940–47

Year	Males						Females				
	Age Groups						Age Groups				
	15–	25–	35–	45–	55 up	All Ages	15–	25–	35–	45 up	All Ages
1940	277	140	131	136	106	202	184	208	274	333	200
1941	110	89	55	78	73	92	73	58	49	—	68
1942	57	46	36	30	29	48	52	51	68	37	52
1943	112	97	94	110	97	103	91	94	122	129	92
1944	51	31	26	33	27	37	25	25	33	—	25
1945	36	23	22	27	65	27	24	26	8	—	24
1946	64	49	40	14	—	55	43	64	38	—	47
1947	61	15	31	45	—	51	43	30	—	—	41

The proportion among men at ages 15–24 was higher in every year than at ages 25–34, while this age-group in turn had higher rates from 1940–46 than the age-group 35–44. No such definite pattern was shown by rates for women. Very few cases of laryngitis were recorded, and since, for cases admitted to hospital, it would be difficult to distinguish clearly between those diagnosed as influenza and those described as common cold, the following tables have been compiled by combining figures for influenza and colds.

TABLE 8

Colds and Influenza. Highest number of weekly admissions and five-weekly averages about the peak week. Persons. 1940–44

Year	Highest weekly admissions		Five-weekly averages of admissions about peak week				
	Week ending	Number of admissions	8–12 weeks before peak	3–7 weeks before peak	2 weeks before —2 weeks after	3–7 weeks after peak	8–12 weeks after peak
1940	Jan. 27 .	761	14	53	562	157	27
1941	Feb. 8 .	310	25	61	230	70	30
1942	Feb. 28 .	82	32	62	76	41	16
1943	Jan. 16 .	122	21	38	92	59	54
1943	Nov. 27.	398	17	61	249	70	39

Table 8 shows the numbers of cases admitted for the two conditions during the 'epidemic' periods of the winters of 1940–44; from 1945–47 the figures showed very little variation from week to week. It will be noted that whereas the peak of the epidemic is usually reached after Christmas, in the winter of 1943–44 the maximum number of weekly admissions occurred during late November. A comparison with Table 9, which gives the numbers of weekly deaths assigned to influenza in 126 Great Towns of England and Wales, shows that in 1943–44 the maximum number of weekly deaths also occurred before Christmas. (Registrar General's Weekly Return of Births, Deaths and Infectious Diseases.)

TABLE 9

Influenza. Highest number of weekly deaths in 126 Great Towns, and five-weekly averages about the peak week, 1940–44

Year	Highest weekly deaths		Five-weekly averages of deaths about peak week				
	Week ending	Number of deaths	8–12 weeks before peak	3–7 weeks before peak	2 weeks before –2 weeks after	3–7 weeks after peak	8–12 weeks after peak
1940	Feb. 24 .	629	29	263	521	165	36
1941	Feb. 15 .	324	31	76	268	121	39
1942	Jan. 31 .	90	30	37	77	69	32
1943	Feb. 13 .	131	31	67	111	68	22
1943	Dec. 11 .	1,148	12	44	809	233	52

There was a less well-marked epidemic period in 1942 than in the other years, both as regards hospital admissions and the deaths in the Great Towns. If curves were drawn for the five-weekly averages shown in Table 8, there would be a skewness of the curve with extension of the descending limb for each year except 1942, and the same trend is apparent for the deaths in Table 9 for the years 1941, 1942 and 1943.

Table 10 shows the distribution of days of in-patient treatment for influenza and for colds; cases in which there was a record of any concurrent disease or injury have been excluded from this table. For influenza, the median period of treatment in hospital for men aged 15–34 and 35–54 was 11 days, while for women aged 15–34 it was 9 days; for colds the median period was 10 days for men in each age group, compared with 8 days for women. That in 1942 the median period was 12 days for men in both age groups may be attributed to the decreased demands on hospital accommodation consequent on the smaller number of cases occurring in that year. The longer durations may be due to defective reporting, the cause of admission only being stated in the case notes, without mention of an accessory disease or complication, or they may be due to cases of post-influenzal debility, which

TABLE 10

Influenza (071) and Colds (072). Periods of In-patient Treatment of cases in which no other pathological condition was recorded

Year	Disease diagnosed	Sex and Age Group	Days of In-patient Treatment											*Median duration
			1–	3–	5–	7–	10–	14–	21–	28–	42–	56–	91 up	
1940	Influenza	Males 15–34	13	65	218	692	840	643	196	101	28	8	4	11
1941			9	52	148	367	378	323	86	49	10	8	3	11
1942			2	15	47	128	133	149	27	28	20	14	5	12
1943			5	46	139	294	325	308	41	37	16	33	4	11
1944			3	17	44	95	75	86	32	20	11	7	4	11
1945			2	13	20	41	51	48	10	7	6	12	6	12
1946			5	8	18	45	54	42	6	8	3	2	2	10
			39	216	634	1,662	1,856	1,599	398	250	94	84	28	11
1940	Influenza	Males 35–54	—	5	24	80	105	61	19	13	3	2	—	11
1941			—	7	17	29	40	43	5	6	3	1	1	11
1942			—	4	10	20	30	27	5	6	1	6	1	12
1943			2	11	33	82	90	75	8	15	5	9	—	11
1944			1	3	8	24	19	17	2	—	1	3	1	10
1945			—	4	5	12	11	16	1	4	2	1	—	12
1946			—	2	1	2	3	6	1	—	—	—	—	12
			3	36	98	249	298	245	41	44	15	22	3	11
1940	Influenza	Females 15–34	2	6	5	20	14	6	3	—	—	1	—	9
1941			—	3	8	15	15	5	—	—	—	—	—	9
1942			2	4	14	19	18	16	5	2	1	3	—	10
1943			4	14	36	67	62	42	9	12	4	1	1	10
1944			2	5	11	17	7	10	3	—	—	—	—	8
1945			2	—	6	4	5	5	1	1	—	—	—	10
1946			—	—	2	7	7	1	2	—	—	—	—	10
			12	32	82	149	128	85	23	15	5	5	1	9

1940	Colds .	Males 15–34	6	13	30	62	71	46	19	3	2	1	—	10
1941			7	24	42	71	80	73	16	14	2	4	1	11
1942			3	20	21	62	55	47	4	4	3	2	3	10
1943			8	23	69	114	91	47	11	12	4	5	1	9
1944			2	17	36	41	39	37	5	3	5	4	—	9
1945			3	15	21	27	33	24	4	5	1	4	5	11
1946			—	12	10	23	20	6	—	2	0	2	0	9
			29	124	229	400	389	280	59	43	17	22	10	10
1940	Colds .	Males 35–54	—	2	—	8	3	—	2	3	—	—	—	8
1941			—	6	5	4	3	6	—	—	—	—	—	8
1942			2	2	4	11	7	8	2	—	—	2	—	11
1943			1	4	9	25	24	17	3	3	—	2	—	10
1944			2	2	4	5	11	10	4	—	1	—	—	13
1945			2	2	4	7	6	6	—	—	—	—	—	9
1946			—	—	—	—	2	4	—	—	—	—	—	16
			7	18	26	60	56	51	11	6	1	4	—	10
1940	Colds .	Females 15–34	—	—	1	—	1	1	—	—	—	—	—	13
1941			—	1	—	2	1	1	—	—	—	—	—	9
1942			3	7	11	12	11	5	2	1	—	1	—	9
1943			2	8	26	30	27	14	2	2	—	—	—	8
1944			1	3	6	6	6	1	—	2	—	—	—	7
1945			1	2	1	11	4	5	2	1	—	—	—	9
1946			—	4	1	4	2	2	—	—	—	—	—	8
			7	25	46	65	52	29	6	6	—	1	—	8

* Adjusted for cases in which the complete period of treatment was not known.

would be coded to the same number as influenza, but would probably require a longer period in hospital.

The disruption caused by influenza and common colds is indicated by the fact that for the men in the 15–34 age group, whose hospital experience is shown in Table 10 during 1940, 2,808 were in hospital with influenza for a total of 37,766 days, an average of 13·4 days per man, while 253 were in for 2,969 days, an average of 11·7 days, with common colds. Corresponding figures for 1941 were, for influenza, 1,433 men for 18,723 days, average 13·1 days and for colds, 334 men for 4,283 days, average 12·8 days.

SCABIES (Short List Number 4)

Scabies, the mite of which is readily transferred by contact or on clothing where people are crowded together, might well become a problem among non-civilian personnel.

TABLE 11

Scabies. Ratio per 1,000 Admissions for Non-infective and Non-respiratory Illnesses, by Sex and Age, 1940–47

Year	Males						Females				
	Age Groups						Age Groups				
	15–	25–	35–	45–	55 up	All	15–	25–	35–	45 up	All
1940	61	46	30	27	47	50	164	50	20	—	123
1941	42	36	26	9	—	36	162	83	37	83	139
1942	17	13	9	12	—	14	89	23	24	—	73
1943	11	5	6	—	—	7	13	2	10	—	11
1944	3	3	2	5	—	3	3	2	—	—	3
1945	5	4	2	2	—	4	4	4	—	—	4
1946	7	8	1	—	—	7	3	—	—	—	2
1947	6	—	—	—	—	5	—	—	—	—	—

Table 11 shows that among men the ratio of admissions for scabies per 1,000 basic admissions declined from 50 in 1940 to 14 in 1942, then varied for the remaining years between 3 and 7, while among women it declined from the high levels of 123 and 139 in 1940 and 1941 respectively to 11 in 1943, afterwards varying between 2 and 4. It is possible that the high rates in the early years of the war were due to people who had brought the infection into the Forces from civilian life, but that once these people had been freed from infestation there was little spread of the disease.

The median period of in-patient treatment for men aged 15–34 varied from year to year between 8 and 11 days; taken over the seven years 1940 to 1946 it was 10 days for this age group and also for men

TABLE 12

Scabies. Periods of In-patient Treatment of cases in which no other pathological condition was recorded, 1940-46

Year	Sex-age group	Days of In-patient Treatment											*Median duration
		1–	3–	5–	7–	10–	14–	21–	28–	56–	91–	182 up	
1940	Males 15–34	25	104	111	212	169	155	73	71	14	2	2	10
1941		25	78	89	168	126	143	44	42	8	3	1	10
1942		7	35	64	60	43	39	8	12	4	1	—	8
1943–46		8	23	27	33	37	43	13	19	7	5	1	11
1940–46		65	240	291	473	375	380	138	144	33	11	4	10
1940	Males 35–54	5	9	9	21	18	12	9	7	1	—	—	10
1941		7	6	13	13	7	14	6	5	3	1	—	9
1942–46		3	7	11	12	11	12	4	9	3	4	—	12
1940–46		15	22	33	46	36	38	19	21	7	5	—	10
1940	Females 15–34	—	6	10	16	9	12	8	2	—	—	—	9
1941		3	23	26	37	26	26	6	7	—	—	—	8
1942		5	30	58	39	21	13	6	5	2	—	—	6
1943–46		—	5	12	20	6	17	7	3	—	—	—	9
1940–46		8	64	106	112	62	68	27	17	2	—	—	8

* Adjusted for cases in which the complete period of treatment was not known.

aged 35–54. The median number of days for women aged 15–34 taken over the seven years was 8. Examination of the numbers of weekly admissions did not show any marked seasonal variation.

OTHER INFECTIVE DISEASES (Short List Group 5)

The group contains, among others, malaria, dysentery, the common infections usually associated with childhood, Vincent's angina and ringworm. From 1940–44 the rates for men under 55 decreased with age, this trend being disturbed during 1945–47 by the influx of large numbers of malaria cases (Table 13). A similar trend was shown

TABLE 13

Other Infective Diseases (Short List Number 5). Ratio per 1,000 Admissions for Non-infective and Non-respiratory Illnesses, by Sex and Age, 1940–47*

Year	Males						Females				
	Age Groups						Age Groups				
	15–	25–	35–	45–	55 up	All	15–	25–	35–	45 up	All
1940	157	68	33	11	—	102	406	634	607	—	467
1941	97	59	25	23	55	67	106	78	37	83	96
1942	98*	56	31	21	—	65	91	104	36	37	91
1943	115	63	38	23	48	75	98	63	106	32	91
1944	194	147	99	68	13	150	110	96	17	—	103
1945	129	195	87	43	32	148	91	75	24	—	83
1946	139	229	117	83	—	169	74	71	78	—	74
1947	136	86	93	—	—	124	136	61	—	—	123

* *See* p. 648 for the composition of this group of diseases.

by women's rates in 1941, 1944, 1945 and 1947. The rates for men and women at all ages were high in 1940, chiefly owing to an increased incidence of rubella in that year, while the high rate for women at all ages in 1944 is attributable to the same cause. Table 14 shows the proportionate composition of admissions assigned to Short List Number 5.

Admissions for malaria, which in the one-in-five sample had been less than 100 annually during 1940-42, increased suddenly in 1944, but declined again by the second half of 1946. The numbers recorded during the ten quarters from January 1944–July 1946 with a primary diagnosis of either benign tertian malaria (M.R.C. No. 0090) or 'other and unspecified malaria' (0094) were as follows:

M.R.C. Code		1944				1945				1946	
		Q1	Q2	Q3	Q4	Q1	Q2	Q3	Q4	Q1	Q2
0090	Benign tertian malaria	213	873	466	234	245	289	224	335	265	87
0094	Other and unspecified malaria . .	129	409	326	135	163	214	180	223	156	49

TABLE 14

Proportionate Composition of Admissions for Short List Group 5, Other Infective Diseases, by Sex, 1940–47

M.R.C. Code	Diagnoses	Males							Females						
		1940	1941	1942	1943	1944	1945	1946–47	1940	1941	1942	1943	1944	1945	1946–47
009	Malaria	17	18	48	94	606	541	442	320	0	0	0	4	0	1
013–016	Dysentery	8	10	34	47	58	98	93	53	3	45	91	67	82	61
060–0	Scarlet Fever	70	77	45	92	37	40	62	55	40	133	103	114	121	102
062	Meningococcal Infn.	65	58	49	17	9	9	22	28	21	28	13	10	16	17
065	Diphtheria	34	68	74	64	34	40	47	48	50	113	65	49	68	67
077	Chicken Pox.	18	36	34	31	19	12	31	24	16	43	63	47	47	45
078	Herpes	26	53	43	38	16	11	13	26	11	14	30	16	13	18
0802	Infectious warts	16	38	38	49	20	18	29	27	5	20	42	45	45	33
082	Measles	51	85	29	56	10	15	25	33	96	79	152	71	139	109
083	Rubella	481	69	34	65	44	17	63	100	597	77	164	372	150	271
084	Mumps	24	53	128	62	22	41	28	46	69	184	91	57	108	98
091	Vincent's infection.	55	234	248	208	49	62	45	112	58	150	101	71	82	91
094 pt.	Ringworm	49	101	72	62	21	23	29	45	0	9	11	16	18	11
	Rest of S.L.5.	86	100	124	115	55	73	71	83	34	105	74	61	111	76
	Totals	1,000	1,000	1,000	1,000	1,000	1,000	1,000	1,000	1,000	1,000	1,000	1,000	1,000	1,000

The estimated total admissions for all forms of malaria in these ten quarters was about 26,000. Of all admissions for malaria during the eight years under review, 49 per cent. occurred in 1944, 33 per cent. in 1945 and 11 per cent. in 1946.

Rubella contributed largely to the admissions for infective diseases of both sexes, a total of 2,388 cases being recorded in the sample, which corresponds to about 12,000 admissions to E.M.S. hospitals altogether. The rate was high for both sexes in 1940 and for women in 1944. A well-marked epidemic trend in weekly admissions was apparent in 1940 and a less pronounced one in 1944 (*See* Table 15).

TABLE 15

Rubella. Highest number of weekly admissions and three-weekly averages about the peak week. Persons, 1940 and 1944

Year	Highest weekly admissions		Three-weekly averages of admissions about peak week				
	Week ending	Number of admissions	5–7 weeks before peak	2–4 weeks before peak	1 week before–1 week after	2–4 weeks after peak	5–7 weeks after peak
1940	Feb. 24	173	16	79	156	107	34
1944	April 15	38	13	27	32	17	7

It will be noticed that the curve for three-weekly averages in 1940 shows a skewness similar to that for influenza admissions in that year.

RHEUMATIC DISEASES (Short List Group 6)

This group includes acute rheumatic fever, arthritis and rheumatism. Table 16 shows that of all admissions for rheumatic diseases during 1940–47, rheumatic fever accounted for a little under one-fifth for

TABLE 16

Proportionate Composition of Admissions for Rheumatic Diseases, by Sex, 1940–47

M.R.C. Code	Diseases	Males Proportion per 1,000	Females Proportion per 1,000	Sex-ratio Males to Females
100	Acute rheumatic fever . .	186	232	7·4
700	Rheumatoid arthritis . .	49	63	7·2
703	Osteo-arthritis . . .	74	29	23·7
701–2, 704–5	Other forms of arthritis .	125	74	15·6
706	Fibrositis, rheumatism, etc. .	566	602	8·7
Totals	Rheumatic diseases . .	1,000	1,000	9·3

men and rather more than one-fifth for women, while for each sex over half were attributed to fibrositis and rheumatism. Further, while between seven and nine times as many men as women were admitted for rheumatic fever, rheumatoid arthritis and rheumatism, twenty-four times as many were admitted for osteo-arthritis and sixteen times for other forms of arthritis.

TABLE 17

Rheumatism, Arthritis and Fibrositis. Proportion per 1,000 Admissions for Non-infective and Non-respiratory Illnesses, by Sex and Age, 1940–47

Year	Males						Females				
	Age Groups						Age Groups				
	15–	25–	35–	45–	55 up	All	15–	25–	35–	45–	All
1940	37	46	90	123	118	51	27	17	78	223	33
1941	33	56	74	114	109	52	25	29	86	—	30
1942	30	48	99	108	131	53	49	59	92	74	53
1943	30	44	78	132	130	48	38	65	123	161	47
1944	30	41	80	120	41	47	31	47	89	143	37
1945	29	33	73	59	65	40	27	32	95	110	32
1946	32	29	50	55	—	33	34	13	115	—	33
1947	23	37	62	45	—	27	—	30	—	—	4

In Table 17 the proportion of admissions attributed to rheumatic diseases per 1,000 non-infective and non-respiratory diseases are shown. From 1940 to 1944 there is no striking annual variation in the rates for men under 55 years of age, while in each year the rates increase with age. At ages 15–24 rheumatic diseases caused less than 4 per cent. of the basic admissions, at ages 25–34 less than 6 per cent., while at age 45 and over they accounted for up to 13 per cent. during 1940–44. Among women the rates at ages 15–34 were considerably less than for those aged 35 and over. Rheumatic fever is known to attack the young rather than those older, while the numbers of deaths from chronic rheumatism (including rheumatoid arthritis) are much higher after age 60 than before. It would appear, therefore, that whatever the actual incidence of rheumatism and fibrositis, the disability caused increases with age.

From Table 18 it is evident that both acute rheumatic fever and muscular rheumatism showed seasonal trends, the admissions for acute rheumatism being highest in either the first or second quarters and those for other rheumatism usually in the first quarter or the fourth quarter of the preceding year. Since there would appear to be a connexion between the period of worst weather conditions and the incidence of rheumatic disease, the question of the provision in workplaces of

TABLE 18

Quarterly Admissions for Acute Rheumatic Fever (M.R.C. Code 100) and Fibrositis, Muscular Rheumatism and Lumbago (M.R.C. Code 706) Males, 1940-1945

M.R.C. Code	Diseases	Season	1940	1941	1942	1943	1944	1945
100	Acute rheumatic fever . .	1st Qtr.	71	80	65	64	71	72
		2nd Qtr.	81	72	44	52	87	97
		3rd Qtr.	46	36	36	30	45	43
		4th Qtr.	55	41	55	41	58	36
706	Rheumatism, fibrositis, etc. .	1st Qtr.	109	233	309	239	219	138
		2nd Qtr.	165	195	206	181	154	99
		3rd Qtr.	193	194	226	171	149	86
		4th Qtr.	224	216	204	195	168	65

facilities for drying clothes becomes pertinent to the problem of preventing this type of disability. Figures from the Survey of Sickness carried out among people aged sixteen and over show that for the period May 1946 to April 1947, the monthly inception rate* for rheumatism and other diseases in M.R.C. Code 706 was 5,301 per 100,000 and the prevalence rate† 16,055 per 100,000. Hence about 1 person out of 19 developed an attack of rheumatism during the average month, while including attacks which began previously, 1 person out of 6 reported suffering from rheumatism at some time during the month. Even where these attacks do not cause absence from work, it is possible that there is a lowering of production efficiency.

For cases in which there was no record of any concurrent disease, the median number of days of in-patient treatment for rheumatism varied between 15 and 20 days for men aged 15–34 and between 19 and 24 days for those aged 35–54. Taken over the seven years 1940–46 the medians were 20 days and 21 days in these two age groups. For women aged 15–34 the median period was about 18 days. The average period of treatment over the years 1942 and 1943 was 37 days for men aged 15–34 and 35 days for those aged 35–54.

In view of the question whether or not rheumatic fever was associated in any way with infection by haemolytic streptococci, 421 case histories of rheumatic fever were examined in detail for mention of scarlet fever, erysipelas, otitis media, streptococcal sore throat and other infections specified as streptococcal. These cases were not selected by any rule, but were the first ones to come to hand. The diagnoses of the 421 cases were as follows:

* Number of diseases beginning in the month, per stated number of people.

† Number of illnesses present in the population at any time during the month, regardless of when they began, per stated number of people.

TABLE 19

Fibrositis, Muscular Rheumatism and Lumbago (706). Periods of In-patient Treatment of cases in which no other pathological condition was recorded

Sex and Age Group	Year	Days of In-patient Treatment										Totals	*Median
		1–	4–	7–	10–	14–	21–	28–	42–	56–	91 up		
Males (15–34) . .	1940	5	20	26	47	81	45	46	20	22	22	334	15
	1941	6	23	37	73	105	36	74	40	35	26	455	19
	1942	11	31	40	60	98	30	42	45	77	42	476	20
	1943	8	24	32	44	97	18	31	20	50	40	364	20
	1944	8	22	20	35	65	34	16	24	32	18	274	19
	1945–46	8	14	25	29	43	15	28	10	30	25	227	20
	1940–46	46	134	180	288	489	178	237	159	246	173	2,130	20
Males (35–54) .	1940	1	6	14	15	34	27	29	20	20	5	171	24
	1941	2	4	19	25	52	18	26	12	16	7	181	19
	1942	7	7	21	24	77	22	30	23	44	19	274	21
	1943	7	10	17	31	67	20	39	23	36	20	270	22
	1944	7	10	23	35	70	28	28	20	36	15	272	20
	1945–46	5	9	11	13	33	15	17	16	25	13	157	22
	1940–46	29	46	105	143	333	130	169	114	177	79	1,325	21
Females (15–34) .	1940–42	4	10	15	10	20	14	8	11	3	7	102	17
	1943	1	7	21	11	29	13	19	12	4	5	122	18
	1944–46	3	11	9	19	42	20	23	5	8	3	143	18
	1940–46	8	28	45	40	91	47	50	28	15	15	367	18

* Adjusted for cases in which the complete period of treatment was not known.

Acute rheumatism .	171	41 per cent.
Sub-acute rheumatism	112	26 per cent.
Rheumatic fever .	105	25 per cent.
Rheumatic carditis .	17	4 per cent.
Others . . .	16	4 per cent.
Totals . .	421	100 per cent

Mention of an attack of scarlet fever was found in 25 cases (5·9 per cent.) and of the presence of streptococci in the throat in 8 cases or 1·9 per cent. Six histories recorded suppurative otitis media and another 10 such conditions as otitis externa or discharging ears. There was no mention of erysipelas. At least one previous attack of acute rheumatism had occurred in 28 per cent. of the cases. The intervals elapsing between the present attack of rheumatic fever and the preceding one, and between attacks of scarlet fever and subsequent rheumatic fever are shown in Table 20.

TABLE 20

Interval between two attacks of Rheumatic Fever and between attacks of Scarlet Fever and Rheumatic Fever in a sample of 421 cases

	Interval in Years							
	Under 1	1–4	5–9	10–14	15–19	20 and over	Not stated	Totals
Rheumatic fever; present attack and preceding one	9	25	34	26	11	8	3	116
Scarlet fever and first attack of rheumatic fever	6	1	6	4	1	1	6	25
Scarlet fever and present attack of rheumatic fever	2	3	5	5	2	2	6	25

The condition of the throat was recorded in 64 per cent. of the cases and in 65 cases (15 per cent.) was stated to be healthy. In some cases rheumatic fever had been very shortly preceded by tonsillitis. There was a past history of sore throats or tonsillitis in 7 per cent. of the cases. In many cases dental sepsis was noted, thus showing the presence of another form of septic focus. The frequency of occurrence of adverse throat conditions is shown in Table 21.

NEOPLASMS, DIABETES, ANAEMIAS AND OTHER GENERAL AND ENDOCRINE DISEASES (Short List Numbers 7–10)

Admissions for these diseases formed a relatively small proportion of the basic total, and except in the case of neoplasms there was very little

TABLE 21

Cases of Rheumatic Fever (M.R.C. Code 100) associated with a throat condition (Sample of 421 cases)

Throat Condition	Acute Rheumatism	Rheumatic Fever	Sub-acute Rheumatism	Rheumatic Carditis	Others
Sore throat immediately preceding attack	34	21	20	6	2
Throat of unhealthy appearance	4	5	3	—	1
Past history of sore throats	3	3	7	—	—
Tonsillitis immediately preceding attack	16	8	7	1	1
Tonsils of unhealthy appearance	11	8	6	1	—
Past history of tonsillitis	9	3	6	—	—
Sore throat and tonsillitis preceding attack	6	2	2	1	—
Both throat and tonsils unhealthy	3	2	—	1	—
Throat stated to be healthy	31	14	17	2	1

variation from year to year. For neoplasms the rates for males showed a general upward trend at all ages and in the three ten-yearly age groups

TABLE 22

Neoplasms. Proportion per 1,000 Admissions for Non-infective and Non-respiratory Illnesses, by Sex and Age, 1940–47

Year	Males						Females			
	Age Groups						Age Groups			
	15–	25–	35–	45–	55 up	All	15–	25–	25–44	All Ages
1940	11	12	13	19	12	12	14	—	59	15
1941	13	14	17	27	91	15	22	24	86	27
1942	15	18	20	32	73	18	23	38	48	28
1943	14	16	23	40	65	17	23	42	111	30
1944	13	18	27	49	122	19	28	40	61	32
1945	17	22	35	109	162	25	31	44	24	35
1946	20	29	44	83	83	27	39	70	192	50
1947	23	46	52	45	166	29	14	30	500	24

under 45. The rates for females also showed a tendency to increase between 1940 and 1946. The ratio of non-malignant neoplasms and those of unspecified nature to those stated to be malignant was as follows:

Ages	15–	25–	35–	45–	55 up	All ages
Males	7·4	4·1	1·5	0·7	0·24	3·0
Females	27·7	12·9	14·3	3	indeterminate	18·1

The most frequently occurring non-malignant neoplasms were those of the skin, bones and cartilage and nasal polyps.

Of the general diseases in Short List Number 10, 39 per cent. of men's admissions were due to lymphadenitis and lymphangitis, 32 per cent. to asthma, 5 per cent. to urticaria and 5½ per cent. to simple and exophthalmic goitre. Taken over the seven years 1940–46, the median period of in-patient treatment for asthma among men aged 15–34 was 21 days, among those aged 35–54, 25 days and for women aged 15–34, 17 days.

TABLE 23

Asthma (211). Periods of In-patient Treatment of cases in which no other pathological condition was recorded, 1940–46

Sex	Age Group	Days of In-patient Treatment												*Median duration
		0–	7–	10–	14–	21–	28–	35–	42–	56–	91–	182–	Total	
Males .	15–34	60	75	98	158	77	63	59	79	93	38	1	801	21 days
Males .	35–54	10	22	17	59	33	31	22	24	27	9	2	256	25 days
Females .	15–34	18	25	16	37	17	15	9	12	9	1	—	159	17 days

* Adjusted for cases in which the complete period of treatment was not known.

DISEASES OF THE NERVOUS SYSTEM (M.R.C. 30–35) AND FUCTIONAL DISORDERS OF THE STOMACH AND INTESTINES (M.R.C. 51) (Short List Numbers 11–13; 16)

The contribution of these diseases to the basic total of causes of admission varied between 10 and 15 per cent.

TABLE 24

Psychoneuroses. Proportion per 1,000 Admissions for Non-infective and Non-respiratory Illnesses, by Sex and Age, 1940–47

Year	Males						Females					
	Age Groups						Age Groups					
	15–	25–	35–	45–	55 up	All	15–	25–	35–	45–	55 up	All
1940	41	46	71	58	35	47	30	8	39	—	—	26
1941	42	51	68	52	18	50	37	54	37	168	—	41
1942	58	67	71	65	14	65	33	83	73	—	—	43
1943	54	71	80	44	16	66	47	48	58	65	—	47
1944	73	92	73	63	13	81	58	83	67	—	—	63
1945	82	119	66	46	32	94	54	65	79	—	—	58
1946	70	71	79	28	—	71	18	13	77	—	—	18
1947	48	34	21	45	—	44	34	—	—	—	—	29

Among men at ages 15–34, the rates for psychoneuroses were highest in 1944 and 1945, coinciding with the opening of the Second Front in Europe, and they were higher than those for men aged 35 and over.

Many of the older men would have gone through the North African campaign, with a resultant weeding out of psychiatric casualties attributable to the fighting in that theatre of war. For women aged 15–24, the rates were also highest in 1944 and 1945. Rates were higher at ages 25–34 than at 15–24, for men in each year from 1940–46 and for women from 1941–45.

TABLE 25

Functional Digestive Disorders. Proportion per 1,000 Admissions for Non-infective and Non-respiratory Illnesses, by Sex and Age, 1940–47.

Year	Males						Females					
	Age Groups						Age Groups					
	15–	25–	35–	45–	55–	All	15–	25–	35–	45–	55–	All
1940	13	17	31	21	47	17	25	42	20	—	—	28
1941	19	28	36	33	55	26	29	19	37	—	—	27
1942	22	31	34	21	—	28	30	25	18	74	—	29
1943	18	22	31	17	—	22	23	23	5	—	—	22
1944	13	20	25	31	13	19	19	12	—	—	—	17
1945	17	22	26	18	32	21	20	11	8	—	—	17
1946	11	14	11	—	—	12	18	25	—	—	—	18
1947	13	15	—	—	—	13	14	—	—	—	—	12

Of admissions for functional digestive disorders (M.R.C. Code 51) among men, 78·8 per cent. were for functional dyspepsia, 16·7 per cent. for constipation and 2·4 per cent. for spastic colon; the corresponding rates for women being 29·9 per cent., 64·9 per cent. and 3·1 per cent. Table 25 shows that, among men, from 1940 to 1945 proportionate rates increased with age between 15 and 44, while with the exception of 1943 the same is true for women aged 15–34.

TABLE 26

Psychoneuroses (Short List Number 11). Proportionate Frequencies in certain Sex-Age Groups, 1940–47

M.R.C. Code	Disease Groups	Males					Females			
		Age Groups					Age Groups			
		15–	25–	35–	45–54	All Ages	15–	25–	35–44	All Ages
331	Abnormal character states . .	91	61	52	18	68	66	40	73	59
3320–3321	Anxiety states .	445	545	514	494	505	358	380	491	370
3322	Obsessional states .	21	28	23	18	25	7	7	—	7
3323	Reactive depression	34	47	68	76	47	116	159	182	132
3324	Hysteria . .	246	197	204	164	214	297	294	163	289
3330	Effort syndrome .	36	35	41	84	37	13	11	—	12
3331–5, 7	Psychoneuroses with somatic symptoms	3	2	3	4	3	5	7	18	6
3336	Nocturnal enuresis . .	56	17	12	27	29	31	4	—	22
3338	Hypochondriasis .	2	5	4	4	4	—	—	—	—
3339	Unspecified psychoneurosis .	66	63	79	111	68	107	98	73	103
		1,000	1,000	1,000	1,000	1,000	1,000	1,000	1,000	1,000

Table 26 shows that, of the psychoneuroses for which men were admitted to hospital, half were described as anxiety states and nearly a quarter as hysteria, while for women nearly two-fifths were ascribed to anxiety states and three-tenths to hysteria. The preponderance of anxiety states (including sexual perversion) made a greater contribution to the among Service doctors. A higher proportion of women than of men had a diagnosis of reactive depression, whereas abnormal character states (including sexual perversion) made a greater contribution to the men's total of psychoneuroses, either due to a greater incidence or because these conditions in the male are perhaps more likely to come to light. Effort syndrome, which includes the condition known during the First World War as soldier's heart, had a comparatively small ratio.

TABLE 27

Psychoneuroses, etc. Proportionate Age Distribution of certain forms. Males, 1940–47

M.R.C. Code	Disease Groups	Age Groups					
		15–	25–	35–	45–	55 up	All
331	Abnormal character states	437	416	142	5	—	1,000
3320–1	Anxiety states	288	501	191	19	1	1,000
3322	Obsessional states	280	529	177	14	—	1,000
3323	Reactive depression	235	464	270	31	—	1,000
3324	Hysteria	376	429	180	15	0	1,000
3330	Effort syndrome	314	436	204	44	2	1,000
3336	Nocturnal enuresis	628	271	80	18	3	1,000
3339	Psychoneurosis unspecified	315	435	218	32	—	1,000
3331–3339	All forms of neurosis	327	465	188	19	1	1,000
340–345	All forms of psychosis	387	398	173	35	7	1,000
5113	Functional dyspepsia	240	472	259	27	2	1,000
5122	Constipation	520	353	114	11	2	1,000

The proportionate age distributions among men of the more frequently occurring forms of neurosis are shown in Table 27, and are compared with similar distributions for psychosis (all forms), functional dyspepsia and constipation. Anxiety and obsessional states and reactive depression appeared much more frequently at age 25–34 than at 15–24. Enuresis, however, was much more frequent as a cause of treatment in those aged 15–24, as might be expected from its incidence in early life and the circumstances of life in the Forces.

Psychoses of all forms were fairly evenly distributed over the two decennial age-groups under 35, an excess of cases of schizophrenia occurring at ages 15–24. Functional dyspepsia showed a distribution very similar to that for reactive depression, while constipation was more frequent as a reason for treatment at ages 15–24.

Of the remaining diseases of the nervous system, the most common was sciatica, a total of 1,658 males and 70 females in the sample having been admitted for this cause during 1940–47, corresponding to around 8,300 actual admissions for men and about 350 for women. The age distribution was as follows:

Ages	15–	25–	35–	45–	55 up	All ages
Males	251	783	542	79	3	1,658
Females	36	32	2	—	—	70

The possible association of sciatica (M.R.C. 323) with a prolapsed intervertebral disc (M.R.C. 726) is one which has come to be increasingly recognised during the last few years. The record cards were examined for cases in which sciatica was stated to be the primary cause of admission, but in which a prolapsed disc was also mentioned, also for those in which a prolapsed disc was given as the primary cause but with mention of sciatica. The results are shown in Table 28 below:

TABLE 28

Association of Sciatica (323) with Prolapsed Intervertebral Disc (726) Males, aged 15–54.

Year	Primary Code 323			Primary Code 726			Primary Code 323 or 726		
	Totals	With mention of 726	Percentage with 726	Totals	With mention of 323	Percentage with 323	Totals	With 323 and 726	Percentage with 323 and 726
Males aged 15–34									
1940	123	2	1·6	1	0	0	124	2	1·6
1941	171	1	0·6	1	0	0	172	1	0·6
1942	192	2	1·0	18	7	38·9	210	9	4·3
1943	167	4	2·4	22	7	31·8	189	11	5·8
1944	171	12	7·0	22	9	40·9	193	21	10·9
1945	158	23	14·6	45	8	17·8	203	31	15·3
1946	43	11	25·6	19	3	15·8	62	14	22·6
1947	9	2	22·2	6	0	0	15	2	13·7
1940–47	1,034	57	5·5	134	34	25·4	1,168	91	13·3
Males aged 35–54									
1940	65	0	0	0	0	0	65	0	0
1941	89	0	0	1	0	0	90	0	0
1942	124	0	0	5	2	40·0	129	2	1·6
1943	86	1	1·2	21	6	28·6	107	7	6·5
1944	126	2	1·6	19	7	36·8	145	9	6·2
1945	116	16	13·8	24	1	4·2	140	17	12·1
1946	14	3	21·4	13	1	7·7	27	4	14·8
1947	1	0	0	2	0	0	3	0	0
1940–47	621	22	3·5	85	17	20·0	706	39	5·5

The order in which the diagnoses were recorded on the card depended on whether the coder considered, from the case history, that the patient was admitted on account of a prolapsed disc or because he had an attack of sciatica. The last column of Table 28 shows that the number of cases in which the two conditions were associated increased year by year until 1946. Taken over the eight years 1940–47, the difference between the percentages in the two age groups is significant. (Difference 7·8. 2 S.E. = 2·6).

Sciatica did not show any variation in seasonal incidence beyond a general tendency to be higher in the winter months. The numbers of men admitted during the four 13-week periods of each year from 1940–45 were as follows:

	1940	1941	1942	1943	1944	1945
1st Quarter	30	86	89	60	74	93
2nd Quarter	43	67	75	57	70	81
3rd Quarter	47	53	75	73	67	54
4th Quarter	65	58	74	66	92	45

Table 29 shows the distribution of days of in-patient treatment and the median number of days' stay for sciatica, the more frequently occurring types of neurosis and functional dyspepsia. For sciatica, the median was 53 days for men aged 15–34, compared with 50 days for those aged 35–54 and 32 days for women at ages 15–34. The younger men had median periods of treatment in excess of those of the older age group for psychophathic personality, anxiety and obsessional states and reactive depression, while for hysteria the medians were the same. In all cases the median was about six or seven weeks. Median periods for women patients were less than those for men except for reactive depression. The median for functional dyspepsia was about three weeks for men and a fortnight for women.

DISEASES OF EYES AND EARS (Short List Numbers 14 and 15)

These two groups of diseases made a comparatively small contribution to the basic total of admissions, the ratios for males of all ages varying, for eye diseases, between 11 and 15 per 1,000 and for ear conditions between 20 and 36, the corresponding figures for females being 7 to 9 and 16 to 28. The rates did not vary greatly from year to year nor as between age groups.

Diseases of the conjunctiva formed 32·4 per cent. of all eye conditions for men and 33·1 per cent. for women, corresponding figures for diseases of the cornea being 27·3 per cent. and 15·8 per cent. and for affections of the lids and lachrymal apparatus 15·6 per cent. and 19·0 per cent. Among women strabismus formed 13·6 per cent. of eye conditions, compared with 3·9 per cent. among men, but possibly women are the more likely to seek treatment for this complaint.

Rather more than three-quarters of all ear diseases, both for men and women, consisted of otitis media with or without mastoiditis. An

TABLE 29

Sciatica. Some Forms of Psychoneuroses and Functional Dyspepsia
Periods of In-Patient Treatment of cases in which no other pathological condition was recorded

Year	Disease diagnosed	Sex-Age Group	Days of In-Patient Treatment														*Median duration
			0–	4–	7–	10–	14–	21–	28–	35–	42–	56–	91–	182–	273–	365 up	
1940–42	Sciatica	Males 15–34	3	8	9	25	52	22	27	26	43	83	60	11	1	—	45
1943–44			5	6	7	10	32	12	15	21	35	47	53	10	1	—	52
1945–46			1	1	4	6	16	9	4	13	22	39	59	19	1	—	77
1940–46			9	15	20	41	100	43	46	60	100	169	172	40	3	—	53
1940–43		Males 35–54	4	3	9	18	41	22	19	20	30	56	47	9	2	—	44
1944–46			4	3	12	10	27	7	8	13	33	58	66	1	1	—	59
1940–46			8	6	21	28	68	29	27	33	63	114	113	10	3	—	50
1940–46		Females 15–34	3	1	4	6	7	5	7	5	7	12	5	—	—	—	32
1940–46	Psychopathic Personality	Males 15–34	3	14	7	17	37	35	35	48	73	73	32	2	—	—	40
1940–46		Males 35–54	2	2	1	2	7	8	7	9	12	11	4	—	—	—	28
1940–46		Females 15–34	—	—	1	1	5	8	5	2	5	10	1	—	—	—	32
1940–41	Anxiety State, not fear reaction	Males 15–34	3	11	12	16	33	41	52	45	72	90	53	4	—	—	42
1942			10	15	18	15	41	48	38	52	89	138	55	5	—	—	45
1943			5	21	14	24	41	28	44	49	114	168	55	2	—	1	48
1944			24	23	23	28	83	73	108	101	200	218	92	1	—	—	43
1945			14	11	11	19	65	95	140	110	261	266	123	5	1	—	47
1946			2	2	6	7	29	23	21	32	47	49	31	3	1	—	42
1940–46			58	83	84	109	292	308	403	389	783	929	409	20	2	1	45

TABLE 29—(contd.)

Sciatica. Some Forms of Psychoneuroses and Functional Dyspepsia
Periods of In-Patient Treatment of cases in which no other pathological condition was recorded

Year	Disease diagnosed	Sex-Age Group	Days of In-Patient Treatment														*Median duration
			0–	4–	7–	10–	14–	21–	28–	35–	42–	56–	91–	182–	273–	365 up	
1940–42		Males 35–54	3	8	11	14	33	28	26	27	59	89	31	2	2	—	46
1943			4	10	9	10	19	20	16	20	46	48	17	2	—	—	42
1944			6	11	3	8	22	28	27	34	45	45	11	—	—	—	37
1945–46			5	4	6	9	22	22	33	25	44	48	25	2	—	—	37
1940–46			18	33	29	41	96	98	102	106	194	230	84	6	2	—	41
1940–46		Females 15–34	6	10	7	17	43	40	34	41	78	62	11	2	—	—	37
1940–46	Obsessional State	Males 15–34	1	1	1	5	14	8	19	14	34	45	28	4	—	1	53
1940–46		Males 35–54	—	—	1	4	1	3	4	7	9	7	8	—	—	—	50
1940–46	Reactive depression	Males 15–34	9	4	6	8	16	25	22	33	61	73	52	1	—	—	48
1940–46		Males 35–54	5	3	5	3	10	16	15	12	20	37	21	—	—	—	43
1940–46		Females 15–34	—	4	5	3	8	12	9	11	23	33	7	2	—	—	45

1940–41	Hysteria	Males 15–34	6	7	10	16	27	16	39	23	58	86	51	2	1	—	48
1942			10	12	7	17	21	17	26	24	48	66	48	6	—	—	46
1943			4	9	10	16	16	21	17	25	51	84	42	1	—	—	51
1944			13	11	6	16	31	29	22	27	61	81	38	4	1	—	46
1945–46			10	15	10	9	24	31	40	31	61	80	26	8	1	—	42
1940–46			43	54	43	74	119	114	144	130	279	397	205	21	3	—	46
1940–46		Males 35–54	6	13	12	15	34	26	39	32	65	106	52	—	—	—	46
1940–46		Females 15–34	12	19	21	21	33	28	28	13	35	35	16	—	—	—	27
1940–41	Functional Dyspepsia	Males 15–34	10	18	22	64	121	76	51	30	45	39	10	1	—	—	21
1942			5	14	37	57	133	36	29	19	32	44	22	—	—	—	19
1943			9	14	19	48	83	24	12	6	18	24	15	—	—	1	18
1944			10	23	24	44	58	25	10	9	14	20	7	—	—	—	16
1945–46			14	28	36	59	65	20	12	7	23	33	12	2	—	—	15
1940–46			48	97	138	272	460	181	114	71	132	160	66	3	—	1	19
1940–46		Males 35–54	19	31	62	92	166	65	56	53	61	61	8	1	—	1	19
1940–46		Females 15–34	2	17	12	16	28	14	5	4	5	3	—	—	—	—	15

* Adjusted for cases in which the complete period of treatment was not known.

estimated total of about 17,500 males and 1,650 females were admitted for this primary cause.

DISEASES OF HEART AND ARTERIES

Service men and women would constitute a highly selected population in respect of heart disease, but for both sexes at all ages about 1 per cent. of the basic total of admissions was due to a condition in M.R.C. code numbers 38–42. The rates rose sharply with age, and for men in the age group 45–54 the ratio varied between 4·3 per cent. and 9·2 per cent. (Table 30).

TABLE 30

Diseases of Heart and Arteries (M.R.C. Codes 38–42)
Proportion per 1,000 Admissions for Non-infective and Non-respiratory Illnesses, 1940–47

Year	Males						Females				
	Age Groups						Age Groups				
	15–	25–	35–	45–	55 up	All	15–	25–	35–	45 up	All
1940	6	7	17	44	107	10	5	25	39	—	13
1941	6	5	8	61	128	7	7	10	49	—	10
1942	7	7	10	45	146	8	11	11	12	37	11
1943	6	6	10	59	97	8	5	12	26	32	7
1944	4	6	13	50	108	8	7	5	11	—	6
1945	6	8	15	43	97	9	6	6	—	—	6
1946	8	10	20	69	251	11	1	19	—	—	4
1947	5	12	31	92	167	8	10	—	—	—	8

Among men the proportion of cases of heart disease believed to be of rheumatic origin, to all cases of heart disease, varied from year to year as follows:

1940	1941	1942	1943	1944	1945	1946–47	1940–47
per cent.	per cent.	per cent.	per cent.	per cent.	per cent.	per cent.	per cent.
36	39	48	45	47	59	44	45

The corresponding proportion for women taken over the whole eight years was 43 per cent. High blood pressure accounted for 23 per cent. of all admissions of men for diseases of the heart and arteries, and 9 per cent. of those of women. Taken over the whole period the number of men admitted in each age group per 10,000 total admissions in that group was as follows:

Age	15–	25–	35–	45–	55 up	All
	3	7	27	122	231	12

In the sample 119 men were admitted during the eight years with diseases of the coronary arteries. Their proportionate age distribution compared with that for all heart disease was:

Ages	15–	25–	35–	45–	55 up	All
Coronary Disease . .	8	210	378	303	101	1,000
All Heart Disease . .	222	306	276	159	37	1,000

DISEASES OF THE VEINS (Short List Number 18)

Admissions for treatment of diseases of the veins, of which the three of most frequent occurrence were varicose veins of the legs, haemorrhoids and varicocele, accounted for a proportion of the basic total varying between 44 and 89 per 1,000 admissions for men and 19 and 41 for women. Table 31 shows that for men the rates were much higher

TABLE 31

Diseases of the Veins
Proportion per 1,000 Admissions for Non-infective and Non-respiratory Illnesses, 1940–47

Year	Males						Females				
	Age Groups						Age Groups				
	15–	25–	35–	45–	55 up	All	15–	25–	35–	45–54	All
1940 . . .	45	97	80	98	94	71	16	33	39	111	24
1941 . . .	58	102	123	108	73	89	14	39	75	—	22
1942 . . .	56	98	105	104	73	85	15	29	61	—	19
1943 . . .	45	92	106	81	113	78	23	51	63	—	29
1944 . . .	47	86	100	73	27	75	29	65	50	71	37
1945 . . .	45	79	75	71	32	66	24	52	32	110	32
1946 . . .	45	77	63	42	167	59	35	51	154	—	41
1947 . . .	38	61	93	45	—	44	5	91	250	—	20

at ages 25 and over than at ages 15–24; from 1941 to 1944 admissions for these diseases accounted for at least 10 per cent. of the basic total of admissions of men aged 35 to 44. Among women, the rates also showed a tendency to increase with age.

Table 32 shows that about 34,000 men are estimated to have been admitted for varicose veins of the legs during the eight years under review, and 25,000 for haemorrhoids. The corresponding figures for women are 2,300 for varicose veins and 900 for haemorrhoids.

RESPIRATORY DISEASES (Short List Numbers 19–21)

Diseases of the respiratory system comprise the diagnostic terms included in the Short List Numbers 19, acute primary pneumonia, 20,

TABLE 32

Varicose Veins. Haemorrhoids and Varicocele. Numbers in sample and Estimated Total Admissions, 1940–47

M.R.C. Code	Disease	Sex	1940	1941	1942	1943	1944	1945	1946–47	Sample total	Estimated total*
430	Varicose veins of lower extremities	M	779	1,210	1,433	1,175	983	890	320	6,790	33,950 ± 412
		F	5	15	53	106	119	122	32	452	2,260 ± 106
431	Haemorrhoids	M	627	1,030	1,005	761	854	635	166	5,078	25,390 ± 356
		F	5	12	24	51	52	31	5	180	900 ± 67
432	Varicocele	M	168	177	127	92	54	38	21	677	3,385 ± 130
		F	—	—	1	—	1	—	—	2	—

* Following the usual convention, the quantities after the ± signs are the approximate standard errors of the quantities preceding these signs.

bronchitis and tracheitis and 21, other respiratory diseases. As these diseases have a marked annual variation and their incidence is affected by such external causes as adverse climatic conditions they have been excluded from the basic total of admissions.

TABLE 33

Respiratory Diseases
Proportion per 1,000 Admissions for Non-infective and Non-respiratory Illnesses, 1940–47

Year	Males						Females			
	Age Groups						Age Groups			
	15–	25–	35–	45–	55 up	All	15–	25–	35–44	All
Acute Primary Pneumonia (Short List. No. 19)										
1940 .	33	24	18	32	23	28	16	17	20	17
1941 .	37	28	22	14	18	30	19	29	12	20
1942 .	42	29	31	44	102	35	21	31	24	23
1943 .	46	32	38	49	32	38	17	14	37	17
1944 .	43	32	33	50	68	37	14	26	17	16
1945 .	63	35	43	46	129	46	27	18	16	24
1946 .	65	39	37	42	83	52	19	6	38	17
1947 .	72	49	72	45	167	68	19	—	—	16
Bronchitis and Tracheitis (Short List No. 20)										
1940 .	47	53	124	197	436	66	52	100	137	75
1941 .	42	50	85	156	363	55	54	97	99	66
1942 .	45	56	84	97	87	58	34	52	73	39
1943 .	40	43	91	151	324	55	32	42	74	36
1944 .	30	34	50	118	68	38	22	36	61	28
1945 .	33	26	45	71	225	33	24	26	32	26
1946 .	25	18	37	28	83	24	27	25	—	27
1947 .	25	12	41	137	—	25	24	30	—	24
Other Respiratory Diseases (Short List No. 21)										
1940 .	37	31	29	37	23	34	25	8	20	20
1941 .	43	33	32	33	18	37	27	49	63	34
1942 .	44	38	32	29	43	39	33	34	6	33
1943 .	52	36	35	31	48	41	29	27	5	29
1944 .	45	37	33	45	41	39	27	34	22	29
1945 .	46	40	32	30	97	41	20	15	39	19
1946 .	50	44	38	—	83	46	42	45	—	41
1947 .	70	52	41	45	167	66	43	—	—	37

Admissions for acute primary pneumonia among men at all ages bore a ratio to the basic total of admissions which increased from 28 per 1,000 in 1940 to 68 per 1,000 in 1947, while for bronchitis and tracheitis the ratio declined from 66 per 1,000 in 1940 to 24 per 1,000 in 1946. For women at all ages the ratios for acute primary pneumonia varied between 16 and 24 per 1,000, without showing a definite trend over the eight years, but for bronchitis and tracheitis they showed a decline from 75 per 1,000 in 1940 to 24 per 1,000 in 1947. The ratios for other respiratory diseases, of which chronic bronchitis showed the highest incidence, increased steadily over the eight years from 34 to 66 per 1,000 for men, while those for women varied between 19 and 41 per 1,000. For males the ratios for acute pneumonia and for the group 'other respiratory diseases' were higher at ages 15–24 than at 25–34, while for bronchitis and tracheitis they were higher at ages 25–34 from 1940 to 1944 but lower than at ages 15–24 from 1945 to 1947. The decline with age in the ratios for 'other respiratory diseases' continued at 35–44, while those for acute pneumonia showed on the whole an increase in this age group over the preceding decennial group. Women's ratios for bronchitis and tracheitis showed a definite upward trend over the three age groups, but for acute penumonia and 'other respiratory diseases' there was considerable variation between age groups and from year to year.

TABLE 34

Pneumonia. Proportionate Constitution of Admissions classed to Short List Group 19. Males, 1940–47

M.R.C. Code	Diagnoses	Year of Admission							
		1940	1941	1942	1943	1944	1945	1946–47	1940–47
450	Lobar pneumonia .	48	53	45	49	52	48	55	50
451	Broncho-pneumonia .	20	21	21	20	23	21	18	21
452	Pneumonia unspecified	32	26	34	31	25	31	27	29
	Pneumonia all forms .	100	100	100	100	100	100	100	100

Table 34 shows the proportions in which lobar, broncho- and unspecified forms of pneumonia were represented in the diagnoses classed to Short List Number 19. Roughly, out of every 10 such admissions, 5 were attributed to lobar, 2 to broncho-pneumonia and 3 to pneumonia not otherwise specified. It is estimated that between 30,670 and 31,460 men and from 1,930 to 2,130 women were admitted to hospital for pneumonia in one or other of its forms during the eight years under review.

Apart from the pneumonias the numbers of admissions were highest for those respiratory diseases shown in Table 35. The total number of men estimated to have been admitted for chronic bronchitis without mention of emphysema was between 28,860 and 30,540 and is therefore slightly less than that for all forms of pneumonia. Acute bronchitis represented two-ninths of all cases coded to bronchitis. The sex-ratio of numbers of admissions of males to females for acute bronchitis was 9·1, for chronic bronchitis 11·4 and for bronchitis with emphysema 100·4. The sex-ratio for pleurisy with effusion was 7·6 whereas for other forms of pleurisy it was 11·5.

TABLE 35

Numbers Admitted to Hospital for Certain Respiratory Diseases (sample) and Estimated Total Numbers Males and Females, 1940–47

M.R.C. Code	Diagnoses	Sex	Year of Admission								Estimated totals
			1940	1941	1942	1943	1944	1945	1946–47	1940–47	
441	Sinusitis	M	138	238	316	286	297	204	98	1,577	8,855
		F	5	10	40	53	54	14	18	194	±210
446	Acute Bronchitis	M	260	298	395	408	219	192	79	1,851	10,270
		F	11	17	53	54	38	21	9	203	±227
447	Chronic Bronchitis without mention of emphysema	M	1,039	1,090	1,210	892	682	520	129	5,562	30,250
		F	27	58	106	135	84	56	22	488	±389
448	Bronchitis with emphysema	M	132	120	165	126	95	57	8	703	3,550
		F	1	1	—	1	2	2	—	7	±133
4540	Pleurisy with effusion	M	89	76	108	98	122	142	95	730	4,130
		F	—	6	23	24	20	16	7	96	±144
4541	Other forms of pleurisy	M	216	227	226	191	227	181	61	1,329	7,225
		F	4	11	24	30	19	19	9	116	±190
458	Bronchiectasis	M	39	39	69	74	78	76	44	419	2,195
		F	—	1	3	4	5	5	2	20	±105

TABLE 36

Quarterly Admissions for Acute Bronchitis, Lobar Pneumonia and Pneumonia Unspecified. Persons, 1940–45

M.R.C. Code	Diseases	Season	1940	1941	1942	1943	1944	1945
446	Acute Bronchitis .	1st Quarter	125	123	205	169	96	92
		2nd Quarter	35	52	90	92	41	43
		3rd Quarter	31	39	45	45	41	21
		4th Quarter	78	98	105	157	78	57
450	Lobar Pneumonia .	1st Quarter	89	147	208	195	201	183
		2nd Quarter	60	119	140	133	140	175
		3rd Quarter	55	71	77	66	82	74
		4th Quarter	82	113	117	144	126	120
452	Pneumonia, unspecified .	1st Quarter	80	81	160	108	82	126
		2nd Quarter	37	59	90	112	69	94
		3rd Quarter	34	36	57	46	52	44
		4th Quarter	50	52	86	102	66	89

Table 36 shows the number of admissions for acute bronchitis, loba, and unspecified pneumonia in periods of thirteen weeks. The seasona fluctuations in these three conditions show in the main similar patterns with highest incidence in the first quarter and lowest in the third. The variation in the number of cases assigned to unspecified forms of pneumonia was not as wide as in the other two diseases. During the winter of 1943–44, the peak number of cases of both acute bronchitis and pneumonia unspecified occurred in the last quarter of 1943, thus resembling the occurrence of the peak of the influenza epidemic of that period. On several occasions the peak number of admissions for two or more of these diseases occurred simultaneously, as may be seen from the following:

Week of occurrence of highest number of weekly admissions

		Influenza	Acute Bronchitis	Lobar Pneumonia	Pneumonia N.O.S.
1940	Week ending	27th Jan.	27th Jan.	2nd Mar.	20th Jan.
1941	Week ending	8th Feb.	8th Feb.	25th Jan.	8th Feb.
1942	Week ending	28th Feb.	7th Mar.	7th Mar.	28th Feb.
1943	Week ending	16th Jan.	23rd Jan.	23rd Jan.	3rd Apr.
1943–44	Week ending	27th Nov.	27th Nov.	25th Mar.	4th Dec.

From Table 37 it would be seen that the median period of in-patient treatment for uncomplicated cases of acute bronchitis varied for men aged 15–34 between 15 and 19 days. If the figures for the seven years 1940–46 be combined, the median period for men aged 15–34 and those aged 35–54 was 17 days, while for women aged 15–34 it was 14 days. It is probable that the large number of men who were in hospital for 70 days of more were suffering from an acute exacerbation of a chronic bronchitis, rather than an attack of acute bronchitis.

TABLE 37

Acute Bronchitis. Periods of In-patient Treatment of cases in which no other pathological condition was recorded

Year	Sex-Age Group	Days of In-patient Treatment																*Median duration
		0–	4–	7–	10–	14–	21–	28–	35–	42–	56–	63–	70–	77–	84–	91 up	Totals	
1940	Males 15–34	1	7	15	39	37	21	8	4	4	5	—	—	1	—	—	142	15
1941		1	7	17	39	63	20	13	8	6	2	1	—	—	—	5	182	16
1942		4	11	24	36	62	26	10	10	21	5	6	1	4	3	7	230	18
1943		3	12	23	46	66	17	14	9	17	4	4	1	4	3	10	233	16
1944		4	10	18	23	29	12	6	10	6	2	2	4	3	1	7	137	17
1945–46		2	6	16	25	47	13	8	10	5	4	2	7	5	7	13	170	19
1940–46		15	53	113	208	304	109	59	51	59	22	15	13	17	14	42	1,094	17
1940–46	Males 35–54	5	12	33	64	89	27	16	18	22	9	8	3	4	2	9	321	17
1940–46	Females 15–34	2	9	28	27	46	11	5	6	6	1	2	1	—	—	—	144	14

* Adjusted for cases in which the complete period of treatment is not known.

During the war years an increasing interest was taken in primary atypical pneumonia. This condition, which was classed to 4514 in the M.R.C. Classification, covers the following diagnostic terms shown in No. 492 in the International Statistical Classification of Diseases, Injuries and Causes of Death, 1948.

Pneumonia, ages 4 weeks and over specified as:
acute interstitial
atypical (primary)
unknown aetiology
virus

Pulmonitis (acute), ages 4 weeks and over
Pulmonitis (unknown aetiology), ages 4 weeks and over

In the one-in-five sample there were 360 men and 44 women admitted with one of these diagnoses, corresponding to a total of about 2,000 admissions during the eight years 1940–47. The distribution of the cases by age and sex is shown below.

TABLE 38

Atypical Pneumonia (M.R.C. Code 4514). Distribution of Admissions by Sex and Age, 1940–47

Year	Males					Females			
	Age Groups					Age Groups			
	15–	25–	35–	45 up	All	15–	25–	35 up	All
1940	2	5	2	—	9	—	—	—	—
1941	24	20	8	1	53	2	—	—	2
1942	4	3	2	1	10	2	—	—	2
1943	16	13	8	1	38	6	1	—	7
1944	58	52	13	3	126	10	1	—	11
1945	40	23	17	1	81	16	2	1	19
1946	16	9	2	—	27	2	1	—	3
1947	15	1	—	—	16	—	—	—	—
Totals	175	126	52	7	360	38	5	1	44

In this series two deaths were recorded, one from virus pneumonia. The second case was of a patient who was also stated to have had tuberculous meningitis. In fourteen cases, or 3·5 per cent., there was mention of pleurisy.

Over the period 1940–46 the term pneumonitis has tended to be replaced by the use of primary atypical or virus pneumonia.

It is difficult to tell from such a small number of cases whether or not there is a seasonal trend in the incidence of this condition; all that can be said from examining the numbers of admissions in periods of

TABLE 39

Atypical Pneumonia. Proportionate Composition of Admissions for M.R.C. Code 4514

Diagnoses	1940	1941	1942	1943	1944	1945	1946	1947	1940–47
Pneumonitis	100	95	83	33	61	10	13	42	47
Pneumonia, primary, atypical	—	5	17	60	38	81	80	50	49
Pneumonia, virus, atypical	—	—	—	7	1	9	7	8	4
	100	100	100	100	100	100	100	100	100

thirteen weeks is that admissions were lowest in the third quarter, except in 1945.

Admissions in Periods of Thirteen Weeks

	1940	1941	1942	1943	1944	1945	1946	1947
1st Quarter	1	11	3	9	28	34	21	10
2nd Quarter	0	16	4	13	40	37	2	4
3rd Quarter	3	11	1	10	29	17	3	1
4th Quarter	5	17	2	13	40	12	4	1

The median period of in-patient treatment was 38 days for men aged 15–34 and 33 days for those aged 35–54. If the mean were taken instead of the median it would give 49 days for the younger and 41 for the older men.

ACUTE HEPATITIS AND JAUNDICE (Short List Number 24)

During the war there was an increased incidence of JAUNDICE, which affected our troops both in this country and overseas. Witts (1944) stated that infective hepatitis was one of the three most important diseases in the Mediterranean theatre, the others being malaria and venereal disease. At home, the increasing prevalence of infective types of jaundice caused the Minister of Health to issue, in 1943, the Jaundice Regulations, by which the notification of catarrhal, toxic and infective jaundice and of acute inflammation, necrosis or atrophy of the liver was made compulsory in the Eastern Region. The Minister was influenced in his choice of district by the existence of a research team working at Cambridge in collaboration with the Medical Research Council. Previous wars had brought epidemics of infective hepatitis in their train, but in this one the use of blood products in the treatment of casualties and the increase in parenteral therapy particularly with arsenical compounds added the problem of jaundice caused by the transference of an

TABLE 40

Atypical Pneumonia. Periods of In-patient Treatment of cases in which no other pathological condition was recorded

Year	Sex-Age Group	Days of In-patient Treatment															*Median duration
		0–	7–	10–	14–	21–	28–	35–	42–	49–	56–	63–	70–	77–	84–	91 up	
1940–47 .	Males 15–34	2	7	14	38	33	22	18	22	13	13	5	5	6	6	41	38
1940–47 .	Males 35–54	—	2	2	7	5	7	4	3	4	2	1	—	1	1	3	33

* Adjusted for cases in which the complete period of treatment is not known.

TABLE 41

Numbers Admitted for Epidemic Hepatitis and Jaundice, and Numbers of Deaths, during 1940–47

M.R.C. Code Nos.	Diagnoses	Males						Females				
		Age Groups					Total deaths	Age Groups				Total deaths
		15–	25–	35–	45–	All		15–	25–	35–	All	
540	Hepatosis (toxic)	27	36	14	—	77	1	3	1	—	4	—
541	'Catarrhal jaundice' (Infective hepatitis)	1,484	1,528	427	23	3,462	9	176	40	6	222	—
542 (pt.)	Cirrhosis of the liver (not alcoholic)	5	7	11	6	29	11	—	—	—	—	—
543	Acute or sub-acute atrophy of the liver	10	4	3	2	19	9	3	1	—	4	1
7606	Jaundice (symptomatic)	113	115	31	3	262	—	16	3	1	20	—
953 (pt.)*	Post-arsphenamine jaundice	59	79	31	4	173	2	—	—	—	—	—

* Including cases admitted primarily for treatment of syphilis, and developing jaundice in hospital after arsenical treatment.

icterogenic agent in the blood from one person to another. The condition known as HOMOLOGOUS SERUM JAUNDICE* had been previously recognised among patients who had received vaccination against yellow fever, the virus used for this purpose being suspended in human serum. Cases had been reported from South America and the United States, as well as in this country. Biological studies of the liver (Dible, McMichael and Sherlock, 1943) showed that the same cytological changes occur in all these instances, so pointing to a like aetiology, and suggesting that these several causes produce a parenchymatous hepatitis.

Table 41 shows that in the sample 4,022 men and 250 women were admitted to E.M.S. hospitals with hepatitis or jaundice during 1940–47, corresponding to a total of about 21,000 cases. These figures do not include cases of jaundice known to have followed blood transfusion, which will be discussed later. Infective hepatitis ('catarrhal jaundice') accounted for 862 out of every 1,000 cases and cases of symptomatic jaundice in which no more definite diagnosis was made before discharge, for another 66 per 1,000. Post-arsphenamine jaundice, toxic hepatosis, cirrhosis of the liver and acute yellow atrophy contributed 41, 19, 7 and 5 per 1,000 respectively.

Among the 4,099 cases admitted other than for arsenical jaundice during the eight years, there were 31 deaths, a case-fatality rate of 7·6 per 1,000. From infective hepatitis alone there were 9 deaths in 3,684 cases, or 2·4 per 1,000. This agrees well with Bradley's surmise of 1 death in 500 cases with icterus (Bradley, 1944). Of 29 patients admitted with cirrhosis, 11 died, a case-fatality rate of 38 per cent., the corresponding rate for acute atrophy of the liver being 43 per cent.

TABLE 42

Acute Hepatitis and Jaundice. Proportion per 1,000 Admissions for Non-infective and Non-respiratory Illnesses, by Sex and Age, 1940–47 (Cases of Post-arsphenamine Jaundice are excluded)

Year	Males						Females			
	Age Groups						Age Groups			
	15–	25–	35–	45–	55 up	All	15–	25–	35–44	All
1940 .	8	6	5	2	—	7	—	—	—	2
1941 .	12	10	5	2	—	10	8	5	—	7
1942 .	26	17	9	9	—	19	14	17	12	14
1943 .	39	32	19	10	—	32	21	24	5	21
1944 .	34	30	20	9	13	29	11	12	11	11
1945 .	39	43	30	9	—	38	14	15	8	15
1946 .	29	33	27	28	—	30	11	19	—	12
1947 .	24	34	10	—	—	24	5	—	—	4

* *See* p. 787.

From Table 42 it will be seen that the proportion of admissions for acute hepatitis and jaundice (M.R.C. codes 540–543 and 7686) per 1,000 admissions for non-infective and non-respiratory illnesses increased for both sexes from 1940–43, declined slightly in 1944 but rose again in 1945, afterwards decreasing in 1946 and 1947. During the latter half of 1943 and the beginning of 1944, the male Service population in this country was increased by the return of a large number of troops from the Mediterranean area. As jaundice had been very rife among our Forces during the North African campaign, it is possible that some of the cases admitted to hospital were already incubating the disease before sailing for home, or were infected during the journey. The increased rates for 1945 may be attributable to cases among the influx of men returning from Sicily, Italy, the Far East and the prison camps of Germany, in all of which there had been a heavy incidence of jaundice. The proportionate rates for men were highest from 1940–44 in the age group 15–24, and these decreased with advancing age, while from 1945 to 1947 they were highest at ages 25–34. Among women, from 1942 to 1946, the rates were highest at ages 25–34. The proportionate rate for males in 1945, the peak year, was five and a half times that for 1940.

The distribution of cases of infective hepatitis by season and region is shown in Table 43. The general trend is towards an autumn-winter maximum and summer minimum, not only for the country as a whole but in the three sub-divisions, Scotland, the six northern counties and Cheshire, and the rest of England and Wales. Despite the fact that the regional distribution of hospital cases is to some extent governed by the number of beds available, it would nevertheless appear that there was a high incidence in the South Eastern Region.

In the years preceding the war, evidence that hepatitis was due to a virus had been accumulating, and in the Sixth Revision of the International Classification of Diseases, Injuries and Causes of Death (1948), infective hepatitis is included in the group of diseases attributable to viruses, instead of in the diseases of the liver. Greenwood (1944) had noted in the case of influenza and encephalitis lethargica, that when influenza increases, there appears to be some increase in encephalitis. Assuming hepatitis to be due to a virus and spread by droplet infection, it would be interesting from the epidemiological point of view, to see whether or not it had any connexion with other respiratory diseases caused by a virus. Table 44 shows the quarterly admissions to E.M.S. hospitals for infective hepatitis and influenza and colds, and the quarterly notifications made to the Registrar General of acute poliomyelitis, cerebro-spinal fever and acute encephalitis lethargica during 1941–46. The highest incidence of influenza and colds occurred in the first quarter of each year except in the winter of 1943–44, when the peak of

TABLE 43

Regional and Seasonal Distribution of Cases of Infective Hepatitis (541) and of Influenza and Colds

Region	Number of Admissions in each Month or Quarter (both sexes)																							
	1941												1942											
	J.	F.	M.	A.	M.	J.	J.	A.	S.	O.	N.	D.	J.	F.	M.	A.	M.	J.	J.	A.	S.	O.	N.	D.
S. East	5	—	3	7	2	3	5	4	5	8	6	2	12	9	9	8	9	8	14	15	15	29	16	23
S. West	1	2	1	1	1	1	—	—	—	2	—	1	2	5	1	3	2	7	1	2	6	2	2	4
East	—	—	—	—	1	1	2	3	3	5	4	2	2	2	4	—	4	2	—	3	3	6	6	6
Midlands	2	1	3	—	3	1	1	3	3	8	4	6	6	5	5	2	2	3	5	6	3	5	10	2
Wales	1	5	—	1	—	—	1	1	—	2	2	2	1	—	2	1	1	1	—	2	5	3	3	4
N. of England	4	5	7	3	9	5	8	4	7	14	13	3	9	18	17	9	6	7	6	7	13	18	14	21
Scotland	—	—	3	2	7	1	1	5	1	4	7	2	4	7	13	5	8	8	6	11	8	13	10	12
N. Ireland	—	—	—	—	—	—	—	—	—	—	—	—	—	—	—	1	—	—	—	—	—	—	—	—
Total Hepatitis	13	13	17	14	23	12	18	20	19	43	36	18	36	46	51	29	32	36	32	46	53	76	61	72
	43			49			57			97			133			97			131			209		
Influenza and Colds	1.554			252			148			373			739			198			136			284		

1943	J.	F.	M.	A.	M.	J.	J.	A.	S.	O.	N.	D.
S. East	25	33	27	38	24	20	24	23	13	28	28	27
S. West	6	4	6	6	4	6	1	1	5	1	3	1
East	7	3	9	5	7	5	5	5	5	13	16	4
Midlands	10	11	7	8	8	9	2	11	7	6	7	5
Wales	5	2	4	3	3	—	1	2	2	3	—	2
N. of England	14	23	14	15	10	12	7	17	20	19	18	23
Scotland	15	16	20	16	11	8	16	10	8	8	8	6
N. Ireland	—	—	—	—	—	—	—	—	—	—	—	2
Total Hepatitis	82	92	87	91	67	60	56	69	60	78	80	70
	261			218			185			228		
Influenza and Colds	848			249			400			1,658		

1944	J.	F.	M.	A.	M.	J.	J.	A.	S.	O.	N.	D.
S. East	32	26	13	20	29	25	8	8	13	10	22	21
S. West	—	1	2	1	2	—	1	—	2	2	2	1
East	24	9	7	15	9	8	4	3	4	7	4	8
Midlands	9	6	8	8	4	6	7	4	6	13	14	9
Wales	2	—	1	1	1	1	4	1	1	—	2	1
N. of England	14	21	11	9	7	12	13	17	14	36	23	10
Scotland	14	15	13	14	8	8	19	3	4	4	9	11
N. Ireland	—	—	—	1	—	—	—	—	—	—	—	—
Total Hepatitis	95	78	55	69	60	60	56	36	44	72	76	61
	228			189			136			209		
Influenza and Colds	463			157			89			244		

1945	J.	F.	M.	A.	M.	J.	J.	A.	S.	O.	N.	D.
S. East	8	15	19	19	25	22	18	17	23	33	19	16
S. West	—	2	—	1	2	2	1	1	—	5	3	—
East	4	3	7	6	6	11	7	3	3	6	3	4
Midlands	12	17	17	10	8	10	6	9	7	14	13	10
Wales	1	—	8	2	1	—	3	2	1	2	7	2
N. of England	17	17	16	18	28	27	22	28	29	36	25	18
Scotland	11	19	9	6	15	8	9	5	4	8	8	6
N. Ireland	—	—	—	—	—	1	—	1	—	—	—	—
Total Hepatitis	53	73	76	62	85	81	66	66	67	104	78	56
	202			228			199			238		
Influenza and Colds	260			97			61			180		

1946	J.	F.	M.	A.	M.	J.	J.	A.	S.	O.	N.	D.
S. East	12	14	12	10	3	3	1	3	3	1	—	2
S. West	3	2	—	—	1	—	—	—	—	—	—	—
East	2	1	1	2	—	—	—	—	—	—	—	—
Midlands	9	4	4	10	1	1	1	3	1	—	—	2
Wales	3	1	1	—	—	1	2	—	—	—	—	—
N. of England	20	9	8	4	7	6	4	7	6	1	2	—
Scotland	5	2	4	—	2	1	1	2	1	1	3	—
N. Ireland	—	—	—	—	—	—	—	—	—	—	—	—
Total Hepatitis	54	33	30	26	14	12	9	15	11	3	5	4
	117			52			35			12		
Influenza and Colds	296			34			17			32		

the epidemic was reached before Christmas. It is apparent from Table 44, that except for an unusually large number of cases in the third quarter of 1945, acute encephalitis lethargica followed the same pattern as influenza, the peak occurring before Christmas during 1943–44. Allowing for the decrease in the number of cases of infective hepatitis in 1946 due to demobilisation, the trend of incidence is similar to that of influenza. On examining the notifications of acute poliomyelitis and acute polio-encephalitis, in which the virus attacks the central nervous system, a maximum incidence in the September and December quarters is observed, while in the case of cerebro-spinal fever, a non-virus disease which affects the central nervous system, the peak incidence occurs in the first quarter of each year. The trend of the winter epidemic of hepatitis was similar to that of influenza during the periods 1941–42, 1942–43, and 1943–44, but during the winters of 1944–45 and 1945–46, jaundice admissions were highest in the fourth quarter and influenza in the following first quarter. The apparent similarity between the incidence curves of influenza and hepatitis may be entirely accidental, the incidence of jaundice having been affected by the opening of the North African and Sicilian campaigns in 1942 and 1943 and of the Western Front in 1944.

Table 45 shows the duration of stay in hospital and the median number of days of treatment. For men aged 15–34 admitted for infective hepatitis, the median period of incapacity varied from year to year between 25 and 36 days, the average over the seven years 1940–46 being 31 days. For men aged 35–54 the median period was 43, while for women in the younger age group it was 20 days. This may be compared with the statement of Witts (1944) that in the Mediterranean theatre the average stay in hospital was about 15 days, with a further month at a convalescent home. Of the younger men, 36 per cent. were in hospital for less than 3 weeks, 55 per cent. for less than 5 weeks, and about 20 per cent. were incapacitated for upwards of 10 weeks. The short duration in hospital in some cases is accounted for by the fact that they were men who had developed jaundice on board ship and were admitted to E.M.S. hospitals on disembarkation. For symptomatic jaundice, the median period was about 4 weeks for men and 3 weeks for women, while for men with arsenical jaundice it was about 6 weeks.

The case histories of 167 patients with infective hepatitis recorded a previous attack of the disease, a re-infection rate of 4·5 per cent. Without a control series it is impossible to conclude whether an attack of infective hepatitis confers any immunity or whether on the contrary it renders the subject more liable to a subsequent attack. The age distribution of patients stated to have had a previous attack of jaundice, with the mean age at attack and the mean interval between the present attack and the preceding one, is shown in Table 46.

TABLE 44

Quarterly Admissions to E.M.S. Hospitals for Acute Infective Hepatitis and Influenza and Colds, and Quarterly Notifications of Acute Poliomyelitis, Cerebro-spinal Fever and Acute Encephalitis Lethargica, 1941–46*

DISEASES	1941				1942				1943			
	Q1	Q2	Q3	Q4	Q1	Q2	Q3	Q4	Q1	Q2	Q3	Q4
Infective Hepatitis	43	49	57	97	133	97	131	209	261	218	185	228
Influenza and Colds	1,554	252	148	373	739	198	136	284	848	249	400	1,658
Acute Encephalitis Lethargica	57	48	32	42	50	39	32	30	17	28	31	31
Acute Poliomyelitis	132	74	359	363	83	82	276	214	69	72	169	157
Cerebro-spinal Fever	5,097	4,066	1,788	1,816	4,329	3,482	1,731	1,531	2,432	1,820	901	874
	1944				**1945**				**1946**			
	Q1	Q2	Q3	Q4	Q1	Q2	Q3	Q4	Q1	Q2	Q3	Q4
Infective Hepatitis	228	189	136	209	202	228	199	238	117	52	35	12
Influenza and Colds	463	157	89	244	260	97	61	180	296	34	17	32
Acute Encephalitis Lethargica	18	28	18	15	21	17	26	12	25	20	18	16
Acute Poliomyelitis	70	98	205	152	58	81	343	369	99	86	262	225
Cerebro-spinal Fever	1,286	906	517	612	815	706	404	382	811	536	331	387

* Port Health Districts not included.
Notifications for 1941–43 inclusive, uncorrected. Notifications for 1944–46 inclusive, partially corrected (i.e., annual corrections not included).

TABLE 45

Acute Hepatitis and Jaundice

Periods of In-patient Treatment of cases in which no other pathological condition was recorded, 1940–46

Year	Diseases diagnosed	Sex-Age Group	Days of In-patient Treatment												*Median duration
			0–	14–	21–	28–	35–	42–	49–	56–	70–	91–	182 up	Totals	
1940–42	Infective hepatitis	Males 15–34	96	195	93	69	63	38	47	46	36	26	2	711	25
1943			67	178	45	42	28	29	33	52	59	47	1	581	28
1944			53	109	38	50	28	22	23	49	70	58	3	503	35
1945–46			77	148	71	70	49	48	34	49	88	98	4	736	36
1940–46			293	630	247	231	168	137	137	196	253	229	10	2,531	31
1940–46		Males 35–54	30	73	29	29	23	32	20	45	44	54	1	380	43
1940–46		Females 15–34	46	75	37	27	24	13	6	7	2	1	—	238	20
1940–46	Cirrhosis of the liver	Males 15–34	—	1	1	—	—	1	—	—	—	2	2	7	102
1940–46		Males 35–54	1	—	—	—	1	2	1	—	1	1	—	7	46
1940–46	Acute yellow atrophy	Males 15–54	3	2	—	2	1	3	—	—	1	—	—	12	29
1940–46		Females 15–34	—	3	—	1	—	—	—	—	—	—	—	4	18
1940–46	Jaundice	Males 15–34	28	47	14	12	17	15	9	19	20	8	1	190	29
1940–46		Males 35–54	4	6	4	4	3	—	2	1	4	2	—	30	28
1940–46		Females 15–34	2	8	1	3	1	—	3	—	—	—	—	18	20
1940–46	Arsenical jaundice	Males 15–54	17	14	16	10	9	11	9	16	24	14	—	140	44

* Adjusted for cases in which the complete period of treatment was not known.

TABLE 46

Age Distribution of patients with a previous attack of jaundice, mean age at previous attack and mean interval between attacks

Age at present attack	Mean age at previous attack, using whole range			Mean age at previous attack, excluding those with over 20 years before the second		
	Number	Mean age	Mean interval	Number	Mean age	Mean interval
Under 20	9	15	2·5	9	15	2·5
22½	57	18·5	4·0	57	18·5	4·0
27½	52	21·8	5·7	49	22·6	4·9
32½	26	23·7	8·8	23	25·7	6·8
37½	20	31·6	5·9	19	33·0	4·5
42½	3	41·0	1·5	3	41·0	1·5

The curve of age at previous attack appears to be bimodal, with maxima in the age groups 10–14 and 20–24. During 1948 there were 928 notifications of 'jaundice' in the Eastern Region (*Report of the Chief Medical Officer on the State of the Public Health for 1948*), with a bimodal age distribution of cases, having maxima at ages 5–9 and 20–24. In the course of an investigation into reasons for absence from school conducted by the Ministries of Health and Education it was found that of 117 children who remembered an attack of jaundice, apart from that of the newborn, 16 were under 5, 71 from 5 to 9 and 30 from 10–14 at the time of the attack.

Ten men who had been treated for venereal disease had had previous attacks of jaundice, but in only one case was the attack dissociated from N.A.B. injections. One patient reported seven attacks between April 1944 and December 1945.

The first symptoms mentioned in 3,615 cases of infective hepatitis occurred in the following order of frequency:

Nausea . .	644	Bile-stained urine	200
Anorexia .	635	Chill, rigor . .	137
Abdominal pain	577	Pyrexia . .	135
Vomiting .	399	Diarrhoea . .	86
Jaundice .	260	Backache . .	78
Headache .	244	Pain in limbs .	58

Influenza . .	58
Constipation .	47
Pale stools . .	34
Sore throat .	19
Coma . .	4

Of the types mentioned by Bradley (1944) there were 31 cases either following or associated with tonsillitis and two with enteritis, while two cases had been preceded at intervals of one week and 10 weeks respectively by an attack of food poisoning. Eleven cases were associated with glandular fever, while in several cases it was noted that there were painful and enlarged glands, although no more definite diagnosis was made.

Certain other symptoms may arise in the course of the illness, and of these the one most frequently observed was pruritus which was stated to be present in 299 cases and absent in 294. It generally increased in intensity at night and was often confined to the lower limbs. Other symptoms were stated to be present (or absent) in the following descending order of frequency; vertigo 100 (11); rash 73 (32); dyspnoea 52 (51); tachycardia 22 (24). Conjunctivitis or other inflammatory conditions of the eyes were recorded in 11 cases, and herpes in 20 cases of which 10 were diagnosed as herpes labialis.

Linsey (1943) has stated that complications of infective hepatitis are supposed to be very rare. Cullinan (1939) refers to a case of parotitis and Maitland and Winner (1939) to one of oöphoritis. In this series there were two patients admitted with a primary diagnosis of mumps with subsequent jaundice and two admitted primarily for jaundice who developed mumps. One man developed orchitis and epididymitis. It is possible that in some cases there may have been an involvement of the pancreas; one case was recorded in this series of chronic hepatitis and chronic pancreatitis, and a second in which the primary cause of admission was pancreatitis, jaundice subsequently developing in hospital. In two cases glycosuria was mentioned, but no record was found of diabetes.

Some virus diseases such as mumps and measles may under certain circumstances attack the nervous system, and it is not surprising to find nervous complications following infective hepatitis. Lescher (1944) has mentioned meningitis, paralysis of the limbs and polyneuritis. While no cases of meningitis were found in this series, there was one case in which facial paralysis occurred and others showing symptoms of involvement of the nervous system, such as weakness in the legs and feet and neck-rigidity.

In all the cases of association of other diseases with infective hepatitis mentioned above, the case histories were examined to see whether there had been a previous attack of jaundice. The only such record was of a case of glandular fever and hepatitis in which an attack of jaundice had occurred ten years previously.

It would be impossible in this survey to attempt to trace a connexion between cases of jaundice. In 279 cases there was no known contact with jaundice and no other cases in the unit, while in 190 cases direct contact or the occurrence of other cases in the same billet, unit or ship was admitted. The periods of time stated to have elapsed between the possibility of contact and the present illness were distributed as follows:

Under 2 weeks	2 wks.	3 wks.	4 wks.	5 wks.	6 wks.	7 wks.	8 wks.	12 wks.
7	11	10	25	7	1	1	1	3

Suggestions have been made that the incidence of hepatitis is greater among commissioned, than among other ranks. Cold has been suggested as one of the predisposing factors to an attack of jaundice, and the high incidence among British air crews, who may be exposed to cold at high altitudes, and among British officers, who undress at night, has been cited. But as Witts (1944) points out, neither American officers nor American flying personnel show an incidence above the normal, and in the R.A.F. steps were taken to prevent chilling at unaccustomed heights. The distribution of infective hepatitis among male commissioned, non-commissioned and other ranks for the three Services combined is shown in Table 47, but it has not been possible to get comparable figures for the population at risk.

TABLE 47

Distribution of Infective Hepatitis by Rank. Males, 1943–45

Rank	1943		1944		1945		1943–45	
	Number	Per cent.	Number	Per cent.	Number	Per cent.	Number	Per cent.
Commissioned	82	11	40	6	16	2	138	6
Non-commissioned	233	31	217	30	263	32	713	31
Other ranks	427	58	459	64	534	66	1,420	63
Totals	742	100	716	100	813	100	2,271	100

The possibility of the disease being acquired through association with rats, as in the case of Weil's disease, has been considered. In this series nineteen men were known to have come into contact with rats or rat-infested premises, while twenty-six stated that there had been no likelihood of such contact.

The distribution by age, civil state and branch of Service of 173 men who developed jaundice following arsenical therapy was as follows:

Age	No.	Percentage	Civil State	No.	Percentage	Branch of Service	No.	Percentage
15–24	59	34	Single	31	18	Army	126	73
25–34	79	46	Married	80	46	Navy	26	15
35–44	31	18	Widowed or Divorced	1	1	Air Force	21	12
45 up	4	2	Not stated	61	35			
Totals	173	100		173	100		173	100

The median period of treatment in hospital was 44 days. Thirty-four per cent. were in hospital for less than 4 weeks, 28 per cent. from 4 to 8 weeks, 29 per cent. from 8 weeks to 3 months and 10 per cent. for 3 months and over.

The first mentioned symptoms in this series of cases were, in descending order of frequency, nausea and bile-stained urine, 18; anorexia, 16; abdominal pain, 14; vomiting, 13; jaundice, 9; others, 14.

The onset of jaundice occurred at varying times during treatment. In 73 cases jaundice appeared as follows:

During the first course	3	After the first course	28
" " second "	19	" " second "	9
" " third "	2	" " third "	8
		" " fourth "	3
		" " eighth "	1

In a further 12 cases in which courses were not distinguished, the number of injections given before jaundice appeared was 1, 2, 3, 5, 6, 8(2), 10, 13, 16, 20, and weekly for two years. The number of cases reported here is too small for any definite conclusion to be drawn. Nevertheless, the appearance of jaundice in a comparatively large number in the earlier stages of treatment would appear to support the view that the disease is due to the introduction into the blood of an infective agent, rather than the toxicity of arsenicals to the liver.

Two patients admitted with a diagnosis of acute atrophy of the liver, one of whom died, had previously had attacks of jaundice following treatment for syphilis, and a third who had previously had arsenical therapy died of portal cirrhosis of the liver.

HERNIA (Short List Number 25)

During the eight years 1940–47, 12,263 males and 98 females in the sample were admitted for hernia. Of these 11,324 men had inguinal hernia without obstruction or strangulation as the primary diagnosis, the corresponding total number of admissions for this cause being from 56 to 57 thousand.

Table 48 shows that as a principal cause of men's admissions to hospital hernia and intestinal obstruction varied between one-tenth of the basic total of admissions in 1940 and one-twentieth in 1947. Between 1941 and 1947 the proportion was highest in the age-group 35–44, while at ages 15–24 it declined steadily from 94 in 1940 to 48 in 1947. Hernia made an insignificant contribution to causes of admission of women.

TABLE 48

Hernia. Proportion per 1,000 Admissions for Non-infective and Non-respiratory Illnesses, by Sex and Age, 1940–47

Year	Males						Females			
	Age Groups						Age Groups			
	15–	25–	35–	45–	55 up	All	15–	25–	35 up	All
1940	94	121	81	84	59	101	5	17	—	7
1941	70	89	100	70	91	83	6	24	—	8
1942	66	64	80	62	14	68	3	3	6	3
1943	59	58	75	64	32	62	3	7	—	4
1944	62	55	69	24	13	60	6	6	17	6
1945	59	58	95	78	32	66	4	1	16	3
1946	52	82	117	111	—	71	3	13	—	4
1947	48	55	82	—	—	50	—	—	—	—

The total numbers of admissions for hernia, with or without obstruction, and the percentages of cases of inguinal, femoral and umbilical hernia described as gangrenous, incarcerated or irreducible or with obstruction or strangulation are shown in Tables 49 and 50.

TABLE 49

Number of Admissions for Hernia, by Sex and Age, 1940–47

M.R.C. Code No.	DIAGNOSES	Males						Females			
		Age Groups						Age Groups			
		15–	25–	35–	45–	55 up	All	15–	25–	35 up	All
5200	Inguinal, without obstruction .	3,956	4,864	2,268	221	15	11,324	51	17	5	73
5201	Inguinal, with obstruction .	195	138	47	3	—	383	1	—	—	1
5210	Femoral, without obstruction .	42	81	57	7	—	187	5	5	2	12
5211	Femoral, with obstruction .	1	6	10	1	—	18	1	1	—	2
5220	Umbilical, without obstruction .	17	22	14	4	—	57	1	—	—	1
5221	Umbilical, with obstruction .	1	2	1	1	—	5	—	—	—	—
523	Incisional . .	30	35	21	3	—	89	3	2	1	6
524	Diaphragmatic .	3	1	2	—	—	6	—	—	—	—
525	Other or Ill-defined .	59	76	49	10	—	194	2	1	—	3

TABLE 50

Percentage of Cases of Inguinal, Femoral and Umbilical Hernia with obstruction, Males, 1940–47

M.R.C. Code Number	Diagnoses	Males					
		Age Groups					
		15–	25–	35–	45–	55 up	All
520	Inguinal	4·7	2·8	2·0	1·3	—	3·3
521	Femoral	2·3	6·9	14·9	12·5	—	8·8
522	Umbilical	5·6	8·3	6·7	20·0	—	8·1

TABLE 51

Inguinal Hernia

Periods of In-patient Treatment of Cases in which no other pathological condition was recorded, 1940–46

Year	Sex-Age Group	Days of In-patient Treatment														*Median duration
		0–	14–	21–	28–	35–	42–	49–	56–	63–	70–	77–	84–	91–	182 up	Total	
1940	Males 15–34	88	275	472	382	189	90	32	36	20	19	10	7	8	6	1,634	27
1941		52	156	221	233	153	136	114	91	67	65	47	39	71	6	1,451	38
1942		26	44	94	98	102	143	148	122	89	99	84	86	179	10	1,324	56
1943		18	15	49	66	63	68	100	75	66	42	54	60	287	8	971	66
1944		26	24	49	52	53	65	65	58	60	34	48	49	309	5	897	69
1945–46		23	48	93	90	73	61	65	74	48	50	24	30	442	17	1,138	69
		233	562	978	921	633	563	524	456	350	309	267	271	1,296	52	7,415	47
1940	Males 35–54	11	31	68	55	16	17	11	3	2	2	2	1	—	1	220	28
1941		8	17	38	42	26	32	30	18	20	14	8	9	28	—	290	46
1942		19	18	19	28	34	43	42	26	27	19	20	11	40	1	347	51
1943		17	11	23	28	19	25	40	19	24	11	9	19	91	2	338	57
1944		20	10	30	17	13	33	28	20	12	17	12	15	106	3	336	63
1945–46		17	25	38	32	35	29	29	29	25	24	16	17	105	6	427	58
		92	112	216	202	143	179	180	115	110	87	67	72	370	13	1,958	50
1940–46	Females 15–34	5	5	11	6	6	8	6	1	2	—	2	—	1	—	53	33

* Adjusted for cases in which the complete period of treatment was not known.

Men aged 15–24 accounted for 35 per cent. of the total admissions for inguinal hernia, and 21 and 29 per cent. of those for the femoral and umbilical forms respectively.

The percentage of men with inguinal hernias with obstruction was greatest at ages 15–24 and decreased with age, while femoral and umbilical hernias showed generally the reverse trend. The difference between the proportion with obstructed inguinal hernia at ages 15–24 and those in the next two decennial age groups is greater than would be due to the chances arising in random sampling, (Difference ±2 S.E. 1·9 ± 1·6; 2·7 ± ·9; 3·4 ± 1·6) but there was no significant difference between the other age groups. Similarly for femoral hernia, the proportion with obstruction was significantly higher at ages 25–34 than at 15–24, while for umbilical hernia there was no significant variation between the age groups. If the proportions of obstructed inguinal and femoral hernias in corresponding age groups be compared, the difference is significant only at ages 35–44 (12·9 ± 8·7).

Table 51 shows that the median period of in-patient treatment among men aged 15–34 increased from 27 days in 1940 to 69 days during 1944 to 1946, the median over the seven years being 47 days. For males aged 35–54 the median duration increased from 28 days in 1940 to 63 days in 1944, and then decreased to 58 days in the last two years. The median period for women was about a fortnight less than for men. Eighteen per cent. of those in the younger age group and 20 per cent. in the older were in hospital for three months or more.

GASTRIC AND DUODENAL ULCERS (Short List Number 26)

The four types of ulcer included in this title are gastric (491), duodenal (492), peptic (493) and gastro-jejunal (494), the term 'peptic' being employable only when it is not specified whether the ulcer was gastric or duodenal. The proportions of the basic total of admissions attributed to ulcers are shown in Table 52.

Among men the highest proportionate admissions for ulcers are found in the age groups 35–44 and 45–54. In 1940 ulcers formed between 9 per cent. and 11 per cent. of the basic total of admissions at ages 35 and over. These high rates, which occurred in the year of the French collapse, declined at all ages during 1941–43, but there was an increase in 1944 and 1945, synchronous with the establishment of a Western Front. There was also an increase in the proportionate rates for women in 1945, especially at ages 25–44. The average number of men admitted during the five quarters January 1943 to March 1944 with a primary diagnosis of gastric, duodenal or peptic ulcer was 225. In the period from April 1944 to September 1945, quarterly admissions exceeded this average by percentages of 47, 13, 31, 75, 69 and 20 for the six quarters respectively. If persons with a certain type of psychological

TABLE 52

Gastric and Duodenal Ulcers. Proportion per 1,000 Admissions for Non-infective and Non-respiratory Illnesses, by Sex and Age, 1940–47

Year	Males						Females			
	Age Groups						Age Groups			
	15–	25–	35–	45–	55 up	All	15–	25–	35–44	All
1940	16	47	110	91	94	43	5	—	39	7
1941	21	46	77	71	36	42	1	10	25	4
1942	19	39	60	65	29	36	2	8	12	3
1943	16	34	53	59	48	32	3	5	11	3
1944	18	44	63	83	68	40	2	5	11	4
1945	51	50	69	78	65	55	7	27	103	16
1946	25	64	89	55	83	47	7	13	—	8
1947	18	49	82	137	167	28	—	—	—	—

constitution are more prone to develop ulcers than their fellows, then it may be that the increase in women's rates was connected with an increase of anxiety about the welfare of their men-folk, while men were mainly affected by the stress of battle.

In the one-fifth sample of admissions there were during 1940–47 1,395 men admitted with gastric, 5,199 with duodenal and 387 with peptic ulcers, corresponding to total admissions of 7,000 for gastric, 26,000 for duodenal and 1,900 for peptic. The ratio of duodenal to gastric ulcers was therefore 3·7, though if individual years be considered it was as high as 4·7 in 1942. While death statistics and hospital studies such as that of the New York hospitals, 1933, have shown a preponderance of gastric over duodenal ulcers, common opinion has been that the proportion of duodenal to gastric ulcers among the general population was five to one or possibly higher. It has been shown that the figures from E.M.S. hospitals and from the Survey of Sickness

TABLE 53

Percentage of gastric and duodenal ulcers with perforation and haemorrhage. Males, 1940–47

M.R.C. Code	Diagnoses	Age groups				
		15–	25–	35–	45–54	All ages
	Gastric ulcer					
4910	with perforation	36·8	26·3	19·4	18·8	24·9
4911	with haemorrhage	4·5	5·4	3·7	5·0	4·6
	Duodenal ulcer					
4920	with perforation	14·0	10·3	9·0	11·3	10·6
4921	with haemorrhage	1·6	2·2	2·6	1·5	2·2

conducted by the Central Office of Information for the General Register Office tend to support this view. (Brooke 1950).

Table 53 shows the percentages of gastric and duodenal ulcers with perforation or haemorrhage in the various age groups. In both cases the proportion of ulcers with perforation is highest at ages 15–24 and decreases with age. This may indicate, not so much that a larger proportion of ulcers perforate among young than among older men, but rather that younger men are less likely to seek hospital treatment for ulcers which are accompanied by neither perforation nor haemorrhage. The differences between the percentages of gastric and duodenal ulcers with perforation or haemorrhage in corresponding age groups are:

	With perforation		*With haemorrhage*	
	Difference	2 × Standard Error	Difference	2 × Standard Error
Age 15–24	22·8	7·62	2·9	2·90
25–34	16·8	3·84	3·2	1·96
35–44	10·4	3·80	1·1	0·96
45–54	7·5	9·84	3·5	5·16

Hence the proportion of gastric ulcers with perforation is significantly greater than that of duodenal in the three age-groups between 15 and 44, while the difference between those with haemorrhage is significant at ages 25–34 and 35–44.

The case-fatality rates per 1,000 among males with gastric ulcers with perforation, haemorrhage, or unqualified were 61, 31 and 2 respectively, the corresponding rates for duodenal ulcers being 47, 35 and 2. These rates are substantially lower than those for the New York Hospitals, 1933, where the overall case-fatality rate for gastric ulcers was 13 per cent. and for duodenal ulcers 7·6 per cent. The difference is partly due to the necessity for sending to hospital men from the Services who under civilian conditions would have been treated at home, and partly to the difference in age structure of the populations at risk.

GASTRO-ENTERITIS, APPENDICITIS AND OTHER DIGESTIVE DISEASES (Short List Numbers 27–29)

The proportion of admissions attributed to gastro-enteritis was fortunately not high, when war-time conditions among Service personnel are considered (*see* Table 54). The rates for males at all ages varied between 11 and 20 per 1,000 basic admissions and for females between 8 and 26.

TABLE 54

Gastro-enteritis. Proportion per 1,000 Admissions for Non-infective and Non-respiratory Illnesses, 1940–47

Year	Males					Females			
	Age Groups					Age Groups			
	15–	25–	35–	45–54	All	15–	25–	35–44	All
1940	11	11	15	15	12	11	42	20	18
1941	10	13	10	12	11	8	15	—	8
1942	18	21	18	24	20	25	27	42	26
1943	17	16	14	10	16	14	12	32	14
1944	18	14	14	14	15	15	14	17	15
1945	20	19	18	14	19	12	13	—	11
1946	18	15	14	14	16	10	—	—	8
1947	15	18	—	—	15	10	30	—	12

Appendicitis accounted for roughly one in twenty of men's basic admissions and from 12 to 24 per cent. of those of women. Table 55 shows that the proportionate rates are highest for both men and women aged 15–24 and lower in the older age groups where many would have already had an appendicectomy.

TABLE 55

Appendicitis. Proportion per 1,000 Admissions for Non-infective and Non-respiratory Illnesses, 1940–47

Year	Males						Females				
	Age Groups						Age Groups				
	15–	25–	35–	45–	55 up	All	15–	25–	35–	45–54	All
1940	73	41	27	14	23	53	253	159	97	111	215
1941	76	45	23	12	—	52	208	146	25	83	186
1942	73	39	23	17	29	48	145	85	42	—	129
1943	74	43	27	21	16	50	138	65	37	65	122
1944	81	45	34	30	27	54	138	102	78	36	128
1945	72	44	36	39	32	52	160	106	79	56	142
1946	85	66	31	55	167	72	174	108	—	—	157
1947	137	80	62	45	—	124	256	182	—	—	242

The M.R.C. classification distinguishes cases of appendicitis complicated by abscess, gangrene or perforation from those which were unqualified or sub-acute. The proportion of such complications occurring in each age group is shown in Table 56 below. From this it appears that a higher proportion of cases were accompanied by gangrene than by perforation or abscess. The proportion of uncomplicated cases was highest in the lower age groups and decreased with age. At ages 15–34,

TABLE 56
Appendicitis. Proportionate Composition of Admissions by Sex and Age, 1940–47

M.R.C. Code No.	Diagnoses	Males					Females			
		Age Groups					Age Groups			
		15–	25–	35–	45 up	All	15–	25–	35 up	All
507	Appendicitis									
5070	with abscess	45	47	72	61	49	19	26	96	22
5071	with gangrene	100	100	99	184	100	26	28	19	26
5072	with perforation	35	33	45	153	37	10	9	—	10
5073	unqualified	820	820	784	602	814	945	937	885	942
	Totals	1,000	1,000	1,000	1,000	1,000	1,000	1,000	1,000	4,000

5·5 per cent. of men and 6·1 per cent. of women were in hospital for less than 10 days, compared with 5·1 per cent. of men aged 35–54.

The case-fatality rate per 1,000 in each sex-age group was as follows:

	Males					*Females*			
	15–24	25–34	35–44	45 up	All	15–24	25–34	35 up	All
With complications	11·3	15·6	37·2	102·6	17·7	14·8	—	—	11·9
Without complications	2·5	0·8	4·4	16·9	2·2	0·9	5·0	21·7	1·8
All forms	4·0	3·4	11·5	51·0	5·0	1·6	4·7	19·2	2·4

Table 57 shows the distribution of days of in-patient treatment for uncomplicated cases of appendicitis (M.R.C. code 5073). The median period of treatment was about four weeks for men in both age groups and three weeks for women. The proportions of men in hospital for less than a fortnight were 13 per cent. and 12 per cent. in the two age groups, compared with 20 per cent. of the women, but nearly a quarter of the men were treated for eight weeks or more, compared with 4 per cent. of the women.

Of the remaining diseases of the digestive system (Short List Number 29, *see* page 648) those occurring with the greater frequency are shown in Table 58. The most important cause of hospitalisation in this group was gastritis, for which in all about 14,500 men and 800 women were admitted to hospital. The sex-ratios of numbers of males to females admitted during the eight years for certain diseases of the digestive system were as follows:

Gastritis	18·4	Appendicitis	3·1	Gastric ulcer	69·8
Duodenitis	103·7	Gastro-enteritis	7·6	Peptic ulcer	91·2

The return of Service men from the Far East brought a number of cases of sprue to the E.M.S. hospitals. In the one-in-five sample 106 males (90 Army and 16 R.A.F.) and 1 female (A.T.S.) were admitted, their diagnoses being sprue 89, tropical sprue 10, recurrent sprue 2, clinical sprue 1, sprue syndrome 2, steatorrhoea 1, idiopathic

TABLE 57

Appendicitis

Periods of In-patient Treatment of Cases in which no other pathological condition was recorded, 1940–46

Year	Sex-Age Group	Days of In-patient Treatment 0–	7–	10–	14–	21–	28–	42–	56–	91–	182–	Total	*Median duration
1940	Males 15–34	22	31	92	338	150	125	43	24	6	—	831	19
1941		22	22	61	256	140	162	109	100	15	4	891	24
1942		17	29	32	173	74	139	136	218	59	3	880	39
1943		16	18	54	145	67	123	100	160	83	4	770	37
1944		19	19	48	123	61	114	92	184	85	—	745	41
1945–46		32	30	103	179	94	106	85	129	135	5	898	29
1940–46		128	149	390	1,214	586	769	565	815	383	16	5,015	28
1940–41	Males 35–54	4	4	10	38	27	18	13	3	1	—	118	21
1942–43		—	2	7	38	32	37	28	32	17	1	194	35
1944–46		11	6	21	40	17	31	22	40	29	—	217	33
1940–46		15	12	38	116	76	86	63	75	47	1	529	29
1940–41	Females 15–34	6	12	60	108	41	22	9	—	—	—	258	16
1942		10	17	45	129	67	85	54	17	4	—	428	21
1943		10	20	39	169	85	121	71	28	2	—	545	23
1944		10	15	67	133	58	83	75	16	2	—	459	21
1945–46		11	21	96	161	67	69	32	9	1	—	467	24
1940–46		47	85	307	700	318	380	241	70	9	—	2,157	20

* Adjusted for cases in which the complete period of treatment was not known.

TABLE 58

Numbers admitted to Hospital for certain Diseases of the Digestive System (sample) and estimated total numbers Males and Females, 1940–47

M.R.C. Code No.	Diagnoses	Sex	Year of Admission								Estimated Totals
			1940	1941	1942	1943	1944	1945	1946–47	1940–47	
480	Hypertrophy of adenoids and tonsils	M.	59	99	205	152	94	52	33	694	3,470 ± 132
		F.	2	10	70	99	72	44	11	308	1,540 ± 88
483	Peritonsillar abscess	M.	169	185	267	351	334	277	113	1,696	8,480 ± 206
		F.	5	5	31	44	40	36	9	170	850 ± 65
484	Other diseases of pharynx and tonsils	M.	101	243	294	288	230	232	105	1,493	7,465 ± 193
		F.	14	26	69	135	116	122	52	534	2,670 ± 116
4900–3	Gastritis	M.	552	694	643	398	337	219	89	2,932	14,660 ± 271
		F.	6	12	38	46	20	31	6	159	795 ± 63
4904	Duodenitis	M.	35	57	72	56	49	33	9	311	1,555 ± 88
		F.	—	—	1	1	—	1	—	3	15 ± 9
508	Other diseases of appendix	M.	24	35	23	17	27	15	7	148	740 ± 61
		F.	3	2	10	18	18	7	4	62	310 ± 39
509	Other diseases of intestines	M.	67	68	78	63	58	36	42	412	2,060 ± 101
		F.	3	2	18	15	20	11	7	76	380 ± 44
532	Anal fistula	M.	66	106	126	101	124	95	37	655	3,275 ± 128
		F.	—	3	3	8	12	5	2	33	165 ± 29
533	Anal fissure	M.	36	49	51	68	60	47	19	330	1,650 ± 91
		F.	—	2	7	15	11	5	5	45	225 ± 34
534	Ischiorectal abscess	M.	68	113	85	97	91	81	45	580	2,900 ± 120
		F.	2	5	7	11	13	7	3	48	240 ± 35
545	Cholecystitis, without mention of calculi	M.	19	23	38	26	18	23	3	150	750 ± 61
		F.	1	3	6	9	8	8	2	37	185 ± 30

steatorrhoea 2 (including the female). The men's age distribution was 15–24, 31; 25–34, 59; 35 and over, 16. Most of the patients had already received treatment abroad, nevertheless their median stay in hospital in this country was 67 days. The median period of treatment from the onset of diarrhoea to discharge from hospital was 9 months. There were two deaths, of which one attributed to sprue occurred 8 months after the initial diarrhoea. The second, in which sprue was complicated by macrocytic anaemia with terminal haemorrhagic broncho-pneumonia, took place 4 months after the onset of diarrhoea. Of the remainder, 38 were discharged from the army, of whom 11 were re-categorised, returned to unit, 4 were sent to other hospitals, 19 were stated to have been discharged from hospital without indication of their future and for 4 there was no information. Anaemia was mentioned as a complication in 4 cases, while 9 cases were accompanied by malaria and 1 by amoebic dysentery.

DISEASES OF THE FEMALE GENITAL ORGANS (Short List Number 30) AND NORMAL AND ABNORMAL CHILDBEARING (Short List Numbers 32, 33)

Table 59 shows that about one-tenth of the basic total of admissions was attributable to diseases of the female genital organs. The proportionate rates were higher on the whole at ages 25–34 than at 15–24.

TABLE 59

Diseases of the Female Genital Organs and Normal and Abnormal Childbearing. Proportions per 1,000 Admissions for Non-infective and Non-respiratory Illnesses, by Age, 1940–47

Year	Diseases of Female Genital Organs					Normal and Abnormal Childbearing			
	Age Groups					Age Groups			
	15–	25–	35–	45 up	All	15–	25–	35–44	All
1940 . .	85	100	118	111	92	27	33	59	31
1941 . .	106	136	99	167	112	25	59	—	29
1942 . .	94	113	159	186	101	41	36	18	39
1943 . .	93	130	101	97	100	37	54	31	39
1944 . .	112	138	185	107	120	70	78	34	70
1945 . .	117	143	134	—	124	66	80	56	69
1946 . .	121	108	115	—	118	45	51	38	46
1947 . .	164	274	—	—	177	48	30	—	45

For all ages together the rates increased up to 1945. Normal and abnormal childbearing caused between 3 and 7 per cent. of the basic total. The rates were highest in 1944 and 1945; in the general population the birth rate reached a maximum in 1944, declined in 1945 and increased in 1946.

TABLE 60

Proportionate Distribution of Diseases of the Female Genital Organs, 1940–47

M.R.C. Code No.	Diagnoses	Total Numbers (Sample)	Proportions
600–603	Diseases of the breast	136	59
605–606	Salpingitis and oöphoritis	202	87
604; 607	Other diseases of ovaries and Fallopian tubes	42	18
608	Diseases of the parametrium	17	7
610	Cervicitis	365	158
611	Genital prolapse	20	9
612–613	Malposition of uterus; chronic subinvolution	111	48
6140	Amenorrhoea	91	39
6141	Dysmenorrhoea	504	218
6142–6144	Menorrhagia	354	153
6145; 616	Other disorders of menstruation and the menopause	127	55
615	Sterility	48	21
617	Diseases of vulva and vagina	192	83
618	Bartholin's glands	68	30
619	Other diseases of female genital organs	35	15
	Totals	2,312	1,000

The proportionate distribution of diseases of the female genitalia is shown in Table 60. Of every 1,000 admissions, 465 were due to disorders of menstruation and menopausal symptoms. The frequency and disabling nature of these conditions is emphasised by figures from the Survey of Sickness, which show that for the period May 1946–April 1947 the monthly inception rate* for this cause was 1,902 per 100,000 women aged 16 and more, and the monthly prevalence rate* was 3,041 per 100,000 (Stocks 1949). Further, 21 per cent. of these illnesses caused either at least one day of incapacity or at least one medical consultation. About 1,800 Service women were admitted for treatment of cervicitis during the eight years.

Table 61 shows the estimated numbers who were treated in E.M.S. hospitals for normal and abnormal childbearing. Since many Service women would seek discharge from the Forces on grounds of pregnancy, and their subsequent history is unknown, these figures may not show a correct ratio of abnormal to normal cases of childbearing. Mackay (1951) has shown that in a sample of hospital discharges, out of 19,800 attributed to pregnancy, childbirth and the puerperium, 11,364 were

* *See* p. 666 for definitions.

TABLE 61

Normal and Abnormal Childbearing. Numbers in sample and estimated total admissions, 1940–47

M.R.C. Code Number	Diagnoses	Total Numbers (Sample)	Estimated total admissions	Proportions
620	Normal pregnancy . . .	117	585 ± 54	111
650	Normal delivery . . .	31	155 ± 28	29
621–638	Abnormal pregnancy . .	111	555 ± 53	105
640–646	Abortion, therapeutic or other, with or without sepsis . .	784	3,920 ± 140	742
651–679	Abnormal delivery and complications of puerperium .	14	70 ± 19	13
620–679	*Totals*	1,057	5,285 ± 163	1,000

due to normal or unqualified childbearing and 8,436 to abnormal, or 57 per cent. and 43 per cent. respectively, but presumably admission to hospital was facilitated if abnormality were recognised or suspected.

OTHER GENITO-URINARY DISEASES (Short List Number 31)

This group comprises diseases of the urinary system and of the male genital organs. They contributed from 4 to 5 per cent. of the basic total of admissions of men and from 2 to 5 per cent. of women (Table 62). These relatively small proportions may be due to the elimination of persons with some forms of kidney disease at the preliminary medical boards. The rates showed no pattern of variation with age except that they were generally lower at ages 15–24 than at 25–34 for both sexes.

TABLE 62

Diseases of the Urinary System and Male Genital Organs Proportions per 1,000 Admissions for Non-infective and Non-respiratory Illnesses, by Sex and Age, 1940–47

Year	Males						Females				
	Age Groups						Age Groups				
	15–	25–	35–	45–	55 up	All	15–	25–	35–	45 up	All
1940 .	37	38	31	29	35	36	19	25	39	—	22
1941 .	46	43	39	35	91	44	41	58	99	83	48
1942 .	43	41	39	53	58	41	43	46	36	—	43
1943 .	39	44	41	47	97	42	41	40	32	97	41
1944 .	42	47	52	40	108	46	43	36	28	71	41
1945 .	43	52	49	48	32	48	38	39	8	—	37
1946 .	48	64	47	111	—	54	33	45	—	—	34
1947 .	40	46	21	—	167	40	34	—	—	—	33

If diseases of the male genitalia be excluded, the proportional composition of admissions for urinary conditions is shown in Table 63. In each year the principal components among men were pyelitis, cystitis and calculi of kidney and ureter, whereas among women pyelitis and cystitis were the principal contributors to the total of urinary diseases. Calculi, which caused 21 per cent. of men's admissions in this disease group accounted for only 6 per cent. of those of women.

TABLE 63

Proportional Composition of Admissions for Diseases of the Urinary System (M.R.C. Code 560–588) by Sex, 1940–47

M.R.C. Code No.	DIAGNOSES	Males							Females	
		1940	1941	1942	1943	1944	1945	1946–7	1940–45	1946–47
560	Acute nephritis .	74	63	37	50	92	89	104	70	20
561–566	Other forms of nephritis .	82	82	121	98	106	174	176	117	34
570	Pyelitis, pyelonephritis, pyelocystitis	166	201	218	199	169	107	116	172	534
574	Cystitis . .	185	191	204	238	187	240	168	206	290
575	Calculi of kidney and ureter .	286	198	195	170	207	192	256	207	59
580	Hydronephrosis	32	42	46	57	67	76	32	54	23
585	Stricture of urethra .	22	16	26	22	31	21	20	23	1
588	Urethritis, etc. .	89	138	102	103	86	68	60	95	18
Rest of 560–588	Other urinary diseases .	64	69	51	63	55	33	68	56	21
		1,000	1,000	1,000	1,000	1,000	1,000	1,000	1,000	1,000

The age distribution for men of cases of acute nephritis, other forms of nephritis, pyelitis, cystitis and calculi is as follows:

	15–	25–	35–	45–	55 up	All ages
Acute nephritis	44	41	13	2	—	100
Other forms of nephritis	32	45	20	3	—	100
Pyelitis	29	48	20	2	1	100
Cystitis	31	45	19	4	1	100
Calculi of kidney and ureter	23	51	24	2	—	100

TABLE 64

Proportional Composition of Admissions for Diseases of the Male Genital Organs, 1940–47, and Estimated Total Admissions

M.R.C. Code Number	Diagnoses	Total Numbers (Sample)	Estimated total admissions	Proportions
590–591	Diseases of the prostate . .	113	565 ± 53	30
592	Hydrocele	814	4,070 ± 143	218
593–594	Haematocele and spermatocele	57	285 ± 38	15
595	Orchitis and epididymitis .	1,115	5,575 ± 167	299
596	Torsion of testis or spermatic cord	22	110 ± 23	6
597	Paraphimosis and phimosis .	1,411	7,055 ± 188	379
598	Other diseases of male genital organs	198	990 ± 70	53
	Totals	3,730	18,650 ± 305	1,000

Acute nephritis caused more hospitalisation among younger men than did the chronic and unspecified forms of this disease, while the other three conditions appeared more frequently in the older men than among those aged 15–24.

It is estimated that about 18,500 men were admitted with a primary diagnosis of disease of the genital organs. Of these roughly 7,000 were treated for phimosis and paraphimosis and 5,500 for orchitis and epididymitis.

DISEASES OF SKIN AND CELLULAR TISSUE (Short List Number 34)

Diseases of the skin and cellular tissue were responsible for a large proportion of the basic total of admissions, the rates for men of all ages varying between 15 and 19 per cent. and for women from 9 to 11 per cent. Table 65 shows that the proportionate rates for men decreased

TABLE 65

Diseases of Skin and Cellular Tissue. Proportion per 1,000 Admissions for Non-infective and Non-respiratory Illnesses, by Sex and Age, 1940–47

Year	Males						Females				
	Age Groups						Age Groups				
	15–	25–	35–	45–	55 up	All	15–	25–	35–	45 up	All
1940 .	228	152	106	84	35	178	88	125	118	111	99
1941 .	224	164	122	105	91	179	110	54	99	83	100
1942 .	190	136	119	105	160	151	91	78	85	111	88
1943 .	206	170	143	139	113	177	98	89	63	65	95
1944 .	209	166	142	160	176	176	115	83	106	71	108
1945 .	183	139	135	119	97	152	109	67	87	167	97
1946 .	189	127	123	125	—	157	109	121	—	—	107
1947 .	210	141	103	92	—	193	87	91	—	—	86

with age, except in 1944. At ages 15–24 admissions for this disease group constituted about one-fifth of the basic total, and at ages 25–34 about one-seventh. While not serious from the point of view of endangering life, these diseases were responsible for a considerable amount of ill-health, and although under civilian conditions the numbers sent to hospital on this account would not be so great as in the sample under review, a considerable amount of incapacity would nevertheless be caused.

Table 66 shows the proportions in which individual skin diseases were represented in the total admissions coded to M.R.C. numbers 680–699. Cellulitis and acute abscess (other than of finger and nail-bed) showed consistently high rates during the eight years, both for men and women. The rate for impetigo, which in 1940 was the most important

TABLE 66

Diseases of Skin and Cellular Tissue. Proportionate Composition of Admissions by Sex, 1940–47

M.R.C. Code No.	DISEASES	Males									Females
		1940	1941	1942	1943	1944	1945	1946	1947	1940–47	1940–47
680	Carbuncles and boils	126	131	139	151	155	148	156	152	142	143
681	Cellulitis, finger and nail-bed	73	91	110	144	163	132	127	163	120	223
682	Cellulitis and acute abscess	212	191	206	233	239	240	296	318	224	218
683	Sycosis barbae	23	22	6	12	18	19	10	10	16	—
684	Impetigo	221	202	179	124	88	82	65	65	146	89
685	Chronic ulcer	19	22	17	24	24	21	19	5	21	18
686	Other local skin infections	26	27	17	19	14	20	18	26	20	9
687	Acne vulgaris	11	11	13	10	10	12	24	26	12	7
688–9	Contact dermatitis, drug rash	6	5	11	8	16	21	12	16	11	14
690	Pruritus, etc.	4	6	8	10	7	8	5	3	7	7
691	Erythematous conditions	5	6	5	5	5	6	4	—	5	11
6920	Eczema	48	49	54	59	48	52	52	23	52	50
6921	Seborrhoeic dermatitis	33	42	40	37	48	74	60	23	45	42
693	Psoriasis	32	29	25	22	24	22	16	5	25	35
694–5	Lichen planus and pemphigus	4	2	2	4	2	5	1	5	3	4
696	Hypertrophy and atrophy of skin	8	8	9	7	5	8	7	5	8	12
6970–3	Diseases of hair	11	9	10	3	5	5	6	—	7	4
6974	Diseases of sweat glands	22	33	33	34	33	29	38	41	32	23
6975	Diseases of nails	42	46	44	41	29	35	45	78	40	37
698–9	Other skin diseases	74	68	72	53	67	61	39	36	64	54
680–699	*Totals*	1,000	1,000	1,000	1,000	1, 000	1,000	1,000	1,000	1,000	1,000

single cause in this group, declined steadily from 221 in that year to 65 in 1946 and 1947. For women, many of whom would be engaged in preparing or serving food, cellulitis of finger and nail-bed showed the highest proportionate rate. Similar high rates obtained for carbuncles and boils. The percentages of carbuncles and boils which appeared on the head and neck were, males 38 per cent.; females 55 per cent. The percentage distribution of cellulitis and acute abscess by site for the two sexes was as follows:

Sex	Head and Neck	Trunk	Arm	Hand	Leg	Foot	Male Genitals	Other and Unspec.	Totals
Males	17	10	11	22	17	20	1	2	100
Females	22	19	8	13	14	23	—	1	100

Examination of the numbers of admissions in 13-weekly periods for non-mycotic sycosis barbae and impetigo (Table 67) showed little seasonal variation except that the total admissions for impetigo in the

TABLE 67

Quarterly Admissions for Sycosis Barbae (M.R.C. Code 683) and Impetigo (M.R.C. Code 684) Persons, 1940–45

M.R.C. Code No.	Diseases	Season	1940	1941	1942	1943	1944	1945
683	Sycosis barbae (non-mycotic)	1st Qtr.	7	20	8	10	20	19
		2nd Qtr.	21	36	7	12	28	20
		3rd Qtr.	41	30	8	12	18	19
		4th Qtr.	24	31	8	19	19	9
684	Impetigo	1st Qtr.	90	272	267	187	152	87
		2nd Qtr.	173	268	166	153	128	83
		3rd Qtr.	300	237	206	148	73	80
		4th Qtr.	326	254	224	182	99	66

second and third quarters were rather less than those for the two winter quarters.

From Table 68 it is apparent that the median period of in-patient treatment for impetigo varied, for men aged 15–34, between 18 and 22 days, the median taken over the seven years 1940–46 being 20 days. Twenty seven per cent. of men in this age group were in hospital for less than 10 days, 41 per cent. from 14–27 days and 32 per cent. for 28 days or more. The median duration of stay for men aged 35–54 was 18 days, 29 per cent. being treated for less than 14 days, 40 per cent. from 14–27 days and 31 per cent. for 28 days or more. The median stay for women aged 15–34 was 15 days. The total number of days of incapacity due to impetigo alone in the 1 in 5 sample was 78,685 for men aged 15–34; 6,681 days for men aged 35–54, and 2,776 days for women aged 15–34. The mean periods in hospital for these three groups were 26, 27 and 19 days respectively.

Of persons admitted with a disease of the skin or cellular tissue assignable to M.R.C. code numbers 68 or 69 as primary diagnosis, 7·3 per cent. also suffered from a second condition in the same group, which was either present on admission or developed during the stay in hospital. The frequency with which such pairs of skin conditions occurred is shown in Table 69. Thus 35 people who suffered from eczema also had carbuncles or boils, while 59 who had impetigo also had cellulitis or acute abscess.

DISEASES OF BONES, JOINTS AND MUSCLES (Short List Number 35)

This group comprises the conditions shown in M.R.C. Code numbers 71 and 72. They caused from 5·3 to 7·5 per cent. of the basic total of men's admissions and from 1·7 to 5·7 of women's. From 1940–45 the proportionate rates for men aged 25–34 were higher than at ages 15–24, and from 1940–44 they then decreased with age. For women also

TABLE 68

Impetigo. Periods of In-patient Treatment of cases in which no other pathological condition was recorded, 1940–46

Year	Sex-Age Groups	Days of In-patient Treatment												*Median Duration
		0–	4–	7–	10–	14–	21–	28–	35–	42–	56–	91 up	Totals	
1940	Males 15–34	2	13	52	90	170	128	75	57	67	36	13	703	22
1941		7	24	48	103	228	101	76	64	55	53	10	769	20
1942		6	15	52	84	181	61	38	34	44	46	15	576	19
1943		2	19	53	71	140	39	27	24	21	27	7	430	17
1944–46		6	16	45	97	142	35	44	32	31	42	19	509	18
1940–46		23	87	250	445	861	364	260	211	218	204	64	2,987	20
1940–46	Males 35–54	—	11	25	34	79	20	14	15	22	18	7	245	18
1940–46	Females 15–34	—	9	18	36	41	23	8	4	8	—	1	148	15

* Adjusted for cases in which the complete period of treatment was not known.

TABLE 69

Distribution of Cases of Two Concurrent Skin Conditions

	M.R.C. Code																					
Carbuncles and boils	680	—																				
Cellulitis of finger	681	99	—																			
Cellulitis and acute abscess	682	208	34	—																		
Sycosis barbae	683	9	4	8	—																	
Impetigo	684	98	29	59	33	—																
Chronic ulcer	685	5	5	30	1	13	1															
Other skin infections	686	30	3	18	4	22	11	—														
Acne vulgaris	687	32	4	21	6	43	—	5	—													
Contact dermatitis	688	5	1	6	2	8	1	3	1	—												
Drug eruptions	689	2	1	1	—	1	—	1	1	—	—											
Pruritus; skin neuroses	690	5	2	2	1	1	—	—	—	—	—	—										
Erythematous conditions	691	4	—	2	—	6	1	—	3	—	—	—	—									
Eczema	6,920	35	5	21	4	74	16	10	7	3	—	7	1	—								
Seborrhoeic dermatitis	6,921	39	6	26	23	87	3	5	20	—	2	6	4	15	—							
Psoriasis	693	15	—	8	4	11	1	4	3	2	1	2	1	15	23	—						
Lichen planus	694	2	1	3	—	1	—	—	—	—	—	—	—	2	1	1	—					
Pemphigus, etc.	695	—	—	—	—	—	—	—	—	—	—	—	—	—	—	—	—	—				
Hypertrophies, atrophies	696	—	—	35	1	1	—	2	4	—	—	—	—	3	—	1	—	—	—			
Hair, sweat glands, nails	697	48	20	224	3	33	1	8	16	1	—	—	2	19	11	4	1	—	10	5		
Anomalies of pigmentation	698	—	—	—	1	—	—	—	—	2	—	—	—	1	—	—	—	—	—	—	—	
Other diseases of skin	699	59	15	86	5	60	17	5	15	—	—	8	4	44	10	8	2	—	2	12	—	—
	M.R.C. Code	680	681	682	683	684	685	686	687	688	689	690	691	6,920	6,921	693	694	695	696	697	698	699

the proportionate rates at ages 25–34 were higher than those at ages 15–24 throughout the eight years under consideration. This may be in some measure due to older people who were unused to physical exertion of a strenuous nature and whose bodies were less supple being re-introduced to physical training and organised games. Internal derangement of the knee joint, which was commonly attributed to one or other of these pastimes, was the primary cause of admission of 3,890 men and 69 women in the sample, corresponding to estimated admissions of about 19,500 men and 350 women. Bursitis and synovitis were responsible for estimated admissions of around 12,000 men and 800 women. Flat foot, hallux valgus and hallux rigidus, conditions which had perhaps been tolerated in civilian life, are calculated to have caused about 6,000 admissions of men and 650 of women.

TABLE 70

Diseases of Bones, Joints amd Muscles (Non-rheumatic). Proportion per 1,000 Admissions for Non-infective and Non-respiratory Illnesses, by Sex and Age, 1940–47

Year	Males						Females				
	Age Groups						Age Groups				
	15–	25–	35–	45–	55 up	All	15–	25–	35–	45 up	All
1940 .	67	90	60	32	23	73	14	33	—	—	17
1941 .	70	81	70	58	36	75	31	39	37	83	33
1942 .	65	82	69	51	14	73	28	39	24	74	30
1943 .	61	79	64	47	32	69	34	51	48	32	37
1944 .	58	71	60	43	41	64	30	38	61	71	33
1945 .	52	57	47	48	129	53	25	31	56	167	28
1946 .	59	57	65	42	83	59	42	51	77	—	45
1947 .	57	55	82	45	167	58	53	91	—	—	57

The proportionate age distribution of men admitted with osteomyelitis, acute infective arthritis, bursitis and synovitis, curvature of the spine or flat foot is as follows:

M.R.C. Code No.	Diseases	Age Groups					
		15–	25–	35–	45–	55 up	All
710, 711	Osteomyelitis . . .	44	38	14	3	1	100
715	Acute infective arthritis .	30	46	19	5	—	100
718	Bursitis and synovitis .	39	44	15	2	0	100
725	Curvature of spine .	34	39	25	2	—	100
727	Flat foot . . .	32	45	21	2	—	100

The proportion of cases of osteomyelitis was higher in the age group 15–24, whereas in the other four conditions the greatest number of cases occurred at ages 25–34.

The M.R.C. code number 729 includes such conditions as bunion, coxa valga or vara, hammer toe and pes cavus. In the 1 in 5 sample 1,348 admissions were assigned to this number. Of these 551 were for hammer toe, the mean stay in hospital for this condition unaccompanied by any complication or concurrent disease being 65 days. There were also 25 cases of cervical rib, with mean duration of 67 days. Three hundred and fifty people in the sample were admitted for treatment of deformities due to previous injuries or diseases.

Sixty-four people were admitted for foot strain, with mean stay of 33 days. *The Lancet* (1942) in a leading article entitled 'Soldier's Foot' comments that 'there are three periods at which pain denoting strain may arise—on enlistment, at physical training and on route marching'. Early recourse to an orthopaedic surgeon is recommended, as otherwise deformities may develop requiring treatment in hospital of from 6–8 weeks. 'The war has shown that a painful foot is a major disability requiring in-patient treatment as out-patient supervision is usually incomplete.'

Another pathological condition brought to notice by Service conditions was that called variously march, fatigue or stress fracture. This is most commonly a break of the second or third metatarsal bone, proximal to the neck, but it may also occur in the upper third of the tibia, though it is uncommon in other sites. Such fractures occur without trauma and may only give rise to slight symptoms such as an aching foot after marching or pain and swelling in the leg. Annan

TABLE 71

Admissions with a Primary Diagnosis of Stress or Fatigue Fracture, 1940–47

Diagnosis	Site of fracture	Sex	Age	Rank	Duration in hospital
March fracture	R. foot	M	22	Private	144 days
March fracture	L. foot	M	31	Private	55 days
March fracture	2nd metatarsal	M	26	Private	88 days
Fatigue fracture	3rd and 4th R. metatarsals	M	18	Private	102 days
Fatigue fracture	2nd R. metatarsal	M	20	Marine	43 days
Fatigue fracture	R. tibia	M	18	Trooper	201 days
Fatigue fracture	R. tibia	M	18	Private	18 days
Fatigue fracture	R. tibia	M	19	Private	36 days
Fatigue fracture	R. tibia	M	18	Private	71+ days
Fatigue fracture	R. tibia	M	18	Private	84 days
Stress fracture	R. tibia	M	18	Private	108 days
Fatigue fracture	R. tibia	M	18	Private	167 days
Fatigue fracture	R. tibia	M	18	Private	125 days
Fatigue fracture	L. tibia	M	19	Private	98 days
Fatigue fracture	L. tibia	M	19	Private	111 days
Fatigue fracture	L. tibia	M	19	Private	130 days
Fatigue fracture	L. tibia	M	18	Rifleman	132 days
Stress fracture	R. fibula	M	21	Private	51 days
March fracture	Not stated	M	22	Sapper	95 days
Fatigue fracture	Not stated	M	25	Private	75 days

(1945) reports 8 cases of shoveller's fracture from a Prisoner-of-War camp in Germany. This is a fracture of the spinous processes of cervical and dorsal vertebrae. He points out that an interesting feature was the premonitory pain in the back present in some cases for a few hours or days before the click in the neck which could be considered to mark the breaking of the bone. No cases of shoveller's fracture were found in this series, but there were in the sample 20 cases described as march fracture or its synonyms; details of these are set out in Table 71.

CONGENITAL MALFORMATIONS (Short List Number 36)

The total number of admissions attributed to this cause in the sample was 768 for men and 51 for women. Their proportionate distribution for men was as follows:

M.R.C. No.	*Disease*	
736–739	Hare lip, cleft palate, congenital pyloric stenosis, imperforate anus and other abnormalities of the digestive system	29 per cent.
741	Undescended testicle	25 per cent.
740; 742	Cystic disease of the kidney and other abnormalities of the genito-urinary system	8 per cent.
743	Clubfoot, congenital deformities of spine, dislocation of hip and other malformations of bones and joints	13 per cent.
Rest of 730–745	Other congenital malformations	25 per cent.

ILL-DEFINED SYMPTOMS (Short List Number 37)

This group, comprising numbers 7600 to 7691 of the M.R.C. code, contains a number of recognised conditions and vague symptoms which may constitute in themselves minor illnesses or may be merely symptomatic of some graver condition as yet either undetected or not manifest. Headache for example may be in itself a minor ailment, perhaps indicating a low state of health or general 'nerviness' or it may be a symptom of hypertension. Similarly praecordial pain and cough can be minor illnesses or they may indicate, among other things, coronary thrombosis and cancer of the lung respectively.

A cause of admission would only be assigned to one of these numbers when:

(a) No more definite diagnosis could be made, no matter what examinations or tests are applied.

(b) The symptom cleared up without a more serious underlying condition being detected.

(c) The patient's discharge occurred before a more definite diagnosis could be made.

It was therefore to be expected that admissions coded to symptoms in M.R.C. group 76 would form a very small proportion of the total of admissions. Table 72 shows that in the present series men's admissions for this cause varied, at all ages, between 2·3 and 5 per cent. of the basic total, and women's between 2·8 and 7·0 per cent.

TABLE 72

Ill-defined Symptoms (except Jaundice) Proportion per 1,000 Admissions for Non-infective and Non-respiratory Illnesses, by Sex and Age, 1940–47

Year	Males						Females				
	Age Groups						Age Groups				
	15–	25–	35–	45–	55 up	All	15–	25–	35–	45 up	All
1940 .	22	21	33	50	47	24	47	25	—	111	39
1941 .	24	21	24	29	36	23	50	34	37	83	46
1942 .	49	48	53	60	73	50	71	68	61	74	70
1943 .	35	33	41	35	32	35	51	48	74	32	51
1944 .	25	24	23	24	41	24	31	32	28	—	31
1945 .	27	23	24	32	65	25	28	31	32	—	28
1946 .	27	26	14	28	83	25	34	13	—	—	29
1947 .	34	55	31	92	—	38	63	30	250	—	61

The proportional rates in the various decennial groups were high for both sexes in 1942 compared with the other years, this being due in greater part to the increased numbers of admissions of both sexes in that year for headache, pain in the chest and abdominal pain, and in the case of women, for diarrhoea. The rates are higher than the average for men aged 55 and over, since in older men such symptoms are more likely to indicate the onset of a serious malady and therefore require hospital investigation.

The fourteen symptoms to which were attributed the highest numbers of admissions, together with the estimated numbers of men with these as primary diagnosis were as follows:

Abdominal pain	4,150 ± 144	Pain in the back	1,050 ± 72
Diarrhoea	3,060 ± 124	Syncope	1,015 ± 71
Headache	1,660 ± 91	Epistaxis	890 ± 67
Pyrexia	1,290 ± 80	Haemoptysis	835 ± 65
Pain in the chest	1,245 ± 79	Haematemesis	810 ± 64
Haematuria	1,120 ± 75	Debility	805 ± 63
Frequency	1,065 ± 73	Vertigo	650 ± 59

That patients with symptomatic diagnoses may nevertheless take up hospital beds for a considerable amount of time is indicated by Table 73, which shows the distribution of days in hospital for eight selected symptoms. The median duration of stay for men with depression was about 8 weeks, while for the remaining conditions it mostly varied between 1½ and 2½ weeks.

TABLE 73

Symptomatic Diagnoses

Periods of In-patient Treatment of Cases in which no other pathological condition was recorded, 1940–46

Symptom diagnosed	Sex-Age Group	Days of In-patient Treatment												*Median duration
		0–	4–	7–	10–	14–	21–	28–	42–	56–	91–	182 up	Totals	
Headache	Males 15–34	13	21	28	31	36	8	14	10	16	2	—	179	13
	Males 35–54	3	4	3	6	5	6	6	—	1	1	—	35	15
	Females 15–34	2	6	9	7	5	3	2	—	—	—	—	34	10
Haemoptysis	Males 15–34	6	4	11	13	20	7	4	7	13	9	—	94	17
	Males 35–54	2	—	—	2	9	2	2	1	3	1	—	22	18
	Females 15–34	—	2	2	1	2	—	—	1	—	1	—	9	10
Dyspnoea	Males 15–34	3	1	3	—	4	2	3	—	—	—	—	16	17
	Males 35–54	—	—	4	—	2	1	—	2	1	—	—	10	17
	Females 15–34	—	1	—	—	1	1	—	—	—	—	—	3	14
Abdominal Pain	Males 15–34	76	84	82	61	86	24	41	25	36	13	—	528	11
	Males 35–54	4	21	13	15	21	7	7	9	6	5	1	109	14
	Females 15–34	14	38	38	20	39	6	15	9	1	—	—	180	10
Diarrhoea	Males 15–34	19	57	63	82	80	18	19	12	16	6	1	373	12
	Males 35–54	8	11	16	22	16	4	8	2	6	7	—	100	12
	Females 15–34	3	5	8	8	6	3	—	—	—	—	—	33	10
Frequency	Males 15–34	2	9	14	16	30	12	12	6	9	8	1	119	17
	Males 35–54	1	1	4	6	17	3	7	1	6	4	—	50	19
	Females 15–34	1	6	3	2	6	1	1	2	—	—	—	22	11
Pyrexia	Males 15–34	10	17	21	26	37	13	15	3	17	7	1	167	10
	Males 35–54	—	2	—	3	2	5	2	3	2	—	—	19	3
	Females 15–34	—	2	6	11	4	5	5	1	1	—	—	35	10
Depression	Males 15–34	2	2	2	2	5	—	3	9	7	5	—	37	53
	Males 35–54	—	3	—	—	1	—	1	1	4	2	1	13	60

* Adjusted for cases in which the complete period of treatment was not known.

Appendix I

CAUSES OF ADMISSION OF SERVICE PATIENTS TO E.M.S. HOSPITALS, 1940

Proportions per 1,000 Non-infective and Non-respiratory Illnesses

Short List Number	Short List Group Title	Males						Females				
		Age Groups					All Ages	Age Groups				All Ages
		15–	25–	35–	45–	55–		15–	25–	35–	45–	
6	Rheumatism, arthritis, fibrositis	37	46	90	123	118	51	27	17	78	223	33
7	Neoplasms	11	12	13	19	12	12	14	—	59	—	15
8	Diabetes	1	2	4	6	—	2	3	—	—	—	2
9	Anaemias	1	1	1	2	12	1	5	8	20	—	7
10	Other general and endocrine diseases	21	23	28	42	47	24	19	17	39	111	22
11	Psychoneuroses	41	46	71	58	35	47	30	8	39	—	26
12	Functional digestive disorders	13	17	31	21	47	17	25	42	20	—	28
13	Other nervous disorders (1)	22	29	40	49	23	28	14	50	—	—	20
14	Diseases of eye, visual defects	12	16	14	10	12	13	5	17	—	—	7
15	Diseases of ear and mastoid	25	19	15	2	—	20	19	33	20	—	22
16	Intracranial vascular lesions	0	0	0	6	12	1	—	—	—	—	—
17	Diseases of heart and arteries	6	7	17	44	107	10	5	25	39	—	13
18	Diseases of veins	45	97	80	98	94	71	16	33	39	111	24
22	Diseases of mouth and teeth	10	8	5	5	—	8	19	8	39	—	18
23	Acute sore throat	140	83	40	21	12	101	171	150	59	—	152
24	Acute hepatitis and jaundice	8	6	5	2	—	7	—	—	—	111	2
25	Hernia	94	121	81	84	59	101	5	17	—	—	7
26	Gastric and duodenal ulcers	16	47	110	91	94	43	5	—	39	—	7
27	Gastro-enteritis	11	11	15	15	35	12	11	42	20	—	18
28	Appendicitis	73	41	27	14	23	53	253	159	97	111	215
29	Other digestive diseases	53	60	82	92	118	61	74	33	59	—	62
30	Diseases of female genital organs	—	—	—	—	—	—	85	100	118	111	92

31	Other genito-urinary diseases ([2])	37	38	31	29	35	36	19	25	39	—	22
32	Normal childbearing	—	—	—	—	—	—	11	—	—	—	7
33	Abnormal childbearing	—	—	—	—	—	—	16	33	59	—	24
34	Diseases of skin and cellular tissue	228	152	106	84	35	178	88	125	118	111	99
35	Diseases of bones, joints, muscles ([3])	67	90	60	32	23	73	14	33	—	—	17
36	Congenital malformations	6	7	1	1	—	6	—	—	—	—	—
37	Ill-defined symptoms ([4])	22	21	33	50	47	24	47	25	—	111	39
6–18 22–37	*Total, non-respiratory and non-infective*	1,000	1,000	1,000	1,000	1,000	1,000	1,000	1,000	1,000	1,000	1,000
1	Tuberculosis	13	13	13	23	47	13	8	25	—	—	11
2	Venereal diseases and sequelae	6	2	5	14	12	5	8	—	—	—	6
3	Colds, influenza, laryngitis	277	140	131	136	106	202	184	208	274	333	200
4	Scabies	61	46	30	27	47	50	164	50	20	—	123
5	Other infective diseases	157	68	33	11	—	102	406	634	607	—	467
19	Pneumonia (acute primary)	33	24	18	32	23	28	16	17	20	—	17
20	Bronchitis and tracheitis	47	53	124	197	436	66	52	100	137	333	75
21	Other respiratory diseases	37	31	29	37	23	34	25	8	20	—	20
1–5 19–21	*Total infective and respiratory diseases*	631	377	383	477	694	500	863	1,042	1,078	666	919
38	Head injuries	49	48	31	34	47	46	22	51	20	—	28
39	Fractures (except of skull)	83	92	81	75	94	86	14	33	20	111	20
40	Acute poisoning	1	1	2	4	—	1	3	—	—	—	2
41	Burns	13	10	9	11	—	11	5	33	—	111	13
42	Other injuries	164	156	120	91	94	152	33	33	—	—	29
38–42	*Total injuries*	310	307	243	215	235	296	77	150	40	222	92
	Total sick and injured	1,941	1,684	1,626	1,692	1,929	1,796	1,940	2,192	2,118	1,888	2,011

([1]) Excluding intracranial vascular lesions (No. 16).
([2]) Non-venereal, including nephritis.
([3]) Non-rheumatic.
([4]) Except jaundice (in No. 24).

APPENDIX I (*contd.*)

CAUSES OF ADMISSION OF SERVICE PATIENTS TO E.M.S. HOSPITALS, 1941

Proportions per 1,000 Non-infective and Non-respiratory Illnesses

Short List Number	Short List Group Title	Males						Females				
		Age Groups					All Ages	Age Groups				All Ages
		15–	25–	35–	45–	55–		15–	25–	35–	45–	
6	Rheumatism, arthritis, fibrositis	33	56	74	114	109	52	25	29	86	—	30
7	Neoplasms	13	14	17	27	91	15	22	24	86	—	27
8	Diabetes	2	2	2	—	—	2	—	—	—	—	—
9	Anaemias	1	1	1	3	—	1	8	10	12	—	8
10	Other general and endocrine diseases	23	24	21	23	—	23	34	29	86	—	37
11	Psychoneuroses	42	51	68	52	18	50	37	54	37	168	41
12	Fuctional digestive disorders	19	28	36	33	55	26	29	19	37	—	27
13	Other nervous disorders ([1])	16	22	33	49	36	22	12	49	49	—	21
14	Diseases of eye, visual defects	15	14	13	17	36	14	6	15	12	—	7
15	Diseases of ear and mastoid	31	22	17	14	—	24	26	10	—	83	22
16	Intracranial vascular lesions	0	0	1	3	—	0	—	—	—	—	—
17	Diseases of heart and arteries	6	5	8	61	128	7	7	10	49	—	10
18	Diseases of veins	58	102	123	108	73	89	14	39	75	—	22
22	Diseases of mouth and teeth	17	11	7	5	18	13	19	—	—	—	14
23	Acute sore throat	107	67	32	23	—	75	102	78	25	—	92
24	Acute hepatitis and jaundice	12	10	5	2	—	10	8	5	—	—	7
25	Hernia	70	89	100	70	91	83	6	24	—	—	8
26	Gastric and duodenal ulcers	21	46	77	71	36	42	1	10	25	—	4
27	Gastro-enteritis	10	13	10	12	—	11	8	15	—	—	8
28	Appendicitis	76	45	23	12	—	52	208	146	25	83	186
29	Other digestive diseases	58	64	72	74	55	63	63	49	25	167	59
30	Diseases of female genital organs	—	—	—	—	—	—	106	136	99	167	112

31	Other genito-urinary diseases (2)	46	43	39	35	91	44	41	58	99	83	48
32	Normal childbearing	—	—	—	—	—	—	6	15	—	—	7
33	Abnormal childbearing	—	—	—	—	—	—	19	44	—	—	22
34	Diseases of skin and cellular tissue	224	164	122	105	91	179	110	54	99	83	100
35	Diseases of bones, joints, muscles (3)	70	81	70	58	36	75	31	39	37	83	33
36	Congenital malformations	6	5	5	—	—	5	2	5	—	—	2
37	Ill-defined symptoms (4)	24	21	24	29	36	23	50	34	37	83	46
6–18 22–37	*Total, non-respiratory and non-infective*	1,000	1,000	1,000	1,000	1,000	1,000	1,000	1,000	1,000	1,000	1,000
1	Tuberculosis	21	16	12	11	18	17	12	10	12	—	12
2	Venereal diseases and sequelae	8	6	7	15	—	7	8	5	—	—	7
3	Colds, influenza, laryngitis	110	89	55	78	73	92	73	58	49	—	68
4	Scabies	42	36	26	9	—	36	162	83	37	83	139
5	Other infective diseases	97	59	25	23	55	67	106	78	37	83	96
19	Pneumonia (acute primary)	37	28	22	14	18	30	19	29	12	—	20
20	Bronchitis and tracheitis	42	50	85	156	363	55	54	97	99	167	66
21	Other respiratory diseases	43	33	32	33	18	37	27	49	63	83	34
1–5 19–21	*Total infective and respiratory diseases*	400	317	264	339	545	341	461	409	309	416	442
38	Head injuries	45	38	27	44	55	39	28	34	25	—	28
39	Fractures (except of skull)	96	84	72	67	36	86	26	34	74	167	32
40	Acute poisoning	2	2	2	—	—	2	1	5	—	—	2
41	Burns	13	11	9	6	—	11	8	—	12	83	7
42	Other injuries	131	101	78	64	91	108	34	59	49	167	41
38–42	*Total injuries*	287	236	188	181	182	246	97	132	160	417	110
	Total Sick and injured	1,687	1,553	1,452	1,520	1,727	1,587	1,558	1,541	1,469	1,833	1,552

(1) Excluding intracranial vascular lesions (No. 16).
(2) Non-venereal, including nephritis.
(3) Non-rheumatic.
(4) Except jaundice (in No. 24).

APPENDIX I (*contd.*)

CAUSES OF ADMISSION OF SERVICE PATIENTS TO E.M.S. HOSPITALS, *1942*.

Proportions per 1,000 Non-infective and Non-respiratory Illnesses.

Short List Number	Short List Group Title	Males						Females				
		Age Groups					All Ages	Age Groups				All Ages
		15–	25–	35–	45–	55–		15–	25–	35–	45–	
6	Rheumatism, arthritis, fibrositis	30	48	99	108	131	53	49	59	92	74	53
7	Neoplasms	15	18	20	32	73	18	23	38	48	148	28
8	Diabetes	2	2	2	2	14	2	0	3	6	—	1
9	Anaemias	1	1	1	2	14	1	6	11	12	—	7
10	Other general and endocrine diseases	24	25	22	27	14	24	34	34	18	37	34
11	Psychoneuroses	58	67	71	65	14	65	33	83	73	—	43
12	Functional digestive disorders	22	31	34	21	—	28	30	25	18	74	29
13	Other nervous disorders (1)	18	23	33	24	14	23	14	20	55	37	17
14	Diseases of eye, visual defects	14	12	10	15	29	12	9	5	12	37	9
15	Diseases of ear and mastoid	31	28	17	21	—	26	25	19	12	—	23
16	Intracranial vascular lesions	0	1	1	5	43	1	1	—	—	37	1
17	Diseases of heart and arteries	7	7	10	45	146	8	11	11	12	37	11
18	Diseases of veins	56	98	105	104	73	85	15	29	61	—	19
22	Diseases of mouth and teeth	13	13	7	6	—	11	15	5	—	—	13
23	Acute sore throat	93	67	33	15	—	69	110	78	42	—	101
24	Acute hepatitis and jaundice	26	17	9	9	—	19	14	17	12	—	14
25	Hernia	66	64	80	62	14	68	3	3	6	—	3
26	Gastric and duodenal ulcers	19	39	60	65	29	36	2	8	12	—	3
27	Gastro-enteritis	18	21	18	24	—	20	25	27	42	37	26
28	Appendicitis	73	39	23	17	29	48	145	85	42	—	129
29	Other digestive diseases	61	68	63	62	58	64	67	60	42	37	64
30	Diseases of female genital organs	—	—	—	—	—	—	94	113	159	186	101

31	Other genito-urinary diseases (2)	43	41	39	53	58	41	43	46	36	—	43
32	Normal childbearing	—	—	—	—	—	—	8	8	6	—	8
33	Abnormal childbearing	—	—	—	—	—	—	33	28	12	—	31
34	Diseases of skin and cellular tissue	190	136	119	105	160	151	91	78	85	111	88
35	Diseases of bones, joints, muscles (3)	65	82	69	51	14	73	28	39	24	74	30
36	Congenital malformations	6	4	2	—	—	4	1	—	—	—	1
37	Ill-defined symptoms (4)	49	48	53	60	73	50	71	68	61	74	70
6–18 22–37	*Total, non-respiratory and non-infective*	1,000	1,000	1,000	1,000	1,000	1,000	1,000	1,000	1,000	1,000	1,000
1	Tuberculosis	30	21	16	23	29	23	26	36	12	—	27
2	Venereal diseases and sequelae	4	4	5	6	—	4	4	4	—	37	4
3	Colds, influenza, laryngitis	57	46	36	30	29	48	52	51	68	37	52
4	Scabies	17	13	9	12	—	14	89	23	24	—	73
5	Other infective diseases	98	56	31	21	—	65	91	104	36	37	91
19	Pneumonia (acute primary)	42	29	31	44	102	35	21	31	24	—	23
20	Bronchitis and tracheitis	45	56	84	97	87	58	34	52	73	74	39
21	Other respiratory diseases	44	38	32	29	43	39	33	34	6	74	23
1–5 19–21	*Total infective and respiratory diseases*	337	263	244	262	290	286	350	335	243	259	332
38	Head injuries	47	42	31	42	29	42	23	27	18	—	23
39	Fractures (except of skull)	113	111	84	102	73	106	35	28	42	—	34
40	Acute poisoning	5	2	1	5	29	3	4	5	—	—	4
41	Burns	13	10	5	11	—	10	13	14	24	—	14
42	Other injuries	106	151	113	77	115	147	61	56	42	74	59
38–42	*Total injuries*	284	316	234	237	246	308	136	130	126	74	134
	Total sick and injured	1,621	1,579	1,478	1,499	1,536	1,594	1,486	1,465	1,369	1,333	1,466

(1) Excluding intracranial vascular lesions (No. 16).
(2) Non-venereal, including nephritis.
(3) Non-rheumatic.
(4) Except jaundice (in No. 24).

APPENDIX I (*contd.*)

CAUSES OF ADMISSION OF SERVICE PATIENTS TO E.M.S. HOSPITALS, *1943*

Proportions per 1,000 Non-infective and Non-respiratory Illnesses

Short List Number	Short List Group Title	Males						Females				
		Age Groups					All Ages	Age Groups				All Ages
		15–	25–	35–	45–	55–		15–	25–	35–	45–	
6	Rheumatism, arthritis, fibrositis	30	44	78	132	130	48	38	65	123	161	47
7	Neoplasms	14	16	23	40	65	17	23	42	111	193	30
8	Diabetes	2	2	4	9	32	3	1	—	—	—	1
9	Anaemias	1	1	1	5	—	1	6	12	11	—	7
10	Other general and endocrine diseases	26	22	24	35	16	24	27	37	42	129	30
11	Psychoneuroses	54	71	80	44	16	66	47	48	58	65	47
12	Functional digestive disorders	18	22	31	17	—	22	23	23	5	—	22
13	Other nervous disorders (1)	16	22	27	30	16	21	6	19	32	—	9
14	Diseases of eye, visual defects	11	11	14	12	16	11	9	10	—	—	9
15	Diseases of ear and mastoid	37	27	18	21	16	29	20	26	16	—	21
16	Intracranial vascular lesions	1	1	1	3	—	1	0	—	—	—	0
17	Diseases of heart and arteries	6	6	10	59	97	8	5	12	26	32	7
18	Diseases of veins	45	92	106	81	113	78	23	51	63	—	29
22	Diseases of mouth and teeth	10	7	5	2	—	7	11	12	—	—	10
23	Acute sore throat	117	78	40	30	—	82	151	66	37	32	133
24	Acute hepatitis and jaundice	39	32	19	10	—	32	21	24	5	—	21
25	Hernia	59	58	75	64	32	62	3	7	—	—	4
26	Gastric and duodenal ulcers	16	34	53	59	48	32	3	5	11	—	3
27	Gastro-enteritis	17	16	14	10	16	16	14	12	32	—	14
28	Appendicitis	74	43	27	21	16	50	138	65	37	65	122
29	Other digestive diseases	61	66	58	45	97	63	75	49	42	—	69
30	Diseases of female genital organs	—	—	—	—	—	—	93	130	101	97	100

No.	Disease											
31	Other genito-urinary diseases (2)	39	44	41	47	97	42	41	40	32	97	41
32	Normal childbearing	—	—	—	—	—	—	6	4	5	—	5
33	Abnormal childbearing	—	—	—	—	—	—	31	50	26	—	34
34	Diseases of skin and cellular tissue	206	170	143	139	113	177	98	89	63	65	95
35	Diseases of bones, joints, muscles (3)	61	79	64	47	32	69	34	51	48	32	37
36	Congenital malformations	5	3	3	3	—	4	2	3	—	—	2
37	Ill-defined symptoms (4)	35	33	41	35	32	35	51	48	74	32	51
6–18 22–37	*Total, non-respiratory and non-infective*	1,000	1,000	1,000	1,000	1,000	1,000	1,000	1,000	1,000	1,000	1,000
1	Tuberculosis	26	16	18	17	16	20	19	14	16	—	18
2	Venereal diseases and sequelae	3	3	3	9	32	3	3	5	16	—	4
3	Colds, influenza, laryngitis	112	97	94	110	97	103	91	94	122	129	92
4	Scabies	11	5	6	—	—	7	13	2	10	—	11
5	Other infective diseases	115	63	38	23	48	75	98	63	106	32	91
19	Pneumonia (acute primary)	46	32	38	49	32	38	17	14	37	32	17
20	Bronchitis and tracheitis	40	43	91	151	324	55	32	42	74	162	36
21	Other respiratory diseases	52	36	35	31	48	41	29	27	5	97	29
1–5 19–21	*Total infective and respiratory diseases*	405	295	323	390	597	342	302	261	386	452	298
38	Head injuries	46	41	31	16	16	40	21	22	11	—	20
39	Fractures (except of skull)	127	112	93	77	48	112	33	33	42	65	34
40	Acute poisoning	3	3	3	2	—	3	3	2	—	—	3
41	Burns	17	11	9	2	—	13	12	15	—	65	12
42	Other injuries	163	153	101	81	65	144	51	41	85	160	51
38–42	*Total injuries*	356	320	237	178	129	312	120	113	138	290	120
	Total sick and injured	1,761	1,615	1,560	1,568	1,726	1,654	1,422	1,374	1,524	1,742	1,418

(1) Excluding intracranial vascular lesions (No. 16).
(2) Non-venereal, including nephritis.
(2) Non-rheumatic.
(4) Except jaundice (in No. 24).

APPENDIX I (*contd.*)

CAUSES OF ADMISSION OF SERVICE PATIENTS TO E.M.S. HOSPITALS, *1944*

Proportions per 1,000 Non-infective and Non-respiratory Illnesses

Short List Number	Short List Group Title	Males						Females				
		Age Groups					All Ages	Age Groups				All Ages
		15–	25–	35–	45–	55–		15–	25–	35–	45–	
6	Rheumatism, arthritis, fibrositis	30	41	80	120	41	47	31	47	89	143	37
7	Neoplasms	13	18	27	49	122	19	28	40	61	107	32
8	Diabetes	2	2	4	3	13	3	1	—	—	—	1
9	Anaemias	2	1	1	2	—	1	3	6	—	—	4
10	Other general and endocrine diseases	31	29	27	30	27	29	26	36	22	143	29
11	Psychoneuroses	73	92	73	63	13	81	58	83	67	—	63
12	Functional digestive disorders	13	20	25	31	13	19	19	12	—	—	17
13	Other nervous disorders (¹)	18	28	31	24	68	25	11	13	6	36	11
14	Diseases of eye, visual defects	14	14	16	21	—	15	9	6	—	—	8
15	Diseases of ear and mastoid	40	33	25	16	—	33	18	16	6	36	18
16	Intracranial vascular lesions	1	1	2	9	27	1	—	1	—	—	0
17	Diseases of heart and arteries	4	6	13	50	108	8	7	5	11	—	6
18	Diseases of veins	47	86	100	73	27	75	29	65	50	71	37
22	Diseases of mouth and teeth	8	7	4	7	13	7	9	10	6	—	9
23	Acute sore throat	95	62	36	23	—	67	96	67	50	36	88
24	Acute hepatitis and jaundice	34	30	20	9	13	29	11	12	11	—	11
25	Hernia	62	55	69	24	13	60	6	6	17	—	6
26	Gastric and duodenal ulcers	18	44	63	83	68	40	2	5	11	36	4
27	Gastro-enteritis	18	14	14	14	—	15	15	14	17	36	15
28	Appendicitis	81	45	34	30	27	54	138	102	78	36	128
29	Other digestive diseases	57	60	57	52	41	58	80	46	50	—	71
30	Diseases of female genital organs	—	—	—	—	—	—	112	138	185	107	120

31	Other genito-urinary diseases (2)	42	47	52	40	108	46	43	36	28	71	41
32	Normal childbearing	—	—	—	—	—	—	8	7	6	—	8
33	Abnormal childbearing	—	—	—	—	—	—	62	71	28	—	62
34	Diseases of skin and cellular tissue	209	166	142	160	176	176	115	88	106	71	108
35	Diseases of bones, joints, muscles(3)	58	71	60	43	41	64	30	38	61	71	33
36	Congenital malformations	5	4	2	—	—	4	2	3	6	—	2
37	Ill-defined symptoms(4)	25	24	23	24	41	24	31	32	28	—	31
6–18 22–37	*Total, non-respiratory and non-infective*	1,000	1,000	1,000	1,000	1,000	1,000	1,000	1,000	1,000	1,000	1,000
1	Tuberculosis	29	26	13	19	13	24	16	16	6	—	15
2	Venereal diseases and sequelae	3	3	4	5	13	3	2	7	—	—	3
3	Colds, influenza, laryngitis	51	31	26	33	27	37	25	25	33	—	25
4	Scabies	3	3	2	5	—	3	3	2	—	—	3
5	Other infective diseases	194	147	99	68	13	150	110	96	17	—	103
19	Pneumonia (acute primary)	43	32	33	50	68	37	14	26	17	36	16
20	Bronchitis and tracheitis	30	34	50	118	68	38	22	36	61	143	28
21	Other respiratory diseases	45	37	33	45	41	39	27	34	22	71	29
1–5 19–21	*Total infective and respiratory diseases*	398	313	260	343	243	331	219	242	156	250	222
38	Head injuries	67	62	39	37	13	58	19	17	22	—	19
39	Fractures (except of skull)	232	218	131	85	55	200	32	21	56	36	30
40	Acute poisoning	2	2	1	—	—	2	2	6	—	—	3
41	Burns	43	36	19	3	—	34	10	14	6	—	11
42	Other injuries	477	387	174	106	13	365	47	60	28	—	48
38–42	*Total injuries*	821	705	364	231	81	659	110	118	112	36	111
	Total sick and injured	2,219	2,018	1,624	1,574	1,324	1,990	1,329	1,360	1,268	1,286	1,333

(1) Excluding intracranial vascular lesions (No. 16).
(2) Non-venereal, including nephritis.
(3) Non-rheumatic.
(4) Except jaundice (in No. 24).

APPENDIX I (*contd.*)

CAUSES OF ADMISSION OF SERVICE PATIENTS TO E.M.S. HOSPITALS, *1945*

Proportions per 1,000 Non-infective and Non-respiratory Illnesses.

Short List Number	Short List Group Title	Males						Females				
		Age Groups					All Ages	Age Groups				All Ages
		15–	25–	35–	45–	55–		15–	25–	35–	45–	
6	Rheumatism, arthritis, fibrositis	29	33	73	59	65	40	27	32	95	110	32
7	Neoplasms	17	22	35	109	162	25	31	44	24	56	35
8	Diabetes	2	4	10	4	32	5	—	5	—	—	1
9	Anaemias	2	1	2	4	—	2	8	8	—	—	7
10	Other general and endocrine diseases	35	29	25	41	—	31	37	36	32	56	36
11	Psychoneuroses	82	119	66	46	32	94	54	65	79	—	58
12	Functional digestive disorders	17	22	26	18	32	21	20	11	8	—	17
13	Other nervous disorders (1)	20	26	41	41	32	27	10	17	32	—	13
14	Diseases of eye, visual defects	12	13	15	7	—	13	9	8	—	—	9
15	Diseases of ear and mastoid	36	29	23	14	—	30	27	27	32	56	28
16	Intracranial vascular lesions	1	1	2	7	—	1	1	1	—	—	1
17	Diseases of heart and arteries	6	8	15	43	97	9	6	6	—	—	6
18	Diseases of veins	45	79	75	71	32	66	24	52	32	110	32
22	Diseases of mouth and teeth	8	7	5	7	—	7	6	6	—	—	6
23	Acute sore throat	82	62	34	14	32	62	62	56	8	—	58
24	Acute hepatitis and jaundice	39	43	30	9	—	38	14	15	8	56	15
25	Hernia	59	58	95	78	32	66	4	1	16	—	3
26	Gastric and duodenal ulcers	51	50	69	78	65	55	7	27	103	56	16
27	Gastro-enteritis	20	19	18	14	—	19	12	13	—	—	11
28	Appendicitis	72	44	36	39	32	52	160	106	79	56	142
29	Other digestive diseases	53	57	47	50	32	54	95	67	79	110	87
30	Diseases of female genital organs	—	—	—	—	—	—	117	143	134	—	124

31	Other genito-urinary diseases ([2])	43	52	49	48	32	48	38	39	8	—	37
32	Normal childbearing	—	—	—	—	—	—	8	5	—	—	7
33	Abnormal childbearing	—	—	—	—	—	—	58	75	56	—	62
34	Diseases of skin and cellular tissue	183	139	135	119	97	152	109	67	87	167	97
35	Diseases of bones, joints, muscles ([3])	52	57	47	48	129	53	25	31	56	167	28
36	Congenital malformations	7	3	3	—	—	5	3	6	—	—	4
37	Ill-defined symptoms ([4])	27	23	24	32	65	25	28	31	32	—	28
6–18 22–37	*Total non-respiratory and non-infective*	1,000	1,000	1,000	1,000	1,000	1,000	1,000	1,000	1,000	1,000	1,000
1	Tuberculosis	28	25	23	14	—	26	30	24	16	—	27
2	Venereal diseases and sequelae	2	3	4	9	—	3	2	1	—	—	2
3	Colds, influenza, laryngitis	36	23	22	27	65	27	24	26	8	—	24
4	Scabies	5	4	2	2	—	4	4	4	—	—	4
5	Other infective diseases	129	195	87	43	32	148	91	75	24	—	83
19	Pneumonia (acute primary)	63	35	43	46	129	46	27	18	16	—	24
20	Bronchitis and tracheitis	33	26	45	71	225	33	24	26	32	111	26
21	Other respiratory diseases	46	40	32	30	97	41	20	15	39	—	19
1–5 19–21	*Total infective and respiratory diseases*	342	351	258	242	548	328	222	189	135	111	209
38	Head injuries	38	28	23	18	—	30	12	6	16	—	11
39	Fractures (except of skull)	136	118	89	62	65	117	19	28	16	111	22
40	Acute poisoning	1	1	1	—	—	1	2	—	—	—	1
41	Burns	12	13	10	5	32	12	11	6	8	56	10
42	Other injuries	140	122	74	68	65	118	32	31	55	—	32
38–42	*Total injuries*	327	282	197	153	162	278	76	71	95	167	76
	Total sick and injured	1,669	1,633	1,455	1,395	1,710	1,606	1,298	1,260	1,230	1,278	1,285

(1) Excluding intracranial vascular lesions (No. 16).
(2) Non-venereal, including nephritis.
(3) Non-rheumatic.
(4) Except jaundice (in No. 24).

APPENDIX I (*contd.*)

CAUSES OF ADMISSION OF SERVICE PATIENTS TO E.M.S. HOSPITALS, 1946

Proportions per 1,000 Non-infective and Non-respiratory Illnesses

Short List Number	Short List Group Title	Males						Females				
		Age Groups					All Ages	Age Groups				All Ages
		15–	25–	35–	45–	55–		15–	25–	35–	45–	
6	Rheumatism, arthritis, fibrositis	32	29	50	55	—	33	34	13	115	—	33
7	Neoplasms	20	29	44	83	83	27	39	70	192	500	50
8	Diabetes	3	7	13	—	—	6	5	—	—	—	4
9	Anaemias	1	1	1	14	—	1	5	13	—	—	7
10	Other general and endocrine diseases	31	27	24	28	—	28	28	45	77	—	33
11	Psychoneuroses	70	71	79	28	—	71	18	13	77	—	18
12	Functional digestive disorders	11	14	11	—	—	12	18	25	—	—	18
13	Other nervous disorders (1)	20	27	34	14	—	24	7	25	—	—	10
14	Diseases of eye, visual defects	12	12	14	—	83	12	8	—	—	—	7
15	Diseases of ear and mastoid	37	31	19	14	—	33	22	13	—	—	20
16	Intracranial vascular lesions	1	2	5	28	—	2	—	—	—	—	—
17	Diseases of heart and arteries	8	10	20	69	251	11	1	19	—	—	4
18	Diseases of veins	45	77	63	42	167	59	35	51	154	—	41
22	Diseases of mouth and teeth	12	11	6	—	—	11	12	6	—	—	11
23	Acute sore throat	105	51	18	14	—	75	87	64	77	—	82
24	Acute hepatitis and jaundice	29	33	27	28	—	30	11	19	—	—	12
25	Hernia	52	82	117	111	—	71	3	13	—	—	4
26	Gastric and duodenal ulcers	25	64	89	55	83	47	7	13	—	—	8
27	Gastro-enteritis	18	15	14	14	—	16	10	—	—	—	8
28	Appendicitis	85	66	31	55	167	72	174	108	—	—	157
29	Other digestive diseases	54	61	68	42	—	58	87	95	77	500	89
30	Diseases of female genital organs	—	—	—	—	—	—	121	108	115	—	118

31	Other genito-urinary diseases ([2])	48	64	47	111	—	54	33	45	—	—	34
32	Normal childbearing	—	—	—	—	—	—	14	—	—	—	11
33	Abnormal childbearing	—	—	—	—	—	—	31	51	38	—	35
34	Diseases of skin and cellular tissue	189	127	123	125	—	157	109	121	—	—	107
35	Diseases of bones, joints, muscles ([3])	59	57	65	42	83	59	42	51	77	—	45
36	Congenital malformations	6	6	4	—	—	6	5	6	—	—	5
37	Ill-defined symptoms ([4])	27	26	14	28	83	25	34	13	—	—	29
6–18 22–37	*Total non-respiratory and non-infective*	1,000	1,000	1,000	1,000	1,000	1,000	1,000	1,000	1,000	1,000	1,000
1	Tuberculosis	38	38	43	28	—	38	15	38	—	—	18
2	Venereal diseases and sequelae	2	5	5	28	—	4	3	6	—	—	3
3	Colds, influenza, laryngitis	64	49	40	14	—	55	43	64	38	—	47
4	Scabies	7	8	1	—	—	7	3	—	—	—	2
5	Other infective diseases	139	229	117	83	—	169	74	71	78	—	74
19	Pneumonia (acute primary)	65	39	37	42	83	52	19	6	38	—	17
20	Bronchitis and tracheitis	25	18	37	28	83	24	27	25	—	500	27
21	Other respiratory diseases	50	44	38	—	83	46	42	45	—	—	41
1–5 19–21	*Total Infective and respiratory diseases*	390	430	318	223	249	395	226	255	154	500	229
38	Head injuries	44	39	24	28	—	40	19	32	—	—	21
39	Fractures (except of skull)	92	87	56	97	83	86	23	39	—	—	25
40	Acute poisoning	2	3	3	—	—	2	7	—	—	—	5
41	Burns	11	9	7	—	—	10	16	6	—	—	14
42	Other injuries	108	77	69	83	—	92	50	25	—	—	45
38–42	*Total injuries*	257	215	159	208	83	230	115	102	—	—	110
	Total sick and injured	1,647	1,645	1,477	1,431	1,332	1,625	1,341	1,357	1,154	1,500	1,339

([1]) Excluding intracranial vascular lesions (No. 16).
([2]) Non-venereal, including nephritis.
([3]) Non-rheumatic.
([4]) Except jaundice (in No. 24).

APPENDIX I (*contd.*)

CAUSES OF ADMISSION OF SERVICE PATIENTS TO E.M.S. HOSPITALS, 1947

Proportions per 1,000 Non-infective and Non-respiratory Illnesses

Short List Number	Short List Group Title	Males						Females				
		Age Groups					All Ages	Age Groups				All Ages
		15–	25–	35–	45–	55–		15–	25–	35–	45–	
6	Rheumatism, arthritis, fibrositis	23	37	62	45	—	27	—	30	—	—	4
7	Neoplasms	23	46	52	45	166	29	14	30	500	—	24
8	Diabetes	4	9	10	—	—	5	—	—	—	—	—
9	Anaemias	—	—	—	—	—	—	10	—	—	—	8
10	Other general and endocrine diseases	26	46	21	137	—	30	19	—	—	—	16
11	Psychoneuroses	48	34	21	45	—	44	34	—	—	—	29
12	Functional digestive disorders	13	15	—	—	—	13	14	—	—	—	12
13	Other nervous disorders (1)	18	34	21	45	166	21	5	30	—	—	8
14	Diseases of eye, visual defects	13	9	10	—	—	12	—	—	—	—	—
15	Diseases of ear and mastoid	39	21	52	45	—	36	19	—	—	—	16
16	Intracranial vascular lesions	—	—	—	—	—	—	—	—	—	—	—
17	Diseases of heart and arteries	5	12	31	92	167	8	10	—	—	—	8
18	Diseases of veins	38	61	93	45	—	44	5	91	250	—	20
22	Diseases of mouth and teeth	13	12	10	—	—	12	—	—	—	—	—
23	Acute sore throat	99	52	62	45	—	89	68	91	—	—	69
24	Acute hepatitis and jaundice	24	34	10	—	—	24	5	—	—	—	4
25	Hernia	48	55	82	—	—	50	—	—	—	—	—
26	Gastric and duodenal ulcers	18	49	82	137	167	28	—	—	—	—	—
27	Gastro-enteritis	15	18	—	—	—	15	10	30	—	—	12
28	Appendicitis	137	80	62	45	—	124	256	182	—	—	242
29	Other digestive diseases	48	76	82	45	—	54	82	—	—	—	69
30	Diseases of female genital organs	—	—	—	—	—	—	164	274	—	—	177

31	Other genito-urinary diseases (2)	40	46	21	—	167	40	34	—	—	1,000	33
32	Normal childbearing	—	—	—	—	—	—	14	30	—	—	16
33	Abnormal childbearing	—	—	—	—	—	—	34	—	—	—	29
34	Diseases of skin and cellular tissue	210	141	103	92	—	193	87	91	—	—	86
35	Diseases of bones, joints, muscles (3)	57	55	82	45	167	58	53	91	—	—	57
36	Congenital malformations	7	3	—	—	—	6	—	—	—	—	—
37	Ill-defined symptoms (4)	34	55	31	92	—	38	63	30	250	—	61
6–18 22–37	*Total non-respiratory and non-infective*	1,000	1,000	1,000	1,000	1,000	1,000	1,000	1,000	1,000	1,000	1,000
1	Tuberculosis	67	123	103	92	—	78	10	30	250	—	16
2	Venereal diseases and sequelae	2	6	—	—	—	2	5	—	—	—	4
3	Colds, influenza, laryngitis	61	15	31	45	—	51	43	30	—	—	41
4	Scabies	6	—	—	—	—	5	—	—	—	—	—
5	Other infective diseases	136	86	93	—	—	124	136	61	—	—	123
19	Pneumonia (acute primary)	72	49	72	45	167	68	19	—	—	—	16
20	Bronchitis and tracheitis	25	12	41	137	—	25	24	30	—	—	24
21	Other respiratory diseases	70	52	41	45	167	66	43	—	—	—	37
1–5 19–21	*Total infective and respiratory diseases*	439	343	381	364	334	419	280	151	250	—	261
38	Head injuries	66	113	41	91	—	73	14	30	—	—	16
39	Fractures (except of skull)	102	166	145	45	333	114	29	—	—	—	24
40	Acute poisoning	3	3	—	—	—	2	—	30	250	—	8
41	Burns	13	21	31	—	—	15	—	30	—	—	4
42	Other injuries	128	131	103	91	—	127	49	30	—	—	46
38–42	*Total injuries*	312	434	320	227	333	331	92	120	250	—	98
	Total sick and injured	1,751	1,777	1,701	1,591	1,667	1,750	1,372	1,271	1,500	1,000	1,359

(1) Excluding intracranial vascular lesions (No. 16).
(2) Non-venereal, including nephritis.
(3) Non-rheumatic.
(4) Except jaundice (in No. 24).

Admissions for Injuries

In the M.R.C. Classification injuries and acute poisoning are considered from three angles. The three- or four-figure numbers from 800–949 are used to show the nature of the injury, e.g. fracture, dislocation, shock, burns, poisoning, etc., the classification being so devised as to distinguish, for local injuries, the part of the body affected. The external cause of the injury is denoted by a suffix, thirty possible numbers being assigned as follows:

0 Railway accident
1 Driver of motor cycle injured on road
2 Driver of other motor vehicle injured on road
3 Passenger or unspecified occupant of motor vehicle
4 Pedestrian injured by motor vehicle
5 Other or unspecified motor vehicle accident on road, including pedal cyclist injured by motor vehicle
6 Pedal cyclist injured on road (not by rail or motor vehicle)
7 Other or unspecified road transport accident
8 Water transport accident
9 Air transport accident (including glider and parachute accident)

0V Accident in mine or quarry
1V Agricultural accident
2V Machinery accident (not included above)
3V Conflagration
4V Bomb injury (including mines, grenades, depth charges and effects of blast)
5V Gunshot injury (including rifle, machine gun and small arms)
6V Other explosive missiles (including mortar, cannon, breech-block weapon burst) and shrapnel (not further defined)
7V Cutting or piercing injuries
8V Cataclysm
9V Injury by animals

0X Fall
1X Crushing, landslide injury
2X Blow
3X Explosion injury (not included elsewhere)
4X Accident during sport
5X Other or unspecified cause of injury in the home
6X Other or unspecified cause of injury at work
7X Other or unspecified cause of injury elsewhere
8X Other cause of injury in unspecified locality
9X Unspecified cause of injury in unspecified locality.

Definitions of these terms may be found on pages 136–41 of the M.R.C. Classification. Broadly speaking, a transport accident for example may be taken to be any accident occurring on or from the type of vehicle involved. Thus a railway accident is any injury (or poisoning) from any cause happening on a railway, or on a tramway where the car was circulating outside a town on its own track, except collisions with motor vehicles. While the M.R.C. Classification worked well for analysing accidents to Service personnel and such types of injuries to civilians as entitled them to treatment in E.M.S. hospitals, nevertheless experience has shown that for making a detailed analysis of external causes of injury it is necessary to define more precisely the terms involved. Railway passenger, goods transport motor vehicle, public highway and pedestrian are examples of such terms calling for careful definition if comparability between statistics is to be obtained, a fact which has been fully recognised in the Sixth Revision of the International Lists of Diseases and Causes of Death.

The third aspect considered in the M.R.C. Classification, that of responsibility for the accident, is denoted by a prefix:

- VX Injury to non-civilian resulting directly from enemy action, including late effects of such action
- VV Injury to civilian directly due to operations of war, including home-guard or fire-guard practices but not other accidents while on civil defence duties unless during enemy operations
- V Self-inflicted injury
- X Injury inflicted intentionally by another person, not in warfare.

No prefix was assigned to injuries which were purely accidental.

In many cases more than one injury was recorded, particularly in aircraft accidents where burns might accompany fractures and bruising or in gunshot injuries where a fracture in one limb might be accompanied by an open wound of another site. In order that the selection of the principal cause of admission should not be left to the choice of the individual coder, a rule was made for selecting as principal cause that injury which is highest in the following list:

Suffocation or immersion	M.R.C. Code 940, 941
Acute poisoning	900–924
Traumatic amputations	817–818
Head injuries	800
Fractures	840–845
Dislocations	846
Burns	930–936
Other effects	Rest of 80–94

Certain code numbers among 80–94 were more commonly used for secondary than for primary coding; thus foreign bodies (812–814) were usually recorded in space II on the record card, i.e. as complications of an open wound recorded as the principle cause of admission in space I. Nerve injuries (82–83) were frequently secondary to fractures. Similarly, conditions assignable to numbers 85–89 might appear in II if related to the primary injury recorded in I. Two other titles, therapeutic misadventures (95) and late complications of therapeutic procedures (96) are only used for primary coding if they occur before admission to hospital, otherwise they are coded as complications.

During the seven years 1940–46, the estimated total number of admissions for injuries and poisoning was 290,000 males and 12,000 females. The ratio of yearly admissions to the 1,000 basic total of admissions is shown in Table 74.

TABLE 74

All Injuries. Ratio per 1,000 Admissions for Non-infective and Non-respiratory Illnesses by Sex and Age, 1940–47 (Service Cases)

Year	Males						Females				
	Age Groups						Age Groups				
	15–	25–	35–	45–	55 up	All	15–	25–	35–	45–54	All
1940 .	310	307	243	215	235	296	77	150	40	222	92
1941 .	287	236	188	181	182	246	97	132	160	417	110
1942 .	344	316	234	237	246	308	136	130	126	74	134
1943 .	356	320	237	178	129	312	120	113	138	290	120
1944 .	821	705	364	231	81	659	110	118	112	36	111
1945 .	327	282	197	153	162	278	76	71	95	167	76
1946 .	257	215	159	208	83	230	115	102	—	—	110
1947 .	312	434	320	227	333	331	92	120	250	—	98

In 1941 the proportionate rates were lower for males in each age group and at all ages than in 1940. At ages under 45 the rates rose to a peak in 1944 when the Second Front in Europe was opened. A decrease followed in 1945 and 1946, but in 1947 the rates in each age group and at all ages were higher than in the previous year, largely due to the return of Service men and prisoners-of-war from the Far East with injuries which required further hospital treatment or stumps which needed treatment prior to limb-fitting. From 1940 to 1946, at ages under 44, the proportional rates for men decreased with age. In 1944, admissions for injuries at ages 15–24 and 25–34 formed 37 per cent. and 35 per cent. of the total admissions for all causes in those age groups, whereas in 1941, when the proportional rates were lowest, they had formed 17 per cent. and 15 per cent. respectively. Proportional rates for women of all ages increased from 92 in 1940 to 134 in 1942, then declined to 76 in 1945, following which there was a rise to 110 in 1946.

HEAD INJURIES (Short List Number 38)

This Short List number includes fractures of the skull (M.R.C. numbers 8400–9) but excludes fractures of skull with fractures of other sites (M.R.C. 8450–1). Table 75 shows the proportionate rates of admission for head injuries.

TABLE 75

Head Injuries. Ratio per 1,000 Admissions for Non-infective and Non-respiratory Illnesses by Sex and Age. 1940–1947 (Service Cases)

Year	Males						Females			
	Age Groups						Age Groups			
	15–	25–	35–	45–	55 up	All	15–	25–	35–44	All
1940	49	48	31	34	47	46	22	51	20	28
1941	45	38	27	44	55	39	28	34	25	28
1942	47	42	31	42	29	42	23	27	18	23
1943	46	41	31	16	16	40	21	22	11	20
1944	67	62	39	37	13	58	19	17	22	19
1945	38	28	23	18	—	30	12	6	16	11
1946	44	39	24	28	—	40	19	32	—	21
1947	66	113	41	91	—	73	14	30	—	16

In the sample 7,161 men and 417 women were admitted with head injuries during the eight years 1940–47, corresponding to about 36,000 men and 2,000 women actually admitted. During 1940–46 the proportionate rates for males declined with age up to 45 years. Among females the rates were higher at ages 25–34 than at 15–24, except in 1944 and 1945. The increase in head injuries in 1944 over the previous years for men aged 15–34 was less pronounced than for all injuries.

Of admissions other than for fracture it will be seen from Table 76 that concussion accounted for 53 per cent. of the men and 59 per cent. of

TABLE 76

Proportionate Distribution of Types of Head Injury, by Sex. 1940–47

M.R.C. Code	Disease Group	Males	Females	M.R.C. Code	Disease Group	Males	Females
8000	Open wounds of scalp	346	258	8400	Fracture, vault of skull	122	110
8001	Bruising, contusion of scalp	35	69	8401	Fracture, base of skull	96	171
8002–4	Extradural, subdural and Subarachnoid Haemorrhage	4	6	8402–3	Fracture, sinuses and orbit	59	146
8005	Cerebral laceration	14	18	8404	Fracture, nasal bones	226	207
8006	Concussion	533	592	8405	Fracture, maxilla, zygoma, malar	114	61
8007–8	Intracranial haemorrhage and other sequelae	43	24	8406	Fracture, lower jaw	224	122
8009	Head injury, unspecified	25	33	8407–8	Fracture, ill-defined, face or skull	77	73
				8409	Multiple fractures of skull	82	110
	Totals	1,000	1,000		Totals	1,000	1,000

TABLE 77

Scalp Wounds, Concussion and Skull Fractures. Periods of In-patient Treatment of Cases in which no other pathological condition was recorded
1940–46

Year	Condition diagnosed	Sex-Age Group	DAYS OF IN-PATIENT TREATMENT											*Median Duration
			0–	4–	7–	10–	14–	21–	28–	42–	56–	91 up	All	
1940–46	Open wound of scalp	Males 15–34	61	64	46	45	74	21	17	10	14	5	357	10
		Males 35–54	9	14	9	15	18	3	6	—	2	—	76	11
		Females 15–34	6	5	5	4	2	3	2	—	—	—	27	7
1940	Concussion . . .	Males 15–34	10	20	23	25	43	26	22	12	11	6	198	16
1941			10	8	20	19	38	20	13	9	12	8	157	17
1942			10	13	28	14	29	17	23	28	29	18	209	26
1943			19	19	15	20	50	12	18	13	26	12	204	18
1944–46			24	35	23	34	48	23	24	12	23	18	264	15
1940–46			73	95	109	112	208	98	100	74	101	62	1,032	18
1940–46		Males 35–54	9	14	9	15	18	13	6	—	2	—	86	13
1940–46		Females 15–34	11	11	12	11	29	9	9	4	5	1	102	14

			DAYS OF IN-PATIENT TREATMENT											
			0–	7–	10–	14–	21–	28–	35–	42–	56–	91–	All	Median
1940–46	Fracture of vault . .	Males 15–34	—	2	2	8	9	7	5	6	7	5	51	32
1940–46	Fracture of base . .	Males 15–34	2	—	1	4	4	1	1	3	2	2	20	22
1940–46	Fracture of nasal bones .	Males 15–34	78	37	47	53	7	11	5	7	5	5	255	11
1940–46		Males 35–54	9	5	3	6	—	2	2	3	—	—	30	10
1940–46		Females 15–34	6	4	1	1	—	—	—	—	—	—	12	6
1940–46	Fracture of maxilla, zygoma or malar bones	Males 15–34	17	12	16	22	10	4	3	6	10	5	105	16
1940–46		Males 35–54	1	—	3	7	1	3	1	1	3	—	20	20
1940–46	Fracture of lower jaw bones	Males 15–34	11	4	8	18	16	14	16	20	49	60	216	56
1940–46		Males 35–54	3	—	2	3	4	2	2	3	5	8	32	38

* Adjusted for cases in which the complete period of treatment was not known.

the women, while a further 35 per cent. and 26 per cent. respectively had open wounds of the scalp. Men were more prone to fracture the vault than the base of the skull, the reverse being true for women. Nearly a quarter of all fractures of skull bones among men were of the nasal bones, the corresponding proportion for women being about one-fifth. For both sexes, fractures of the lower jaw were about twice as common as those of the upper jaw bones. It is estimated that about 8,500 men and 430 women were admitted for open wounds of the scalp, and 13,200 men and 990 women for concussion. Whereas women's admissions for head injuries, other than fractures, were 6·4 per cent. of the total admissions, for fracture of the skull bones they were only 3·6 per cent. of the total admissions.

Table 77 shows the distribution of days of in-patient treatment and the median number of days in hospital for certain types of head injury. The median period of treatment of scalp wounds was 10 to 11 days for men and a week for women. For concussion the median period for younger men varied in different years between 15 and 26 days, while over the seven years 1940–46 it was 18 days. For older men the median was 13 days and for women 14 days. Rather more than 32 per cent. of the younger men were treated for 28 days or more, the corresponding proportions of older men and women being 9 per cent. and 18 per cent. Fractures of the vault of the skull in this series required an average of 32 days in hospital, compared with 22 days for fractures of the base. The median period of treatment for fractures of the nasal bones was 10–11 days for men and 6 days for women. Of 255 men aged 15–34 admitted for this disability, 30 per cent. were in hospital for less than 4 days. Fractures of the lower jaw bone necessitated 56 days median duration of in-patient treatment among men of 15–34 years and 38 days for those aged 35–54. Twenty-eight per cent. of the younger men were in hospital for periods of three months or over.

The record cards of 2,179 persons of both sexes admitted during 1942–46, primarily for head injuries, but with one or more other conditions recorded, were examined; 1,484 had primary diagnoses assigned to M.R.C. numbers 8000–8009 and 695 had fractures of the skull in 8400–8409. These cases form a large proportion of admissions with multiple causes; some cases which came in late are not included. The complications and accessory acute conditions shown in Table 78 are those which might be assumed to be related to the primary diagnosis of head injury.

TABLE 78

Head Injuries. Principal Diagnosis in relation to Complications (II) or Accessory Acute Conditions (III) for cases with record of more than one clinical condition (P = Total of II and III as a percentage of total in the diagnostic group)

Complication of Primary Cause of Admission (II) or Accessory Acute Condition (III)	Principal Cause of Admission: Scalp Wound			Bruising Scalp			Haemorrhage (brain)			Cerebral Laceration			Concussion			Sequelae of Injury			Head Injury (unspecified)		
	II	III	P.	II	III	P.	II	III	P.	II	III	P.	II	III	P.	II	III	P.	II	III	P.
Concussion	319	1	51·9	38	—	74·5	5	—	41·7	8	—	18·6	—	—	—	1	—	1·6	17	—	33·3
Shock	41	—	6·6	1	—	2·0	1	—	8·3	4	—	9·3	26	—	4·0	—	—	—	3	—	5·9
Foreign bodies in head	46	—	7·5	—	—	—	—	—	—	6	—	14·0	1	1	0·3	2	—	3·3	—	—	—
Epilepsy (including Jacksonian)	2	—	0·3	—	1	2·0	—	—	—	—	—	—	5	1	0·9	13	—	21·3	—	—	—
Psychoses	—	—	—	—	—	—	—	—	—	—	—	—	2	—	0·3	1	—	1·6	—	—	—
Neuroses	2	3	0·8	—	1	2·0	—	—	—	—	—	—	20	13	6·6	15	2	27·9	1	1	3·9
Abnormal Character States	—	1	0·2	—	—	—	—	—	—	—	—	—	2	2	0·6	2	1	4·9	—	—	—
Nerve Injuries	—	3	0·5	—	—	—	—	1	8·3	—	—	—	2	1	0·5	—	—	—	3	—	5·9
Haemorrhage (brain)	—	—	—	—	—	—	—	—	—	2	—	4·7	—	—	—	—	—	—	—	—	—
Total cards with more than one condition recorded	616			51			12			43			650			61			51		

	Fracture of Vault			Fracture of Base			Fracture of Sinus or Orbit			Fracture of Nasal Bones			Fracture of Upper Jaw			Fracture of Lower Jaw			Fracture skull ill-defined			Multiple Fracture of Skull		
	II	III	P.	II	III	P.	II	III	P.	II	III	P.	II	III	P.	II	III	P.	II	III	P.	II	III	P.
Concussion	39	—	36·1	35	—	37·6	16	—	28·6	23	—	24·0	17	—	27·9	14	—	10·4	20	—	27·4	18	—	24·7
Haemorrhage (brain)	5	—	4·6	4	—	4·3	1	1	3·6	—	—	—	—	—	—	—	—	—	7	—	9·6	—	—	—
Cerebral laceration	17	1	16·7	16	—	17·2	4	—	7·1	—	—	—	—	—	—	—	1	0·7	11	—	15·1	15	—	20·5
Shock	2	—	1·9	8	—	8·6	3	—	5·4	2	—	2·0	1	—	1·6	3	—	2·2	5	—	6·8	4	—	5·5
Foreign bodies in head	11	—	10·1	2	—	2·2	4	—	7·1	1	—	1·0	6	—	9·8	15	1	11·9	2	—	2·7	7	—	9·6
Epilepsy (including Jacksonian)	2	—	1·9	—	—	—	—	—	—	—	—	—	—	—	—	—	—	—	—	—	—	—	—	—
Psychoses	—	—	—	—	—	—	—	—	—	—	—	—	—	—	—	—	—	—	—	—	—	—	—	—
Neuroses	—	1	0·9	—	—	—	—	1	1·8	—	1	1·0	—	—	—	—	1	0·7	1	—	1·4	—	—	—
Abnormal character states	—	—	—	—	—	—	—	—	—	—	—	—	—	—	—	—	—	—	—	—	—	—	—	—
Nerve injuries	1	1	1·9	2	2	4·3	1	—	1·8	—	1	1·0	3	1	6·6	2	2	3·0	2	1	4·1	2	2	5·5
Total cards with more than one condition recorded	108			93			56			96			61			135			73			73		

FRACTURES, OTHER THAN SKULL (Short List Number 39)

In the one in five sample, 19,465 men and 646 women were admitted with a primary diagnosis of fracture other than of skull bones only; the corresponding estimated total of admissions was around 97,000 men and 3,200 women. The proportionate representation of the chief sites in every 1,000 fractures was as follows:

	Spinal Column	Trunk (except Spine)	Upper Limb	Lower Limb	Multiple Sites	Totals
Males	35	47	320	494	104	1,000
Females	39	39	363	514	45	1,000

There was little difference between the sexes as regards spinal fractures, but men showed a higher proportion of fractures of trunk bones of multiple sites, while women had a higher proportion of fractures of either upper or lower limbs. The very much higher proportion of fractures of multiple sites among men is due in part to their greater exposure to injury by high explosives, especially shrapnel.

TABLE 79

Fractures, other than Skull. Ratio per 1,000 Admissions for Non-infective and Non-respiratory Illnesses, by Sex and Age, 1940–1947

Year	Males						Females				
	Age Groups						Age Groups				
	15–	25–	35–	45–	55 up	All	15–	25–	35–	45–54	All
1940	83	92	81	75	94	86	14	33	20	111	20
1941	96	84	72	67	36	86	26	34	74	167	32
1942	113	111	84	102	73	106	35	28	42	—	34
1943	127	112	93	77	48	112	33	33	42	65	34
1944	232	218	131	85	55	200	32	21	56	36	30
1945	136	118	89	62	65	117	19	28	16	111	22
1946	92	87	56	97	83	86	23	39	—	—	25
1947	102	166	145	45	333	114	29	—	—	—	24

It will be seen from Table 79 that for men the ratio of the number of admissions for fractures to the basic total of admissions was 8·6 per cent. in 1940 and 1941, rising to 20 per cent. in 1944 and declining to 8·6 per cent. in 1946. The subsequent increase to 11·4 per cent. in 1947 was due to admissions of returned prisoners-of-war and casualties from the Far East. This pattern of increasing rates up to 1944, a decrease in 1945–46 followed by a further increase in 1947 is observable for each age group under 45 years. During 1941–46 the proportionate rate for fractures decreased with age in the three groups under 45 years. Among women, fractures formed from 2 to 3·4 of the basic total of admissions, and there was little variation from this level in the two age groups under 35.

(a) *Fractures and Fracture-Dislocations of the Vertebral Column*

Admissions for fracture of the vertebral column during 1940–46 were 711 in the sample, or about 3,500 estimated total admissions, of which 96 per cent. were male cases. The M.R.C. Classification distinguishes four groups of vertebrae, 7 cervical, 12 thoracic, 5 lumbar and the sacral process, and separate code numbers are assigned to distinguish cases in which the fracture was accompanied by an injury to the spinal cord. In coding, where the fracture involved vertebrae in two or more of these groups, as for instance the frequent combination of twelth thoracic and first lumbar, the assignment was to the group first mentioned above.

TABLE 80

Proportionate Composition of Admissions for Fractures of Vertical Column. (Sexes combined, 1940–46)

Part of Vertebral Column Injured	1940	1941	1942	1943	1944	1945–6	1940–46
Cervical spine . .	10	13	10	9	12	12	11
Thoracic spine .	13	11	15	21	27	29	20
Lumbar spine . .	60	65	61	57	49	46	55
Sacral spine or coccyx	15	8	10	9	10	7	10
Vertebral column, ill-defined . .	3	3	4	4	2	6	4
Vertebral column (all parts) . .	100	100	100	100	100	100	100

Table 80 shows the proportionate distribution of fractures among the four regions, the numbers for males and females being combined because of the small proportion of females with this type of injury. During the seven years, over half the total spinal fractures were in the lumbar region, one-fifth in the thoracic, one-tenth each in the cervical and sacral regions, while in 4 per cent. the exact position in the spine in which the injury occurred was not defined.

The proportion of fractures in which there was mention of injury to the spinal cord is shown in Table 81. Rather less than a quarter of the fractures of the cervical spine were accompanied by damage to the cord, 30 per cent. of those in the thoracic region and less than one-tenth of those in the lumbar region. For all parts of the vertebral column there was damage to the cord in 15 per cent. of the cases. The years 1944–45,

TABLE 81

Percentage of Spinal Fractures with mention of Spinal Cord Lesion (Sexes combined, 1940–46)

Part of Vertebral Column Injured	1940 %	1941 %	1942 %	1943 %	1944 %	1945–6 %	1940–46 %
Cervical spine	25	9	25	8	33	29	23
Thoracic spine	30	30	24	19	44	23	30
Lumbar spine	2	0	6	9	16	18	9
Sacral spine	0	0	0	9	6	12	4
Vertebral column, ill-defined	0	0	20	0	50	29	19
Vertebral column (all parts)	8	4	10	11	25	21	15

when many injuries were received in fighting on the Second Front, show the highest percentages of fractures with spinal cord lesion, due to the greater frequency of gunshot and shrapnel wounds penetrating into the spinal canal.

More detailed information about spinal cord injuries was obtained by examining the case records of 256 Service men and women who had applied for War Pensions on the grounds of incapacity due to damage to the vertebral column. For its own statistical purposes the Ministry of Pensions prepares a record sheet relating to each new applicant, showing the nature of the disability on which the claim is based. By searching these sheets for records of cases with spinal cord involvement it is possible to refer back to the original medical documents. As cases are reviewed periodically for assessment of the amount of residual disability, it is possible to follow up the medical history for a considerable time. The disadvantage of this survey is that, since the injuries occurred in different years but the investigation had to be completed in one operation, the 'follow-ups' extend over varying periods of time. Nevertheless the following tables are presented, subject to the condition that rigorous conclusions should not be drawn from them.

The region of the spine in which the fracture had occurred in the 256 cases examined was:

	Cervical	Thoracic	Lumbar	Sacral	Not stated	Totals
Numbers	35	130	70	2	19	256
Percentage	14	51	27	1	7	100

The over-all figures of cases who had survived up to the time of the last examination are as follows:

	Cervical	Thoracic	Lumbar	Sacral	Not stated	Totals
Cases	35	130	70	2	19	256
Survivors	34	83	61	2	19	199
Percentage Surviving	97	64	87	100	100	77

The percentage of cases with thoracic injury who survived is significantly lower than that for injury to either the cervical or lumbar vertebrae, the differences being 33 ± 10·2 and 23 ± 11·6 respectively, whereas the difference between the percentages surviving with cervical or lumbar injury is 10 ± 9·8. Table 82 shows, in six monthly intervals, the period between date of injury and either the date of death or the last date for which information was recorded; the latter would in general be the date of the last Medical Board prior to the survey under discussion. Thus, of persons with injury in the thoracic region who were last examined at a period of 2 years but less than 2

TABLE 82

Spinal Cord Injury. Period between date of injury and last date for which information recorded, or date of death.

Site of Spinal Fracture	Survived or Died	Period in Months												
		0–	6–	12–	18–	24–	30–	36–	42–	48–	54–	60–	66–71	All
Cervical	Survived	—	1	2	3	3	8	5	3	2	1	5	1	34
	Died	—	1	—	—	—	—	—	—	—	—	—	—	1
Thoracic	Survived	3	—	3	11	20	11	18	7	6	1	2	1	83
	Died	3	14	12	7	5	4	1	1	—	—	—	—	47
Lumbar	Survived	1	1	3	7	10	11	7	10	8	3	—	—	61
	Died	1	—	4	—	2	—	—	1	1	—	—	—	9
Sacral	Survived	—	—	—	—	—	2	—	—	—	—	—	—	2
	Died	—	—	—	—	—	—	—	—	—	—	—	—	—
Not stated	Survived	—	1	—	2	3	4	3	2	1	1	2	—	19
	Died	—	—	—	—	—	—	—	—	—	—	—	—	-

years 6 months from the date of injury, 20 were alive at the time of examination whereas 5 had died. Forty-nine of the 57 who died were paralysed at the time of death and of those who had survived some were completely paralysed in the lower limbs with little or no control over the urinary system at the time of the last examination recorded. The numbers of such cases, distributed according to the period between injury and either death or last date of examination, are shown in Table 83.

Deaths occurring in this group of paraplegics, while having as underlying cause the initial spinal injury, fall mainly into two groups as regards secondary causes; those due to pyelonephritis and other disorders of the urinary tract, and those due to septicaemia from infected bedsores. Of the 57 deaths in this series, two were not stated to be due to the fracture of the spine, one being due to an anaesthetic misadventure during tooth extraction and the other to pulmonary tuberculosis. A further nine deaths were assigned to 'war operations',

TABLE 83

Spinal Cord Injury. Cases with Total Paralysis at last recorded date or at death

Site of Spinal Injury	Survived or Died	Period since Injury (Months)												
		0–	6–	12–	18–	24–	30–	36–	42–	48–	54–	60–	66–71	All
Cervical	Survived	—	1	—	1	1	2	—	1	—	—	—	—	6
	Died	—	—	—	—	—	—	—	—	—	—	—	—	—
Thoracic	Survived	3	—	2	3	14	5	9	4	3	1	1	—	45
	Died	3	12	12	6	5	2	1	1	—	—	—	—	42
Lumbar	Survived	—	1	—	1	4	4	3	2	1	—	—	—	16
	Died	1	—	4	—	1	1	—	—	—	—	—	—	7
Sacral	Survived	—	—	—	—	—	—	—	—	—	—	—	—	—
	Died	—	—	—	—	—	—	—	—	—	—	—	—	—
Not stated	Survived	—	—	—	—	1	1	1	1	—	—	—	—	4
	Died	—	—	—	—	—	—	—	—	—	—	—	—	—
Total paralysed and under In-patient treatment		3	1	1	4	17	5	5	4	1	1	—	—	42

but in four cases the medical notes referred to trophic or gangrenous bedsores, while in addition one case reported transverse myelitis and another pyelonephritis. Pyelonephritis was stated as the secondary cause in 14 cases, pyelitis in 3, pyelonephrosis in 1 and cystitis in 1, while in 2 cases urinary tract infection was stated; 21 cases therefore, or 37 per cent., had a disorder of the urinary tract as secondary cause of death. Septicaemia or pyaemia was the terminal cause of 17 deaths, following in 11 cases upon trophic ulcers or bedsores. Transverse myelitis was the secondary cause of 2 deaths, and the remainder were attributable to pulmonary oedema, general cachexia, pyopneumothorax, perforated ulcer with peritonitis, and severe asthma respectively, each of these conditions being attributed to paraplegia.

(b) *Fracture of trunk bones, other than spine*

An estimated total of 4,700 persons was admitted for treatment of fractures of the trunk bones other than spine during 1940–46, 97 per cent. being men. In 55 per cent. of the cases one or more ribs were fractured, and in a further 40 per cent. the pelvis was fractured. The proportionate admissions for fractures at each site in males is shown in Table 84, the number of females being too small to warrant inclusion.

TABLE 84

Proportionate Admissions for Fracture of Trunk Bones (not Spine). Males, 1940–46

M.R.C. Code	Type of Injury	1940	1941	1942	1943	1944	1945	1946	1940–6
8420–1	Fracture of one or more ribs . .	61	67	62	49	51	48	35	55
8423–4	Fracture of pelvis .	33	32	34	39	46	49	59	40
8422; 8425–7	Fracture of sternum and ill-defined or multiple fractures	6	1	4	12	3	3	6	5
	Totals	100	100	100	100	100	100	100	100

For admissions during 1942–46, 298 cards with record of more than one pathological condition were examined. The principal complications or accessory acute conditions mentioned were shock, haemothorax, nerve injuries and respiratory diseases. The frequency with which they occurred was as follows:

Complication or Accessory Acute Condition	Fracture of Ribs		Fracture of Pelvis		Fracture of Sternum and ill-defined fractures of Trunk Bones	
	Number	Percentage	Number	Percentage	Number	Percentage
Shock	12	7·5	15	12·0	—	—
Haemothorax	12	7·5	—	—	2	13·3
Injury to sacral, sciatic or peroneal nerve	—	—	12	9·7	—	—
Pneumonia (all forms)	14	8·8	5	4·0	—	—
Empyema	4	2·5	—	—	—	—
Pleurisy	14	8·8	1	0·8	—	—
Spontaneous pneumothorax	1	0·6	—	—	—	—
Pulmonary collapse	4	2·5	1	0·8	1	6·7
Total cards examined	159		124		15	

(c) *Fractures of Upper Limb or Limbs*

During 1940–46 the sample number of admissions primarily for fracture of the upper limbs was 6,283 males and 235 females, corresponding to an estimated total of from 31,020 to 31,810 males and 1,100 to 1,250 females actually admitted. The frequencies with which the various sites were represented in each 1,000 fractures were:

Highest Frequencies				*Lowest Frequencies*			
Males		*Females*		*Males*		*Females*	
Radius	218	Radius	497	Carpal	84	Radius and ulna	60
Phalanges	149	Humerus	98	Ulna	73	Metacarpals	47
Humerus	146	Ulna	81	Radius and ulna	48	Carpal	34
Metacarpals	129	Clavicle	72	Scapula	32	Scapula	30
Clavicle	119	Phalanges	72	Ill-defined	9	Ill-defined	9

Fractures of the radius were commonest in both males and females, accounting for over one-fifth of all fractures of the upper limbs among men and for nearly a half of those of women. Fractures of the bones of the hand were more frequent among males than females, while fractures of the ulna were commoner among the latter.

Table 85 shows the yearly number of admissions for fractures of an upper limb in the sample and the estimated total admissions, the figures for 1944 being shown for two six-monthly periods. The total number of fractures in 1944 and the first half of 1945 was 35 per cent.

TABLE 85

Fractures of Upper Limb or Limbs. Numbers in sample and estimated total admissions, 1940–46.

M.R.C. Code	Site of Fracture	Sex	1940	1941	1942	1943	1944		1945	1946	Sample totals	Estimated totals
							Jan.–June	July–Dec.				
8430	Clavicle	M.	91	120	121	145	76	87	82	21	743	3,715±136
		F.	2	1	3	4	2	—	3	2	17	85
8431	Scapula	M.	23	23	34	26	21	41	29	1	198	990± 70
		F.	—	—	1	3	3	—	—	—	7	35
8432	Humerus	M.	89	83	116	129	118	217	134	23	909	4,545±151
		F.	1	1	1	10	5	2	3	—	23	115
8433	Ulna	M.	50	39	64	51	65	93	82	13	457	2,285±107
		F.	—	1	7	2	1	3	3	2	19	95
8434	Radius (including Colles's and Smith's)	M.	120	201	296	248	112	164	170	46	1,357	6,785±184
		F.	2	2	28	44	10	15	13	3	117	585± 54
8435	Radius and ulna	M.	29	31	35	47	35	74	40	8	299	1,495± 86
		F.	1	1	3	1	—	2	5	1	14	70
8436	Carpal	M.	41	71	116	101	44	63	76	18	530	2,650±115
		F.	—	—	4	3	1	—	—	—	8	40
8437	Metacarpals (including Bennett's)	M.	90	112	135	114	103	138	85	27	804	4,020±142
		F.	—	—	2	7	1	1	—	—	11	55
8438	Phalanges	M.	74	127	200	172	109	158	71	18	929	4,645±152
		F.	1	2	2	8	2	—	2	—	17	85
8439	Upper limb, ill-defined	M.	10	8	5	7	14	4	5	4	57	285± 38
		F.	—	—	—	—	2	—	—	—	2	10
8430–9	Totals	Persons	624	823	1,173	1,122	724	1,062	803	187	6,518	32,590±404

of the total for the whole seven years from 1940–46, while the number in 1944 alone showed an increase of 56 per cent. on the average of the two preceding years. The period of hostilities in Western Europe was therefore characterised by a considerable increase in the number of admissions for fractures. Among men, the increase was particularly marked in the case of fractures of scapula, humerus, and ulna with or without radius, for the numbers of admissions for the twelve months July 1944–June 1945 bore ratios to the corresponding averages for 1942 and 1943 of 2·0, 2·6, 2·5 and 2·6 respectively, and this does not take into account the large number which would have occurred between D-day, June 6, 1944 and the end of June of that year.

The proportionate distribution of admissions of Servicemen by age is shown for certain fractures in Table 86, the fractures chosen being those for which a large number of admissions were reported and which might be regarded as among the more disabling. If the period when the

TABLE 86

Fractures of Radius, Humerus and Clavicle. Proportionate Distribution of Admissions by Age, 1940–43 and 1944–45. (Males)

Nature of Injury	Year of Admission	Age Groups				
		15–	25–	35–	45 up	All
Fracture of Radius	1940–43	460	387	126	27	1,000
	1944–45	393	437	157	13	1,000
Fracture of Humerus	1940–43	410	408	151	31	1,000
	1944–45	399	460	122	19	1,000
Fracture of Clavicle	1940–43	423	470	99	8	1,000
	1944–45	425	408	155	12	1,000

greater number of injuries were coming in from the Western Front be compared with 1940–43, there was a shift in maximum age incidence from the 15–24 age group to 25–34 for fractures both of the radius and of the humerus. Fractures of the humerus occurred less frequently at ages 35–44 during the second period, while fractures of the radius and of the clavicle were more frequent in that age-group during this period. The proportion of fractures of the clavicle which occurred at ages 25–34 was greater during 1940–43 than in 1944–45.

The records of admissions during 1944 and 1945 were examined for mention of certain complications of the primary fracture; these two years were chosen because they gave a good proportion of the total admissions during 1940–46 and also because the coders employed on injury cases had gained considerable experience by the time work on these cases was being done and would be less likely to omit any of the pathological conditions mentioned. The complications which it was felt would be most likely to arise were nerve injuries, paralysis due to nerve injury and loss of muscular or joint function; other possible complications of trauma such as tetanus or gas gangrene were effectively prevented by prophylactic inoculations. Surgical amputations were recorded, however, since the coding rules ordained that the original injury should be entered as the primary cause of admission and the surgical amputation recorded in the second diagnosis space on the card in the same way as with complications. The results, shown as numbers and as rates per 1,000 fractures of each site, are shown in Table 87.

In the total of 2,510 fractures of an upper limb examined, there were 97 records of amputations, an over-all rate of 39 per 1,000. The highest amputation rates were for fractures of phalanges—142 per 1,000, metacarpals—58 per 1,000, humerus—41 per 1,000, and radius and ulna—40 per 1,000. According to the site of amputation, 9 per 1,000 were through the upper arms, 3 per 1,000 through the forearm, and 26 per 1,000 were partial amputations of the hand. Injuries to nerves were recorded for 83 per 1,000 total fractures of an upper limb, the greatest rates occurring in the case of fractures of the humerus—209 per 1,000, radius and ulna—174 per 1,000, and the ulna alone—167 per 1,000. The nerves most frequently affected were the radial nerve, in 35 cases per 1,000 fractures, the ulnar nerve, 29 per 1,000, and the median nerve, 14 per 1,000. Of other possible sequelae, loss of joint function occurred in 4 per 1,000 of all fractures of the upper limb.

The distribution of periods of in-patient treatment for uncomplicated fractures of the upper limb is shown in Table 88. For fractures of the clavicle the median period of treatment for younger men, aged 15–34, was 34 days and for older men, aged 35–54, 44 days. The corresponding period for women was 13 days, but this result is based on very few cases. The median periods for fractures of the scapula were 53 days for younger men, and 40 days for those older. For fractures of the humerus men in the younger age group required 12 weeks treatment, compared with 9 weeks for older men and 38 days for women. For fractures of the ulna men of both age-groups needed in-patient treatment for about 9 weeks, and the few women who were treated had a median period of 18 days. The average number of days in hospital for fractures of the radius for younger men increased from 20 days in 1940–41 up to 54 days in 1944–46, the average over the seven years 1940–46 being 44 days. For older men the median period was 46 days and for women 18 days. Fractures of both radius and ulna required 92 and 127 days for the two age-groups of men and 46 days for women. The greater duration for males than females was due to the more serious character of their injuries.

TABLE 87

Fractures of Upper Limb. Frequency of Certain Complications (numbers and rates per thousand) for Males admitted in 1944 and 1945

M.R.C. Code	Nature of Complication	Site of Fracture: Clavicle	Scapula	Humerus	Ulna	Radius	Radius and Ulna	Carpal	Meta-carpals	Phalanges	Upper Limb (ill-defined)	All sites
	Amputation:											
7900	Upper arm	—	—	19	2	—	1	—	—	—	—	22
	Rate per 1,000	—	—	41	8	—	7	—	—	—	—	9
7901	Forearm	—	—	—	1	—	5	—	—	—	1	7
	Rate per 1,000	—	—	—	4	—	34	—	—	—	43	3
7902	Hand, complete	—	—	—	—	—	—	—	—	2	—	2
	Rate per 1,000	—	—	—	—	—	—	—	—	6	—	1
7903	Hand, partial	—	—	—	1	—	—	—	19	46	—	66
	Rate per 1,000	—	—	—	4	—	—	—	58	136	—	26
7900–3	Total	—	—	19	4	—	6	—	19	48	1	97
	Rate per 1,000	—	—	41	17	—	40	—	58	142	43	39
	Nerve Injuries:											
829	Brachial plexus	—	3	4	—	—	—	—	—	—	—	7
	Rate per 1,000	—	33	9	—	—	—	—	—	—	—	3
830	Circumflex nerve	1	—	—	—	—	—	—	—	—	—	1
	Rate per 1,000	4	—	—	—	—	—	—	—	—	—	0
831	Median nerve	—	—	8	4	11	7	4	2	—	—	36
	Rate per 1,000	—	—	17	17	25	47	22	6	—	—	14
832	Ulnar nerve	—	—	21	34	4	9	—	4	—	1	73
	Rate per 1,000	—	—	45	142	9	60	—	12	—	43	29
833	Radial nerve	—	1	65	2	9	10	—	—	—	—	87
	Rate per 1,000	—	11	139	8	20	67	—	—	—	—	35
834	Digital nerve	—	—	—	—	—	—	—	3	1	—	4
	Rate per 1,000	—	—	—	—	—	—	—	9	3	—	2
829–34	Total	1	4	98	40	24	26	4	9	1	1	208
	Rate per 1,000	4	44	209	167	54	174	22	28	3	43	83
895	Persistent paralysis due to nerve injury	—	—	1	1	—	—	—	—	—	—	2
	Rate per 1,000	—	—	2	4	—	—	—	—	—	—	1
896	Loss of muscular function due to tendon injury	—	—	—	—	—	1	—	1	1	—	3
	Rate per 1,000	—	—	—	—	—	7	—	3	3	—	1
898	Loss of joint function following recent injury	1	1	1	2	—	—	1	2	1	2	11
	Rate per 1,000	4	11	2	8	—	—	5	6	3	87	4
Totals	All Complications above	2	5	119	47	24	33	5	31	51	4	321
	Rate per 1,000	8	55	254	196	54	221	27	95	151	174	129

TABLE 88

Fractures of Upper Limb. Period of In-patient Treatment for cases in which no other pathological condition was recorded. 1940–46.

Year	Diagnoses	Sex-Age Group	DAYS OF IN-PATIENT TREATMENT												*Median Duration
			0–	7–	14–	21–	28–	35–	42–	56–	70–	91–	182–	All	
1940–46	Fracture of clavicle	Males 15–34	47	45	73	60	56	48	63	44	44	42	7	529	34
1940–46		Males 35–54	3	7	5	6	5	1	7	5	7	10	—	56	44
1940–46		Females 15–34	3	4	1	2	2	1	—	—	—	—	—	13	13
1940–46	Fracture of scapula .	Males 15–34	5	5	11	9	7	4	16	9	13	16	4	99	53
1940–46		Males 35–54	1	1	2	2	1	1	1	2	2	3	—	16	40
1940–46	Fracture of humerus	Males 15–34	12	16	18	10	13	10	30	43	34	119	41	346	85
1940–46		Males 35–54	5	9	4	3	4	3	5	6	8	9	6	62	64
1940–46		Females 15–34	3	3	—	2	1	1	2	1	1	4	1	19	38
1940–46	Fracture of ulna .	Males 15–34	13	20	19	6	6	8	16	20	25	48	11	192	63
1940–46		Males 35–54	2	6	2	1	1	1	2	3	1	13	—	32	65

1940–46		Females 15–34	1	3	5	2	—	1	—	2	—	2	—	16	18
1940–41	Fracture of radius	Males 15–34	55	28	17	14	8	13	24	17	9	13	2	200	20
1942			29	21	17	9	12	10	25	26	30	31	1	211	47
1943			22	16	16	6	2	7	20	23	17	34	4	167	52
1944–46			40	22	12	14	12	9	28	30	24	56	12	259	54
1940–46			146	87	62	43	34	39	97	96	80	134	19	837	44
1940–46		Males 35–54	35	12	13	6	1	4	16	14	20	17	8	146	46
1940–46		Females 15–34	28	16	7	8	9	5	10	8	4	3	—	98	18
1940–46	Fracture of radius and ulna	Males 15–34	11	6	8	4	4	1	13	10	9	44	23	133	92
1940–46		Males 35–54	—	2	—	1	1	—	—	1	1	9	4	19	127
1940–46		Females 15–34	1	—	4	—	1	—	2	—	—	2	3	13	46

* Adjusted for cases in which the complete period of treatment was not known.

For males aged 15–34, the percentage of cases of fracture of the upper limb requiring in-patient treatment for 10 weeks or longer was:

	Per cent.		Per cent.		Per cent.
Clavicle	18	Scapula	67	Humerus	56
Ulna	44	Radius	28	Radius and ulna	57

(d) *Fractures of the Lower Limbs*

Admissions for fractures of a lower limb formed 49 per cent. of admissions for all fractures other than those of skull alone among men patients and 51 per cent. among women. An estimated total of about 48,000 men and 1,660 women were admitted for this cause during 1940–46. The frequencies with which various sites were represented in each 1,000 lower limb fracture cases for either sex were:

Highest				*Lowest*			
Males		*Females*		*Males*		*Females*	
Ankle	206	Ankle	440	Femur (not neck)	97	Phalanges	39
Tibia and fibula	192	Tarsal and metatarsal	145	Phalanges	81	Patella	27
Tarsal and metatarsal	133	Fibula	127	Patella	41	Os calcis	9
Fibula	112	Tibia and fibula	117	Os calcis	29	Femur (not neck)	6
Tibia	101	Tibia	90	Femoral neck	8	Femoral neck	0

Fractures of the ankle, which constituted one-fifth of the fractures of the lower limb among males and over two-fifths among women, were the commonest among both men and women; fractures of the neck of the femur were least common among men and did not occur at all among females.

Table 89 shows the number of yearly admissions for fractures of a lower limb found in the one-in-five sample and the estimated total admissions of men and, in the case of fractures of the ankle, of women. The total admissions for these fractures increased annually during 1940–42, decreased slightly in 1943, increased again during 1944 and then declined sharply during 1945–46. Men's admissions during the latter half of 1944 and the first half of 1945 showed an increase of 44 per cent. on the average for the years 1942 and 1943. The increase was most marked for fractures of the femoral neck, other parts of the femur, the tibia with or without a fracture of the fibula and the tarsals and metatarsals, the ratio of admissions for the twelve months from July 1944 to June 1945 to the average number for 1942 and 1943 being 4, 2, 1·8, 1·8 and 1·5 respectively. Fractures of the ankle showed a decreased ratio of 0·8.

TABLE 89

Fractures of Lower Limb. Numbers in sample and estimated total admissions, 1940–46

M.R.C. Code	Site of Fracture	Sex	1940	1941	1942	1943	1944		1945	1946	Sample totals	Estimated totals
							Jan.–June	July–Dec.				
8440	Femoral neck . . .	M.	8	6	10	6	10	18	20	—	78	390± 44
		F.	—	—	—	—	—	—	—	—	—	
8441	Femur, other than neck .	M.	70	90	88	103	127	250	178	28	934	4,670±153
		F.	—	—	1	1	—	—	—	—	2	
8442	Patella .	M.	53	50	67	51	39	49	60	22	391	1,955± 99
		F.	—	—	1	3	2	2	1	—	9	
8443	Tibia .	M.	115	115	155	126	116	147	161	39	974	4,870±156
		F.	2	2	8	7	5	2	2	2	30	
8444	Fibula	M.	147	158	218	176	108	116	127	28	1,078	5,390±164
		F.	—	4	11	13	4	5	5	—	42	
8445	Tibia and fibula (excluding Pott's and Dupuytren's) .	M.	173	224	272	287	200	310	289	81	1,836	9,180±214
		F.	2	3	6	10	5	6	4	3	39	
8446	Ankle (including Pott's and Dupuytren's) . . .	M.	209	307	407	357	202	235	190	74	1,981	9,905±223
		F.	3	9	32	41	15	15	24	7	146	730± 60
8447	Os calcis	M.	23	23	70	45	27	29	52	5	274	1,370± 83
		F.	—	—	—	3	—	—	—	—	3	
8448	Tarsal bones and metatarsals	M.	114	157	217	207	170	214	157	44	1,280	6,400±179
		F.	1	5	8	13	4	7	8	2	48	
8449	Phalanges . .	M.	56	91	169	163	89	114	75	25	782	3,910±140
		F.	—	—	6	1	2	2	2	—	13	
8440–9	Totals	Persons	976	1,244	1,746	1,613	1,125	1,521	1,355	360	9,940	48,770±499

TABLE 90

Fractures of Ankle, Tibia and Fibula, and Femur. Proportionate Distribution of Admissions by Age. 1940–43 and 1944–45 (Males)

Nature of Injury	Year of Admission	Age Groups				
		15–	25–	35–	45 up	All
Fracture of Ankle	1940–43	360	446	171	23	1,000
	1944–45	359	441	190	10	1,000
Fracture of Tibia and Fibula	1940–43	407	433	141	19	1 000
	1944–45	365	491	136	8	1,000
Fracture of Femur	1940–43	461	419	100	20	1,000
	1944–45	424	461	110	5	1,000

In Table 90 the proportionate age-distributions of men admitted for fractures of the ankle, tibia and fibula and femur (other than femoral neck) during 1940–43 are compared with similar distributions for 1944 and 1945. For fractures of the ankle there is little difference between the proportions falling in age-groups 15–24 and 25–34, but the proportion occurring at ages 35–44 was greater during 1944–45. The proportion of fractures of tibia and fibula at ages 15–24 was greater during 1940–43, whereas the proportion at ages 25–34 was 491 in the second period compared with 433 in the first. This shift in maximum incidence from the younger to the older age group which was also apparent for fractures of the femur, had previously been noticed for fractures of the humerus and radius. When all admissions for diseases are considered, the proportionate age distribution is as follows:

Year of Admission	Age Groups				
	15–	25–	35–	45 up	All
1940–1943	398	414	160	28	1,000
1944–1945	352	429	197	22	1,000

A corresponding shift is noticeable here and one explanation of this may be a changed age distribution of those at risk, due to a more complete call-up of men aged 30–35.

As in the case of fractures of the upper limbs, the records of admissions during 1944 and 1945 for fractures of the lower limbs were examined for complications of the primary fracture, surgical amputations, as explained above, being treated as complications of the primary injury. The results are shown in Table 91.

TABLE 91

Fractures of Lower Limb. Frequency of Certain Complications (numbers and rates per 1,000) for Males admitted in 1944 and 1945

M.R.C. Code	Nature of Complication	Site of Fracture										
		Femoral neck	Femur, other	Patella	Tibia	Fibula	Tibia and Fibula	Ankle	Os calcis	Tarsals, Meta-tarsals	Phalanges	All sites
	Amputation:											
7910	Thigh	—	23	1	—	—	10	1	—	—	—	35
	Rate per 1,000	—	41	7	—	—	13	2	—	—	—	9
7911	Leg	—	15	2	14	1	36	7	3	2	—	80
	Rate per 1,000	—	27	14	33	3	45	11	28	4	—	21
7912	Foot, complete	—	—	—	—	—	—	—	—	2	—	2
	Rate per 1,000	—	—	—	—	—	—	—	—	4	—	1
7913	Foot, partial	—	—	—	—	—	—	—	1	5	16	22
	Rate per 1,000	—	—	—	—	—	—	—	9	9	58	6
7910–3	Total	—	38	3	14	1	46	8	4	9	16	139
	Rate per 1,000	—	68	20	33	3	58	13	37	17	58	36
	Nerve Injuries:											
836	Sciatic nerve	4	32	—	3	5	4	—	—	—	—	48
	Rate per 1,000	83	58	—	7	14	5	—	—	—	—	12
837	Peroneal nerve	—	3	1	4	6	6	—	—	1	—	21
	Rate per 1,000	—	5	7	9	17	8	—	—	2	—	5
838	Tibial nerve	1	1	—	2	1	2	—	—	1	—	8
	Rate per 1,000	21	2	—	5	3	3	—	—	2	—	2
836–8	Total	5	36	1	9	12	12	—	—	2	—	77
	Rate per 1,000	104	65	7	21	34	15	—	—	4	—	20
895	Persistent paralysis due to	—	4	—	—	2	5	—	—	—	—	11
	nerve injury	—	7	—	—	7	6	—	—	—	—	3
896	Loss of muscular function	—	—	—	—	—	—	—	—	—	—	—
	due to tendon injury	—	—	—	—	—	—	—	—	—	—	—
898	Loss of joint function,	—	4	—	2	1	—	2	—	—	—	9
	following recent injury	—	7	—	5	3	—	3	—	—	—	2
Totals	All Complications above	5	82	4	25	16	63	10	4	11	16	236
	Rate per 1,000	104	148	27	59	46	79	16	37	20	58	61

TABLE 92

Fractures of Lower Limb. Period of In-patient Treatment for cases in which no other pathological condition was recorded. 1940–46.

Year	Diagnoses	Sex-Age Group	Days of In-patient Treatment										*Median duration
			0–	14–	28–	42–	56–	70–	91–	182–	273–	All	
1940–46	Fracture, femoral, neck . .	Males 15–54	2	2	1	4	1	4	10	7	2	33	147
1940–46	Fracture, femur, other than neck	Males 15–34	16	12	9	7	17	22	94	90	55	322	171
1940–46		Males 35–54	2	2	3	2	1	1	15	16	3	45	176
1940–46	Fracture, patella . . .	Males 15–34	13	16	13	12	7	28	74	31	8	202	103
1940–46		Males 35–54	6	5	2	1	8	0	8	1	1	32	60
1940–46	Fracture, tibia . . .	Males 15–34	49	41	24	24	38	49	196	75	19	515	112
1940–46		Males 35–54	5	7	3	7	2	5	22	11	2	64	94
1940–46		Females 15–34	6	1	2	1	1	4	7	—	—	22	68
1940–46	Fracture, fibula . . .	Males 15–34	106	101	51	76	90	90	159	11	4	688	59
1940–46		Males 35–54	25	19	11	9	12	17	35	5	1	134	63
1940–46		Females 15–34	13	7	3	7	2	3	2	—	1	38	20

1940–42	Fracture, tibia and fibula	Males 15–34	38	15	20	18	13	19	110	81	28	342	145
1943			11	11	2	6	2	8	48	62	15	165	181
1944			10	10	3	3	4	14	74	68	31	217	180
1945–46			12	10	4	5	3	7	40	59	26	166	190
1940–46			71	46	29	32	22	48	272	270	100	890	163
1940–46		Males 35–54	8	9	7	3	7	9	49	56	15	163	170
1940–46		Females 15–34	7	2	1	1	1	4	7	4	—	27	77
1940–46	Fracture, os calcis	Males 15–34	9	8	8	18	9	10	49	12	5	128	94
1940–46		Males 35–54	3	4	6	3	—	6	19	5	3	49	97
1940–41	Fracture, ankle, including Pott's and Dupuytren's	Males 15–34	85	49	33	40	34	37	41	8	—	327	41
1942			31	22	22	27	19	43	82	16	2	264	77
1943			28	20	9	17	19	34	94	16	—	237	86
1944–46			43	35	18	25	29	62	149	24	3	388	85
1940–46			187	126	82	109	101	176	366	64	5	1,216	71
1940–46		Males 35–54	59	24	17	24	14	39	91	18	3	289	71
1940–46		Females 15–34	33	12	9	11	11	15	26	—	—	117	48

* Adjusted for cases in which the complete period of treatment was not known.

In examining the case histories of 3,879 patients admitted for fracture of a lower limb, records of 139 amputations were found, an over-all rate of 36 per 1,000. The highest amputation rate was 68 per 1,000 in cases of fracture of femur other than femoral neck; the rates for fractures of tibia and fibula and of phalanges were each 58 per 1,000. According to the site of amputation for fractures of lower limbs in this series, 9 per 1,000 had an amputation above the knee. Injuries to nerves were recorded in 1 out of every 50 cases; in 1 out of 10 cases of fracture of the femoral neck and in about 1 in 15 cases of fractures of femur other than neck. The sciatic nerve was injured in 83 cases per 1,000 fractures of the femoral neck and 58 per 1,000 cases of other fractures of the femur. Fractures of these two sites also had the highest over-all rates of incidence for the types of complication under discussion.

Table 92 shows the distribution of periods of in-patient treatment for fractures of the lower limbs, and the median period in hospital for cases in which no pathological condition but the fracture was recorded. The median period of treatment for males aged 15–54 with fractures of the femoral neck was 21 weeks, and for other fractures of the femur a little under 6 months. Fractures of the patella required 103 days on an average for men aged 15–34 and 60 days for older men. Fractures of the tibia necessitated hospital treatment for over 3 months for men in each age group and about 10 weeks for women. The median period for fractures of both tibia and fibula was around six months for men but only 77 days for women, while fractures of os calcis also required an average of 3 months in-patient treatment.

For males aged 15–34, the percentage of cases of certain fractures of lower limbs requiring in-patient treatment for six months or more was as follows:

	Per cent.		Per cent.
Femur (other than neck)	44	Fibula	8
Patella	19	Tibia and fibula	42
Tibia	18	Os calcis	13
Ankle, including Pott's and Dupuytren's fractures			6

(e) *Multiple Fractures*

The M.R.C. Classification provides combination code numbers for fractures of multiple sites. (Numbers 8450–8459.) Admissions for multiple fractures in the sample numbered 2,023 males and 29 females; the estimated total number of men admitted for this cause lies around 10,000. The sample number of admissions and the estimated total numbers for various combinations of sites are shown in Table 93.

The principal causes of admission in this group were fractures involving either both lower or both upper limbs or upper and lower limbs.

TABLE 93

Multiple Fractures. Numbers in Sample and estimated total admissions. Males. 1940–46

M.R.C. Code	Site of Fractures	1940	1941	1942	1943	1944		1945	1946	Sample Totals	Estimated Totals
						Jan.–June	July–Dec.				
8450	Skull and trunk bones	3	5	10	6	9	2	7	2	44	220 ± 33
8451	Skull and limb or limbs	23	29	39	43	29	38	36	13	250	1,250 ± 79
8452	Spine and other trunk bones	3	7	8	5	4	12	6	4	49	245 ± 35
8453	Spine and limb or limbs	2	4	8	10	6	6	16	6	58	290 ± 38
8454	One or both upper limbs (except radius and ulna)	33	37	54	54	52	94	54	9	387	1,935 ± 98
8455	Upper limb and lower limb	37	34	34	55	48	69	53	19	349	1,745 ± 93
8456	Upper limb and trunk bones, other than spine	11	10	29	15	14	27	27	9	142	710 ± 60
8457	One or both lower limbs (except tibia and fibula)	48	55	69	90	87	157	112	17	635	3,175 ± 126
8458	Lower limb and trunk bones, other than spine	3	4	6	6	4	14	10	3	50	250 ± 35
8459	Other or ill-defined	3	11	13	10	3	10	5	4	59	295 ± 38
	Totals	166	196	270	294	256	429	326	86	2,023	10,115 ± 225

While such fractures may not be among those most dangerous to life they present an important problem from the point of view of possible loss of working power, so that in addition to ordinary hospital treatment it is necessary to provide rehabilitation centres and training courses for instruction in new methods of earning a living. This question applies in greater or less degree to all fractures and led to the undertaking of a follow-up of certain fracture cases, the results of which will be presented in the next section.

The proportionate distribution of admissions for multiple fractures over the seven years is as follows, males only being considered:

1940	1941	1942	1943	1944	1945	1946	Total
82	97	133	145	339	161	43	1,000

Half the admissions for multiple fractures therefore occurred in 1944–45.

The number of admissions for multiple fractures during the 12 months July 1944–June 1945 bore the following proportions to the average admissions during 1942 and 1943 for fractures of the same combination of sites.

Skull and trunk bones	0·9	Upper limb and lower limb	2·4
Skull and limb or limbs	1·5	Upper limb and trunk (not spine)	2·2
Spine and other trunk bones	2·5	One or both lower limbs, except tibia or fibula	2·9
Spine and limb or limbs	1·9	Lower limb and trunk (not spine)	3·7
One or both upper limbs, except radius and ulna	2·4	Other or ill-defined	1·1

Except for fractures of the skull and trunk bones there was an increase in the number of admissions during the period of fighting on the Western Front over the average for the two years prior to 1944. This excess was particularly marked in cases in which the lower limbs were involved.

Table 94 shows the amputation rates for Servicemen admitted with multiple fractures involving either upper or lower limbs or both. Of 515 cases admitted for multiple fractures of one or both lower limbs, 18 had both legs or feet amputated and a further 83 lost one leg or foot; thus roughly one in five of these cases required an amputation.

(f) *Follow-up of Cases of Fracture of either an Upper or a Lower Limb*

In the hope of obtaining some information about the period of disability due to fractures of either an arm or a leg, 1,000 cases of such fractures admitted to E.M.S. hospitals during 1944 and 1945 were followed up by letters of enquiry sent out during the latter half of

TABLE 94

Amputation Rates per 1,000 Service Males admitted for Multiple Fractures during 1942–45

Multiple Fractures causing admission to hospital	Nature of Amputation and M.R.C. Code Number														No. of cases Admitted
	One arm or hand 7900–3		One leg or foot 7910–3		Both arms or hands 7920–4		Both legs or feet 7930–4		One arm or one leg 7940–3		Others 7950–1		Total of Amputations		
	No.	Rate	No.	Rate	No.	Rate	No.	Rate	No.	Rate	No.	Rate	No.	Rate	
Skull and limb or limbs .	1	5	4	22	—	—	—	—	—	—	—	—	5	27	185
Spine and limb or limbs .	—	—	—	—	—	—	—	—	—	—	—	—	—	—	46
One or both upper limbs, except radius and ulna .	36	117	—	—	—	—	—	—	—	—	—	—	36	117	308
Upper limb and lower limb	11	42	19	73	—	—	—	—	1	4	—	—	31	120	259
Upper limb and trunk bones (not spine) . .	1	9	—	—	—	—	—	—	—	—	—	—	1	9	112
One or both lower limbs, except tibia and fibula .	—	—	83	161	—	—	18	35	—	—	1	2	102	198	515
Lower limb and trunk bones (not spine) . .	—	—	1	25	—	—	—	—	—	—	—	—	1	25	40

1946 and the beginning of 1947. The letter of enquiry informed the patient that for research purposes information was being collected about the number of weeks of incapacity following certain kinds of fractures and he was assured that the information was to be used for statistical purposes only. The questions asked were:

(1) Name of Hospital from which you received your discharge.
(2) Date of leaving that hospital.
(3) Occupation before entering the Service.
(4) Date of resuming that or a similar occupation or
Date of commencing a lighter occupation.
(5) Date when certified as fit to resume your former occupation or
Date when certified as fit for a lighter occupation.

The first two questions helped in correctly identifying the subject of a record card with the appropriate questionnaire in cases where there were two or more people with the same name and injury. In the interests of accuracy the remaining questions were made as simple as possible.

In all 566 usable replies were received. When the patients' files were being searched for their most recent address, it was noticed that a great many had had several changes of residence, and it is therefore probable that in addition to those forms which were returned to the central office marked 'Unknown', there were others which failed to reach the subject of the enquiry because he had moved away. It may be that this mobility was in some measure due to the housing shortage obliging people to live in rooms, thus making them less stable than if they were living in houses. In any case the problem of tracing those who move from one address to another is a serious one for anyone attempting a follow-up by postal enquiry. A second reason for failure to answer the questions may have been a fear that the answers could be used in some way as a means of reducing the assessment of disability pension. Whether those who were still seriously handicapped or those who had recovered full use of their limb would be more likely to reply is a matter for speculation.

In Table 95 the numbers who were certified as fit for work and those who resumed work are shown according to the type of work undertaken or for which they were judged suitable. Under the heading 'None' on the left-hand side of the table are included those who had not resumed work, some who were still in hospital or under treatment and those who did not reply to question 4 above, while on the right-hand side under 'None' are entered those who had not been certified as fit for work and those who did not answer question 5. Where a patient first started a lighter occupation and later resumed his old one, the former

TABLE 95

Follow-up of Fracture Cases. Numbers who resumed previous or lighter occupations and numbers certified as fit for resuming work

Site of Fracture	Number of Cases	Type of work Resumed			Type of Work for which Certified Fit		
		Lighter	Same	None	Lighter	Same	None
Humerus	71	47	16	8	44	11	16
Ulna	21	15	3	3	15	2	4
Radius (including Colles's, Smith's)	7	6	1	—	6	1	—
Radius and ulna	17	9	6	2	10	3	4
Carpal bones	4	3	—	1	4	—	—
Metacarpal bones	6	5	1	—	5	1	—
Phalanges	2	1	1	—	—	1	—
Total, Arm and Hand	128	86	28	14	84	19	24
Percentage	100	67	22	11	66	15	19
Femoral neck	4	2	1	1	3	—	1
Femur, other than neck	193	110	55	28	110	44	39
Patella	8	5	3	—	4	3	1
Tibia	64	33	26	5	31	16	17
Fibula	14	8	6	—	7	3	4
Tibia and Fibula	153	85	54	14	71	35	47
Tarsals and Metatarsals	2	1	1	—	—	1	1
Total, Leg and Foot	438	244	146	48	226	102	110
Percentage	100	56	33	11	52	23	25

has been counted for the purpose of this survey. Furthermore, in analysing these cases according to the site of the fracture which was the principal cause of admission to hospital, it has not been found possible to take into account other concurrent diseases or injuries such as for example open wounds, burns or dislocations.

Sixty-seven per cent. of those with fractures of an upper limb took up a lighter occupation than they had had before their service with the Forces, compared with 56 per cent. with fractures of a lower limb. The difference between these proportions is significant. (Difference 11; 2.SE = 9·5.) Sixty-six per cent. with fractures of an arm or hand and 52 per cent. with fractures of a leg or foot were certified as fit for a lighter occupation, the difference between these results also being significant. (Difference 14; 2.SE = 9·6.) There were 8 people with fractures of the arm or hand and 20 with fractures of leg or foot who were either still in hospital or attending for out-patient treatment so often that it was impossible for them to work. A number of those who had been certified fit for a light occupation but had not yet started working were awaiting admission to a training centre. Twenty-two per cent. with fractures of an upper limb and thirty-three per cent. with fractures of a lower limb were able to resume their pre-war occupation.

TABLE 96

Follow-up of Fracture Cases. Period from Date of Injury to Date when certified fit for work

Site of Fracture	Under 6 m (,, 182 d)	6 mo– (182 d–)	9 mo– (273 d–)	1 yr– (365 d–)	1 yr 3 m– (456 d–)	1 yr 6 m– (547 d–)	1 yr 9 m– (638 d–)	2 yr– (730 d–)	2 yr 3 m– (821 d–)	2 yr 6 m– (912 d–)	2 yr 9 m up (1,003 d–)	Totals	Median Duration
Humerus	5	10	14	6	7	3	3	4	2	—	1	55	337 days
Ulna	2	4	4	1	1	2	2	1	—	—	—	17	321 days
Radius	—	1	1	3	1	—	—	—	1	—	—	7	404 days
Radius and ulna	—	3	2	4	2	—	2	—	—	—	—	13	397 days
Carpal bones	—	1	—	—	1	—	—	—	—	1	—	3	543 days
Metacarpals	—	3	—	—	1	—	1	—	—	—	—	5	239 days
Phalanges	—	—	1	—	—	—	—	—	—	—	—	1	—
Total, Arm and Hand	7	22	22	14	13	5	8	5	3	1	1	101	357 days
Femoral neck	—	1	1	—	—	—	—	1	—	—	—	3	349 days
Femur, other	5	10	32	32	20	23	8	13	5	2	—	150	438 days
Patella	1	2	3	—	—	—	—	1	—	—	—	7	312 days
Tibia	2	5	7	10	9	4	2	3	2	1	—	45	437 days
Fibula	1	2	3	1	1	1	—	—	—	—	1	10	310 days
Tibia and fibula	1	8	31	20	13	11	13	4	3	2	—	106	405 days
Tarsals and metatarsals	—	—	—	1	—	—	—	—	—	—	—	1	—
Total, Leg and Foot	10	28	77	64	43	39	23	22	10	5	1	322	421 days

In Table 96 are shown the periods from date of injury to date when certified fit for work, and the median periods of incapacity. For 55 cases of fracture of the humerus the median period was about 48 weeks and 23 per cent. of the cases were incapacitated for 18 months or more. Taking all fractures of an upper limb together, the median time of unfitness for work was 357 days. Fractures of the femur other than the femoral neck showed a median period of 438 days or rather less than 15 months, based on 150 cases, and fractures of tibia and fibula a median period of 405 days or about 59 weeks, based on 106 cases. For fractures of the tibia alone the median time of incapacity based on 45 cases was also just under 15 months. If all the 322 fractures of leg or foot be considered the median period was 421 days or about 60 weeks. Since the majority of fractures (75 per cent. and 73 per cent. for upper and lower limb respectively) were due to operations of war, of which the chief would involve bombs, mortars, gunshot and various kinds of high explosives, it is possible that the fractures under consideration would involve greater bone damage than many of the fractures to which a civilian population would be subject in peace-time, and hence that the periods of incapacity shown here are greater than would normally be expected.

The distribution of periods from date of injury to date of starting work is shown in Table 97. For fractures of an upper limb the median periods were longer than the corresponding ones in the preceding table, except for fractures of the carpal bones, the number of which is very small in any case. The median time before starting work for those with fractures of arm or hand was 6–7 weeks longer than the median time before being certified as fit for work. For fractures of a lower limb the median time from injury to starting work exceeded the time until certification of fitness for work when the femoral neck, the fibula or both tibia and fibula were involved, but was less for fractures of other parts of the femur, the patella or the tibia. Taking all fractures of the lower limb, there was little difference between the two intervals. Many of those who had had fractures subsequently spent as much as six months in a Government Training Centre learning a new occupation, and in some of these cases there was time spent in awaiting admission to the Centres, facts which will partially explain the differences between the periods shown in Tables 96 and 97.

Table 98 shows that 446 patients out of 1,000 with fractures of either an upper or a lower limb started work not more than one week after being certified as fit to resume their occupation; 38 per cent. of those with fractures of an upper and 47 per cent. of those with fractures of a lower limb are included in this total. Eight per cent. of those with fractures of arm or hand and 7 per cent. of those with fractures of leg or foot started work before being certified as fit; in this connexion the

TABLE 97

Follow-up of Fracture Cases. Period from Date of Injury to Date of starting work

Site of Fracture	Under 6 m (,, 182 d)	6 mo– (182 d–)	9 mo– (273 d–)	1 yr– (365 d–)	1 yr 3 m– (456 d–)	1 yr 6 m– (547 d–)	1 yr 9 m– (638 d–)	2 yr– (730 d–)	2 yr 3 m– (821 d–)	2 yr 6 m– (912 d–)	2 yr 9 m– (1,003 d–)	Totals	Median Duration
Humerus . .	2	12	13	7	11	2	5	5	4	—	1	62	426 days
Ulna . .	1	5	4	3	1	2	—	1	1	—	—	18	344 days
Radius . .	—	1	1	3	—	2	—	—	—	—	—	7	444 days
Radius and ulna.	—	—	4	5	1	2	2	1	—	—	—	15	431 days
Carpal bones .	—	1	—	—	1	—	—	—	—	1	—	3	500 days
Metacarpals .	—	3	—	—	—	—	1	—	—	—	—	4	248 days
Phalanges . .	—	—	2	—	—	—	—	—	—	—	—	2	—
Total, Arm and Hand . .	3	22	24	18	14	8	8	7	5	1	1	111	404 days
Femoral neck .	—	—	2	—	—	—	—	1	—	—	—	3	352 days
Femur, other .	5	13	31	39	18	23	13	11	8	3	—	164	424 days
Patella . .	—	3	3	1	1	—	—	—	—	—	—	8	307 days
Tibia . .	2	10	12	9	12	5	3	2	3	—	1	59	420 days
Fibula . .	1	3	4	2	2	1	—	—	—	—	1	14	335 days
Tibia and fibula.	2	11	33	29	23	14	15	6	4	2	—	139	430 days
Tarsals and metatarsals .	—	—	—	2	—	—	—	—	—	—	—	2	—
Total, leg and Foot . .	10	40	85	82	56	43	31	20	15	5	2	389	417 days

TABLE 98

Folllow-up of Fracture Cases. Period between Date of Certification as fit for work and Date on which work commenced

Site of Fracture	Work begun before Certification								Work begun after Certification										Totals
	Period in weeks								Period in weeks										
	Over 52	–52	–39	–26	–13	–8	–4	–2	0–1	–2	–4	–6	–8	–13	–26	–39	–52	Over 52	
Humerus	—	—	—	—	—	—	—	—	18	6	10	3	4	5	2	2	—	—	50
Ulna	—	—	1	—	—	1	—	—	5	1	2	—	1	3	—	—	—	—	14
Radius	—	1	—	—	—	—	1	1	3	—	—	—	—	—	1	—	—	—	7
Radius and ulna	—	—	—	1	—	—	—	—	3	—	3	3	—	—	1	—	—	—	11
Carpal bones	—	—	—	—	—	1	—	—	2	—	—	—	—	—	—	—	—	—	3
Metacarpals	—	—	—	—	—	—	—	—	3	—	—	—	1	—	1	—	—	—	5
Phalanges	—	—	—	—	—	—	—	—	1	—	—	—	—	—	—	—	—	—	1
Femoral neck	—	—	—	—	—	—	—	—	1	—	—	—	1	1	—	—	—	—	3
Femur, other	—	—	4	1	2	—	1	1	65	15	13	7	7	6	13	2	3	—	140
Patella	1	—	—	—	—	—	—	—	3	—	—	—	2	—	—	1	—	—	7
Tibia	1	—	—	2	—	1	—	1	19	4	2	4	3	2	3	2	—	—	44
Fibula	—	—	—	—	—	—	—	—	5	1	1	2	1	—	—	—	—	—	10
Tibia and fibula	—	3	—	—	1	2	—	—	47	10	7	10	4	5	2	5	2	—	98
Tarsals and metatarsals	—	—	—	—	—	—	—	—	1	—	—	—	—	—	—	—	—	—	1
Proportions	5	10	13	10	8	13	5	8	446	94	96	74	61	56	58	30	13	—	1,000

TABLE 99

Follow-up of Fracture Cases. Proportionate Distribution of Periods between Date of Injury and (a) Date of leaving hospital, (b) Date of certification as fit for work and (c) Date of starting work

Site of Fracture		Under 6 m (,, 182 d)	6 mo– (182 d–)	9 mo– (273 d–)	1 yr– (365 d–)	1 yr 3 m– (456 d–)	1 yr 6 m– (537 d–)	1 yr 9m– (638 d–)	2 yr– (730 d–)	2 yr 3 m– (821 d–)	2 yr 6 m– (912 d–)	2 yr 9 m– (1,003 d–)	Totals	Median Duration
Humerus	(a)	214	342	143	86	86	29	29	57	14	—	—	1,000	225 days
	(b)	91	182	254	109	127	55	55	73	36	—	18	1,000	337 days
	(c)	32	194	209	113	177	32	81	81	65	—	16	1,000	426 days
Femur, not neck	(a)	156	240	297	115	99	21	36	16	5	10	5	1,000	298 days
	(b)	33	67	214	214	133	153	53	87	33	13	—	1,000	438 days
	(c)	30	79	190	238	110	140	79	67	49	18	—	1,000	424 days
Tibia and fibula	(a)	156	286	313	116	75	27	7	20	—	—	—	1,000	287 days
	(b)	9	75	292	189	123	104	123	38	28	19	—	1,000	405 days
	(c)	14	79	238	209	165	101	108	43	29	14	—	1,000	430 days

possibility that the answers to questions 4 and 5 of the enquiry sheet were interchanged must be taken into account. Four weeks after the date of being certified fit for work, only 292 per 1,000 were not employed; six months after certification only 43 per 1,000 were still not at work.

For the sites of the three largest numbers of fractures in this series, a comparison is made in Table 99 of the proportionate distribution of periods of in-patient treatment and incapacity for work and of non-working periods. The median period of treatment in hospital for fractures of the humerus was 7½ months, of the femur other than the femoral neck 10 months and of tibia and fibula 9½ months. The periods of incapacity in these three cases were approximately 1½, 1½ and 1·4 times as long as the periods in hospital, while the median periods from injury to resumption of occupation were 1·9, 1·4 and 1·5 times as long as the median periods of in-patient treatment.

As the number of returns (566) was less than had been hoped for, it was not considered advisable to attempt any analysis by occupation, especially as from the point of view of fitness for work, a very detailed break-down would be required.

ACUTE POISONING (Short List Number 40)

This Short List Number comprises acute poisoning by toxins and substances other than gases, poisoning and other injury by gases and late effects of acute poisoning. The number of admissions in the sample during the eight years 1940–47 for these conditions was 357 males and 60 females, giving an estimated total number of from 1,980 to 2,185 persons admitted. The ratio of admissions for this cause to 1,000 admissions for non-infective and non-respiratory diseases in the eight years was:

	1940	1941	1042	1943	1944	1945	1946	1947
Males . .	1	2	3	3	2	1	2	2
Females . .	2	2	4	3	3	1	5	8

The rates for males did not rise above 3 per 1,000 in any year and those for females only rose above 4 per 1,000 in 1946 and 1947 when the total number of women admitted was small.

The principal causes of admission in this group for the whole period, with sample numbers of patients and estimated totals were as follows:

	Males	Females	Estimated Totals
Food Poisoning:			
by bacterial toxins	60	6	
botulism; other agents	8	—	
Totals	68	6	370 ± 43
Acute Poisoning:			
by narcotic, analgesic or soporific drugs .	40	32	
by corrosive substances . . .	16	6	
by other substances (not gases) . .	57	13	
Totals	113	51	820 ± 64
Poisoning and Other Injury by Gases:			
carbon monoxide	72	3	
war gases; screen smokes	15	—	
vesicants	49	—	
others	22	—	
other gases	14	—	
Totals	172	3	875 ± 66
Late Effects of Acute Poisoning . . .	4	—	

BURNS (Short List Number 41)

The M.R.C. code provides a dual classification for burns, the third digit indicating the agent causing the burn and the fourth digit the part of the body involved. During 1940–47 the sample number of males admitted with a primary diagnosis of burns was 2,555, and of females 252; it is estimated therefore that about 12,800 men and 1,340 women were admitted for this cause. Sunburn (M.R.C. Code 936) is excluded from these figures.

TABLE 100

Burns. Ratio per 1,000 Admissions for Non-infective and Non-respiratory Illnesses, by Sex and Age. 1940–47 (Service Cases)

Year	Males					Females				
	Age Groups					Age Groups				
	15–	25–	35–	45–54	All	15–	25–	35–	45–54	All
1940 .	13	10	9	11	11	5	33	—	111	13
1941 .	13	11	9	6	11	8	—	12	83	7
1942 .	13	10	5	11	10	13	14	24	—	14
1943 .	17	11	9	2	13	12	15	—	65	12
1944 .	43	36	19	3	34	10	14	6	—	11
1945 .	12	13	10	5	12	11	6	8	56	10
1946 .	11	9	7	—	10	16	6	—	—	14
1947 .	13	21	31	—	15	—	30	—	—	4

Table 100 shows that among Servicemen the ratio of admissions for burns to the basic total of admissions varied between 1 per cent. and 3·4 per cent., the maximum ratio occurring in 1944, whereas for women the ratio varied from 0·4 to 1·4 per cent. Among males the rates for burns tended to decrease with age except for 1947. The highest ratios, 43 and 36 per 1,000 were for men aged 15–24 and 25–34 in 1944.

An analysis of the total admissions for burns by the part of the body affected is shown in Table 101. About one quarter of men's admissions for burns were included in group 6, the face, head, neck and limbs

TABLE 101

Burns. Total Admissions for 1940–47, by Part of Body affected

M.R.C. Suffix	Site of Involvement	Males		Females	
		Numbers	Proportion	Numbers	Proportion
0	Face, head and neck .	267	105	29	115
1	Trunk	36	14	5	20
2	Upper limb or limbs .	254	99	27	107
3	Hand or hands . .	392	153	21	83
4	Lower limb or limbs .	472	185	116	461
5	Face, head and neck, trunk and limbs .	118	46	4	16
6	Face, head and neck, limbs . . .	650	254	20	79
7	Trunk and limbs .	96	38	11	44
8	Other and unqualified areas . . .	270	106	19	75
0–8	Totals . . .	2,555	1,000	252	1,000

being involved, while in a further 19 per cent. the lower limbs only were affected. Forty-six per cent. of women's admissions were for burns of the lower limbs only, and 12 per cent. involved injury to the sites in group 0. In 1944, the year in which the number of men admitted for burns was greatest, 29 per cent. had involvement of the sites in group 6, 13 per cent. of those in group 4 and 17 per cent. of one or both hands.

An analysis of burns by their causative agent is shown in Table 102. Nearly half the burns among men were caused by fire or hot objects and roughly another 20 per cent. by hot liquids or vapours; 64 per cent. of women's burns were due to scalding and 14 per cent. to fire or hot objects. The case records of 400 patients admitted for burns during 1942 and 1943 were examined in detail, and it was found that of 170 burns caused by fire and hot objects, 43 per cent. were due to burning petrol, 25 per cent. to flames from fires, blow-lamps, cookers, etc., 13 per cent. to incendiary bombs and other instruments of war. (Brooke,

TABLE 102

Burns. Sample Total Admissions for 1940–47, by Causative Agent

M.R.C. Code	Causative Agent	Males		Females	
		Numbers	Proportion	Numbers	Proportion
930	Fire or hot objects .	1,272	498	35	139
931	Hot liquids or vapours .	496	194	161	638
932	Corrosive liquids .	59	23	9	36
933	Various forms of radiations . .	2	1	1	4
934	Electric currents .	27	11	3	12
935	Other agents, or unqualified . .	699	273	43	171
930–5	Totals . .	2,555	1,000	252	1,000

1945.) There seems little doubt that many of the admissions for this cause were due to avoidable accidents.

In the sample of 400 cases, it was found that the distribution of burns according to degree was as follows:

	1st degree	*2nd degree*	*3rd degree*	*Not stated*	*All Types*
Males	9·6	42·8	6·8	40·8	100
Females	22·2	37·8	0	40·0	100

For men the median number of days treatment, including any period of treatment at the unit before admission to hospital, for burns to face, head, neck and limbs was 18 days for first degree burns, 20 days for second degree, 30 for third degree and 19 for all burns of this site including those whose degree was not stated. Women with burns of the lower limbs required 15 days treatment for those of the first degree, 35 days for those of the second degree and 26 days for all burns of this site.

OTHER INJURIES (Short List Number 42)

This group includes open wounds (except of scalp), bruising and contusions with intact skin surface, foreign bodies where admission was primarily for their removal, crushing injuries and traumatic amputations. It also contains a number of conditions which are sequelae of trauma, general effects of external causes, therapeutic misadventures and late complications of therapeutic procedures. In such conditions there is a very wide range in degree of severity so that tables of duration of treatment in hospital would tend to reflect the gravity of the injury rather than give a picture of the amount of hospital time required for restoring the patient to health. For this reason, no attempt is made here

TABLE 103

Open Wounds. Admissions of Servicemen, 1940–47

Nature of Open Wound	1940	1941	1942	1943	1944		1945	1946–7	Totals 1940–47	Proportions per 1,000
					Jan.–June	July–Dec.				
Face and Neck	279	258	414	364	306	372	191	89	2,273	171
Trunk (superficial)	187	50	65	74	215	444	53	11	1,099	82
Upper Limbs	430	249	387	336	471	909	236	108	3,126	235
Lower Limbs	549	248	322	317	492	929	207	61	3,125	234
Open wounds with internal injury of chest	5	6	18	12	29	78	37	—	185	14
Open wounds with internal injury of abdomen	15	4	24	26	31	89	28	5	222	17
Multiple or unqualified	554	324	259	277	524	1,059	206	90	3,293	247
Totals	2,019	1,139	1,489	1,406	2,068	3,880	958	364	13,323	1,000
Proportions	152	85	112	106	155	291	72	27	1,000	

TABLE 104

Sprains and Strains. Admissions of Servicemen, 1940–47

Site of Sprain or Strain	1940	1941	1942	1943	1944	1945	1946–47	1940–47	Proportions
Shoulder, elbow or wrist	33	46	91	51	45	14	7	287	64
Knee	147	213	551	280	237	128	52	1,608	357
Ankle	207	285	429	368	378	188	62	1,917	425
Spine or sacro-iliac region	28	24	50	35	24	13	4	178	39
Other and ill-defined sprains	67	85	134	75	106	33	19	519	115
Totals	482	653	1,255	809	790	376	144	4,509	1,000

to show anything beyond the numbers of men admitted to hospital each year for those of the injuries in this Short List Group which occurred most frequently.

In the one-in-five sample there were 13,323 men and 321 women admitted with a principal diagnosis of open wounds; hence the estimated total number of Servicemen admitted to E.M.S. hospitals for this cause was about 66,600. Table 103 shows that wounds of one upper limb, one lower limb, and of multiple sites each comprised just under a quarter of the total number. Admissions for this cause in the second half of 1944 and in 1945 formed 36 per cent. of the total admissions in the eight years.

The most frequent cause of admission after open wounds was sprains or strains, and from Table 104 it may be seen that the commonest sites were knees and ankles. The greatest number of sprains or strains occurred in 1942 which might be regarded as pre-eminently a training year with the Armed Forces. Taking the three age groups 15–24, 25–34, 35 and over, the percentage of sprains in each group was:

Knee, 41, 45, 14; Ankle, 43, 44, 13; Other sites, 42, 40, 18

The proportion of sprains occurring at ages 25–34 was therefore higher for injuries to ankle or knee than for other sites. If to the 1,608 men with sprained knees be added the 3,890 whose primary cause of admission was internal derangement of the knee joint, a sample total of 5,498 admissions is obtained, to which corresponds an estimated total of 27,500.

Another large group of admissions was attributable to bruising, contusion or haematoma, with intact skin surface. For this cause 3,802 men and 229 women in the sample were admitted to hospital, the number of yearly admissions being shown in Table 105. Bruising of the trunk and of a lower limb or hip together accounted for half the total admissions for this cause, and the highest yearly number of cases occurred, as in the case of sprains or strains, in 1942.

The numbers treated primarily for dislocations (Table 106) also showed a maximum in 1942. The site most commonly affected was the shoulder, this being the part affected in nearly two-fifths of all dislocations.

For the group of conditions shown in number 94 of the M.R.C. Classification, under the title of 'General Effects of External Causes', 1,593 men in the sample were admitted; an analysis of these admissions is shown in Table 107. More than half these patients were admitted with a diagnosis assignable to M.R.C. number 9496, and of the 818 men admitted for this reason in 1944, the majority were suffering from Battle Exhaustion, a syndrome brought on by the stress of conditions

TABLE 105

Bruising, Contusion or Haematoma. Admissions of Servicemen. 1940–47. Numbers in Sample and Proportions per 1,000

Bruising, Contusion or Haematoma	1940	1941	1942	1943	1944	1945	1946–47	1940–47	Proportions
Face	46	39	95	41	58	32	13	324	85
Trunk	119	140	211	156	104	55	32	817	215
Genital Organs	17	28	45	24	22	9	3	148	39
Bruising unqualified	55	80	52	51	72	30	26	366	96
Upper Limb or Shoulder	37	73	100	60	53	29	11	363	95
Lower Limb or Hip	116	168	259	209	201	84	41	1,078	284
Foot	34	55	89	68	62	24	11	343	90
Haemarthrosis of knee joint	8	21	28	19	20	8	5	109	29
Other bruising and haemarthroses	41	39	51	42	57	14	10	254	67
Totals	473	643	930	670	649	285	152	3,802	1,000

TABLE 106

Dislocations. Admissions of Servicemen, 1940–47. Numbers in Sample and Proportion per 1,000 Dislocations

Site of Dislocation	1940	1941	1942	1943	1944	1945	1946–47	1940–47	Proportions
Shoulder	41	68	75	73	60	35	19	371	390
Elbow	19	18	31	32	31	33	10	174	183
Finger or thumb	14	20	17	14	23	12	10	110	115
Knee	12	15	25	18	17	10	11	108	113
Other or unqualified	20	25	44	34	32	22	13	190	199
Totals	106	146	192	171	163	112	63	953	1,000

TABLE 107

General Effects of External Causes. Admissions of Servicemen, 1940–47

M.R.C. No.	General Effects of External Causes	1940	1941	1942	1943	1944	1945	1946–7	1940–47	Proportions
941	Drowning and immersion	10	12	15	18	15	4	—	74	46
942	Hunger or thirst*	—	—	—	—	—	254	12	266	167
943	Excessive cold, including frostbite	8	7	4	1	11	81	5	117	73
947	Bites and stings of venomous animals	17	15	30	13	24	10	7	116	73
9496	Other or unspecified effects†	48	6	4	10	818	17	1	904	568
Rest of 94	Other general effects	24	19	21	22	17	6	7	116	73
	Totals	107	59	74	64	885	372	32	1,593	1,000

* This title includes malnutrition in returning prisoners-of-war.
† This title includes 'battle exhaustion'.

of warfare on the Western Front. A detailed analysis of the records of 500 such cases, who were not at the same time suffering from either trauma or disease has already been presented (Brooke, 1945). The age distribution of these patients showed no marked difference from that of all injury cases. The median period in hospital for men aged 15–34 was 54 days, which is 9 days longer than for a random group of patients with non-combat neurosis. It was further noticed that men with less than 2 or more than 4 years' service were the more likely to break down. As regards family influence, it was found that nearly three-quarters of those whose family history had been recorded had one or more unstable first degree relatives while many of the patients who broke down had shown such predisposing traits as 'nervy or neurotic, fears, somatic symptoms, shy, solitary or moody'. Cases did not appear to occur more frequently in active than in passive units and the general conclusion was that an inherited predisposition to instability rather than an external factor was the causative agent of the breakdown.

In 1945 a number of returned prisoners-of-war in a serious state of undernourishment were admitted to E.M.S. hospitals. The diagnosis in these cases was coded to M.R.C. 942, since it was felt that these men were suffering from deprivation of food rather than malnutrition in the sense in which it is implied in M.R.C. number 269. In all 266 men in the sample were admitted for this condition, or about 1,330 actual admissions.

The remaining group of importance in Short List Number 42, is that of complications of trauma where these were primary causes of admission. From Table 108 it will be seen that nearly half the admissions in this group were due to loss of joint function following recent injury, the estimated total admitted for this cause being between 2,845 and 3,085.

HOMOLOGOUS SERUM JAUNDICE (*See* p. 690)

Though not generally appearing as a primary cause of admission, a condition which caused great concern was jaundice or hepatitis following the administration of blood, plasma or serum. (M.R.C. Code 963.) The appearance of hepatitis in patients who received inoculation with blood products was not an occurrence peculiar to the Second World War, but the increase in the number of casualties so treated, with a resulting increase in the number developing homologous serum jaundice served to focus attention on the problem. Oliphant (1944) gives a chronological list in which the earliest report was that of Hirsch (1883–84), recording the vaccination of 1,289 persons with humanised lymph in glycerine, as a result of which 191 people developed jaundice, the incubation period varying from several weeks to 2 months. Further cases were reported following the administration of convalescent

TABLE 108

Complications of Trauma. Admissions of Servicemen, 1940–47

M.R.C. No.	Nature of Complication of Trauma	1940	1941	1942	1943	1944	1945	1946–7	1940–47	Proportions
892	Delayed healing of wounds . .	6	7	10	20	26	23	1	93	73
893	Persistent sinus following injury .	8	9	16	54	78	36	10	211	166
895	Persistent paralysis due to nerve injury	2	10	12	9	14	4	1	52	41
896	Loss of muscular function due to tendon injury	7	12	16	20	28	16	4	103	81
897	Symptoms from scars of traumatic origin.	—	12	35	42	57	34	10	190	150
898	Loss of joint function following recent injury	31	41	62	177	194	67	21	593	468
Rest of 89	Other complications of trauma . .	3	0	1	5	13	3	2	27	21
	Totals	57	91	152	327	410	183	49	1,269	1,000

measles serum (MacNalty, 1937), Yellow Fever vaccine (Findlay and MacCullum, 1938; Soper and Smith, 1938; Fox and others, 1942), blood transfusion, mumps convalescent serum (Ministry of Health, 1943), citrated blood and pooled plasma (Beeson, 1943) and serum, plasma or both (Morgan and Williamson, 1942). If when pooled blood products are used, one donor has contributed an icterogenic agent, any or all of the recipients of this blood are liable to infection. Further, Bradley, Loutit and Maunsell (1944) have shown that in their series of cases the clinical features and biochemical findings in homologous serum jaundice were indistinguishable from those of infective hepatitis, so that diagnosis must depend on a history of injection or transfusion. It is not possible to detect by laboratory or animal tests the presence of an icterogenic agent in blood intended for transfusion, which makes accurate recording of batch or bottle numbers desirable. The distinguishing feature of homologous serum jaundice is its long incubation period of 2–3 months as compared with 20–40 days in the case of infective hepatitis.

In an attempt to estimate the incidence of serum jaundice all case histories in the sample of E.M.S. hospital admissions which had already been coded to jaundice were re-examined for mention of blood transfusion or inoculation. At the same time all incoming records were examined and information was recorded about the three following groups:

(i) injured patients who were transfused.
(ii) sick patients who were transfused.
(iii) injured patients who were not transfused.

The size this investigation would assume was not anticipated at the start, or the records of blood transfusion jaundice got from re-examining jaundice cases would have been kept separate from those obtained from incoming records. The following tables, while not covering all cases in the three groups admitted during 1940–45, give some indication of the incidence and case-fatality rates among Servicemen under observation for 3 months or more after injury or transfusion.

TABLE 109

Incidence of Jaundice following Blood Transfusion, 1940–45, among Servicemen under observation for 3 months or more after transfusion or injury

Group whose hospital records were examined	Total number of patients whose records were examined	Numbers who developed jaundice during observation	Number of these who died subsequently to jaundice	Incidence rate per 1,000 in observation period (and standard error)
Injured patients who were transfused .	1,316	124	17	94±8
Sick patients who were transfused .	82	16	7	195±49
Injured patients who were not transfused .	6,350	6	0	0·9±0·3

Table 109 shows that in all 7,748 records were examined in the three groups and that of 1,398 sick or injured patients who were transfused, 140 subsequently developed jaundice of whom 24 died. The overall incidence and case-fatality rates in the transfused group were 100 and 171 per 1,000 respectively. Among injured patients who were not transfused there were 6 cases of jaundice of whom none died, the incidence rate being therefore 0·9 per 1,000. The incidence rate among injured patients who were transfused was 94 per 1,000 and the case-fatality rate 137 per 1,000. The case-fatality rates when compared with that of 2·4 per 1,000 for cases of infective hepatitis show a much higher death-rate among cases of homologous serum jaundice.

Jaundice was known to be rife among both Allied and enemy forces in North Africa, hence it might be that where a record of blood transfusion and of a subsequent attack of jaundice occurred in a case from the Mediterranean theatre of war, it was by a coincidence that they occurred to the same patient. The 7,666 cases of injury were therefore analysed according to the theatre of war in which the injury was received, and the results are shown in Table 110.

TABLE 110

Incidence of Jaundice following Blood Transfusion. Admissions for injuries analysed by Theatre of War in which injury occurred

	Transfused			Not Transfused		
	Total examined	Jaundice developed	Died after jaundice	Total examined	Jaundice developed	Died after jaundice
Mediterranean	308	55	6	905	0	0
Western Europe	613	55	9	2,133	0	0
Far East	30	5	1	80	0	0
United Kingdom	107	8	1	1,240	3	0
Not stated	258	1	0	1,992	3	0
Totals	1,316	124	17	6,350	6	0

Jaundice therefore occurred in 179 per 1,000 of those who were injured in the Mediterranean theatre and subsequently received a blood transfusion, whereas there was no instance of jaundice reported among 905 men injured in that theatre but not transfused. In Western Europe 90 per 1,000 of those injured and transfused developed jaundice, but no mention of jaundice occurred in the records of 2,133 men who were injured but not transfused. The incidence of jaundice was greater, for every theatre of war, among the transfused than among those who had not received transfusion.

In considering the incidence of jaundice in the cases discussed above, no attention has been paid to the period between transfusion and onset of jaundice. In some instances the administration of blood of an incompatible group produced a reaction within up to 14 days; allowing therefore for delay in recording, it might be assumed that where jaundice was stated to have appeared in less than 10 days from the transfusion, it was haemolytic, rather than homologous serum jaundice which was observed. In cases which appeared to have a short incubation period, the possibility that the patient was experiencing an attack of an infective hepatitis contracted before the transfusion was given cannot be ruled out.

The search for cases in which jaundice followed blood transfusion was continued after the above tables had been made, and altogether 175 cases were found. The intervals between transfusion and the appearance of jaundice showed the following distribution, two or more periods being recorded where more than one transfusion was given. (The left-hand number of each pair shows the number of days elapsing; the second number gives the frequency.)

Days	F.	Days	F.	Days	F.	Days	F.	Days	F.	Days	F.	Days	F.	Days	F.	Days	F.	Days	F.
1	4	19	1	48	2	62	3	75	4	88	6	101	3	116	1	132	1	176	1
3	2	23	1	49	2	63	5	76	5	89	3	102	1	117	1	133	2	181	1
4	1	27	1	50	1	64	5	77	3	90	5	103	3	118	1	134	2	203	1
5	2	28	3	52	3	65	2	78	4	91	3	104	2	119	2	142	2	209	1
6	1	30	2	53	1	66	2	79	3	92	4	105	1	120	1	143	1	215	1
8	2	31	1	54	1	67	3	80	1	93	2	106	3	121	2	147	2	243	1
9	1	32	3	55	2	68	3	81	4	94	3	107	4	122	5	153	1	283	1
11	1	33	1	56	1	69	4	82	3	95	5	108	3	123	3	156	4	285	1
12	2	35	1	57	3	70	4	83	5	96	3	109	3	124	1	158	1	288	1
13	1	38	2	58	4	71	3	84	2	97	1	111	3	125	1	161	1	290	1
16	2	42	1	59	2	72	4	85	3	98	3	112	1	128	3	166	1		
17	1	44	1	60	3	73	7	86	6	99	3	114	3	130	1	170	1		
18	1	46	1	61	3	74	2	87	2	100	2	115	3	131	1	173	1		

2 less than 12, 1 not more than 76,
1 not more than 77; one more than 92.

Of the cases in which the periods were stated exactly, 13 had intervals of less than 10 days and there were 276 with intervals of 10 days or more. If those cases with less than 10 days' interval be regarded as haemolytic jaundice, the median interval for the remaining cases is 85 days, the lower quartile being 65 days and the upper quartile 107 days.

In 152 cases there was a record of either blood or plasma or both having been given; the total quantities administered to each patient were estimated and the distribution is shown in Table 111. In all 54 people received blood only and 27 received plasma only, while the remainder received varying quantities of each. In addition 4 people received serum only, 2 serum and blood and 1 had serum, blood and plasma.

In records of infective hepatitis the most frequently mentioned first symptoms were:

nausea 18 per cent. anorexia 18 per cent.
abdominal pain 16 per cent. vomiting 11 per cent.

The same symptoms were among the first five most frequently mentioned in cases of homologous serum jaundice, with frequencies:

nausea 14 per cent. anorexia 16 per cent.
abdominal pain 17 per cent. vomiting 18 per cent.

TABLE III

Jaundice following Blood Transfusion. Distribution of Total Quantities of blood and plasma given to each patient

	Plasma (pints)											
		0	1	2	3	4	5	6	7	8	N.S.	All
Blood (pints)	0	—	6	8	3	2	1	—	2	1	4	27
	1	12	7	3	3	1	—	—	—	—	2	28
	2	12	1	6	2	2	—	1	—	—	—	24
	3	6	6	4	2	3	2	—	—	—	1	24
	4	4	—	2	—	—	—	—	—	—	—	6
	5	—	—	—	—	2	1	1	—	—	—	4
	6	5	1	—	1	—	—	—	—	—	1	8
	7	2	1	—	—	—	—	—	—	—	—	3
	8	2	1	1	—	—	—	—	—	—	—	4
	9	—	1	—	—	—	—	—	1	—	—	2
	10	—	1	—	1	—	—	—	—	—	—	2
	11	1	1	1	—	—	—	—	—	—	—	3
	12	1	1	—	—	—	—	—	—	—	1	3
	N.S.	9	—	—	—	—	—	—	—	—	5	14
	All	54	27	25	12	10	4	2	3	1	14	152

In the latter, however, bile-stained urine was the first symptom mentioned in 18 per cent. of the cases, compared with 6 per cent. in cases of infective hepatitis.

While the investigation was being carried out the question was raised of whether the administration of pentothal was in any way connected with the incidence of jaundice. The records of those who had had homologous serum jaundice were therefore re-examined for mention of pentothal, and this was found in 63 cases or 36 per cent. The intervals between administration of pentothal and onset of jaundice were distributed:

Days	F.	Days	F.	Days	F.	Days	F.	Days	F.	Days	F.	Days	F.	Days	F.	Days	F.
4	1	40	1	57	2	69	1	79	1	92	1	109	2	122	1	161	1
10	1	44	1	59	2	70	4	81	1	94	2	110	1	123	1	218	1
13	1	49	1	60	1	73	2	82	2	95	2	111	1	130	1	289	1
26	1	50	1	63	2	74	2	83	1	100	1	114	1	132	1	327	1
30	1	51	1	64	1	75	2	84	1	101	1	117	1	135	1		
31	1	52	1	65	2	76	1	88	4	104	3	118	1	136	1		
34	1	53	1	67	1	77	2	89	2	106	1	119	2	142	1		
39	1	55	1	68	3	78	4	90	4	107	3	121	1	159	1		

The median interval was 82 days, the lower quartile 57 days and the upper quartile 106 days. The distribution was very similar to that for intervals between blood transfusion and jaundice. Such a similarity would however be expected since it was usually shortly after injury that the patient was anaesthetised while his injuries were being dressed and then also that he received blood transfusions. It was not possible at the time to select a series of cases from which all other possible jaundice-causing factors were absent and in which some had and others had not had pentothal.

There were 23 deaths in the series, but the cause of death was not stated in every case. Among the eighteen in which the cause was defined, 3 were attributed to acute yellow atrophy following infective hepatitis, 3 to necrosis of the liver, 3 to toxic hepatitis, 2 to liver failure due to infective hepatitis and 1 to jaundice and cerebral abscess.

EXTERNAL CAUSES OF ACCIDENTS

The external causes of accidents are classified in the M.R.C. List in three main groups, traffic accidents, those chiefly likely to occur in the course of an occupation, whether civilian or with the Services, and other accidents such as falls, blows, injuries at sport, etc. (Detailed list p. 740.) Accidents treated in E.M.S. hospitals are further classified according to whether they were stated in the records to be due to enemy action or not so stated; the number ascribed to operations of war may therefore be an understatement of the true figure. The proportions of total admissions assigned to M.R.C. numbers 80–96 which were ascribed to enemy action in the seven years 1940–46 were as follows:

	1940	1941	1942	1943	1944	1945	1946	1940–46
Percentage	27	5	3	9	48	25	2	23

In the sample only 494 traffic accidents were assigned to enemy action, of which 233 occurred in water transport and 159 in air transport. It is estimated that about 65,000 Servicemen were admitted for traffic accidents not due to operations of war. The annual proportionate composition of admissions for these reasons, together with the estimated total admissions for the whole seven years are shown in Table 112.

The largest group involved in traffic accidents were drivers of motorcycles injured on the road, about 23,000 being admitted to E.M.S. hospitals. Admissions of motor cycle drivers varied between 29 per cent. and 38 per cent. of all traffic accidents in the seven years and formed 35 per cent. of all traffic accidents other than those due to war operations during 1940–46. Passengers or unspecified occupants of motor vehicles formed the second largest group, about 11,500 being estimated to have been admitted, with annual proportionate rates varying between 15 per cent. and 21 per cent. of the total in each year. Admissions for water transport accidents were estimated to be about 2,200 but these would in all probability be due to accidents occurring round our shores; further, a good proportion of men would go to one or other of the Royal Naval Hospitals, while those incurring accidents during long voyages

TABLE 112

Proportionate Composition of Admissions due to Traffic Accidents (not due to Operations of War) among Male Service Personnel, 1940–46

M.R.C. Code Suffix	External Cause	Proportions per 1,000 Admissions								Estimated Total Admissions
		1940	1941	1942	1943	1944	1945	1946	1940–46	
0	Railway accident	23	17	29	14	15	30	37	21	1,380 ± 83
1	Driver of motor cycle injured on road	381	360	345	374	358	291	327	353	22,795 ± 338
2	Driver of other motor vehicle injured on road	27	24	30	27	23	23	29	26	1,665 ± 91
3	Passenger or unspecified occupant of motor vehicle	185	187	156	153	190	188	208	177	11,460 ± 239
4	Pedestrian injured by motor vehicle	101	111	101	67	64	72	53	85	5,475 ± 165
5	Other or unspecified motor vehicle accident on road (including pedal cyclist injured by motor vehicle)	95	83	90	73	96	117	139	93	6,010 ± 173
6	Pedal cyclist injured on road, not by rail or motor vehicle	26	40	78	95	64	84	49	64	4,120 ± 144
7	Other or unspecified road transport accident	75	63	54	72	70	98	98	71	4,600 ± 152
8	Water transport accident	24	30	27	35	47	41	30	34	2,185 ± 105
9	Air transport accident (including glider and parachute accidents)	63	85	90	90	73	56	30	76	4,895 ± 156
	Totals	1,000	1,000	1,000	1,000	1,000	1,000	1,000	1,000	64,585 ± 568

would have been treated on board and in all probability not need hospital treatment on reaching their destination.

TABLE 113

Proportionate Composition by Nature of Injury of Admissions due to certain types of Traffic Accidents (including those due to Operations of War) among Male Service Personnel, 1940–46

M.R.C. Code	Nature of Injury	M.R.C. Suffix for External Cause of Accident							
		1	2	4	5	6	7	8	9
800	Head Injuries (not fractures) .	145	226	272	236	228	220	87	173
840	Fractures of skull . . .	51	68	55	85	90	85	31	60
	Total head injuries . .	196	294	327	321	318	305	118	233
801	Open wounds, face and neck .	40	55	41	76	93	73	42	57
804	Open wounds, lower limbs .	56	15	27	35	13	22	51	22
807	Open wounds, multiple or N.O.S.	54	52	71	76	65	73	48	112
Rest 80	Open wounds, other sites .	14	18	13	19	22	20	55	29
	Total open wounds (not head).	164	140	152	206	193	188	196	220
810–1	Bruising, contusions, haematoma . . .	64	104	99	78	67	86	72	45
841	Fractures, vertebral column .	10	40	13	15	7	12	25	43
842	Fractures, other trunk bones .	13	46	32	36	14	29	25	13
843	Fractures, upper limb . .	117	116	51	92	178	86	99	69
844	Fractures, lower limb . .	273	103	205	128	74	138	128	112
845	Fractures, multiple . .	88	57	52	61	31	65	31	77
	Total fractures (not skull only)	501	362	353	332	304	330	308	314
846–7	Dislocations, sprains and strains	47	60	34	32	73	40	69	46
93	Burns	2	7	—	5	4	3	97	84
Rest 80–96	Other types of injury . .	26	33	35	26	41	48	140	58
	Total Injuries	1,000	1,000	1,000	1,000	1,000	1,000	1,000	1,000

Table 113 shows the types of injury incurred by the chief groups of victims of traffic accidents. Half the men involved in accidents on railways had a principal diagnosis of fracture, the legs being most commonly affected, and about a further 20 per cent. had head injuries, of which a quarter were fractures of the skull. Nearly 30 per cent. of the injured drivers of motor cycles received head injuries, fractures of the skull and other head injuries occurring in the proportion 7:23. A further 36 per cent. had fractures, the upper and lower limbs being the most frequently involved sites. Among pedestrians injured by motor vehicles, 33 per cent. had head injuries and 35 per cent. fractures other than of skull. Burns formed a higher proportion of the total injuries in both water and air transport accidents than in any other form of traffic accident, the percentages being 10 and 8 respectively.

The proportionate annual composition of admissions attributed to bombs and the effects of blast, gunshot and other explosive missiles is shown in Table 114.

Taken over the seven years, the number of bomb injuries attributed to war operations was 2·8 times those not so ascribed; corresponding

TABLE 114

Annual Proportionate Distribution of Admissious due to Injury by Bombs and Effect of Blast, Gunshot and Other Explosive Missiles, among Male Service Personnel, 1940–46

M.R.C. Code Suffix	External Cause	Proportions per 1,000 Admissions								Estimated Total Admissions
		1940	1941	1942	1943	1944	1945	1946	1940–46	
Due to Operations of War										
4V	Bombs (including mines, grenades, depth charges and effects of blast) .	160	63	41	81	566	89	0	1,000	12,360±249
5V	Gunshot (including rifle, machine gun and small arms)	148	10	27	69	618	125	3	1,000	18,900±307
6V	Other explosives (including mortar, cannon, breechblock, weapon burst and shrapnel) .	123	7	10	38	724	97	1	1,000	25,270±355
Not due to Operations of War										
4V	Bombs, etc., and effects of blast . . .	53	67	225	222	283	133	17	1,000	4,420±149
5V	Gunshot, etc. . . .	152	110	179	143	287	109	20	1,000	9,485±218
6V	Shrapnel, etc. . . .	110	61	137	176	403	90	23	1,000	3,760±137

TABLE 115

Proportionate Composition by Nature of Injury of Admissions due to Injury by Bomb, Gunshot and Other Explosive Missiles. Male Service Personnel, 1940–46

M.R.C. Code Number	Nature of Injury	External Cause of Injury					
		Bombs and Effects of Blast		Gunshot		Other Explosive Missiles	
		War Operation	Not War Operation	War Operation	Not War Operation	War Operation	Not War Operation
800	Head Injury (not fracture) .	70	38	17	14	32	45
840	Fracture of Skull . . .	21	27	23	19	18	24
		91	65	40	33	50	69
801	Open wounds, face and neck .	57	94	28	42	42	47
802	Open wounds, trunk . .	34	32	61	72	79	81
803	Open wounds, upper limb .	50	52	116	150	127	129
804	Open wounds, lower limb .	70	78	154	198	136	136
805–6	Open wounds, with internal injuries to chest or abdomen . .	18	14	30	38	24	12
807	Open wounds, multiple or N.O.S. . .	177	172	121	65	163	185
801–7	Total open wounds (not head) .	406	442	510	565	571	590
810–1	Bruising, Contusion, Haematoma	23	23	1	2	1	9
817–18	Traumatic Amputations . .	76	28	11	19	22	29
841	Fracture, vertebral column .	12	3	8	5	7	3
842	Fracture, trunk . . .	12	5	16	12	12	4
843	Fracture, upper limb . .	62	62	118	122	78	69
844	Fracture, lower limb . .	94	95	132	145	117	66
845	Fracture, multiple . . .	68	42	52	25	47	17
841–5	Total fractures (not skull). .	248	207	326	309	261	159
87	Shock	12	10	2	1	2	4
93	Burns	19	139	11	5	2	40
Rest, 80–96	Other types of injury . .	125	86	99	66	91	100
80–96	Total Injuries.	1,000	1,000	1,000	1,000	1,000	1,000

ratios for gunshot and for shrapnel and other explosive injuries were 2·0 and 6·7. Of injuries attributed in the records to war operations 57 per cent. of the seven year total due to the effects of bombs or blast, 62 per cent. of those due to gunshot and 72 per cent. of those due to shrapnel and other explosives caused admissions in the year 1944. Twenty-two per cent. of bomb injuries not attributed to enemy action occurred in each of 1942 and 1943, and a further 28 per cent. in 1944, but 40 per cent. of shrapnel injuries caused admissions in this year which suggests that more of such injuries should have been attributed to war operations. In all about 56,500 missile injuries were ascribed to war operations and 17,700 not so ascribed.

Table 115 shows a comparison of the nature of the injuries caused by these missiles, those due to war operations being distinguished from the others. Gunshot caused fractures of the skull rather than other types of head injury, whereas the reverse was true for bombs and shrapnel. Bombs and blast and shrapnel caused more open wounds of multiple sites but gunshot wounds were more frequent in the lower limbs.

Of the injuries caused by shrapnel in war operations, 26 per cent. were fractures other than of skull, compared with 16 per cent. of those not stated to be due to enemy action.

Among the remaining types of external cause, included under suffixes 0X-9X, 5X and 7X-9X provide for the classification of causes about which information is not precise. Such accidents as falls, crushing, blows and accidents during sport would be likely to occur in civilian life, but under Service conditions some of the injuries caused might be more likely to result in admission to hospital whereas normally they would be treated at home or in the Out-patients' Department. As shown in Table 116 it is estimated that nearly 20,000 men were admitted with injuries received during sport during 1940–46, in addition to which a

TABLE 116

Annual Proportionate Distribution of Admissions due to Falls, Blows and other External Causes with M.R.C. suffix 0X–9X (not due to Operations of War) among Male Service Personnel, 1940–46

M.R.C. Code Suffix	External Cause	Proportions per 1,000 Admissions								Estimated Total Admissions
		1940	1941	1942	1943	1944	1945	1946	1940–46	
0X	Fall	107	132	274	191	161	101	34	1,000	26,680 ± 365
1X	Crushing	73	127	197	216	259	109	19	1,000	8,545 ± 207
2X	Blow	100	135	212	212	203	99	39	1,000	12,310 ± 248
3X	Explosion (not included elsewhere)	58	90	130	181	352	152	36	1,000	1,385 ± 83
4X	Accident during sport	104	176	238	178	156	110	38	1,000	19,940 ± 316
6X	Unclassified or unspecified cause of injury on duty	93	143	193	214	227	105	25	1,000	18,650 ± 305
5X; 7X–9X	Other causes of injury in the home, or elsewhere	113	139	220	171	211	106	40	1,000	46,545 ± 482
0X-9X		103	142	226	189	199	106	35	1,000	134,055 ± 819

proportion of the 18,650 estimated admissions ascribed to suffix 6X would be due to injuries received during physical training. Nearly a quarter of the total injuries causing admission which were received during sport occurred in 1942. In this year also 27 per cent. of the injuries due to falls occurred, the estimated total number of admissions due to this cause during 1940–46 being about 26,700. If the small number of admissions during 1946 be deducted, the average number of admissions over the remaining six years is nearly 21,000 a year, and the amount of time lost to service, coupled with that during which hospital beds were occupied suggests that every effort should be made to reduce the number of accidents ascribed to these causes.

Table 117 shows the proportionate composition by nature of injury of admissions attributable to falls, crushing, blows, injuries during

TABLE 117

Proportionate Composition by Nature of Injury of Admissions due to Falls, Blows, Crushing, Injuries at Sport and Injuries incurred while on duty, but not otherwise specified, 1940–46

M.R.C. Code	Nature of Injury	M.R.C. Suffix for External Cause (*See* Table 116)				
		0X	1X	2X	4X	6X
800	Head Injury (not fracture)	89	8	172	44	29
840	Fracture of skull	34	13	133	43	19
	Total head injuries	123	21	305	87	48
801	Open wounds, face and neck	27	6	78	10	23
803	Open wounds.	13	90	19	2	29
804	Open wounds, lower limbs	15	22	22	10	13
807	Open wounds, multiple or N.O.S.	7	4	7	1	9
802, 5, 6	Open wounds, other sites	3	3	2	1	4
	Total open wounds (not head)	65	125	128	24	78
810–1	Bruising, Contusions, Haematoma	128	101	221	130	60
815–6	Crushing Injuries	3	91	4	4	5
841	Fracture, vertebral column	25	15	12	6	13
842	Fracture, other trunk bones	25	37	17	11	8
843	Fracture, upper limbs	202	195	105	131	120
844	Fracture, lower limbs	192	304	142	257	255
845	Fracture, multiple	32	27	9	3	19
	Total fractures (not skull)	476	578	285	408	415
846–7	Dislocations, sprains and strains	187	23	36	331	203
93	Burns	4	1	1	2	100
Rest, 80–96	Other types of injury	14	60	20	14	91
80–96	*Totals*	1,000	1,000	1,000	1,000	1,000

sport and those incurred while on duty but not otherwise specified. Twelve per cent. of the injuries caused by falls involved the head and another 19 per cent. were dislocations, sprains and strains. Half the crushing injuries resulted in either a fractured arm or leg, compared with 39 per cent. in the case of falls, 25 per cent. for blows, 39 per cent. for injuries at sport and 38 per cent. for injuries on duty. Dislocations, sprains and strains were 33 per cent. of the injuries received during sport.

Part II. Civilian Patients

Four main groups of civilian patients were entitled to treatment in E.M.S. hospitals:

(a) Merchant Navy officers and men, sick and injured.
(b) Evacuee children, refugees from Gibraltar and the Channel Islands, sick civilians moved from target areas, transferred war workers and those in agricultural and forestry camps.
(c) Civilians, including regular Police, suffering from war injuries and injuries incurred in the performance of Civil Defence duties.
(d) Cases of fractures and certain other types of injury occurring among manual workers in factories and full-time Civil Defence workers.

ADMISSIONS FOR DISEASES

In the one-fifth sample of admissions to E.M.S. hospitals 14,421 males and 8,852 females were admitted during 1940–46 for treatment of diseases, the estimated total admission being about 72,000 men and boys and 44,000 women and girls. The proportions admitted in individual years from 1940 to 1946 were:

	1940	1941	1942	1943	1944	1945	1946	1940–46
Males .	309	284	107	76	162	47	15	1,000
Females	344	233	58	46	264	53	2	1,000

Fifty-nine per cent. of the males and 58 per cent. of the females were admitted during 1940 and 1941; the annual proportions decreased in 1942–43, increased again in 1944 and then further declined in 1945–46, for both sexes.

The proportionate age and sex composition of the two groups was:

Ages	0–	1–	5–	10–	15–	25–	35–	55–	75 up	All
Males										
Numbers .	54	202	275	458	2,179	3,109	5,276	2,424	444	14,421
Proportion	4	14	19	32	151	216	365	168	31	1,000
Females .										
Numbers .	53	163	212	303	1,412	1,393	2,568	2,033	715	8,852
Proportion	6	18	24	34	160	157	290	230	81	1,000
Males per 100 Females .	102	124	130	151	154	223	205	119	62	163

The preponderance of males over females admitted at ages 15–54 is attributable to admissions of merchant seamen and men engaged in Civil Defence duties.

Appendix II(a) (page 814) shows the proportions per 1,000 total admissions for illness in each year from 1940 to 1945, the diseases in M.R.C. numbers 00-76 being divided into 15 groups, following the arrangement shown on pages 17–19 of the M.R.C. Classification, but grouping together congenital malformations and diseases peculiar to the first year of life. The groups showing the highest proportional rates for males and females at all ages in the six years 1940–45 were as follows:

	1940		1941		1942		1943		1944		1945	
	Males											
1	Digestive	251	Digestive	203	Digestive	247	Digestive	247	Digestive	259	Digestive	244
2	Nervous, sense organs	156	Infective, parasitic	202	Infective, parasitic	205	Nervous, sense organs	170	Infective, parasitic	202	Nervous, sense organs	215
3	Infective, parasitic	147	Nervous, sense organs	189	Nervous, sense organs	123	Infective, parasitic	155	Nervous, sense organs	190	Infective, parasitic	206
4	Respiratory	81	Bones, organs of movement	99	Skin, cellular tissue	101	Bones, organs of movement	113	Skin, cellular tissue	79	Respiratory	95
5	Bones, organs of movement	81	Skin, cellular tissue	93	Bones, organs of movement	99	Skin, cellular tissue	101	Respiratory	73	Skin, cellular tissue	71
	Females											
1	Nervous, sense organs	329	Nervous, sense organs	319	Nervous, sense organs	253	{ Infective, parasitic	171	Nervous, sense organs	387	Nervous, sense organs	552
2	Digestive	125	Digestive	164	Digestive	162	{ Nervous, sense organs	171	Digestive	157	Infective, parasitic	102
3	Infective, parasitic	118	Infective, parasitic	111	Infective, parasitic	135	{ Skin, cellular tissue	143	Infective, parasitic	84	Digestive	82
4	Circulatory	85	Skin, cellular tissue	72	Ill-defined, symptomatic	81	{ Bones, organs of movement	143	Skin, cellular tissue	72	{ Genito-urinary	61
5	Respiratory	79	Pregnancy, Childbirth, etc.	68	{ Respiratory { Circulatory	63 63	Digestive	114	Ill-defined, symptomatic	60	{ Bones, organs of movement	61

The disparity in the size of the groups of diseases is one factor in determining their order of relative frequency. Hence it is to be expected that diseases of the digestive system, a group covering numbers 47–55 of the M.R.C. Classification, will have a high frequency, and for males it was the most important group in each year, accounting for from 20–26 per cent. of the annual admissions. Among females, diseases of the digestive system were second in importance to those of the nervous system and sense organs during 1940 to 1942 and in 1944, whereas in 1943 they were fifth in order of frequency and third in 1945. This group accounted for percentages of the total admissions for diseases varying from 8 per cent. in 1945 to 16 per cent. in 1941 and 1942. The most important group responsible for females' admissions was that affecting the nervous system and sense organs, and the proportion of admissions for this cause varied from 17 per cent. in 1943 up to 55 per cent. in 1945. Infective and parasitic diseases, and diseases of the respiratory system, of bones, joints and organs of movement, and of skin and cellular tissue were also among the groups occurring most frequently.

Of all admissions of males for diseases of the digestive system, hernia accounted for 39 per cent., diseases of the intestines for 20 per cent., of stomach and duodenum for 15 per cent. and of the pharynx and oesophagus for 15 per cent. Among women's admissions for diseases of this system, diseases of the intestines (notably appendicitis) accounted for 39 per cent., of the pharynx and oesophagus for 25 per cent. and

TABLE 118

Civilian Patients admitted to E.M.S. Hospitals, 1940–45. Proportions per 1,000 total admissions for illness in each age group, for infective and parasitic diseases, diseases of nervous system and sense organs, and those of digestive system

Year	Males							Females						
	Age Groups							Age Groups						
	0–	15–	25–	35–	55–	75 up	All	0–	15–	25–	35–	55–	75 up	All
Infective and Parasitic														
1940	269	259	198	103	17	—	147	261	208	103	81	40	—	118
1941	250	306	280	135	34	—	202	53	278	102	20	34	—	111
1942	100	296	202	190	91	—	205	250	186	167	—	91	—	135
1943	667	260	118	143	31	—	155	—	91	384	—	—	—	171
1944	143	200	286	179	115	—	202	500	50	222	—	—	—	84
1945	500	301	264	121	73	—	206	—	124	250	63	—	—	102
Nervous System and Sense Organs														
1940	39	86	138	176	242	333	156	130	208	277	460	600	133	329
1941	71	83	150	251	311	200	189	158	148	245	492	484	714	319
1942	200	111	98	116	273	—	123	250	116	233	456	454	—	253
1943	—	123	219	161	187	—	170	—	181	—	250	1,000	—	171
1944	143	147	174	213	262	—	190	500	200	499	445	545	—	387
1945	—	107	165	302	293	1,000	215	—	250	500	749	778	—	552
Digestive System														
1940	154	225	293	291	156	—	251	217	291	173	54	—	—	125
1941	196	185	220	231	139	—	203	368	296	61	102	104	—	164
1942	500	241	231	260	205	1,000	247	—	350	67	45	—	—	162
1943	333	260	237	262	187	—	247	—	182	77	125	—	—	114
1944	428	348	199	257	197	200	259	—	500	56	74	—	—	157
1945	500	252	290	215	171	—	244	—	187	—	—	111	—	82

hernia for 13 per cent. The principal causes of admission among diseases of the nervous system for both men and women were contained in numbers 330–3324 of the M.R.C. Classification, the proportion of all nervous diseases classified to these numbers being 65 per cent. for males and 60 per cent. for females. The principal individual diseases were anxiety states, depression and hysteria. The two main groups of infective and parasitic diseases causing admission of males were venereal disease and diseases in 090–098, particularly scabies and pediculosis, each being 30 per cent. of the total of all infective and parasitic diseases. The persons admitted for venereal disease were mainly merchant seamen of various nationalities.

Table 118 shows the proportionate admissions in each age group during 1940–45. Infective and parasitic diseases formed on the whole smaller proportions of the men's total admissions for sickness at ages 35 and over, than at ages under 35. A similar falling off in the proportions for digestive diseases occurred at ages of 55 and upwards. Women at ages 35 and upwards had larger proportionate rates of diseases of the nervous system.

ADMISSIONS FOR INJURIES

Injuries to civilians are divided into two chief categories in the M.R.C. Classification:

(i) Those directly due to operations of war (Prefix VV) including

(a) accidents due to home-guard or fire-guard practices but not other accidents while on civilian war duties unless during actual operations of war.

(b) all kinds of injury or poisoning attributable to enemy action but not to civil rioting.

(ii) Those not stated to be due to operations of war (No prefix).

Since assignment between these two categories in the E.M.S. coding depended on the information given in the case histories, it is possible that some accidents actually due to war operations, especially those due to bombs or the effects of blast, have been included erroneously in the second group because they were not stated in the medical records to have been due to enemy action.

The number of civilians in the sample admitted for injuries was 19,575, the estimated total admissions being about 98,000. The distribution between males and females, according to whether the accident was stated to be due to war operations or not was as follows:

	Stated to be due to War Operations		Not stated to be due to War Operations	
	Number in Samples	Estimated Totals	Number in Samples	Estimated Totals
Males .	9,303	46,515±482	2,001	10,005±224
Females	8,043	40,215±448	228	1,140± 76
Persons	17,346	86,730±655	2,229	11,145±528

The ratio of male to female casualties due to war operations was 1·2, and for those not so ascribed, 8·8.

TABLE 119

Civilian Casualties due to Operations of War. Admissions during 1940–1945, by war-time duty, and childhood or adult status.

CLASS OF PERSON INJURED	Males and Females under 15	Males 15 Years and over	Females 15 Years and and over	All
Ordinary Civilians .	1,441	6,991	7,342	15,774
Civil Defence Personnel .	1	1,002	49	1,052
Merchant Navy Personnel	—	517	2	519
Totals . . .	1,442	8,510	7,393	17,345
Proportion . .	83	491	426	1,000

The aggregate civilian admissions due to operations of war have been sub-divided in Table 119 according to whether the patient was a merchant seaman (including passengers carried in merchant ships), a member of the Civil Defence services or an ordinary civilian. In the latter class there were 1,441 children under 15, 6,991 adult males and 7,342 adult females. Among civil defence personnel more than 20 times as many men as women were admitted, the nature of their duties exposing them to greater risk of injury by enemy action. Of every 1,000 persons with injuries due to war operations, 83 were children under 15, 491 adult males and 426 adult women.

The annual admissions due to enemy action of these three groups of patients are shown in Table 120. The greatest sample numbers of ordinary civilians to be admitted to E.M.S. hospitals were 5,849 in 1940 and 4,167 in 1941, compared with 3,674 in 1944, at the time of the V1 and V2 missiles.

TABLE 120

Civilian Casualties due to Operations of War. Annual Admissions during 1940–45, by war-time duty and childhood or adult status

		Males and Females under 15 years	Males, 15 years and over	Females, 15 and over	All
1940	Ordinary Civilians	483	2,740	2,626	5,849
	Civil Defence .	—	365	17	382
	Merchant Navy .	—	241	1	242
		483	3,346	2,644	6,473
1941	Ordinary Civilians	324	2,151	1,692	4,167
	Civil Defence .	1	322	16	339
	Merchant Navy .	—	163	1	164
		325	2,636	1,709	4,670
1942	Ordinary Civilians	81	361	312	754
	Civil Defence .	—	130	2	132
	Merchant Navy .	—	53	—	53
		81	544	314	939
1943	Ordinary Civilians	79	278	307	664
	Civil Defence .	—	84	3	87
	Merchant Navy .	—	28	—	28
		79	390	310	779
1944	Ordinary Civilians	376	1,264	2,034	3,674
	Civil Defence .	—	97	11	108
	Merchant Navy .	—	23	—	23
		376	1,384	2,045	3,805
1945	Ordinary Civilians	98	197	371	666
	Civil Defence .	—	4	—	4
	Merchant Navy .	—	9	—	9
		98	210	371	679

The civilian admissions for injury were attributable to external causes according to the list of suffixes on p. 740 as follows:

	Suffix	Males	Females
Transport	0–9	1,096	83
Occupational or due to missiles, etc.	0V–9V	8,751	7,979
Falls, blows and miscellaneous .	0X–9X	1,457	209
Totals		11,304	8,271

Ninety-seven out of every 1,000 males were admitted following a transport injury, and 10 out of every 1,000 females. Of 1,096 men admitted for this type of accident, 670 or 61 per cent. had received

TABLE 121

Civilians admitted to E.M.S. Hospitals for Transport Accidents, (M.R.C. Suffix. 0–9). 1940–45

Year	Accidents due to Operations of War											Per 1,000	Accidents not ascribed to Operations of War											Per 1,000
	0	1	2	3	4	5	6	7	8	9	All		0	1	2	3	4	5	6	7	8	9	All	
Males																								
1940	1	2	—	1	4	1	—	—	226	2	237	478	—	24	6	14	14	11	11	13	40	6	139	232
1941	1	—	—	—	—	—	—	2	150	—	153	309	3	19	3	26	14	18	11	13	51	5	163	272
1942	—	2	1	1	1	—	—	—	47	—	52	105	—	27	3	16	7	9	10	9	41	3	125	208
1943	—	1	2	—	—	1	—	2	20	2	28	56	—	17	2	8	3	4	8	4	21	6	73	122
1944	1	—	—	1	—	—	—	—	15	1	18	36	—	19	—	6	4	4	3	4	23	2	65	108
1945	—	—	—	—	—	—	—	—	8	—	8	16	—	1	—	3	—	—	—	1	28	2	35	58
	3	5	3	3	5	2	—	4	466	5	496	1,000	3	107	14	73	42	46	43	44	204	24	600	1,000
Females																								
1940	—	—	1	—	—	—	—	—	3	1	5	227	—	2	1	2	1	2	3	2	2	1	16	262
1941	1	—	—	—	—	—	—	—	2	3	6	273	1	—	—	1	3	1	2	—	—	6	14	230
1942	—	2	—	—	—	1	1	—	—	3	7	319	—	2	1	—	2	1	3	1	—	2	12	197
1943	—	1	—	—	—	—	—	1	—	1	3	136	1	5	—	—	—	—	1	1	—	2	10	164
1944	—	—	—	—	—	—	—	—	—	—	—	—	—	1	—	2	—	—	—	—	—	2	5	82
1945	—	—	—	1	—	—	—	—	—	—	1	45	—	—	—	1	1	—	—	—	—	2	4	65
	1	3	1	1	—	1	1	1	5	8	22	1,000	2	10	2	6	7	4	9	4	2	15	61	1,000

Suffix

0 Railway.
1 Motor cycle driver.
2 Driver, other motor vehicle.
3 Motor vehicle passenger.
4 Pedestrian, by motor vehicle.
5 Other motor vehicle, including injury to pedal cyclist.
6 Pedal cyclist, not by motor vehicle.
7 Other road transport.
8 Water transport.
9 Air transport, including glider and parachute.

TABLE 122

Civilians admitted to E.M.S. Hospitals for Occupational, Missile and other Injuries (M.R.C. Suffix 0V–9V) 1940–45

Year	Accidents due to Operations of War								Accidents not ascribed to Operations of War							
	0V–3V	4V	5V	6V	7V	8V–9V	All	Per 1,000	0V–3V	4V	5V	6V	7V	8V–9V	All	Per 1,000
Males																
1940	—	3,297	17	11	1	—	3,326	388	2	—	21	3	11	—	37	202
1941	—	2,596	28	11	2	—	2,637	307	6	4	5	3	10	—	28	153
1942	—	441	13	10	4	—	468	55	4	11	15	3	7	—	40	219
1943	1	349	3	12	—	2	367	43	5	10	11	5	5	1	37	202
1944	—	1,506	6	12	—	—	1,524	178	1	11	10	4	6	—	32	175
1945	—	242	1	3	—	—	246	29	—	4	2	3	—	—	9	49
Totals	1	8,431	68	59	7	2	8,568	1,000	18	40	64	21	39	1	183	1,000
Per 1,000	0	984	8	7	1	0		1,000	98	219	350	115	213	5		1,000
Females																
1940	—	2,815	8	3	3	—	2,829	355	1	—	—	—	—	—	1	83
1941	—	1,820	1	4	1	1	1,827	229	1	—	—	—	—	—	1	83
1942	1	328	—	2	—	—	331	42	—	2	1	1	—	1	5	417
1943	—	326	1	2	1	—	330	41	—	3	—	—	—	—	3	250
1944	—	2,227	—	4	—	—	2,231	280	—	—	1	—	1	—	2	167
1945	—	418	—	1	—	—	419	53	—	—	—	—	—	—	—	—
Totals	1	7,934	10	16	5	1	7,967	1,000	2	5	2	1	1	1	12	1,000
Per 1,000	0	996	1	2	1	0		1,000	167	417	167	83	83	83		

0V Mine or Quarry.
1V Agriculture.
2V Other machinery not in 0V or 1V.
3V Conflagration.
4V Bombs and effects of blast.
5V Gunshot.
6V Other explosives, shrapnel, etc.
7V Cutting or piercing.
8V Cataclysm.
9V Injury by animals.

TABLE 123

Civilians admitted to E.M.S. Hospitals for Falls, Blows, Crushing, Accidents at Sport and other external causes in M.R.C. Suffixes 0X–9X, 1940–45

Year	Accidents due to Operations of War												Accidents not ascribed to Operations of war											
	0X	1X	2X	3X	4X	5X	6X	7X	8X	9X	All	Per 1,000	0X	1X	2X	3X	4X	5X	6X	7X	8X	9X	All	Per 1,000
Males																								
1940	24	2	3	—	—	—	34	2	—	2	67	280	81	10	23	2	3	—	39	16	7	46	227	186
1941	9	—	4	2	—	2	16	1	2	4	40	167	125	8	32	3	21	—	67	22	13	57	348	286
1942	16	10	6	2	—	—	31	3	—	1	69	289	94	15	27	4	20	1	26	18	19	48	272	223
1943	14	3	1	4	—	—	15	1	1	—	39	163	56	3	24	2	10	1	22	9	11	29	167	137
1944	1	1	1	—	—	—	13	1	1	3	21	88	40	10	15	2	10	1	23	11	9	26	147	121
1945	1	—	1	—	—	—	1	—	—	—	3	13	12	3	8	2	1	1	7	4	4	15	57	47
Totals	65	16	16	8	—	2	110	8	4	10	239	1,000	408	49	129	15	65	4	184	80	63	221	1,218	1,000
Proportion	272	67	67	33	—	8	461	33	17	42		1,000	335	40	106	12	53	3	152	66	52	181		1,000
Females																								
1940	6	2	—	—	—	—	—	1	—	—	9	167	21	1	2	1	1	1	1	4	1	7	40	258
1941	3	1	1	—	—	—	1	—	—	1	7	130	11	—	3	—	1	—	5	8	—	9	37	239
1942	4	3	—	—	—	—	1	1	2	2	13	240	16	1	1	1	—	1	3	2	2	10	37	239
1943	5	2	2	—	—	—	1	—	—	2	12	222	8	—	2	—	—	—	1	—	1	—	12	77
1944	1	4	1	—	—	1	1	—	—	3	11	204	10	2	1	—	—	—	1	1	2	6	23	148
1945	—	1	—	—	—	—	—	—	—	1	2	37	—	—	—	—	—	—	—	—	2	4	6	39
Totals	19	13	4	—	—	1	4	2	2	9	54	1,000	66	4	9	2	2	2	11	15	8	36	155	1,000
Proportion	351	241	74	—	—	19	74	37	37	167		1,000	425	26	58	13	13	13	71	97	52	232		1,000

0X Fall.
1X Crushing, landslide.
2X Blow.
3X Explosion (not included elsewhere).
4X Accident at sport.
5X Unspecified accident at home.
6X Unspecified accident at work.
7X Unspecified accident elsewhere.
8X Other cause of injury in unspecified locality.
9X Unspecified cause of injury in unspecified locality.

injuries in water transport, and 112 or 10 per cent. were drivers of motor cycles injured on the roads. Table 121 shows the annual admissions for transport accidents, whether ascribed to war operations or not, according to external cause. It will be noticed that the number of admissions for water transport accidents due to operations of war declined from 229 in the 1940 sample to 8 in 1945. Several women who received injuries in air transport accidents were engaged in ferrying aircraft from the factories to the flying stations.

Among injuries due to the external causes listed in M.R.C. suffixes 0V–9V, the greatest number were due to bombs and effects of blast. Table 122 shows that 8,431 males and 7,934 females in the sample had been injured in this way by enemy action; the corresponding estimated total admissions being about 42,000 males and 40,000 females. Among males admitted for injuries due to bombs or effects of blast during the six years 1940–45, 39 per cent. and 31 per cent. entered hospital in 1940 and 1941 respectively, the corresponding percentages of women's admissions being 35 per cent. and 23 per cent. Only 18 per cent. of the males' admissions occurred in 1944 compared with 28 per cent. of the women's.

The numbers of admissions attributable to other external causes are shown in Table 123. Among men's admissions stated to be due to operations of war, accidents on duty formed the largest group, falls being the next most important cause. Falls were also responsible for 33·5 per cent of men's admissions in this group not ascribed to operations of war, and were the chief cause of women's admissions, whether due to war operations or not. If all thirty external causes of injury be considered together the main causes in descending order of magnitude were:—

	Males		*Percentage of all males admitted for injuries*
4V	Bombs and effects of blast .	8,471	75
8	Water transport .	670	6
OX	Falls	473	4
6X	Accidents on duty . .	294	3
9X	Unspecified accidents .	231	2
2X	Blows	145	1

	Females		*Percentage of all females admitted for injuries*
HV	Bombs and effects of blast .	7,939	96
OX	Falls	85	1

Table 124 shows the nature of the injuries for which civilian casualties were admitted to hospital each year, a distinction being made between

TABLE 124

Civilians admitted to E.M.S. Hospitals for Injuries, 1940–45. Nature of Injury and whether or not attributed to Operations of War

M.R.C. Code Number	Nature of Injury	Accidents due to Operations of War								Accidents not due to Operations of War							
		1940	1941	1942	1943	1944	1945	Totals	Proportions	1940	1941	1942	1943	1944	1945	Totals	Proportions
Males																	
800	Head Injuries	435	337	58	51	259	59	1,199	129	50	67	68	49	38	11	283	142
801	Open wounds, face and neck	224	190	42	29	201	34	720	77	27	17	30	18	12	4	108	54
802	trunk	86	60	17	13	27	3	206	22	5	2	1	2	2	—	12	6
803	upper limbs	113	84	34	21	68	10	330	35	9	16	13	6	8	8	60	30
804	lower limbs	204	157	36	28	99	9	533	57	26	17	10	10	19	2	84	42
805	chest injuries	15	8	10	3	6	1	43	5	—	—	2	—	—	—	2	1
806	abdominal injuries	24	14	7	4	1	—	50	5	1	1	5	3	—	—	10	5
807	multiple or N.O.S.	768	545	81	68	398	77	1,937	208	25	27	15	12	12	4	95	47
810–1	Bruising, Contusion, Haematoma	197	174	40	26	82	11	530	57	36	46	40	12	19	10	163	82
812–4	Foreign Bodies	17	20	7	1	6	2	53	6	3	2	5	3	—	1	14	7
815–6	Crushing Injuries	12	17	6	5	5	1	46	5	2	8	6	2	3	1	22	11
817–8	Traumatic Amputations	35	28	5	10	10	—	88	9	—	6	4	1	4	2	17	8
840	Fractures, skull	137	120	24	20	34	2	337	36	22	35	33	16	7	4	117	59
841	vertebral column	32	15	7	5	9	1	69	7	2	9	8	3	1	3	26	13
842	trunk bones	95	92	15	8	24	7	241	26	19	26	10	3	8	4	70	35
843	upper limbs	150	160	30	16	41	4	401	43	31	40	27	17	15	6	136	68
844	lower limbs	266	204	44	39	59	7	619	67	51	99	57	48	50	17	322	161
845	multiple	141	118	31	19	25	1	335	36	20	27	17	12	5	1	82	41
846	Dislocations	12	7	—	3	3	—	25	3	9	7	3	4	1	—	24	12
847	Sprains and Strains	27	25	8	5	9	1	75	8	18	34	35	19	10	4	120	60
87	Haemorrhage, Shock, etc.	301	188	16	12	154	16	687	74	3	3	5	1	5	—	17	8
90–92	Poisoning	39	7	3	—	5	—	54	6	14	9	4	2	6	3	38	19
93	Burns and Scalds	192	163	24	16	25	4	424	46	15	32	22	21	12	10	112	56
94	General Effects of External Causes	105	80	18	7	7	2	219	24	14	5	3	2	3	—	27	13
Rest of 80–96	Other injuries	3	17	26	25	6	5	82	9	1	4	14	11	4	6	40	20
	Totals	3,630	2,830	589	434	1,563	257	9,303	1,000	403	539	437	277	244	101	2,001	1,000
	Proportions	390	304	63	47	168	28		1,000	201	269	218	139	122	51		1,000

TABLE 124—(*contd.*)

Civilians admitted to E.M.S. Hospitals for Injuries, 1940–45. Nature of Injury and whether or not attributed to Operations of War

M.R.C. Code Number	Nature of Injury	Accidents due to Operations of War								Accidents not due to Operations of War							
		1940	1941	1942	1943	1944	1945	Totals	Pro-portions	1940	1941	1942	1943	1944	1944	Totals	Pro-portions
Females																	
800	Head Injuries	369	298	49	41	314	55	1,126	140	9	11	11	5	4	1	41	180
801	Open wounds, face and neck	189	121	35	34	262	66	707	88	2	1	—	1	3	2	9	39
802	trunk	47	22	4	8	27	4	112	14	1	—	2	—	—	—	3	13
803	upper limbs	85	49	10	15	81	9	249	31	2	1	—	—	1	—	4	18
804	lower limbs	124	73	17	14	143	10	381	47	2	3	3	2	2	1	13	57
805	chest injuries	4	1	—	3	2	—	10	1	—	—	—	—	—	—	—	—
806	abdominal injuries	16	5	5	—	3	—	29	4	—	—	—	—	—	—	—	—
807	multiple or N.O.S.	583	372	66	70	575	149	1,815	225	2	1	—	2	1	—	6	26
810–1	Bruising, Contusion, Haematoma	218	153	28	21	143	24	587	73	3	3	9	5	6	2	28	123
812–4	Foreign Bodies	9	8	2	5	9	4	37	5	—	1	—	—	—	—	1	4
815–6	Crushing Injuries	14	10	7	9	7	2	49	6	—	—	—	—	—	—	—	—
817–8	Traumatic Amputations	13	8	1	2	2	1	27	3	—	1	—	—	—	—	1	4
840	Fractures, skull	87	70	11	11	35	7	221	27	3	2	3	1	1	—	10	44
841	vertebral column	28	16	1	3	6	2	56	7	—	1	1	—	—	—	2	9
842	trunk bones	52	45	13	5	24	4	143	18	1	1	—	—	1	—	3	13
843	upper limbs	106	88	21	25	74	9	323	40	11	6	—	—	1	1	19	83
844	lower limbs	134	90	15	19	33	12	303	38	12	8	8	4	4	1	37	163
845	multiple	94	62	12	13	15	5	201	25	—	—	1	2	1	—	4	18
846	Dislocations	11	5	—	—	4	1	21	3	1	1	1	—	—	—	3	13
847	Sprains and Strains	18	11	3	3	3	1	39	5	3	2	2	1	2	—	10	44
87	Haemorrhage, Shock, etc.	528	264	29	29	439	45	1,334	165	1	—	3	—	1	—	5	22
90–92	Poisoning	13	1	—	1	—	—	15	2	2	—	1	—	—	—	3	13
93	Burns and Scalds	92	48	4	6	26	5	181	23	2	7	8	1	2	2	22	97
94	General Effects of External Causes	4	9	2	2	11	3	31	4	—	—	—	1	—	—	1	4
Rest of 80–96	Other injuries	5	11	16	6	4	4	46	6	—	2	1	—	—	—	3	13
	Totals	2,843	1,840	351	345	2,242	422	8,043	1,000	57	52	54	25	30	10	228	1,000
	Proportions	353	229	44	43	279	52		1,000	250	228	236	110	132	44		1,000

those which were stated to be due to operations of war and the remainder. The types of injury which occurred most frequently and their proportionate rates as shown in Table 124 were as follows:

Attributed to War Operations		*Not Attributed to War Operations*	
Males			
Multiple open wounds	208	Head injuries, including fractured skull	201
Head injuries, including fractured skull	165	Fractures of lower limbs	161
Open wounds, face and neck	77	Bruising, contusion and haematoma	82
Haemorrhage, shock, etc.	74	Fractures of upper limbs	68
Females			
Multiple open wounds	225	Head injuries, including fractured skull	224
Head injuries, including fractured skull	167	Fractures of lower limbs	163
Haemorrhage, shock	165	Bruising, contusion and haematoma	123
Open wounds of face and neck	88	Burns and scalds	97

The distribution of days of in-patient treatment for casualties suffering only from shock without mention of any other disease or injury was as follows:

Days of In-patient Treatment

	0–	3–	5–	7–	10–	14–	21–	28–	35–	42–	56-	91 up	All	Average
Males	270	57	45	31	23	21	14	9	3	2	1	1	477	6 days
Females	531	116	74	80	59	55	28	25	5	13	8	7	1,001	7 days
Persons	801	173	119	111	82	76	42	34	8	15	9	8	1,478	7 days

Fifty-four per cent. of the patients were in hospital for only one or two days. The average period of in-patient treatment for men was 6 days and for women 7 days.

APPENDIX II(a)

CAUSES OF ADMISSION (DISEASES) OF CIVILIAN PATIENTS TO E.M.S. HOSPITALS, 1940

Proportions per 1,000 Total Admissions for Illness

M.R.C. Code Number	Disease Group Title	Males							Females						
		Age Groups							Age Groups						
		0–	15–	25–	35–	55–	75 up	All	0–	15–	25–	35–	55–	75 up	All
00–101	Infective and Parasitic Diseases	269	259	198	103	17	—	147	261	208	103	81	40	—	118
11–20	Neoplasms	—	17	9	18	34	—	16	87	—	—	81	80	67	46
21–26	General Diseases	—	—	17	24	87	—	26	—	—	—	27	—	—	7
27–28	Diseases of Blood, Blood-forming Organs and Lymphoid Tissue	38	17	—	12	52	—	16	—	—	34	—	—	—	7
29	Chronic Poisoning and Intoxication	—	—	—	—	—	—	—	—	—	—	—	—	—	—
30–37	Diseases of Nervous System and Sense Organs	39	86	138	176	242	333	156	130	208	277	460	600	133	329
38–43	Diseases of Circulatory System	—	17	9	30	69	333	30	—	83	34	27	160	334	85
44–46	Diseases of Respiratory System	115	69	78	73	103	167	81	174	42	103	54	—	133	79
47–55	Diseases of Digestive System	154	225	293	291	156	—	251	217	291	173	54	—	—	125
56–61	Diseases of Genito-Uurinary System and Breast	154	34	26	24	69	—	40	—	42	69	27	—	—	26
62–67	Pregnancy, Childbirth and their Complications	—	—	—	—	—	—	—	—	42	139	27	—	—	39
68–69	Diseases of Skin and Cellular Tissue	154	225	103	79	34	—	102	43	42	—	27	40	67	33
70–72	Diseases of Bones and Organs of Movement	—	34	86	97	103	167	81	44	—	34	81	40	133	53
73–75	Congenital Malformations and diseases of the First Year of Life	39	—	9	6	—	—	7	—	—	—	—	—	—	—
76	Ill-defined Conditions and Symptoms	38	17	34	67	34	—	47	44	42	34	54	40	133	53
	Total Illnesses	1,000	1,000	1,000	1,000	1,000	1,000	1,000	1,000	1,000	1,000	1,000	1,000	1,000	1,000

APPENDIX II(a) (*contd.*)

CAUSES OF ADMISSION (DISEASES) OF CIVILIAN PATIENTS TO E.M.S. HOSPITALS, 1941

Proportions per 1,000 Total Admissions for Illness

M.R.C. Code Number	Disease Group Title	Males							Females						
		Age Groups							Age Groups						
		0–	15–	25–	35–	55–	75 up	All	0–	15–	25–	35–	55–	75 up	All
00–101	Infective and Parasitic Diseases	250	306	280	135	34	—	202	53	278	102	20	34	—	111
11–20	Neoplasms	18	9	5	16	46	—	16	158	—	41	102	69	—	58
21–26	General Diseases	—	—	5	8	34	—	8	—	37	20	20	—	—	19
27–28	Diseases of Blood, Blood-forming Organs and Lymphoid Tissue	54	9	20	12	11	—	17	—	19	—	—	—	—	5
29	Chronic Poisoning and Intoxication	—	—	—	4	—	—	1	—	—	—	—	—	—	—
30–37	Diseases of Nervous System and Sense Organs	71	83	150	251	311	200	189	158	148	245	492	484	714	319
38–43	Diseases of Circulatory System	18	28	45	52	139	200	55	—	—	—	61	34	143	24
44–46	Diseases of Respiratory System	196	74	65	52	34	200	69	105	19	102	61	34	—	58
47–55	Diseases of Digestive System	196	185	220	231	139	—	203	368	296	61	102	104	—	164
56–61	Diseases of Genito-Urinary System and Breast	36	19	10	20	23	—	18	53	55	20	41	34	—	39
62–67	Pregnancy, Childbirth and their Complications	—	—	—	—	—	—	—	—	37	245	—	—	—	68
68–69	Diseases of Skin and Cellular Tissue	125	185	65	80	69	—	93	52	74	123	61	34	—	72
70–72	Diseases of Bones and Organs of Movement	—	83	130	115	57	200	99	—	37	—	20	69	—	24
73–75	Congenital Malformations and Diseases of the First Year of Life	—	—	—	—	—	—	—	53	—	—	—	—	—	5
76	Ill-defined Conditions and Symptoms	36	19	5	24	103	200	30	—	—	41	20	104	143	34
	Total Illnesses	1,000	1,000	1,000	1,000	1,000	1,000	1,000	1,000	1,000	1,000	1,000	1,000	1,000	1,000

APPENDIX II(a) (*contd.*)

CAUSES OF ADMISSION (DISEASES) OF CIVILIAN PATIENTS TO E.M.S. HOSPITALS, 1942

Proportions per 1,000 Total Admissions for Illness

M.R.C. Code Number	Disease Group Title	Males							Females						
		Age Groups							Age Groups						
		0–	15–	25–	35–	55–	75 up	All	0–	15–	25–	35–	55–	75 up	All
00–101	Infective and Parasitic Diseases	100	296	202	190	91	—	205	250	186	167	—	91	—	135
11–20	Neoplasms	—	19	11	21	68	—	21	500	—	33	45	91	—	45
21–26	General Diseases	—	9	17	16	—	—	13	—	—	—	45	—	—	9
27–28	Diseases of Blood, Blood-forming Organs and Lymphoid Tissue	—	—	17	11	—	—	10	—	—	—	—	—	—	—
29	Chronic Poisoning and Intoxication	—	9	—	—	—	—	2	—	—	—	—	—	—	—
30–37	Diseases of Nervous Systems and Sense Organs	200	111	98	116	273	—	123	250	116	233	456	454	—	253
38–43	Diseases of Circulatory System	—	9	23	32	91	—	29	—	70	67	—	91	1,000	63
44–46	Diseases of Respiratory System	—	37	69	79	91	—	66	—	23	133	45	91	—	63
47–55	Diseases of Digestive System	500	241	231	260	205	1,000	247	—	350	67	45	—	—	162
56–61	Diseases of Genito-Urinary System and Breast	—	19	11	21	45	—	19	—	93	33	45	—	—	54
62–67	Pregnancy, Childbirth and their Complications	—	—	—	—	—	—	—	—	23	133	45	—	—	54
68–69	Diseases of Skin and Cellular Tissue	100	130	103	95	45	—	101	—	23	—	45	182	—	36
70–72	Diseases of Bones and Organs of Movement	—	55	149	101	23	—	99	—	23	67	92	—	—	45
73–75	Congenital Malformations and Diseases of the First Year of Life	—	—	—	5	—	—	2	—	—	—	—	—	—	—
76	Ill-defined Conditions and Symptoms	100	65	69	53	68	—	63	—	93	67	137	—	—	81
	Total Illnesses	1,000	1,000	1,000	1,000	1,000	1,000	1,000	1,000	1,000	1,000	1,000	1,000	1,000	1,000

APPENDIX II(a) (*contd.*)

CAUSES OF ADMISSION (DISEASES) OF CIVILIAN PATIENTS TO E.M.S. HOSPITALS, 1943

Proportions per 1,000 Total Admissions for Illness

M.R.C. Code Number	Disease Group Title	Males							Females						
		Age Groups							Age Groups						
		0–	15–	25–	35–	55–	75 up	All	0–	15–	25–	35–	55–	75 up	All
00–101	Infective and Parasitic Diseases	667	260	118	143	31	—	155	—	91	384	—	—	—	171
11–20	Neoplasms	—	12	—	12	63	—	13	—	—	—	125	—	—	29
21–26	General Diseases	—	12	36	12	—	—	18	—	—	—	—	—	—	—
27–28	Diseases of Blood, Blood-forming Organs and Lymphoid Tissue	—	—	9	—	—	—	3	—	91	—	—	—	—	29
29	Chronic Poisoning and Intoxication	—	12	9	—	—	—	5	—	—	—	—	—	—	—
30–37	Diseases of Nervous System and Sense Organs	—	123	219	161	187	—	170	—	181	—	250	1,000	—	171
38–43	Diseases of Circulatory System	—	37	36	50	93	1,000	49	—	—	—	—	—	—	—
44–46	Diseases of Respiratory System	—	74	55	50	63	—	57	—	91	77	—	—	—	57
47–55	Diseases of Digestive System	333	260	237	262	187	—	247	—	182	77	125	—	—	114
56–61	Diseases of Genito-Urinary System and Breast	—	12	9	31	63	—	23	—	—	—	125	—	—	29
62–67	Pregnancy, Childbirth and their Complications	—	—	—	—	—	—	—	—	—	77	125	—	—	57
68–69	Diseases of Skin and Cellular Tissue	—	99	118	99	63	—	101	1,000	182	154	—	—	—	143
70–72	Diseases of Bones and Organs of Movement	—	62	127	130	125	—	113	—	182	154	125	—	—	143
73–75	Congenital Malformations and Diseases of the First Year of Life	—	—	—	—	—	—	—	—	—	—	—	—	—	—
76	Ill-defined Conditions and Symptoms	—	37	27	50	125	—	46	—	—	77	125	—	—	57
	Total Illnesses	1,000	1,000	1,000	1,000	1,000	1,000	1,000	1,000	1,000	1,000	1,000	1,000	1,000	1,000

APPENDIX II(a) (*contd.*)

CAUSES OF ADMISSION (DISEASES) OF CIVILIAN PATIENTS TO E.M.S. HOSPITALS, 1944

Proportions per 1,000 Total Admissions for Illness

M.R.C. Code Number	Disease Group Title	Males							Females						
		Age Groups							Age Groups						
		0–	15–	25–	35–	55–	75 up	All	0–	15–	25–	35–	55–	75 up	All
00–101	Infective and Parasitic Diseases	143	200	286	179	115	—	202	500	50	222	—	—	—	84
11–20	Neoplasms	—	20	6	7	33	200	14	—	—	111	—	—	250	36
21–26	General Diseases	—	13	12	15	33	—	15	—	50	—	—	91	—	24
27–28	Diseases of Blood, Blood-forming Organs and Lymphoid Tissue	143	—	19	7	—	—	9	—	50	—	—	—	—	12
29	Chronic Poisoning and Intoxication	—	—	6	—	—	—	2	—	—	—	—	—	—	—
30–37	Diseases of Nervous System and Sense Organs	143	147	174	213	262	—	190	500	200	499	445	545	—	387
38–43	Diseases of Circulatory System	—	13	31	55	33	200	38	—	—	—	74	91	250	48
44–46	Diseases of Respiratory System	—	73	62	77	65	400	73	—	—	—	—	91	250	24
47–55	Diseases of Digestive System	428	348	199	257	197	200	259	—	500	56	74	—	—	157
56–61	Diseases of Genito-Urinary System and Breast	—	60	50	18	33	—	37	—	—	56	74	—	—	36
62–67	Pregnancy, Childbirth and their Complications	—	—	—	—	—	—	—	—	—	—	37	—	—	12
68–69	Diseases of Skin and Cellular Tissue	143	93	62	77	98	—	79	—	100	—	148	—	—	72
70–72	Diseases of Bones and Organs of Movement	—	13	62	77	115	—	61	—	—	56	37	91	250	48
73–75	Congenital Malformations and Diseases of the First Year of Life	—	—	—	—	—	—	—	—	—	—	—	—	—	—
76	Ill-defined Conditions and Symptoms	—	20	31	18	16	—	21	—	50	—	111	91	—	60
	Total Illnesses	1,000	1,000	1,000	1,000	1,000	1,000	1,000	1,000	1,000	1,000	1,000	1,000	1,000	1,000

APPENDIX II(a) (*contd.*)

CAUSES OF ADMISSION (DISEASES) OF CIVILIAN PATIENTS TO E.M.S. HOSPITALS, 1945

Proportions per 1,000 Total Admissions for Illness

M.R.C. Code Number	Disease Group Title	Males							Females						
		Age Groups							Age Groups						
		0–	15–	25–	35–	55–	75 up	All	0–	15–	25–	35–	55–	75 up	All
00–101	Infective and Parasitic Diseases . .	500	301	264	121	73	—	206	—	124	250	63	—	—	102
11–20	Neoplasms	—	10	17	13	73	—	19	—	63	—	—	—	—	20
21–26	General Diseases	—	19	—	—	24	—	7	—	—	125	—	111	—	41
27–28	Diseases of Blood, Blood-forming Organs and Lymphoid Tissue. .	—	19	8	—	24	—	9	—	—	—	—	—	—	—
29	Chronic Poisoning and Intoxication .	—	—	8	7	—	—	5	—	—	—	—	—	—	—
30–37	Diseases of Nervous System and Sense Organs.	—	107	165	302	293	1,000	215	—	250	500	749	778	—	552
38–43	Diseases of Circulatory System . .	—	10	33	47	98	—	38	—	—	—	—	—	—	—
44–46	Diseases of Respiratory System . .	—	87	66	114	146	—	95	—	63	—	—	—	—	20
47–55	Diseases of Digestive System . .	500	252	290	215	171	—	244	—	187	—	—	111	—	82
56–61	Diseases of Genito-Urinary System and Breast	—	10	41	20	—	—	21	—	63	—	125	—	—	61
62–67	Pregnancy, Childbirth and their Complications	—	—	—	—	—	—	—	—	63	—	—	—	—	20
68–69	Diseases of Skin and Cellular Tissue .	—	117	50	67	49	—	71	—	63	125	—	—	—	41
70–72	Diseases of Bones and Organs of Movement	—	29	41	47	49	—	40	—	124	—	63	—	—	61
73–75	Congenital Malformations and Diseases of the First Year of Life. . .	—	10	—	—	—	—	2	—	—	—	—	—	—	—
76	Ill-defined Conditions and Symptoms .	—	29	17	47	—	—	28	—	—	—	—	—	—	—
	Total Illnesses	1,000	1,000	1,000	1,000	1,000	1,000	1,000	—	1,000	1,000	1,000	1,000	—	1,000

APPENDIX II(b)

CAUSES OF ADMISSION (INJURIES) OF CIVILIAN PATIENTS TO E.M.S. HOSPITALS, 1940–46

Proportions per 1,000 Total Admissions for Injury

Year	Injury Group	Males										Females									
		Age Groups										Age Groups									
		0–	1–	5–	10–	15–	25–	35–	55–	75 up	All	0–	1–	5–	10–	15–	25–	35–	55–	75 up	All
1940	Head Injuries	200	189	210	205	149	159	141	184	184	160	278	185	158	121	167	140	170	160	174	162
	Fractures	100	122	136	213	160	181	231	225	96	200	—	55	88	165	122	138	177	176	114	151
	Acute Poisoning	—	27	—	8	11	13	15	11	8	13	—	19	—	22	4	9	5	3	—	5
	Burns	—	27	49	16	85	66	54	20	—	51	55	74	53	121	32	35	30	28	—	32
	Other Injuries	700	635	605	558	595	581	559	560	712	576	667	667	701	571	675	678	618	633	712	650
	Totals	1,000	1,000	1,000	1,000	1,000	1,000	1,000	1,000	1,000	1,000	1,000	1,000	1,000	1,000	1,000	1,000	1,000	1,000	1,000	1,000
1941	Head Injuries	83	194	267	152	158	165	155	180	196	165	375	182	213	209	209	176	181	221	209	198
	Fractures	—	83	250	171	195	219	251	280	103	231	—	121	128	149	139	163	220	182	98	172
	Acute Poisoning	—	—	—	—	2	6	5	7	—	4	—	—	—	—	—	—	2	—	—	1
	Burns	167	28	50	38	67	70	67	28	28	58	—	30	64	45	38	39	24	17	20	29
	Other Injuries	750	695	433	639	578	540	522	505	673	542	625	667	595	597	614	622	573	580	673	600
	Totals	1,000	1,000	1,000	1,000	1,000	1,000	1,000	1,000	1,000	1,000	1,000	1,000	1,000	1,000	1,000	1,000	1,000	1,000	1,000	1,000
1942	Head Injuries	—	111	67	309	188	176	177	158	150	178	500	—	385	—	178	113	188	224	250	182
	Fractures	—	333	133	143	188	275	266	230	150	241	—	125	154	231	178	183	197	171	71	175
	Acute Poisoning	—	—	—	—	6	12	8	7	—	8	—	—	—	—	14	—	—	—	—	2
	Burns	—	—	67	24	41	45	53	36	50	45	—	125	—	—	68	14	25	26	—	30
	Other Injuries	1,000	556	733	524	577	492	496	569	650	528	500	750	461	769	562	690	590	579	679	611
	Totals	1,000	1,000	1,000	1,000	1,000	1,000	1,000	1,000	1,000	1,000	1,000	1,000	1,000	1,000	1,000	1,000	1,000	1,000	1,000	1,000

1943	Head Injuries	500	—	—	119	174	192	205	216	172	192	1,000	200	267	333	106	130	144	146	179	155
	Fractures	—	—	111	190	141	292	265	248	207	239	—	—	133	83	258	148	231	195	71	190
	Acute Poisoning	—	—	—	—	—	8	—	8	—	3	—	—	—	—	15	—	—	—	—	3
	Burns	—	333	222	71	54	8	71	40	—	52	—	—	133	—	30	19	10	12	—	19
	Other Injuries	500	667	667	620	631	500	459	488	621	514	—	800	467	584	591	703	615	647	750	633
	Totals	1,000	1,000	1,000	1,000	1,000	1,000	1,000	1,000	1,000	1,000	1,000	1,000	1,000	1,000	1,000	1,000	1,000	1,000	1,000	1,000
1944	Head Injuries	53	231	203	130	140	196	163	220	219	184	200	231	212	177	132	104	159	171	189	157
	Fractures	53	38	85	43	64	160	135	126	86	115	—	26	—	139	46	52	68	88	80	69
	Acute Poisoning	—	—	—	—	—	12	—	9	—	4	—	—	—	—	—	—	—	—	—	—
	Burns	53	—	—	58	25	25	17	13	8	18	—	—	19	—	25	16	18	2	9	12
	Other Injuries	841	731	712	769	771	607	685	632	687	679	800	743	769	684	797	823	755	739	722	762
	Totals	1,000	1,000	1,000	1,000	1,000	1,000	1,000	1,000	1,000	1,000	1,000	1,000	1,000	1,000	1,000	1,000	1,000	1,000	1,000	1,000
1945	Head Injuries	—	454	133	188	59	286	259	288	214	234	—	154	—	211	106	140	167	182	129	148
	Fractures	—	91	—	—	88	57	86	135	—	77	—	—	77	158	61	80	71	111	32	78
	Acute Poisoning	—	—	—	—	—	—	—	—	—	—	—	—	—	—	—	—	—	—	—	—
	Burns	333	91	—	—	59	—	12	—	—	19	—	—	—	—	—	40	24	—	—	12
	Other Injuries	667	364	867	812	794	657	643	577	786	670	1,000	846	923	631	833	740	738	707	839	762
	Totals	1,000	1,000	1,000	1,000	1,000	1,000	1,000	1,000	1,000	1,000	1,000	1,000	1,000	1,000	1,000	1,000	1,000	1,000	1,000	1,000
1946	Head Injuries	—	—	—	1,000	143	71	384	—	—	196	—	—	—	—	—	—	—	—	—	—
	Fractures	—	—	—	—	286	215	308	500	—	283	—	—	—	—	1,000	—	—	—	—	333
	Acute Poisoning	—	—	—	—	—	—	—	—	—	—	—	—	—	—	—	—	—	—	—	—
	Burns	—	—	—	—	143	357	77	—	—	174	—	—	—	—	—	—	—	—	—	—
	Other Injuries	—	—	—	—	428	357	231	500	—	347	—	—	—	—	—	—	1,000	—	—	667
	Totals	—	—	—	1,000	1,000	1,000	1,000	1,000	—	1,000	—	—	—	—	1,000	—	1,000	—	—	1,000

Conclusion

In hospital morbidity statistics there are, among others, three groups which merit consideration:

(i) The number of admissions and the conditions causing them, irrespective of whether the same person appears more than once.

(ii) The number of different individuals who are hospitalised, irrespective of the number of times each one is admitted.

(iii) The total number of different morbid conditions and the contribution of each to the total pool of hospital morbidity.

In this study only the first of these groups has been considered. In the material available, for second or higher order admissions the envelopes containing the case histories were pinned together. Apart from the likelihood of their becoming detached, there was the possibility of error in the alphabetical order of filing, especially where names were identical and only regimental numbers differed, hence it will be apparent that there would have been considerable difficulty in obtaining reliable results as to the number of different individuals hospitalised. With the more widespread use of the unit system of keeping medical records and the increased efficiency in record departments, it should be possible to provide valuable information on the second point listed above.

The third item is also one which presents some difficulty. On the E.M.S. record cards provision was made for recording four diagnoses, and instructions were given that any further pathological conditions should be recorded on the back of the card. It was found that in this way, where the hospital notes were copious, that as many as eleven conditions might be recorded, but how far some of these should be regarded as symptomatic of others would be difficult to say. A clear distinction would also need to be drawn between morbid conditions found in hospital patients and morbid conditions for which treatment was given during the period of in-patient stay.

Even allowing for the war-time difficulties experienced by all working in hospitals, it is apparent that the divergence in the completeness and quality of clinical notes is very great. One of the principal difficulties in this work is the interpretation of medical reporting, and experience has suggested that there is a tendency in case records for emphasis to be laid on what requires treatment, rather than to record all that the patient is suffering from with a view to building up a picture of morbidity in hospitalised patients, related to underlying causes. The figures and percentages shown in Table 78 on page 747 have an interest in this connexion. Since it is probable that most head injuries are accompanied by some degree of concussion, the proportions here seem to be small especially since they are related only to those cases in which multiple causes are reported and not to all head injuries. Thus in cases of bruised scalp the secondary diagnosis was concussion in 75 per cent. of the cases, compared with 36 per cent. and 38 per cent. in fractures of the vault and base respectively, suggesting that in the former case it was on concussion that the treatment was concentrated, whereas in the latter emphasis was on treating the fracture. Similarly the highest proportions of mental diseases are shown here as sequelae of unspecified forms of head injury, suggesting that it was for the mental condition, rather than for the injury, that treatment was required. From the clinician's point of view the condition requiring treatment is undoubtedly the most important, and it has considerable value also for the hospital administrator. From the rather wider aspect of preventive medicine, complete assessment of morbidity is more important, but for this it is essential that underlying causes should also be considered. One of the problems that emerges from the present study is how far it is possible accurately to obtain the two purposes simultaneously and with a minimum of effort.

It seems that a preliminary to good statistics of hospital-treated sickness is an improvement in medical records. For collecting statistical material for tabulation by a central statistical office, a form which relies as little as possible on writing and in which every section requires some answer seems the best method; this avoids the impossibility of telling whether a blank denotes that the clinician has made a certain examination and found nothing adverse, or whether he has not made the examination at all. Time and labour may be saved if the form of the statistical record is followed in designing the front sheet of the case history.

A further vexed question is whether or not any useful purpose is served by asking the patient's occupation. The kind of replies received in the follow-up of fracture cases showed the great difficulty of associating the nature of a disease or injury with occupation. In many cases it is impossible to get an exact statement, especially when the patient himself is unable to answer questions; many wives, for example, do not know what their husband's work is, but only who he works for. To elicit a satisfactory reply the services of a trained investigator are needed in which case it is doubtful if the results justify the expense. In so far as occupation can be used as an indication of social status its recording could be useful as some deductions might be made about the connexion between social class and hospitalised sickness. But to determine whether or not a certain occupation has a particular risk, it seems better to start with a group of people following that occupation rather than to hope that hospital statistics will throw some light on the question.

In presenting information about periods of in-patient stay, all cases in which a complication or other morbid condition was mentioned have been excluded, and the median has been given rather than the mean as not being so influenced by a few excessively short or unduly long stays. In future studies further experiments will need to be made before the most satisfactory method of recording this information can be evolved.

Little attention has been paid here to deaths among E.M.S. hospital patients, and in general some difficulty is experienced in obtaining precise information as to the cause of death as stated by the certifying medical practitioner. The whole question of case fatality rates in hospital patients is one requiring research; to take the number of deaths occurring among patients admitted for certain diseases overlooks the possibility of death being due to an intercurrent cause.

In conclusion it may be stated that since hospital statistics are in their infancy, all that can be done at present is to make available such information as can be put together, so that the magnitude and difficulties of the problems involved may inspire the finding of a solution.

REFERENCES

Annan, J. H. (1945), *Lancet*, I, 174.

Brooke, E. M. (1945), *Brit. Med. J.*, I, 259; (1946), *Brit. Med. J.*, II, 491; (1950), *Brit. Med. J.*, I, 560.

Bradley, W. H. (1944), *Monthly Bulletin of Min. of Health*, *3*, 46. H.M. Stationery Office, London.

Cullinen, E. R. (1939), *Proc. R. Soc. Med.*, *32*, 933.

Deardorff, M. R. and Fraenkel, M. (1942, 1943). An analysis of 576, 623 patients discharged from hospitals in New York in 1933. *Hospital Discharge Study*, *1933*, I and II. Welfare Council of New York City, New York.

Dible, J. H., McMichael, J. and Sherlock, S. P. V. (1943), *Lancet*, II, 402.

Greenwood, M. (1944), *Practitioner*, CLIII, No. 918, 323.

Health, Ministry of (1950), *Report for the year ended 31st March, 1949, including the Report of the Chief Medical Officer on the State of the Public Health for the year ended 31st December, 1948*. H.M. Stationery Office, London.

Lancet (1942), Soldier's Foot, II, 312.

Lescher, G. (1944), *Brit. Med. J.*, I, 554.

Linsey, A. A. (1943), *Proc. R. Soc. Med.*, *37*, 165.

Mackay, D. (1951), *Hospital Morbidity Statistics:* Studies on Medical and Population Subjects, No. 4. H.M. Stationery Office, London.

Maitland, E. M. and Winner, A. L. (1939), *Lancet*, I, 161.

Medical Research Council (1944). A Provisional Classification of Diseases and Injuries for use in compiling Morbidity Statistics, *Sp. Rep. Ser.*, No. 248.

Registrar General (1940–44), *Weekly Returns*. H.M. Stationery Office, London; (1949–50), *Quarterly Returns*, Nos. 402, 403, 404, 405, Tables A–H. H.M. Stationery Office, London.

Stocks, P. (1949), *Sickness in the Population of England and Wales in 1944–47:* Studies on Medical and Population Subjects, No. 2. H.M. Stationery Office, London.

War Office (1948), *Statistical Report on the Health of the Army, 1943–45*. H.M. Stationery Office, London.
Witts, L. J. (1944), *Brit. Med. J.*, I, 739.
World Health Organization (1948), *Manual of the International Statistical Classification of Diseases, Injuries and Causes of Death*, I. H.M. Stationery Office, London.

ANNEXURE

Strength and Casualties of the Armed Forces and Auxiliary Services of the United Kingdom 1939 to 1945

Presented by the Prime Minister and the Minister of Defence to Parliament by Command of His Majesty June 1946

H.M.S.O.
Cmd. 6832 (Out of print)

27*CMS

INTRODUCTION

This paper gives statistics of the number of men and women who served in the Armed Forces and auxiliary services of the United Kingdom and of the casualties suffered during the war. The figures relate only to British subjects usually domiciled in Great Britain and Northern Ireland and to those British subjects and other persons elsewhere who individually enlisted and served in the Armed Forces and Auxiliary Services of the United Kingdom. They do not include men and women who served in units and contingents of His Majesty's Forces, other than those of the United Kingdom, or in Allied units and contingents under British or Allied Commands.(1)

SECTION I.—NUMBERS SERVING IN THE ARMED FORCES AND AUXILIARY SERVICES OF THE UNITED KINGDOM

Armed Forces

2. On August 31, 1939, the strength of the Armed Forces of the United Kingdom (Royal Navy, Army and Royal Air Force) was 681,000 men. Including reservists mobilised, a further 5,215,000 men were taken into the Services between August 31, 1939 and June 30, 1945, making a total of 5,896,000 men who served in the Armed Forces during the war. Of this total 923,000 men served in the Royal Navy, 3,788,000 in the Army, and 1,185,000 in the Royal Air Force.(2) This intake was sufficient, not only to meet casualties and discharges on medical and other grounds, but also to raise the total serving strength of the Armed Forces from 681,000 men at the outbreak of the war to 2,223,000 by June 1940, and to a peak of 4,683,000 men in June 1945.

3. Most of these men were drawn from the younger age groups between 18 and 30. Three out of every five men born between 1905 and 1927 and seven out of every ten born between 1915 and 1927 served in the Armed Forces.

Women's Auxiliary Services

4. The strength of the Women's Auxiliary Services (Women's Royal Naval Service, Auxiliary Territorial Service, Women's Auxiliary Air

(1) The total strength of the British Commonwealth and Empire Armed Forces (excluding Women's Services) was 8,845,000 at the middle of 1945. If allowance is made for the number who became casualties and who were discharged on medical and other grounds the total number of men who served during the war was over 10 millions.

(2) To avoid duplication, men or women who transferred from one Service to another have been excluded from the intake figure of the Service to which they were later transferred.

Force and the Nursing Services) at the beginning of the war was 21,000.

Between August 31, 1939 and June 30, 1945, 619,000 women entered the Women's Auxiliary Services, so that a total of 640,000 women served during the war. From the beginning of the war to June 30, 1945, 86,000 women served in the Women's Royal Naval Service, 307,000 in the Auxiliary Territorial Service, 219,000 in the Women's Auxiliary Air Force and 28,000 in the Nursing Services.([1]) This rate of intake made it possible to raise the total serving strength of the Women's Auxiliary Services from 21,000 at the beginning of the war to a maximum of 466,000 in 1944. Although the mobilization of women was directed mainly to the replacement of men in industry, one in every nine women born between 1915 and 1927 served in the Women's Auxiliary Services.

Other Services

5. In addition to the men and women serving in the Armed Forces and the Women's Auxiliary Services, a large number of men served in the Merchant Navy and many men and women were recruited for service, whole-time or part-time, in Civil Defence,([2]) the Royal Observer Corps, and the Home Guard.

6. *Whole-time.*—At June 1944, when the strength of the Armed Forces was 4,544,000, there were 417,000 men serving whole-time in Civil Defence, the Merchant Navy and the Royal Observer Corps. In addition to the 466,000 women in the Women's Auxiliary Services at this date there were 61,000 women serving whole-time in Civil Defence and the Royal Observer Corps.

7. *Part-time.*—At June 1944, there were 3,002,000 men giving part-time service. Of this total 1,253,000 were in Civil Defence (excluding Fire Guards), 1,727,000 in the Home Guard and 22,000 in the Royal Observer Corps. In addition there were 391,000 women performing part-time duties in these three Services.

Peak of Mobilization

8. The peak of mobilization of the Armed Forces, Auxiliary and other Services taken together was reached in June 1944, when the liberation of Europe began. The numbers actually serving at that date were as follows:

([1]) Queen Alexandra's Royal Naval Nursing Service, Queen Alexandra's Imperial Military Nursing Service, Territorial Army Nursing Service, Princess Mary's Royal Air Force Nursing Service and members of Voluntary Aid Detachments serving with the Armed Forces.

([2]) Civil Defence General Services (including the Casualty Services and the Civil Defence Reserve), National Fire Service, Regular Police and Auxiliary Police. Members of the Fire Guard service, other than those engaged in supervisory duties, are excluded.

Men		Women	
Armed Forces	*Thousands*	*Women's Auxiliary Services*	*Thousands*
Royal Navy	790	W.R.N.S.	74
Army	2,742	A.T.S.	199
Royal Air Force	1,012	W.A.A.F.	174
		Nursing Services	19
Total	4,544	Total	466
Other Services		*Other Services*	
Whole-time		*Whole-time*	
Civil Defence	231	Civil Defence	58
Merchant Navy	180	Royal Observer Corps	3
Royal Observer Corps	6		
Total	417	Total	61
Part-time		*Part-time*	
Civil Defence	1,253	Civil Defence	358
Royal Observer Corps	22	Royal Observer Corps	2
Home Guard	1,727	Home Guard	31
Total	3,002	Total	391

SECTION II.—STRENGTH OF INDIVIDUAL SERVICES

Armed Forces

9. Table I shows the expansion of the Armed Forces of the United Kingdom from 1939 to 1945. The figures include men locally enlisted abroad in United Kingdom Forces (of whom there were 30,000 at June 1945) and men from overseas who enlisted in the United Kingdom to serve in the United Kingdom Forces.

STRENGTH OF THE ARMED FORCES OF THE UNITED KINGDOM

TABLE I — Thousands

End of month	Total Armed Forces	Royal Navy	Army	Royal Air Force
August, 1939	681	161	402	118
June, 1940	2,223	276	1,656	291
June, 1941	3,291	405	2,221	665
June, 1942	3,815	507	2,468	840
June, 1943	4,332	671	2,692	969
June, 1944	4,544	790	2,742	1,012
June, 1945	4,683	789	2,931	963

10. The figures relate only to men actually serving at the dates shown. They exclude men:

(a) on deferred service

(b) on reserve

(c) temporarily released to industry or released on compassionate grounds

(d) reported prisoners of war or missing

(e) members of the Home Guard.

11. The total strength of the Armed Forces reached its peak of 4,683,000 in June 1945. Of this total strength 666,000 were engaged in the war against Japan in South-East Asia and the Far East and 4,017,000 were serving in other overseas theatres and at home. The numbers in each service were:

	Against Japan	*Others*
Royal Navy	224,000	565,000
Army	315,000	2,616,000
Royal Air Force . . .	127,000	836,000

12. *Royal Navy.*—The strength of the Royal Navy rose from 161,000 at the beginning of the war to 789,000 in June 1945. The figures given include the Royal Marines, the Naval Air Arm and merchant seamen serving with the Royal Navy on special agreements (T.124 agreements and variants). In June 1945, the strength of the Naval Air Arm was 79,802, of whom 8,350 were trained aircrew and 4,283 aircrew in training. The strength of the Royal Marines was 78,000 and the number serving under T.124 agreements (and variants) was 13,000.

13. *Army.*—The strength of the Army was raised rapidly from 402,000 at August 31, 1939 to 1,656,000 in June 1940, and then increased each year to a peak of 2,931,000 in June 1945. This latter figure included some 108,000 men who were formerly prisoners of war in Germany. The figures for the Army exclude the British component of the Indian Army amounting to about 18,000 at June 30, 1945. At the end of the war over one and three-quarter million men of the Army were serving abroad.

14. *Royal Air Force.*—The strength of the Royal Air Force was 118,000 at the beginning of the war. This was raised steadily to a peak of 1,012,000 by the middle of 1944 declining slightly to 963,000 in June 1945. The numbers shown exclude all Dominion Air Forces serving under their own Commands or placed at the disposal of the Royal Air Force and also exclude Allied Air Forces serving under their own or under British Commands. At the end of the war 316,000 men of the Royal Air Force were serving abroad.

Women's Auxiliary Services

15. The total strength of the Women's Auxiliary Services, including the Nursing Services, rose steadily from 21,000 at the beginning of the war to 466,000 at the middle of 1944. At this date there were 74,000

women serving in the Women's Royal Naval Service, 199,000 in the Auxiliary Territorial Service, 174,000 in the Women's Auxiliary Air Force, and 19,000 in the Nursing Services. About 37,000 members of the Women's Services were serving abroad at the end of the war.

STRENGTH OF THE WOMEN'S AUXILIARY SERVICES OF THE UNITED KINGDOM

TABLE 2 — Thousands

End of month	Total	W.R.N.S.	A.T.S.	W.A.A.F.	Nursing Services
August, 1939	21	—	18	2	1
June, 1940	56	6	32	12	6
June, 1941	105	15	43	37	10
June, 1942	307	29	140	126	12
June, 1943	461	53	210	182	16
June, 1944	466	74	199	174	19
June, 1945	437	72	191	153	21

Civil Defence

16. Grouped under this heading are the Civil Defence General Services (including the Casualty Services and the Civil Defence Reserve), National Fire Service, Regular Police and Auxiliary Police. These services exclude members of the Fire Guard Service other than those engaged in supervisory duties.

The total strength of the Civil Defence Services was raised rapidly by the middle of 1940 to 1,742,000, of whom 349,000 were serving whole-time. The number of men serving whole-time increased to 330,000 in 1941 and then declined to 231,000 by the middle of 1944. The number of both men and women serving part-time, however, rose between 1940 and 1944 so that the total strength of the Civil Defence Services reached its peak of 1,900,000 at the middle of 1944.

STRENGTH OF THE CIVIL DEFENCE SERVICES OF THE UNITED KINGDOM

TABLE 3 — Thousands

End of month	Total			Whole-time			Part-time		
	Total	Men	Women	Total	Men	Women	Total	Men	Women
June, 1939	83	83	—	83	83	—	—(1)	—	—
June, 1940	1,742	1,401	341	349	296	53	1,393	1,105	288
June, 1941	1,834	1,487	347	390	330	60	1,444	1,156	288
June, 1942	1,728	1,399	329	391	311	80	1,337	1,088	249
June, 1943	1,881	1,472	409	331	260	71	1,550	1,212	338
June, 1944	1,900	1,484	416	289	231	58	1,611	1,253	358
June, 1945(2)	411	369	42	131	116	15	280	253	27

(1) Considerable numbers were enrolled for part-time duty, but only limited numbers were required to perform regular duties in June 1939.

(2) Only the National Fire Service, Regular Police and Auxiliary Police were still performing active duties at the end of June 1945.

Home Guard and Royal Observer Corps

17. The appeal for men to enrol in the Local Defence Volunteers, which was re-named the Home Guard, was made in May 1940. By the end of June 1940, the strength of the Home Guard was 1,456,000. This strength was raised to 1,784,000 by the middle of 1943 and maintained at about one and three-quarter million until the end of 1944. In 1943 women were enrolled in the Home Guard for non-combatant duties and 31,000 were serving at the middle of 1944.

The Royal Observer Corps was created to ensure the rapid detection of enemy aircraft attacking the United Kingdom and to provide navigational help to the Royal Air Force operating from the United Kingdom. By June 1940, there were 28,000 men and women serving in the Royal Observer Corps, of whom 2,000 were serving whole-time and 26,000 part-time. The strength was increased to 33,000 in 1941 and maintained at about this level throughout the war.

STRENGTH OF THE HOME GUARD AND ROYAL OBSERVER CORPS

TABLE 4 — Thousand

End of month	Home Guard		Royal Observer Corps				
				Whole-time		Part-time	
	Men	Women	Total	Men	Women	Men	Women
June, 1940 .	1,456	—	28	2	—	26	—
June, 1941 .	1,603	—	33	4	—	29	—
June, 1942 .	1,565	—	34	5	—	28	1
June, 1943 .	1,784	7	33	6	1	25	1
June, 1944 .	1,727	31	33	6	3	22	2

SECTION III.—CASUALTIES

18. The figures given in this section relate to the casualties suffered during the war by the Armed Forces and auxiliary services enumerated in Section II and to casualties suffered by the civilian population of the United Kingdom. In the case of the Armed Forces, casualty figures are subject to continuous revision and a final statement cannot be issued until the fate of all men still reported missing is determined. Four categories of casualties to the Armed Forces and the Women's Auxiliary Services are distinguished—killed, missing, wounded and prisoners of war.

(a) *Killed*. The numbers recorded as killed include those who have died of wounds or injuries, those missing presumed dead and those who have died in captivity. The Royal Navy include deaths from disease attributable to war service and the Royal Air Force include suicides. All other deaths from natural causes are excluded.[1]

(b) *Missing*. Men reported missing and then subsequently reported killed, wounded or prisoners of war have been transferred from 'missing' to the other category. The figures for missing shown in the tables include men reported missing who subsequently rejoined their units as well as those who were still missing on February 28, 1946.

(c) *Wounded*. The number of wounded recorded by the Army is limited to injuries classified as battle casualties, which are defined as comprising injuries caused by enemy action, accidental injuries occurring in action or in proximity to the enemy and injuries caused by fixed apparatus laid as defences against the enemy. The figures relate to wounds requiring treatment at a hospital or field dressing station. The other two Services use the term in a wider sense which embraces all injuries sustained on war service. The Royal Air Force also include accidents occurring during training. The figures for all Services exclude absence from duty due to sickness.

(d) *Prisoners of War*. The figures include men interned in neutral countries. They also include prisoners of war who have been repatriated or who have escaped, but they exclude prisoners who have died in captivity. Reported deaths in captivity are transferred from 'prisoners of war' to 'killed'. For prisoners in Europe the figures are based partly on official notifications received from Germany and Italy. For prisoners in Japanese hands the figures are based partly on official notifications and partly on information received from prisoners themselves.

19. The figures relate to the gross number of casualties and not to the number of men who became casualties. A man who was reported missing, wounded or prisoner of war more than once has been counted as a casualty on each occasion so reported. Men reported missing or prisoners of war are deducted from the figures of strength when so reported and are included again in the figures of strength if and when they rejoin their units.

20. The total casualties suffered during the war by the Armed Forces, the Auxiliary Services and the civilian population of the United Kingdom were 950,794. Of these 357,116 were killed, 369,267 were wounded, 178,332 were prisoners of war or internees and 46,079 were missing.

(1) In addition to the casualty figures given in Table 5; the following numbers of men died from natural causes during the war while serving in the Armed Forces: Royal Navy 6,950, Army 19,935, Royal Air Force 4,386, Total 31,271.

CASUALTIES SUFFERED DURING THE WAR BY THE ARMED FORCES, THE AUXILIARY SERVICES AND THE CIVILIAN POPULATION OF THE UNITED KINGDOM FROM SEPTEMBER 3, 1939 TO AUGUST 14, 1945 AS REPORTED TO FEBRUARY 28, 1946

TABLE 5 Number

	Total	Armed Forces	Women's Auxiliary Services	Home Guard	Merchant Navy and Fishing Fleet	Civilians
Killed . .	357,116	264,443	624	1,206	30,248	60,595
Missing . .	46,079(1)	41,327	98	—	4,654	—
Wounded . .	369,267	277,077	744	557	4,707	86,182
Prisoner of war and internees .	178,332	172,592	20	—	5,720	(2)
Total . .	950,794	755,439	1,486	1,763	45,329	146,777

(1) Including 6,244 still missing at February 28, 1946 and 39,835 who rejoined their units.
(2) The number of United Kingdom civilians interned in enemy occupied countries is not known.

Armed Forces

21. Table 6 shows the casualties to each of the three Services of the Armed Forces of the United Kingdom(1) during the war. The Royal Navy suffered 73,642 casualties including 50,758 killed and 14,663 wounded. The 569,501 casualties to the Army included 144,079 killed and 239,575 wounded. In the Royal Air Force total casualties amounted to 112,296, including 69,606 killed and 22,839 wounded.

CASUALTIES TO ALL RANKS OF THE ARMED FORCES OF THE UNITED KINGDOM DURING THE WAR AS REPORTED TO FEBRUARY 28, 1946

TABLE 6 Number

	Total	Royal Navy	Army	Royal Air Force
Killed . .	264,443	50,758	144,079	69,606
Missing(1) .	41,327	820	33,771	6,736
Wounded .	277,077	14,663	239,575	22,839
Prisoners of war	172,592	7,401	152,076	13,115
Total .	755,439	73,642	569,501	112,296

(1) Including the following who were still missing on February 28, 1946; Royal Navy 340, Army 2,267, Royal Air Force 3,089; Total 5,696.

22. In Tables 7 and 8, the casualties in the war against Japan are distinguished from casualties in the war against Germany and Italy.

(1) The figures include casualties to men from overseas serving in the United Kingdom Forces, in particular from Newfoundland and Southern Rhodesia. They exclude casualties to the Armed Forces of the Dominions, India and the Colonies. Casualties to all ranks of the Armed Forces of the Dominions, India and the Colonies reported up to the end of the war were 490,768, of whom 108,929 were killed, 37,805 missing, 197,980 wounded and 146,054 prisoners of war

They show that the Armed Forces suffered 90,332 casualties in the war against Japan—about 12 per cent. of the total casualties of 755,439.

CASUALTIES TO ALL RANKS OF THE ARMED FORCES OF THE UNITED KINGDOM IN THE WAR AGAINST GERMANY, AS REPORTED TO FEBRUARY 28, 1946

TABLE 7 Number

	Total	Royal Navy	Army	Royal Air Force
Killed	234,475	46,911	121,484	66,080
Missing(1)	35,075	416	29,255	5,404
Wounded	260,548	14,360	224,427	21,761
Prisoners of war	135,009	5,518	119,764	9,727
Total	665,107	67,205	494,930	102,972

(1) Including the following still missing on February 28, 1946: Royal Navy nil, Army 671, Royal Air Force 2,109; Total 2,780.

CASUALTIES TO ALL RANKS OF THE ARMED FORCES OF THE UNITED KINGDOM IN THE WAR AGAINST JAPAN, AS REPORTED TO FEBRUARY 28, 1946

TABLE 8 Number

	Total	Royal Navy	Army	Royal Air Force
Killed	29,968	3,847	22,595	3,526
Missing(1)	6,252	404	4,516	1,332
Wounded	16,529	303	15,148	1,078
Prisoners of war	37,583	1,883	32,312	3,388
Total	90,332	6,437	74,571	9,324

(1) Including the following still missing on February 28, 1946: Royal Navy 340, Army 1,596, Royal Air Force 980; Total 2,916.

23. Table 9 shows the total number of prisoners of war in each of the Services reported captured in the war against Germany and against Japan and the numbers reported killed or died in captivity. The total

TOTAL NUMBER OF PRISONERS OF WAR OF THE ARMED FORCES OF THE UNITED KINGDOM CAPTURED BY THE ENEMY AS REPORTED TO FEBRUARY 28, 1946

TABLE 9 Number

	Total	Royal Navy	Army	Royal Air Force
Captured by Germany and Italy				
Total reported captured	142,319	5,629	126,811	9,879
Killed or died in captivity	7,310	111	7,047	152
Captured by Japan				
Total reported captured	50,016	2,304	42,610	5,102
Killed or died in captivity	12,433	421	10,298	1,714

number of prisoners captured by Germany and Italy was 142,319, of whom 7,310 died in captivity; but of a total of 50,016 prisoners captured by Japan, 12,433 died in captivity.

The difference between the total number of prisoners captured and the number who died in captivity is identical with the numbers shown as prisoners of war in Tables 7 and 8, in which those who died in captivity are included in the numbers killed.

Women's Auxiliary Services

24. The Women's Auxiliary Services suffered 1,486 casualties. Of these 624 women were killed and 744 wounded.

CASUALTIES TO THE WOMEN'S AUXILIARY SERVICES DURING THE WAR AS REPORTED TO FEBRUARY 28, 1946

TABLE 10 — Number

	Total	Women's Royal Naval Service	Auxiliary Territorial Service and Army Nursing Services	Women's Auxiliary Air Force
Killed	624	102	335	187
Missing	98	—	94(1)	4
Wounded	744	22	302	420
Prisoners of war	20	—	20	—
Total	1,486	124	751	611

(1) Including 18 women who were still missing at February 28, 1946.

Civil Defence and Civilian Casualties

CASUALTIES TO UNITED KINGDOM CIVILIANS DUE TO ENEMY ACTION AS REPORTED TO JULY 31, 1945

TABLE 11 — Number

	Total Civilian Casualties					Casualties to Civil Defence workers(1) on duty (included in civilian casualties)		
	Total	Men	Women	Children under 16	Unidentified	Total	Men	Women
Killed and missing believed killed	60,595	26,923	25,399	7,736	537	2,379	2,148	231
Injured and detained in hospital	86,182	40,738	37,822	7,622	—	4,459	4,072	387
Total	146,777	67,661	63,221	15,358	537	6,838	6,220	618

(1) Civil Defence General Services, National Fire Service, Regular and Auxiliary Police.

25. There were 146,777 civilian casualties in the United Kingdom due to enemy action. Of these 60,595 were killed or missing believed killed and 86,182 were injured and detained in hospital. These figures include 6,838 casualties suffered by Civil Defence workers while on duty of whom 6,220 were men and 618 women.

Merchant Navy and Fishing Fleet

26. The Merchant Navy and Fishing Fleet sustained 45,329 casualties during the war. Of these 30,248 were fatal (including deaths presumed in missing ships and deaths while interned), and 4,707 were wounded. There were 4,654 men reported missing of whom 530 had not been accounted for on February 28, 1946; in addition 5,720 men were reported as internees. The figure for deaths, missing, and internees, include all British subjects and nationals of allied countries who served in British registered ships and fishing boats as well as British subjects who served in foreign ships chartered by the United Kingdom during the war.

Home Guard

27. Members of the Home Guard suffered 1,763 casualties attributable to service. Of these 1,206 died of wounds, injury or illness attributed to service and 557 were wounded (excluding accidental injuries or illness).

INDEX

www.ingramcontent.com/pod-product-compliance
Lightning Source LLC
Chambersburg PA
CBHW050521300426
44113CB00012B/1913

* 9 7 8 1 4 7 4 5 3 6 0 6 6 *